VOLUME · ONE
STRUCTURE *of* ANTIGENS

M.H.V. Van Regenmortel

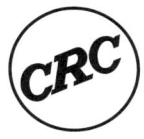

CRC Press
Boca Raton   Ann Arbor   London   Tokyo

Library of Congress Cataloging-in-Publication Data

Structure of antigens / edited by M. H. V. Van Regenmortel.
    p. cm.
   Includes bibliographical references and index.
   ISBN 0-8493-8865-1
   1. Antigens--Structure.   I. Van Regenmortel, M. H. V.
   [DNLM: 1. Antigens--analysis. 2. Antigens--immunology.
   3. Molecular Structure. 4. Proteins--analysis. 5. Proteins-
-immunology.   QW 573 S927]
QR186.5S76   1992
591.2'92--dc20
DNLM/DLC
for Library of Congress   91-29193
                                                                                                   CIP

Developed by Telford Press.

    This book represents information obtained from authentic and highly regarded sources. Reprinted material is quoted with permission, and sources are indicated. A wide variety of references are listed. Every reasonable effort has been made to give reliable data and information, but the author and the publisher cannot assume responsibility for the validity of all materials or for the consequences of their use.

    All rights reserved. This book, or any parts thereof, may not be reproduced in any form without written consent from the publisher.

    Direct all inquiries to CRC Press, Inc., 2000 Corporate Blvd., N.W., Boca Raton, Florida 33431.

© 1992 by CRC Press, Inc.

International Standard Book Number 0-8493-8865-1

Library of Congress Card Number 91-29193

Printed in the United States of America 1 2 3 4 5 6 7 8 9 0

PREFACE

The structural basis of antigenicity is an issue of considerable interest to biologists for two reasons. Most biologically important antigens are proteins and it is expected that an elucidation of their antigenic structure could throw considerable light on the general mechanisms of immunological recognition and specificity. Thus, the first motivation for studying protein antigens is the wish to understand how the immune system is able to recognize individual molecules amidst the enormous diversity of proteins. A second more utilitarian motive arises from the realization that knowledge of the structure of antigens has many applications in molecular biology and biomedicine. Examples of such applications are the preparation of immunological reagents to study the structure, conformation, and cellular expression of proteins, as well as the development of new vaccines and better diagnostic reagents for a variety of infectious agents.

In the present two-volume work, several chapters are devoted to the analytical methods used to elucidate the structure of antigens. Since the antigenic determinants of molecules recognized by the immune system are relational entities, recognizable only by the binding of complementary antibody combining sites, several chapters in Volumes 1 and 2 are devoted to the structure of antibodies. Antigenic determinants and antibody combining sites are relational partners that can be defined only in an operational sense by the occurrence of a binding reaction. The binding pocket of an antibody is in fact a functional concept and not solely a structural entity. In the realm of biological recognition phenomena, the elucidation of structure should never be dissociated from measurements of functional binding activity. Since any binding measurement is always subject to operational constraints, it is important also to consider which physicochemical parameters affect the structure of an immunoassay. Therefore, several chapters are devoted to the principles underlying modern immunoassays and the measurement of antibody binding affinity.

Twelve of the chapters of Volume 1 and two chapters of Volume 2 deal with physicochemical principles and methodological aspects. The other chapters are concerned with some major groups of antigens distinguished by their functional activity and biological role (drugs, autoantigens, snake toxins, allergens, etc.) or by their association with particular biological systems (antigens of microorganisms, viruses, etc.).

The book is intended for researchers and graduate students in all fields of biological science who wish to have an overview of our current understanding of antigenic specificity.

M. H. V. Van Regenmortel
June 1991

THE EDITOR

Marc H. V. Van Regenmortel, Ph. D., is Head of the Immunochemistry Department, Institute of Molecular and Cellular Biology, Strasbourg, France.

Dr. Van Regenmortel received his Ph.D. degree in 1961 from the University of Cape Town, South Africa. He was an International Fellow of the U.S. Public Health Service at the University of California, Berkeley from 1965 to 1966 and held professorial appointments at the University of Stellenbosch, South Africa (1967 to 1970) and the University of Strasbourg, France (1970 to 1972). He was Professor and Head of the Department of Microbiology at the University of Cape Town from 1973 to 1977 and, since 1978, Research Director at the Institute of Molecular and Cellular Biology in Strasbourg, France.

Dr. Van Regenmortel has written and edited a number of books in virology and immunochemistry and published over 200 original papers and reviews in the fields of general virology, plant virology, immunochemistry of viral proteins, histones and synthetic peptides, and immunodiagnosis of viral and autoimmune diseases.

He is currently Editor for *Archives of Virology, FEMS Microbiology Immunology, Research in Virology,* and *World Journal of Microbiology and Biotechnology,* and serves on the editorial boards of *Advances in Virus Research, Applied Virology Research, Biologicals, Immunological Investigations, Journal of Molecular Recognition, Molecular Immunology,* and *Seminars in Virology.*

He has served as Vice Chairman (1984 to 1987) and Chairman (1987 to 1990) of the Virology Division of the International Union of Microbiological Societies (IUMS) and is presently Secretary General of IUMS.

CONTENTS

Chapter 1	Molecular Dissection of Protein Antigens **Marc H. V. Van Regenmortel**	1
Chapter 2	Structure of Protein Epitopes Deduced from X-Ray Crystallography **Eduardo A. Padlan**	29
Chapter 3	Antigen Mimicry with Synthetic Peptides **S. Vuilleumier and M. Mutter**	43
Chapter 4	Antigen Mimicry with Anti-Idiotypic Antibodies **Neil S. Greenspan**	55
Chapter 5	Prediction of T Cell-Recognized Epitopes in Proteins **Shan Lu, Victor E. Reyes, Christopher M. Bositis, Thomas G. Goldschmidt, Valery Lam, Christopher H. Sorli, Rochelle R. Torgerson, Robert A. Lew, and Robert E. Humphreys**	81
Chapter 6	Antigen-Antibody Reactions **Carel J. van Oss**	99
Chapter 7	Measurement of Antibody Affinity **Robert Karlsson, Danièle Altschuh, and Marc H. V. Van Regenmortel**	127
Chapter 8	Maturation of the Immune Response **Claudia Berek**	149
Chapter 9	Immunoadjuvants **Arlette Adam and Vongthip Souvannavong**	159
Chapter 10	Precipitation and Agglutination **Carel J. van Oss**	179
Chapter 11	The Behavior of Antigens and Antibodies Immobilized on a Solid Phase **John E. Butler**	209
Chapter 12	Drugs as Antigens **Johan Hoebeke and A. Donny Strosberg**	261

Chapter 13	Snake Toxins as Antigens **André Ménez, Laurence Pillet, Michel Léonetti, François Bontems, and Bernard Maillère**	293
Chapter 14	Antibody Subclasses **Roy Jefferis**	321
Chapter 15	Histocompatibility Antigens **Béatrice Perarnau, Hélène Gournier, Claude Barra, Razqallah Hakem, and François A. Lemonnier**	339
Chapter 16	Vaccine Antigens **Gordon L. Ada**	367

Index   393

Chapter 1

Molecular Dissection of Protein Antigens

Marc H. V. Van Regenmortel
Institut de Biologie Moléculaire et Cellulaire, CNRS
Strasbourg, France

ANTIGENIC DETERMINANTS OF PROTEINS

The antigenic specificity of a protein resides in restricted areas of the molecule, known as antigenic determinants or epitopes, which are recognized by the combining sites or paratopes of certain immunoglobulin molecules. The precision of steric and chemical fit between epitope and paratope necessary for achieving this type of immunological "recognition" is highly variable since different antibodies may have affinity constants in the range of 10^3 to 10^{11} L/mol.

The most common way of classifying epitopes consists in distinguishing continuous and discontinuous epitopes (Atassi and Smith, 1978). The label continuous epitope is given to any short linear peptide fragment of the antigen that is able to bind to antibodies raised against the intact protein. Usually these antibodies cross-react only weakly with the peptide and the continuous epitope identified in this manner is unlikely to mimic exactly the conformation and structure of the corresponding epitope in the intact protein. The peptide fragment probably does not retain the conformation present in the folded protein, and, furthermore, it is likely to represent only a portion of a more complex epitope.

The second type of epitope, known as discontinuous epitope, is believed to correspond to the vast majority of epitopes found in proteins. They are made up of residues that are not continuous in sequence but are brought

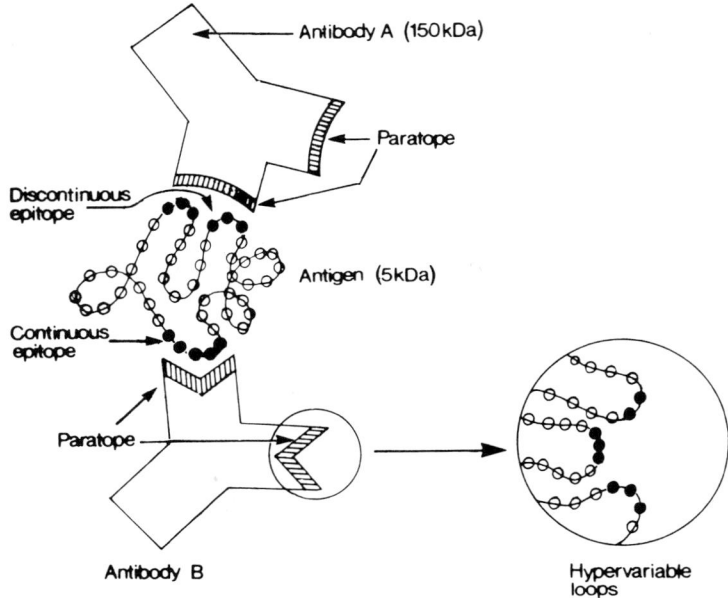

Figure 1. Schematic representation of two antibodies interacting with a continuous and a discontinuous epitope of a protein antigen. Contact residues are indicated in black. (From Van Regenmortel, 1986.)

together by the folding of the polypeptide chain (Fig. 1). Most antibodies to discontinuous epitopes will bind to the protein only if the molecule is intact and its conformation is preserved. When the protein is fragmented into a number of peptides, the various residues that made up the discontinuous epitope are scattered and each component is no longer individually recognized by the antibody. It is generally accepted today that the majority of monoclonal antibodies (MAbs) raised against intact proteins are specific for discontinuous epitopes, and it is believed that this explains why such MAbs usually do not react with any linear peptide fragment derived from the antigen. However, it is also true that a certain percentage of the MAbs raised against intact proteins, usually of the order of 10%, do react with linear peptide fragments of the protein. Since the range of specificities observed with a panel of MAbs is very similar to that found in a polyclonal antiserum to the same antigen (Quesniaux et al., 1990), it is reasonable to assume that about 10% of the antibodies present in an antiserum are also able to recognize so-called continuous epitopes of the protein antigen.

In recent years, some authors have challenged the view that *native* proteins possess continuous epitopes. Laver et al. (1990), for instance, suggested that all continuous epitopes represent "unfoldons," i.e., unfolded regions of the antigen that cross-react only with antibodies specific for the denatured protein. Such antibodies may be present in antisera raised against the protein because some of the antigen molecules used for immunization were denatured (Scibienski, 1973; Lando and Reichlin, 1982; Jemmerson, 1987a). Similarly, antibodies obtained by immunization with linear peptides may also be specific for unfoldons and may recognize the parent protein only because of the presence of denatured protein molecules in the preparation used in the immunoassay. Although it is true that in many immunoassays in current use, the protein antigen is at least partly denatured, it seems nevertheless too extreme a view to maintain that all reported cases of cross-reactivity between proteins and peptides are due to antibodies specific only for the denatured form of the protein. The most compelling argument against this view lies in the ability of some antipeptide antibodies to neutralize certain biological activities associated with the native state of proteins. For instance, in the case of many different viruses, it has been firmly established that immunization with peptides can lead to the formation of antibodies that neutralize virus infectivity (Anderer and Schlumberger, 1965; Bittle et al., 1982; DiMarchi et al., 1986; Emini et al., 1985; McCray and Werner, 1987; Parry et al., 1988; Roehrig et al., 1989; Smyth et al., 1990). These findings imply that the antipeptide antibodies recognize the native state of the viral protein present in infectious particles. Such findings do not mean that the linear peptide reproduces exactly the epitope in the intact protein but only that it resembles the cognate structure in the parent protein sufficiently to allow antibody cross-reactivity.

Although only a small fraction of the total immune response against a protein leads to the formation of antibodies that cross-react with linear peptides, there is considerable interest in unravelling the structural basis of this cross-reactivity. The main impetus for these studies lies in the many practical applications that would arise if protein antigens could be replaced by synthetic peptides (Lerner, 1984; Walter, 1986).

ANTIGENIC CROSS-REACTIVITY

Antigenic cross-reactivity is a consequence of the fact that the relationship between an antigen and its antibody is never of an exclusive nature. Cross-reactivity may be observed because two multideterminant antigens share one or more identical epitopes recognized by distinct antibody subpopulations present in a polyclonal antiserum. This type of cross-reactivity, which may be described as *shared reactivity*, arises because a particular antibody recognizes the same epitope in two different proteins and is of little relevance in the present context (Berzofsky and Schechter, 1981). For instance, when a panel of MAbs raised against a multideterminant protein is tested against two antigenically related proteins, it is frequently observed that certain MAbs react in an identical fashion with the two antigens, obviously because they recognize the same epitope (Briand et al., 1982). A totally different type of cross-reactivity, which has been termed *true cross-reactivity* (Berzofsky and

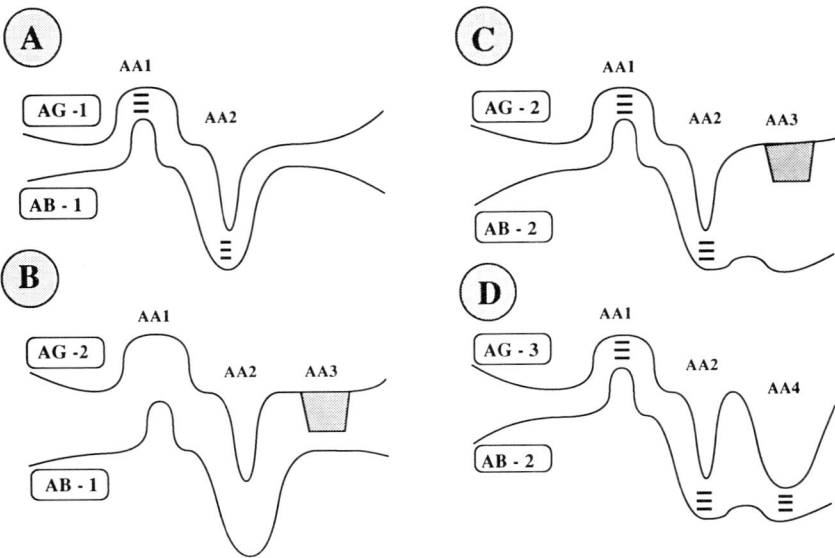

Figure 2. Schematic representation of epitope-paratope interfaces. In A, the energetic epitope of antigen 1 consists of two residues (AA1 and AA2) hydrogen-bonded to residues of the paratope of antibody 1. In B, the same energetic epitope of antigen 1 seems to be present, but a bulky substitution in a third residue (AA3) prevents H-bond formation with antibody 1. The influence of a substitution of AA3 might lead to the conclusion that this residue is implicated in the epitope of antigen 1, although its contribution is limited to the establishment of shape complementarity. In C, the energetic epitope in antigen 2 is again found to interact once the necessary complementarity in shape has been reestablished with antibody 2. In D, antibody 2 is able to show increased (i.e., heterospecific) binding with the modified epitope in antigen 3.

Schechter, 1981), arises when a particular antibody recognizes an epitope that is different but structurally related to the epitope used to raise the antibody. In most cases, the paratope will react with higher affinity with the homologous epitope used for immunization, although it is not uncommon for a paratope to bind more strongly to certain other epitopes than to the one against which it was raised (see Fig. 2). This phenomenon, known as heterospecificity (or heteroclitic binding), is commonly found whenever it is looked for, i.e., when the antibody is tested against a range of antigens closely related structurally to the immunogen (Al Moudallal et al., 1982; Harper et al., 1987; Mäkelä, 1965, Underwood, 1985).

True cross-reactivity occurs, for instance, when a peptide fragment of a protein cross-reacts with an epitope of the intact protein. Since the initial protein conformation present before fragmentation is unlikely to be retained in a peptide fragment, an antibody raised against the protein reacts with the peptide with a lower affinity. In addition, the linear peptide fragment usually represents only part of a more complex discontinuous epitope, which means that there will be fewer contact points between the paratope and the cross-reacting peptide than with the homologous protein. Whereas all six complementarity determining regions (CDR) of the antibody may have contributed some contact residues to the paratope that recognized the intact protein, it is possible that a smaller number of CDRs are involved in the binding observed with the cross-reactive peptide.

When there are only few contact points between paratope and epitope, the possibility arises that the CDRs that are not involved in the binding with a particular epitope will be able to bind to a totally dissimilar epitope. In this case the antibody, by the involvement of different subregions of the paratope, will be able to cross-react with two epitopes that have no structural similarity whatsoever. Such cross-reactions are probably responsible for the finding that MAbs sometimes react in a nonspecific manner with certain antigens. This reactivity is enhanced when the antigen presents a high local concentration of repeated epitopes or when it is used at a high density in solid phase or immunoblotting assays (Ghosh and Campbell, 1986). In both cases, the high local density of epitopes favors bivalent binding with IgG-type antibodies which facilitates the detection of weak cross-reactions shown by antibodies of low affinity. When IgM antibodies are used, the multivalence effect is further amplified (Hirayama et al., 1985), which makes irrelevant cross-reactions that are not based on a structural similarity in the epitope even more common (Ghosh and Campbell, 1986).

The study of cross-reactions between intact proteins and linear peptide fragments has led to the identification of large numbers of so-called continuous epitopes of proteins. Not every residue in the linear stretch of 5 to 8 residues that is believed to constitute a continuous epitope is, in fact, a contact residue interacting with the paratope. Usually some residues in the continuous epitope can be replaced by any of the other 19 amino acids without impairing the antigenic reactivity of the peptide (Geysen, 1985). This means that the linear peptide is, in fact, antigenically discontinuous and that the distinction between continuous and discontinuous epitopes is somewhat artificial (Van Regenmortel, 1987). There is no consensus at present about the minimum number of residues necessary for giving rise to a process that could properly be described as immunological recognition as opposed to chemical recognition. Obviously, the minimum number is one residue and there is, in fact, published evidence that a highly accessible, single C-terminal residue can be recognized with a certain degree of specificity by antibodies (Anderer and Schlumberger, 1966). This should come as no surprise in view of the existence of antibodies capable of recognizing as small a structure as dinitrophenol. There are 400 possible adjacent pairings of the 20 common amino acids, and studies by Geysen et al. (1986) have shown that certain MAbs are able to preferentially recognize some of these amino acid pairs. Since the immunoassay used to detect such antibody reactivity employs a high density of rod-coupled peptides, bivalent antibody binding is favored. This allows antibodies that have only a low intrinsic affinity for the dipeptide to be detected. When the dipeptide is extended at both ends by additional residues, some of the tetra- and hexapeptides that are obtained will be recognized by the MAb even better. When a particular residue is added to the dipeptide, it is sometimes found that it can be placed at more than one position and still increase the binding reaction. For instance, Geysen et al. (1986) reported that a MAb, which reacted weakly with the dipeptide Met-Lys, showed increasingly better reactivity with Try-Met-Lys, with Try-Met-Lys-His, and even better with Try-Gln-Met-Arg-His-Ser. This type of result implies that a variety of contacts can be established between epitope and paratope residues and that peptides of increasing size are able to readjust themselves to different subregions of the paratope (Edmundson et al., 1987).

In view of the multispecificity of antibodies, there is no guarantee that building up an epitope in this way (a "mimotope" according to Geysen's terminology) will produce a structure that is antigenically equivalent to the immunogen used to raise the test antibody. Until now there is no good evidence that immunization with such mimotopes produces antibodies able to recognize the structure being mimicked.

There is evidence that sequences of three residues can be recognized by certain antibodies of low affinity (Geysen et al., 1986; Trifilieff et al., 1991). It is also possible that longer peptides of 4 to 8 residues bind to an antibody because of the presence in the peptide of a few contact residues interspersed with noninteracting residues playing the role of scaffold. In such a case the systematic replacement of each residue of the peptide by other amino acids would show that the three contact residues are essential for binding while the other residues may be replaceable by virtually any amino acid (Schoofs et al., 1988). The minimum number of contacts or chemical bonds necessary for specific antibody recognition cannot be defined in an a priori manner. Furthermore, the minimum level of affinity required for calling the binding of an immunoglobulin "specific" and for considering that such an immunoglobulin is an "antibody" for the ligand depends on the context and on the type of assay used (Van Regenmortel, 1989a).

At the other end of the scale, it is equally meaningless to speak of perfect fit between epitope and paratope. It is clearly impossible to rule out that an antibody may show improved heterospecific binding with a structural relative of the epitope. In practice, it seems that *discrimination potential* is a more useful concept than *specificity* for describing the binding pattern of an antibody. It is the particular need of the investigator to differentiate between two entities that provides the necessary criterion for deciding whether an antibody is specific or not. Specificity is only meaningful with respect to a desired level of discrimination and this depends on the particular task at hand. The same antibody may thus be called specific or nonspecific, depending on the context.

TABLE 1.
Methods Used for Localizing Protein Epitopes

Method	Type of Epitope Recognized	Criterion for Residue Allocation
X-ray crystallography of antigen-Fab complexes	Discontinuous epitope reacting with homologous antibody	Contact with epitope-paratope interface
Use of peptide fragments as cross-reactive antigenic probes 1. Free peptides 2. Peptides adsorbed to solid-phase 3. Peptides conjugated to carrier 4. Peptides attached to support used for synthesis	Continuous epitope cross-reacting with heterologous antibody	Residual binding of linear fragment above threshold of assay
Identification of critical residues in peptide fragment by systematic replacement studies	Continuous epitope containing essential residues interspersed with irrelevant residues	Abrogation or decrease of cross-reactivity by replacement of functionally essential residue
Use of fusion proteins and peptides 1. Prokaryotic expression vectors 2. Chimeras	Continuous epitope	Residual binding above threshold of assay
Use of antipeptide antibodies	Continuous epitope cross-reacting with heterologous antibody	Induction of cross-reactive antibodies
Study of mutants, analogs and homologous proteins	Discontinuous epitopes	Abrogation or decrease of cross-reactivity
Topographic mapping by competitive binding assay	Only relative position of epitopes is defined	

METHODS USED FOR LOCALIZING EPITOPES

Methods used for identifying epitopes in proteins have been described in several reviews (Atassi, 1984; Benjamin et al., 1984; Berzofsky, 1985; Jemmerson and Paterson, 1986; Van Regenmortel, 1984, 1989a). The different approaches that have been used are summarized in Table 1. As discussed elsewhere (Van Regenmortel, 1989b), the only method that is truly based on a structural analysis is X-ray crystallography of antigen-antibody complexes. This analysis describes the spatial relationships observed at the two interacting surfaces and tends to emphasize the static aspects of the contact points once a stable complex has been formed. It should be noted that the identification of a contact residue contributing to the structure of an epitope is not at all straightforward since different definitions of what constitutes a contact have been given (Getzoff et al., 1988). For instance, contact residues can be defined as residues within Van der Waals contact, residues buried to a certain radius probe sphere, or residues with their side chains interacting directly. The five epitopes that have so far been analyzed by X-ray crystallography were found to comprise 15 to 22 contact residues, a size considerably larger than what has been traditionally regarded as being the size of an epitope, i.e., 5 to 6 residues.

All other methods listed in Table 1 are based on binding measurements and introduce the fourth dimension of time as a component of what is being observed. Binding assays take the form of activity measurements and correspond to a functional analysis of antigen-antibody interaction (Van Regenmortel, 1989b). Such analysis incorporates dynamic aspects that are not directly perceptible in a structural picture describing the bound state at equilibrium. Furthermore, most methods based on binding assays listed in Table 1 analyze the cross-reactive binding properties of antibodies, i.e., the ability of antibodies to cross-react with related structures that may differ considerably in conformation from the intact homologous antigen used to raise the antibody. Therefore, much of the information that is obtained in this way relates to rather incomplete and adulterated versions of the original epitopes existing in the native protein. These methods have led to the conclusion that only 3 to 8 residues of the antigen are critical to antibody binding. The epitope defined in a functional sense thus appears to involve fewer residues than the epitope defined in structural terms. Recently, an attempt has been made to compute how many of the residues allocated to various epitopes actually contribute to the binding energy of interaction (Novotny et al., 1989). By calculating the relative binding contributions of individual residues in the epitope defined in structural terms, it was found that most of the free energy contribution came from as few as 3 to 5 residues. This makes it possible to define a so-called "energetic epitope" in which the energetics of complex formation are emphasized and which has a size similar to that of epitopes defined by binding assays. The additional residues present in the structural epitope can then be viewed as playing a scaffolding role necessary to keep the critical, interacting residues in their proper position and orientation.

An important conclusion, therefore, is that different analytical approaches lead to different perceptions of what constitutes a protein epitope. As illustrated schematically in Fig. 2, an energetic epitope may, for instance, be viewed as comprising two residues (AA1 and AA2 in Fig. 2A) which are hydrogen-bonded to residues of the paratope. Although both residues are retained in antigen 2 (Fig. 2B), a bulky substitution at AA3 located outside the energetic epitope would eliminate the binding potential of the energetic epitope for antibody 1. If the epitope had been mapped in terms of which substitutions affect binding, residue AA3 would have been included in the epitope of antigen 1. On the other hand, when tested with respect to antibody

2, the energetic epitope in antigen 2 is again able to bind (Fig. 2C). Furthermore, another substitution (AA4 in antigen 3, Fig. 2D) may give rise to heterospecific binding by antibody 2. Clearly, epitope-paratope pairs are relational partners that should be defined only in terms of each other and not in the absolute. Like all relational concepts (e.g., father, brother) an epitope exists only by virtue of its relationship with a complementary partner, i.e., a particular paratope.

Crystallographic Analysis of Protein-Antibody Complexes

During the last 5 years, our knowledge of the structural basis of antigen-antibody interaction has been considerably advanced by X-ray diffraction studies of complexes of monoclonal antibody Fab fragments with their protein antigens (Colman, 1988; Davies et al., 1988; Mariuzza et al., 1987). Five epitopes have been analyzed by this method, three of lysozyme (Amit et al., 1986; Padlan et al., 1989; Sheriff et al., 1987) and two of influenza neuraminidase (Colman et al., 1987; Tulip et al., 1989). In all five cases, a large area of the protein surface (700 to 800 $Å^2$, comprising between 15 to 22 amino acid residues was identified as being in contact with residues of the antibody combining site. In all cases there was so much complementarity in shape between the interacting surfaces of antigen and antibody that water was almost entirely excluded from the interface (see Chapter 2).

All epitopes identified by X-ray crystallography so far are clearly discontinuous. The epitopes recognized by the antilysozyme D1.3 and HyHEL-5 antibodies consist essentially of two stretches of the lysozyme polypeptide chain (residues 18 to 27 and 116 to 129 for D1.3, and 41 to 53 and 67 to 70 for HyHEL-5), whereas the lysozyme HyHEL-10 epitope consists of the exposed surface of a helix (residues 88 to 99) together with residues from several lysozyme segments (residues 15 to 16, 20 to 21, 63, and 74 to 75). The two neuraminidase epitopes are also discontinuous. The NC41 epitope consists of segments 368 to 370, 400 to 403, 430 to 434 and portions of 325 to 350 (Colman et al., 1987), whereas the NC10 epitope involves five segments of the polypeptide chain.

The three lysozyme paratopes are made up of residues from all six CDRs of the antibody, whereas the two neuraminidase paratopes utilize residues from only four CDRs (antibody NC10) or five CDRs (antibody NC41). In addition, some framework residues are also involved in the binding interaction.

In the lysozyme-antibody complexes, no large conformational changes were observed in the lysozyme as a result of the binding to antibody. However, movement of the backbone atoms of as much as 2 Å at the point of contact have been recorded (Davies et al., 1988). It is a matter of debate whether such small adjustments are in favor of the "induced fit" mechanism proposed for antigen-antibody interaction or whether they are compatible with the "lock-and-key" model (Mariuzza et al., 1987; Van Regenmortel, 1989a). It is clear that readjustment of side chains does occur but movement of the backbone atoms is more difficult to establish unambiguously. The magnitude of the motions observed in the segmental mobility of the peptide chain is only of the order of 1 to 2 Å and the functional significance of such small movements is a matter of interpretation. Recently, a small rearrangement (0.5 to 0.7 Å) of the V_H and V_L domains of the paratope of antilysozyme antibody D1.3 was found to occur upon complex formation with the antigen and this was interpreted in terms of induced fit (Bhat et al., 1990).

The two explanatory models of antigen-antibody interaction, the lock-and-key and induced fit models, are sometimes presented as mutually exclusive, although it is clear that both models are useful to describe some aspects of epitope-paratope recognition. In a similar vein, the opposition between static and dynamic views of antigenicity seems somewhat artificial (Novotny et al., 1987a). The debate on whether the location of epitopes in proteins is better "explained" by the static surface accessibility of certain regions or by their segmental mobility (Novotny et al., 1986; Sasaki et al., 1988; Tainer et al., 1985; Westhof et al., 1984) is clouded by the fact that the accessibility and mobility of short segments of polypeptide chains are not independent variables but represent interconnected aspects of the folding pattern of globular proteins. Loops and turns, for instance, are mostly surface projections and also tend to possess higher than average mobility. Attempts to find the best correlation between these properties and the antigenicity of ill-defined "continuous" epitopes have given rise to much debate and contradictory claims (Geysen et al., 1987a; Hopp, 1986; Novotny et al., 1987b; Thornton et al., 1986). Unfortunately, the search for correlations has not yet produced an effective method for predicting the location of epitopes in proteins.

Preliminary X-ray data of crystal structures of complexes of peptides with antipeptide Fab have been published (Schulze-Gahmen et al., 1988; Stura et al., 1989). In one study, the detailed structure of a complex between peptide 67 to 89 of myohemerythrin and a Fab fragment obtained by immunization with the peptide was presented (Stanfield et al., 1990). Surprisingly, the N-terminal part of the peptide was found to adopt a β-turn conformation in the antibody-peptide complex, although the same region in native myohemerythrin was in a helical conformation. However, since the Mab used to prepare the Fab had been screened for reactivity with solid-phase plate-bound myohemerythrin (Fieser et al., 1987) it is possible that the helical conformation was absent in the plate-bound antigen. The authors reported that solution-phase myohemerythrin was able to compete with the solid-phase protein in ELISA and suggested that this unusual finding was brought about by a conformational change due to "unknown causes" (Stanfield et al., 1990). It is not clear to what extent induced fit phenomena may be responsible for these observations (Crumpton, 1986; Wilson et al., 1985).

Studies with Peptides as Antigenic Probes

The most widely used method for localizing protein epitopes consists in identifying which natural or synthetic peptide fragments of the molecule are able to cross-react with antibodies raised against the intact protein. Any peptide that is able to bind to the protein antibodies is said to contain a continuous epitope. Peptides of decreasing size may be tested to determine which is the smallest peptide that retains a significant level of antigenic reactivity (Benjamini, 1977). The degree of antigenic cross-reactivity observed with small peptides is mostly very low with the exception of peptides corresponding to chain termini. In a majority of proteins, the terminal segments are surface-oriented (Thornton and Sibanda, 1983) and are also more mobile than internal sections of the polypeptide chain. Both features may explain why the cross-reactivity observed with short terminal peptides tends to be much higher than with internal peptides (Absolom and Van Regenmortel, 1977; Milton and Van Regenmortel, 1979; Tainer et al., 1985; Walter, 1986; Westhof et al., 1984).

Free Peptides and Peptide Conjugates

As a result of rapid developments in the technique of solid-phase peptide synthesis (Atherton and Sheppard, 1989; Houghten, 1985; Kent and Clark-Lewis, 1985; Plaué, 1990; Van Regenmortel et al., 1988), synthetic peptides have virtually replaced natural peptide fragments as antigenic probes. After synthesis, the peptides are cleaved from the resin and are tested either as free peptides in solution, as immobilized peptides adsorbed to a solid phase, or as peptide-carrier conjugates. The different immunoassay formats used to determine the antigenic reactivity of peptides have recently been reviewed (Van Regenmortel et al., 1988). It should be stressed that the antigenic reactivity of peptides is highly dependent on the assay format (Muller et al., 1986). Sometimes the free peptide in solution is most active (Altschuh and Van Regenmortel, 1982; Nestorowicz et al., 1985), but in other cases the activity is higher when the peptide is conjugated to a carrier (Al Moudallal et al., 1985). In such cases the microenvironment at the surface of the carrier protein probably induces the peptide to adopt a more suitable conformation for antibody recognition. It should also be recognized that peptides corresponding to inner sequences of a polypeptide chain possess ionizable groups at their termini which are absent in the protein because of the formation of peptide bonds. The presence of the additional charged groups could lower any potential antigenic cross-reactivity with the intact protein. On the other hand, when the free α-carboxyl group of the terminal COOH is replaced by an amide group, the antigenicity of the peptide may also be altered drastically (Gras-Masse et al., 1986; Hodges et al., 1988). It must be recognized, therefore, that the detection of cross-reactivity with the parent protein can be adversely affected both if the extraneous charges of the peptide are retained or if the charges are removed by amidation or acetylation.

The binding of a peptide to antiprotein antibodies may be facilitated by the induction of a native-like conformation in the peptide during formation of the peptide-antibody complex (Crumpton, 1986; Getzoff et al., 1987, 1988). The use of longer peptides does not necessarily lead to a higher level of cross-reactivity since longer peptides may adopt a conformation different from that present in the native protein (Jemmerson, 1987b; Wilson et al., 1984). Shorter peptides may also fold more easily into the proper orientation required for binding to the antibody (Hodges et al., 1988). A variety of approaches have been used to increase the level of conformational mimicry between peptide and intact protein (see Chapter 3). Cyclization of the peptide has frequently been used for this purpose (Arnon et al., 1971; Dorow et al., 1985; Dreesman et al., 1982; Fourquet et al., 1988; Jemmerson and Hutchinson, 1990; Schulze-Gahmen et al., 1986), although it appears that information on the three-dimensional structure of the epitope is required to achieve the best results (Muller et al., 1990; Plaué, 1990). Other strategies for stabilizing certain peptide backbone conformations have also been proposed (Gras-Masse et al., 1988; Mutter, 1988; Satterthwait et al., 1989).

The antigenic cross-reactivity of peptides may be tested by measuring their capacity to inhibit the reaction of the protein with its homologous antibodies, or simply by adsorbing the peptides to a solid phase and measuring their ability to be recognized by antiprotein antibodies. In the latter case, it may be necessary to try a variety of buffers (Geerligs et al., 1988) and to prevent the peptide solution from drying up during the test (Norrby et al., 1987). It has been suggested that in order to establish the specific nature of a cross-reaction, it is necessary to include controls in which the liquid-phase protein is allowed to compete with plate-bound antigen and to show that inhibition to a level approaching 100% occurs (Jemmerson, 1987a). However, it cannot be excluded that a genuinely cross-reacting antigen reacts with antibodies so weakly that a complete inhibition cannot be observed at experimentally achievable concentrations (Berzofsky and Schechter, 1981).

Peptides Attached to Support Used for Synthesis

Peptides can be tested for antigenic activity without prior cleavage from the support used during synthesis (Hurrell et al., 1977; Shi et al., 1984). The pepscan method developed by Geysen et al. (1984, 1987b) allows the concurrent synthesis of hundreds of peptides on polyethylene pins. The pins are assembled into a polyethylene holder with the format and spacing of a microtiter plate. This allows the peptides to be tested by an enzyme immunoassay while they remain attached to the pin. After each test the pins can be freed of bound antibody by sonication and retested with different antibody preparations as many as 30 times. The pepscan method is ideally suited for the systematic testing of all possible overlapping peptides of a protein, starting from the N-terminal residue down to the C-terminal one. Usually 6 to 10 residue-long peptides are analyzed in this fashion (Geysen et al., 1987b). Covalent attachment of the peptide to the solid support may, in some cases, impair its antigenic activity and it is thus possible to miss certain peptides that would be revealed as antigenically active in a different type of immunoassay. Another problem encountered with the pepscan technique is that some peptide sequences tend to give rise to nonspecific binding. The high concentration of peptide on the pins favors bivalent binding of antibody and facilitates the detection of very low levels of cross-reactivity. As a result, di- or tripeptide sequences may give rise to observable cross-reactions in this technique (Geysen et al., 1986; Trifilieff et al., 1991).

Identification of Critical Residues by Replacement Studies

The pepscan technique is also frequently used to determine the contribution of individual amino acids to the binding interaction between peptide and antibody (Getzoff et al., 1988). This is achieved by analyzing peptide replacement sets in which each residue of the peptide is, in turn, replaced by the other 19 possible amino acids. In this way some residues are found to be essential for binding since they cannot be replaced by any residue without impairing the antigenic reactivity. Presumably they correspond to critical residues that contribute to the energy of interaction. Other residues can be replaced by all common amino acids without affecting binding and their role may be limited to that of a scaffold. By analyzing the pattern of replaceability linked to retention of antibody binding in 103 continuous epitopes of various proteins, Geysen et al. (1988) found that, on average, only five out of six residues in hexapeptides were essential for activity.

Studies with Fusion Proteins and Peptides

Epitopes can be identified by expressing parts of the protein in a prokaryotic expression system and measuring the antigenic activity of the expression product (Lenstra et al., 1990). For instance, in the pEX expression system, the product of an inserted DNA fragment becomes the C-terminal portion of a hybrid galactosidase protein which precipitates in the cell. The hybrid protein is solubilized in sodium dodecyl sulfate (SDS) and transferred to a nitrocellulose filter for testing its antigenicity (Stanley, 1983). In recent years a number of expression vector systems have been developed (Charbit, 1991; Mehra et al., 1986; Young and Davis, 1983). Viral chimeras, in which the epitopes of one virus are inserted by recombinant DNA techniques into the particles of another virus, are also increasingly used (Clarke et al., 1987; Delpeyroux et al., 1986; Michel et al., 1988). The recombinant approach to epitope analysis has been reviewed by Hofnung and Charbit (1992).

Studies with Antipeptide Antibodies

In these studies, synthetic peptides are used for immunization and the resulting antipeptide antibodies are tested for their ability to cross-react with the intact protein. A positive cross-reaction is taken as an indication that the peptide approximates to an epitope of the protein. Although it has repeatedly been claimed (Green et al., 1982; Lerner, 1984; Niman et al., 1983) that immunization with peptides leads to a very high frequency of induction of antibodies able to recognize the *native* protein, it is now generally accepted that these claims arose because the antipeptide antibodies reacted with denatured protein molecules present in solid-phase immunoassay (Jemmerson, 1987a; Jemmerson and Blankenfeld, 1989; Van Regenmortel, 1989a). It is now widely recognized that proteins become at least partly denatured when they are adsorbed to plastic during a solid-phase assay (Darst et al., 1988; Friguet et al., 1984; Soderquist et al., 1980) which explains why antipeptide antibodies frequently react quite well with plate-bound protein antigens (see Chapter 11).

The contention that antibodies against a highly disordered state (the peptide) are mostly able to recognize the highly ordered state (the folded protein in its native conformation), although the reverse is not necessarily the case, has been called the order-disorder paradox (Dyson et al., 1988). In an attempt to resolve this paradox, it was suggested that a preferred conformation of the peptide present in solution becomes stabilized at the surface of the carrier protein or when the peptide binds to the B-cell receptor during immune stimulation. However, if a process of induced fit is able to influence the conformation of the immunogenic form of the peptide, one would expect that a similar induction of conformation would occur when the peptide interacts with antiprotein antibodies. In other words, antibodies against the ordered state should also be able to recognize at high frequency the disordered peptide, which was in fact not observed (Green et al., 1982). The paradox simply vanishes, however, if it is accepted that the extent of cross-reactivity between peptides and native protein is always rather low, irrespective of whether antiprotein or antipeptide antibodies are tested. This low level of cross-reactivity is illustrated by the finding that intact cytochrome c was able to activate only a small fraction of peptide-primed B lymphocytes (Jemmerson and Blankenfeld, 1989).

In order to produce antipeptide antisera, it is customary to couple peptides of less than 10 to 15 residues to a carrier protein (Briand et al., 1985; Palfreyman et al., 1984; Van Regenmortel et al., 1988). Since the method of conjugation may strongly influence the type of antipeptide antibodies that are produced (Bahraoui et al., 1987; Dyrberg and Oldstone, 1986; Mariani et al., 1987; Schaaper et al., 1989), it is advisable to use more than one conjugation procedure and immunization schedule. An approach which avoids the formation of antibodies to a carrier protein is the multiple-antigen peptide (MAP) system introduced by Tam (1988). The MAP consists of a core matrix made up of three levels of lysine residues and eight amino terminals for anchoring peptide antigens. Although the MAP system enhances the immunogenicity of peptides and leads to high levels of peptide antibodies in immunized animals, the antibodies do not always cross-react strongly with the cognate protein.

Studies with Mutants and Analogs

In this method the antigenic cross-reactivity between related proteins presenting known amino acid substitutions is studied by means of MAbs. If the substitution leads to a change in antibody binding, it is assumed that the mutated residue is involved in the structure of an epitope (Hornbeck and Wilson, 1984). In general, it seems that single substitutions at the surface of a protein only cause a local change with no long-range structural alterations (Benjamin et al., 1984). This is demonstrated by the fact that usually other MAbs directed against neighboring epitopes of the protein are unaffected by the one substitution. There are exceptions, however, and certain mutations may alter the antigenicity by an indirect distal conformational effect (Al Moudallal et al., 1982; Barnett et al., 1989; Blondel et al., 1986; Collawn et al., 1988; Hurrell et al., 1977).

Since the number of available substitutions in a series of homologous proteins is always limited, a more extensive analysis may require generating protein variants by site-directed chemical modification (Cooper et al., 1987; Oertle et al., 1989) or by site-directed mutagenesis (Smith et al., 1991). This latter approach has the added advantage that multiple substitutions can be examined for any given amino acid. In this case, a residue is defined as a contact residue if the substitution leading to decreased binding does not significantly increase the side-chain volume (Smith and Benjamin, 1991). Such a precondition is introduced because substitution of a small noncontact residue by a bulky side chain could alter binding by preventing antibody from establishing normal bond distances with other contact residues (Fig. 2C).

Instead of inferring the position of epitopes from the ability of MAbs to distinguish between protein variants, it is possible in the case of infectious agents to select nonneutralizable mutants by the immunological selection pressure of neutralizing MAbs (Pollock et al., 1984). By growing a virus in the presence of neutralizing MAbs, escape mutants can be selected that are then sequenced to identify the substitution which rendered the mutant neutralization-resistant (Air and Laver, 1986; Wiley and Skehel, 1987).

Topographic Epitope Mapping

Competitive bindings assays with pairs of MAbs can be used to determine the relative position of epitopes on the surface of a protein (Berzofsky, 1984). However, two epitopes are recognized as different only if they are far enough apart to allow simultaneous binding of the two MAbs. Because of the bulkiness of antibody molecules, considerable steric hindrance may occur and MAbs directed against distinct but neighboring epitopes could thus be presented from binding simultaneously to the antigen surface. Although a single Fab antibody fragment covers about 700 $Å^2$ of the surface of an antigen, this does not mean that the epitope necessarily extends over the same area. Incidentally, this makes the argument for the exclusive existence of discontinuous epitopes in proteins (Barlow et al., 1986) less compelling, since a MAb recognizing, for instance, a continuous epitope of only three residues would still cover an area of about 700 Å^2 of the antigen surface.

When the number of MAbs used in epitope mapping is large, one often observes a continuum of epitopes that can no longer be subdivided into discrete, separate antigenic domains (Mathews and Roehrig, 1984; Underwood, 1982). Instead of blocking binding, a competing antibody may actually enhance the binding of a second antibody presumably by an allosteric effect (Cecilia et al., 1988; Heinz et al., 1984). Such enhancement of binding may be caused by only one of two antibodies (unidirectional enhancement) or it may be bidirectional (Heinz, 1986).

THE PREDICTION OF CONTINUOUS EPITOPES

Many attempts have been made to correlate the location of continuous epitopes in a few well-characterized proteins with parameters such as the hydrophilicity, accessibility, and mobility of short segments of their polypeptide chains. All prediction calculations are based on propensity scales for each of the 20 amino acids. These scales describe the tendency of each residue to be associated with properties such as surface accessibility or hydrophilicity. Usually a window of seven residues is used in the analysis. The corresponding value of the scales is introduced for each of the seven residues and the arithmetical mean of the seven values assigned to the center of the window.

Various algorithms for predicting secondary structure have also been applied to the prediction of continuous epitopes. Whereas the core of proteins usually contains a combination of helices and sheets, their surface is replete with turns and loops (Rose et al., 1985a). The success rate of secondary structure prediction algorithms is limited since at most 55 to 70% of the structural elements are correctly predicted (Fasman, 1989; Kabsch and Sander, 1983). The predictive value of eight scales has been compared, using as a criterion of success the number of residues correctly predicted to be antigenic in four well-studied proteins (Van Regenmortel and Daney de Marcillac, 1988). It was found that none of the methods achieved a high level of correct prediction, although the hydrophilicity scale of Parker et al. (1986) and the segmental mobility scale of Karplus and Schulz (1985) were slightly more successful than the others (Fig. 3).

In a recent study, the validity of 22 different scales for predicting antigenicity was analyzed using 9 proteins containing 54 identified continuous epitopes (Pellequer et al., 1991). The method of analysis calculated how many residues of each protein were correctly or wrongly predicted to be antigenic. The results obtained with 10 of the scales are summarized in Table 2. From the ratio of correctly over wrongly predicted residues it was found that various hydrophobicity and hydrophilicity scales gave 51 to 57% correct predictions. The accessibility scales gave 46 to 52% correct predictions, whereas the scales that predict turns gave a slightly higher level of correct prediction (53 to

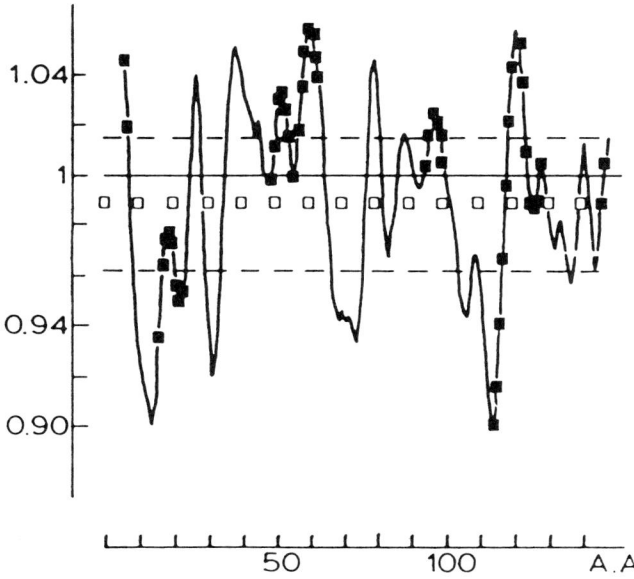

Figure 3. Prediction of continuous epitopes in proteins. Segmental mobility profile of myoglobin calculated with the scale of Karplus and Schulz (1985). The smoothing procedure of Van Regenmortel and Daney de Marcillac (1988a) was used. The black squares correspond to amino acids that are part of known continuous epitopes of myoglobin. The white squares represent the average value of the mobility parameter over the entire sequence and the two horizontal broken lines represent ±0.7 SD from the mean. Such an interval corresponds to 50% of the population.

61%). These results again confirm earlier studies (Getzoff et al., 1988; Van Regenmortel and Daney de Marcillac, 1988) which showed that none of the algorithms in current use give a high level of correct prediction.

CONCLUSION

The different analytical approaches used to delineate protein epitopes lead to different perceptions of the nature of protein antigenicity. The structural approach of X-ray crystallography concentrates on the relative position of atoms at the antigen-antibody interface and identifies epitopes as structural entities of 15 to 22 residues. In contrast, the functional approach based on cross-reactive binding measurements introduces the additional dimension of time and leads to the view that only about five residues are implicated in epitopes defined in a functional way. Furthermore, binding measurements are unavoidably submitted to operational constraints and different immunoassays or different types of probes (for instance, free peptide, conjugated peptide, or solid-phase peptide) point to different residues as being critical in an

TABLE 2.
Comparative Value of 10 Antigenicity Prediction Scales Applied to Nine Proteins of Known Antigenic Structure

	Correctly Predicted Residues[a]	Wrongly Predicted Residues[a]	Ratio[b]	Percentage Correct Prediction[c]
Inverted hydrophobicity scale of Kyte and Doolittle, 1982	180	171	1.05	51
Inverted hydrophobicity scale of Rose et al., 1985b	150	134	1.11	53
Hydrophilicity scale of Hopp and Woods 1981	150	147	1.02	51
Hydrophilicity scale of Parker et al., 1986	190	145	1.31	57
Accessibility scale of Chotia, 1976	180	167	1.07	52
Acrophilicity scale of Hopp, 1984	142	124	1.14	53
Flexibility scale of Karplus and Schulz, 1985	152	138	1.10	52
Antigenicity scale of Welling et al., 1985	133	236	0.56	36
Scale for turns of Chou and Fasman, 1978	151	111	1.36	58
Scale for turns of Levitt, 1976	169	108	1.56	61

[a] The columns correctly predicted and wrongly predicted correspond to the number of correctly predicted and wrongly predicted amino acids, respectively, above the cut-off level ($+ 0.7 \times SE$).
[b] Ratio of correctly predicted/wrongly predicted amino acids.
[c] Ratio [correctly predicted/(correctly predicted + wrongly predicted)] expressed as percentage correct prediction.

Adapted from Pellequer et al., 1991.

epitope. Structural and functional analyses have been termed "two different ways of seeing" (Lambert and Hughes, 1988), and these two approaches lead to complementary models of biological and immunological reality.

Epitopes are relational entities since they can be recognized only by the binding of complementary paratopes. An epitope is thus not an intrinsic feature of a protein molecule existing independently of its paratope partner. Epitopes and antigens can be defined only in terms of the emerging properties and relationships that arise in an immunological system.

The molecular dissection of protein antigens should thus not be confused with an attempt to reduce biology to chemistry. The distinction between an immunochemical interaction and a simple chemical one remains valid also when the binding reaction between two immunological reactants is analyzed in molecular terms.

REFERENCES

Absolom, D., and Van Regenmortel, M. H. V. (1977) Purification by immunoadsorption and immunochemical properties of histone H3. *FEBS Lett.* 81:419—422.

Air, G. M., and Laver, W. G. (1986) The molecular basis of antigenic variation in influenza virus. *Adv. Vir. Res.* 31:53—102.

Al Moudallal, Z., Briand, J. P., and Van Regenmortel, M. H. V. (1982) Monoclonal antibodies as probes of the antigenic structure of tobacco mosaic virus. *EMBO J.* 1:1005—1010.

Al Moudallal, Z., Briand, J. P., and Van Regenmortel, M. H. V. (1985) A major part of the polypeptide chain of tobacco mosaic virus protein is antigenic. *EMBO J.* 4:1231—1235.

Altschuh, D., and Van Regenmortel, M. H. V. (1982) Localization of antigenic determinants of a viral protein by inhibition of enzyme-linked immunosorbent assay (ELISA) with tryptic peptides. *J. Immunol. Meth.* 50:99—108.

Amit, A. G., Mariuzza, R. A., Phillips, S. E. V., and Poljak, R. J. (1986) Three-dimensional structure of an antigen-antibody complex at 2.8 Å resolution. *Science* 233:747—753.

Anderer, F. A., and Schlumberger, H. D. (1965) Properties of different artificial antigens immunologically related to tobacco mosaic virus. *Biochim. Biophys. Acta* 97:503—509.

Anderer, F. A., and Schlumberger, H. D. (1966) Cross-reactions of antisera against the terminal amino acid and dipeptide of tobacco mosaic virus. *Biochim. Biophys. Acta* 115:222—224.

Arnon, R., Maron, E., Sela, M., and Anfinsen, C. B. (1971) Antibodies reactive with native lysozyme elicited by a completely synthetic antigen. *Proc. Natl. Acad. Sci. U.S.A.* 68:1450—1455.

Atassi, M. Z. (1984) Antigenic structures of proteins. Their determination has revealed important aspects of immune recognition and generated strategies for synthetic mimicking of protein binding sites. *Eur. J. Biochem.* 145:1—20.

Atassi, M. Z., and Smith, J. A. (1978) A proposal for the nomenclature of antigenic sites in peptides and proteins. *Immunochemistry* 15:609—610.

Atherton, E., and Sheppard, R. C. (1989) *Solid Phase Peptide Synthesis. A Practical Approach.* IRL Press, Oxford, 203.

Bahraoui, E., El Ayeb, M., Granier, C., and Rochat, H. (1987) Immunochemistry of scorpion toxins. Immunogenicity of peptide 19—28 a model of an accessible and relatively rigid region. *Eur. J. Biochem.* 167:371—375.

Barlow, D. J., Edwards, M. S., and Thornton, J. M. (1986) Continuous and discontinuous protein antigenic determinants. *Nature (London)*, 322:747—748.

Barnett, P. V., Ouldridge, E. J., Rowlands, D. J., Brown, F., and Parry, N. R. (1989) Neutralizing epitopes of type 0 foot-and-mouth disease virus. I. Identification and characterization of three functionally independent, conformational sites. *J. Gen. Virol.* 70:1483—1491.

Benjamin, D. C., Berzofsky, J. A., East, I. J., Gurd, F. R. N., Hannum, C., Leach, S. J., Margoliash, E., Michael, J. G., Miller, A., Prager, E. M., Reichlin, M., Sercaz, E. E., Smith-Gill, S. J., Todd, P. E., and Wilson, A. C. (1984) The antigenic structure of proteins: a reappraisal. *Annu. Rev. Immunol.* 2:67—101.

Benjamini, E. (1977) Immunochemistry of the tobacco mosaic virus protein. In *Immunochemistry of Proteins*, Vol. 2 (M. Z. Atassi, ed.), Plenum Press, NY, pp. 265—310.

Berzofsky, J. A. (1984) Monoclonal antibodies as probes of antigenic structures. In *Monoclonal and Anti-idiotypic Antibodies: Probes for Receptor Structure and Function* (J. C. Venter, C. M. Fraser, and J. Lindstrom, eds.), Alan R. Liss, NY, pp. 1—19.

Berzofsky, J. A. (1985) Intrinsic and extrinsic factors in protein antigenic structure. *Science* 229:932—940.

Berzofsky, J. A., and Schechter, A. N. (1981) The concepts of crossreactivity and specificity in immunology. *Mol. Immunol.* 18:751—763.

Bhat, T. N., Bentley, G. A., Fischmann, T. O., Boulot, G., and Poljak, R. J. (1990) Small rearrangements in structures of Fv and Fab fragments of antibody D1.3 on antigen binding. *Nature (London)* 347:483—485.

Bittle, J. L., Houghten, R. A., Alexander, H., Shinnick, T., Sutcliffe, J. G., Lerner, R. A., Rowlands, D. J., and Brown, F. (1982) Protection against foot-and-mouth disease by immunization with a chemically synthesized peptide predicted from the viral nucleotide sequence. *Nature (London)* 298:30—33.

Blondel, B., Crainic, R., Fichot, O., Dufraisse, G., Candrea, A., Diamond, D., Girard, M., and Horaud, F. (1986) Mutations conferring resistance to neutralization with monoclonal antibodies in type 1 poliovirus can be located outside or inside the antibody-binding site. *J. Virol.* 57:81—90.

Briand, J. P., Al Moudallal, Z., and Van Regenmortel, M. H. V. (1982) Serological differentiation of tobamoviruses by means of monoclonal antibodies. *J. Virol. Meth.* 5:293—300.

Briand, J. P., Muller, S., and Van Regenmortel, M. H. V. (1985) Synthetic peptides as antigens: pitfalls of conjugation methods. *J. Immunol. Meth.* 78:59—69.

Cecilia, D., Gadkari, D. A., Kedarnath, N., and Ghosh, S. N. (1988) Epitope mapping of Japanese encephalitis virus envelope protein using monoclonal antibodies against an Indian strain. *J. Gen. Virol.* 69:2741—2747.

Charbit, A. (1991) Expression de peptides étrangers sous forme de fusions génétiques de protéines chez les bactéries et les bactériophages. *Bull. Inst. Pasteur* 89:17—49.

Chothia, C. (1976) The nature of the accessible and buried surfaces in proteins. *J. Mol. Biol.* 105:1—14.

Chou, P. Y., and Fasman, G. D. (1978) Prediction of secondary structure of proteins from amino acid sequence. *Adv. Enzymol. Relat. Subj. Biochem.* 47:45—148.

Clarke, B. E., Newton, S. E., Carroll, A. R., Francis, M. J., Appleyard, G., Syred, A. D., Highfield, P. E., Rowlands, D. J., and Brown, F. (1987) Improved immunogenicity of a peptide epitope after fusion to hepatitis B core protein. *Nature (London)* 330:381—384.

Collawn, J. F., Wallace, C. J. A., Proudfoot, A. E. I., and Paterson, Y. (1988) Monoclonal antibodies as probes of conformational changes in protein-engineered cytochrome c. *J. Biol. Chem.* 263:8625—8634.

Colman, P. M. (1988) Structure of antibody-antigen complexes: implications for immune recognition. *Adv. Immunol.* 43:99—132.

Colman, P. M., Laver, W. G., Varghese, J. N., Baker, A. T., Tulloch, P. A., Air, G. M., and Webster, R. G. (1987) Three-dimensional structure of a complex of antibody with influenza virus neuraminidase. *Nature (London)* 326:358—363.

Cooper, H. M., Jemmerson, R., Hunt, D. F., Griffin, R., Yates, J. R., Shabanowitz, J., Zhu, N. Z., and Paterson, Y. (1987) Site-directed chemical modification of horse cytochrome c results in changes in antigenicity due to local and long-range conformational perturbations. *J. Biol. Chem.* 262:11591—11597.

Crumpton, M. J. (1986) The importance of conformation and of equilibria in the interaction of globular proteins and their fragments with antibodies. *Ciba Found. Symp.* 119:93—106.

Darst, S. A., Robertson, C. R., and Berzofsky, J. A. (1988) Adsorption of the protein antigen myoglobin affects the binding of conformation-specific monoclonal antibodies. *Biophys. J.* 53:533—539.

Davies, D. R., Sheriff, S., and Padlan, E. A. (1988) Antigen-antibody complexes. *J. Biol. Chem.* 263:10541—10544.

Delpeyroux, F., Chenciner, N., Lim, A., Malpiece, Y., Blondel, B., Crainic, R., Van der Werf, S., and Streeck, R. E. (1986) A poliovirus neutralization epitope expressed on hybrid hepatitis B surface antigen particles. *Science* 233:472—475.

DiMarchi, R., Brooke, G., Gale, C., Cracknell, V., Doel, T., and Mowat, N. (1986) Protection of cattle against foot-and-mouth disease by a synthetic peptide. *Science* 232:639—641.

Dorow, D. S., Shi, P. T., Carbone, F. R., Minasian, E., Todd, P. E. E., and Leach, S. J. (1985) Two large immunogenic and antigenic myoglobin peptides and the effects of cyclisation. *Mol. Immunol.* 22:1255—1264.

Dreesman, G. R., Sanchez, Y., Ionescu-Matiu, I., Sparrow, J. T., Six, H. R., Peterson, D. L., Hollinger, F. B., and Melnick, J. L. (1982) Antibody to hepatitis B surface antigen after a single inoculation of uncoupled synthetic HBsAg peptides. *Nature (London)* 295:158—160.

Dyrberg, T., and Oldstone, M. B. A. (1986) Peptides as antigens. Importance of orientation. *J. Exp. Med.* 164:1344-1349.

Dyson, H. J., Lerner, R. A., and Wright, P. E. (1988) The physical basis for induction of protein-reactive antipeptide antibodies. *Ann. Rev. Biophys. Biophys. Chem.* 17:305—324.

Edmundson, A. B., Ely, K. R., Herron, J. N., and Cheson, B. D. (1987) The binding of opioid peptides to the Mcg light chain dimer: flexible keys and adjustable locks. *Mol. Immunol.* 24:915—935.

Emini, E. A., Hughes, J. V., Perlow, D. S., and Boger, J. (1985) Induction of hepatitis A virus-neutralizing antibody by a virus-specific synthetic peptide. *J. Virol.* 55:836—839.

Fasman, G. D. (1989) *Prediction of Protein Structure and the Principles of Protein Conformation,* Plenum Press, NY.

Fieser, T. M., Tainer, J. A., Geysen, H. M., and Houghten, R. A. (1987) Influence of protein flexibility and peptide conformation on reactivity of monoclonal antipeptide antibodies with a protein α-helix. *Proc. Natl. Acad. Sci. U.S.A.* 84:8568—8572.

Fourquet, P., Bahraoui, E., Fontecilla-Camps, J. C., Van Rietschoten, J., Rochat, H., and Granier, C. (1988) Immunochemistry of scorpion toxins. Synthesis and antigenic properties of a model of a loop region specific to alpha-toxins. *Int. J. Peptide Protein Res.* 32:81—88.

Friguet, B., Djavadi-Ohaniance, L., and Goldberg, M. E. (1984) Some monoclonal antibodies raised with a native protein bind preferentially to the denatured antigen. *Mol. Immunol.* 21:673—677.

Geerligs, H. J., Weijer, W. J., Bloemhoff, W., Welling, G. W., and Welling-Wester, S. (1988) The influence of pH and ionic strength on the coating of peptides of herpes simplex virus type 1 in an enzyme-linked immunosorbent assay. *J. Immunol. Meth.* 106:239—244.

Getzoff, E. D., Geysen, H. M., Rodda, S. J., Alexander, H., Tainer, J. A., and Lerner, R. A. (1987) Mechanisms of antibody binding to a protein. *Science* 235:1191—1196.

Getzoff, E. D., Tainer, J. A., Lerner, R. A., and Geysen, H. M. (1988) The chemistry and mechanism of antibody binding to protein antigens. *Adv. Immunol.* 43:1—98.

Geysen, H. M. (1985) Antigen-antibody interactions at the molecular level: adventures in peptide synthesis. *Immunol. Today* 6:364—369.

Geysen, H. M., Mason, T. J., and Rodda, S. J. (1988) Cognitive features of continuous antigenic determinants. *J. Mol. Recognition* 1:32—41.

Geysen, H. M., Meloen, R. H., and Barteling, S. J. (1984) Use of peptide synthesis to probe viral antigens for epitopes to a resolution of a single amino acid. *Proc. Natl. Acad. Sci. U.S.A.* 81:3998—4002.

Geysen, H. M., Rodda, S. J., and Mason, T. J. (1986) A priori delineation of a peptide which mimics a discontinuous antigenic determinant. *Mol. Immunol.* 23:709—715.

Geysen, H. M., Rodda, S. J., Mason, T. J., Tainer, J. A., Alexander, H., Getzoff, E. D., and Lerner, R. A. (1987a) Antigenicity of myohemerythrin. *Science* 238:1584—1586.

Geysen, H. M., Rodda, S. J., Mason, T. J., Tribbick, G., and Schoofs, P. G. (1987b) Strategies for epitope analysis using peptide synthesis. *J. Immunol. Meth.* 102:259—274.

Ghosh, S., and Cambell, A. M. (1986) Multispecific monoclonal antibodies. *Immunol. Today* 7:217—222.

Gras-Masse, H. S., Jolivet, M. E., Audibert, F. M., Beachey, E. H., Chedid, L. A., and Tartar, A. L. (1986) Influence of CONH2 or COOH as C-terminus groups on the antigenic characters of immunogenic peptides. *Mol. Immunol.* 23:1391—1395.

Gras-Masse, H., Jolivet, M., Drobecq, H., Aubert, J. P., Beachey, E. H., Audibert, F., Chedid, L., and Tartar, A. (1988) Influence of helical organization on immunogenicity and antigenicity of synthetic peptides. *Mol. Immunol.* 25:673—678.

Green, N., Alexander, H., Olson, A., Alexander, S., Shinnick, T. M., Sutcliffe, J. G., and Lerner, R. A. (1982) Immunogenic structure of the influenza virus hemagglutinin. *Cell* 28:477—487.

Harper, M., Lema, F., Boulot, G., and Poljak, R. J. (1987) Antigen specificity and cross-reactivity of monoclonal anti-lysozyme antibodies. *Mol. Immunol.* 24:97—108.

Heinz, F. X. (1986) Epitope mapping of flavivirus glycoproteins. *Adv. Vir. Res.* 31:103—168.

Heinz, F. X., Mandl, C., Berger, R., Tuma, W., and Kunz, C. (1984) Antibody-induced conformational changes result in enhanced avidity of antibodies to different antigenic sites on the tick-borne encephalitis virus glycoprotein. *Virology* 133:25—34.

Hirayama, A., Takagaki, Y., and Karush, F. (1985) Interaction of monoclonal anti-peptide antibodies with lysozyme. *J. Immunol.* 134:3241—3247.

Hodges, R. S., Heaton, R. J., and Parker, J. M. (1988) Antigen-antibody interaction. Synthetic peptides define linear antigenic determinants recognized by monoclonal antibodies directed to the cytoplasmic carboxyl terminus of rhodopsin. *J. Biol. Chem.* 263:11768—11775.

Hofnung, M., and Charbit, A. (1992) Expression of antigens as recombinant proteins. In *Structure of Antigens* (M. H. V. Van Regenmortel ed.), Vol. 2, Telford Press, Boca Raton, FL, in press.

Hopp, T. P. (1984) Protein antigen conformation: folding patterns and predictive algorithms; selection of antigenic and immunogenic peptides. *Ann. Sclavo* 2:47—60.

Hopp, T. P. (1986) Protein surface analysis. Methods for identifying antigenic determinants and other interaction sites. *J. Immunol. Meth.* 88:1—18.

Hopp, T. P., and Woods, K. R. (1981) Prediction of protein antigenic determinants from amino acid sequence. *Proc. Natl. Acad. Sci. U.S.A.* 78:3824—3828.

Hornbeck, P. V., and Wilson, A. C. (1984) Local effects of amino acid substitutions on the active site region of lysozyme: a comparison of physical and immunological results. *Biochemistry* 23:998—1002.

Houghten, R. A. (1985) General method for the rapid solid-phase synthesis of large numbers of peptides: specificity of antigen-antibody interaction at the level of individual amino acids. *Proc. Natl. Acad. Sci. U.S.A.* 82:5131—5135.

Hurrell, J. G. R., Smith, J. A., Todd, P. E., and Leach, S. J. (1977) Cross-reactivity between mammalian myoglobins: linear vs. spacial antigenic determinants. *Immunochemistry* 14:283—288.

Jemmerson, R. (1987a) Antigenicity and native structure of globular proteins: low frequency of peptide reactive antibodies. *Proc. Natl. Acad. Sci. U.S.A.* 84:9180—9184.

Jemmerson, R. (1987b) Polypeptide fragments of horse cytochrome c activate a small subset of secondary B lymphocytes primed against the native protein. *J. Immunol.* 139:1939—1945.

Jemmerson, R., and Blankenfeld, R. (1989) Affinity consideration in the design of synthetic vaccines intended to elicit antibodies. *Mol. Immunol.* 26:301—307.

Jemmerson, R., and Hutchinson, R. M. (1990) Fine manipulation of antibody affinity for synthetic epitopes by altering peptide structure: antibody binding to looped peptides. *Eur. J. Immunol.* 20:579—585.

Jemmerson, R., and Paterson, Y. (1986) Mapping antigenic sites on proteins: implications for the design of synthetic vaccines. *BioTechniques* 4:18—31.

Kabsch, W., and Sander, C. (1983) How good are predictions of protein secondary structure? *FEBS Lett.*, 155:179—182.

Karplus, P. A., and Schulz, G. E. (1985) Prediction of chain flexibility in proteins. *Naturwissenschaften* 72:212—213.

Kent, S., and Clark-Lewis, I. (1985) Modern methods for the chemical synthesis of biologically active peptides. In *Synthetic Peptides in Biology and Medicine* (K. Alitalo, P. Partanen, and A. Vaheri, eds.), Elsevier, NY, pp. 29—57.

Kyte, J., and Doolittle, R. F. (1982) A simple method for displaying the hydropathic character of a protein. *J. Mol. Biol.* 157:105—132.

Lambert, D. M., and Hughes, A. J. (1988) Keywords and concepts in structuralist and functionalist biology. *J. Theor. Biol.* 133:133—145.

Lando, G., and Reichlin, M. (1982) Antigenic structure of sperm whale myoglobin. II. Characterization of antibodies preferentially reactive with peptides arising in response to immunization with the native protein. *J. Immunol.* 129:212—216.

Laver, W. G., Air, G. M., Webster, R. G., and Smith-Gill, S. J. (1990) Epitopes on protein antigens: misconceptions and realities. *Cell* 61:553-556.

Lenstra, J. A., Kusters, J. G., and Van der Zeijst, B. A. M. (1990) Mapping of viral epitopes with prokaryotic expression products. *Arch. Virol.* 110:1—24.

Lerner, R. A. (1984) Antibodies of predetermined specificity in biology and medicine. *Adv. Immunol.* 36:1—44.

Levitt, M. (1976) A simplified representation of protein conformations for rapid simulation of protein folding. *J. Mol. Biol.* 104:59—107.

Mäkelä, O. (1965) Single lymph node cells producing heteroclitic bacteriophage antibody. *J. Immunol.* 95:378—386.

Mariani, M., Bracci, L., Presentini, R., Nucci, D., Neri, P., and Antoni, G. (1987) Immunogenicity of a free synthetic peptide: carrier-conjugation enhances antibody affinity for the native protein. *Mol. Immunol.* 24:297—303.

Mariuzza, R. A., Phillips, S. E. V., and Poljack, R. J. (1987) The structural basis of antigen-antibody recognition. *Annu. Rev. Biophys. Chem.* 16:139—159.

Mathews, J. H., and Roehrig, J. T. (1984) Elucidation of the topography and determination of the protective epitopes on the E glycoprotein of Saint Louis encephalitis virus by passive transfer with monoclonal antibodies. *J. Immunol.* 132:1533—1537.

McCray, J., and Werner, G. (1987) Different rhinovirus serotypes neutralized by antipeptide antibodies. *Nature (London)* 329:736—738.

Mehra, V., Sweetser, D., and Young, R. A. (1986) Efficient mapping of protein antigenic determinants. *Proc. Natl. Acad. Sci. U.S.A.* 83:7013-7017.

Michel, M. L., Mancini, M., Sobczak, E., Favier, V., Guetard, D., Bahraoui, E. M., and Tiollais, P. (1988) Induction of anti-human immunodeficiency virus (HIV) neutralizing antibodies in rabbits immunized with recombinant HIV-hepatitis B surface antigen particles. *Proc. Natl. Acad. Sci. U.S.A.* 85:7957—7961.

Milton De, L. R. C., and Van Regenmortel, M. H. V. (1979) Immunochemical studies of tobacco mosaic virus. III. Demonstration of five antigenic regions in the protein subunit. *Mol. Immunol.* 16:179—184.

Muller, S., Plaué, S., Couppez, M., and Van Regenmortel, M. H. V. (1986) Comparison of different methods for localizing antigenic regions in histone H2A. *Mol. Immunol.* 23:593—601.

Muller, S., Plaué, S., Samama, J. P., Valette, M., Briand, J. P., and Van Regenmortel, M. H. V. (1990) Antigenic properties and protective capacity of a cyclic peptide corresponding to site A of influenza virus haemagglutinin. *Vaccine* 8:308—314.

Mutter, M. (1988) Nature's rules and chemist's tools: a way for creating novel proteins. *Trends Biochem. Sci.* 13:260—265.

Nestorowicz, A., Tregear, G. W., Southwell, C. N., Martyn, J., Murray, J. M., White, D. O., and Jackson, D. J. (1985) Antibodies elicited by influenza virus hemagglutinin fail to bind to synthetic peptides representing putative antigenic sites. *Mol. Immunol.* 22:145—154.

Niman, H. L., Houghten, R. A., Walker, L. A., Reisfeld, R. A., Wilson, I. A., Hogle, J. M., and Lerner, R. A. (1983) Generation of protein-reactive antibodies by short peptides is an event of high frequency: implications for the structural basis of immune recognition. *Proc. Natl. Acad. Sci. U.S.A.* 80:4949—4953.

Norrby, E., Mufson, M. A., Alexander, H., Houghten, R. A., and Lerner, R. A. (1987) Site-directed serology with synthetic peptides representing the large glycoprotein G of respiratory syncytial virus. *Proc. Natl. Acad. Sci. U.S.A.* 84:6572—6576.

Novotny, J., Bruccoleri, R. E., Carlson, W. D., Handschumacher, M., and Haber, E. (1987b) Antigenicity of myohemerythrin. *Science* 238:1584—1586.

Novotny, J., Bruccoleri, R. E., and Saul, F. A. (1989) On the attribution of binding energy in antigen-antibody complexes McPC 603, D1.3, and HyHEL-5. *Biochemistry* 28:4735—4749.

Novotny, J., Handschumacher, M., Haber, E., Bruccoleri, R. E., Carlson, W. B., Fanning, D. W., Smith, J. A., and Rose, G. D. (1986) Antigenic determinants in proteins coincide with surface regions accessible to large probes (antibody domains). *Proc. Natl. Acad. Sci. U.S.A.* 83:226—230.

Novotny, J., Handschumacher, M., and Bruccoleri, R. E. (1987a) Protein antigenicity: a static surface property. *Immunol. Today* 8:26—31.
Oertle, M., Immergluck, K., Paterson, Y., and Bosshard, H. R. (1989) Mapping of four discontiguous antigenic determinants on horse cytochrome c. *Eur. J. Biochem.* 182:699—704.
Padlan, E. A., Silverton, E. W., Sheriff, S., and Cohen, G. H. (1989) Structure of an antibody-antigen complex: crystal structure of the HyHEL-10 Fab-lysozyme complex. *Proc. Natl. Acad. Sci. U.S.A.* 86:5938—5942.
Palfreyman, J. W., Aitcheson, T. C., and Taylor, P. (1984) Guidelines for the production of polypeptide specific antisera using small synthetic oligopeptides as immunogens. *J. Immunol. Meth.* 75:383—393.
Parker, J. M. R., Guo, D., and Hodges, R. S. (1986) New hydrophilicity scale derived from high-performance liquid chromatography peptide retention data: correlation of predicted surface residues with antigenicity and X-ray-derived accessible sites. *Biochemistry* 25:5425—5432.
Parry, N. R., Syred, A., Rowlands, D. J., and Brown, F. (1988) A high proportion of anti-peptide antibodies recognize foot-and-mouth disease virus particles. *Immunology* 64:567—572.
Pellequer, J. L., Westhof, E., and Van Regenmortel, M. H. V. (1991) Overview of methods for predicting the location of continuous epitopes in proteins from their primary structures. *Meth. Enzymol.,* 203:176—201.
Plaué, S. (1990) Synthesis of cyclic peptides on solid support. Application to analogs of hemagglutinin of influenza virus. *Int. J. Pept. Protein Res.* 35:510—517.
Pollock, R. P., Teillaud, J. L., and Scharff, M. D. (1984) Monoclonal antibodies: a powerful tool for selecting and analyzing mutations in antigens and antibodies. *Annu. Rev. Microbiol.* 38:389—417.
Quesniaux, V. F. J., Schmitter, D., Schreier, M. H., and Van Regenmortel, M. H. V. (1990) Monoclonal antibodies to cyclosporine are representative of the major antibody populations present in antisera of immunized mice. *Mol. Immunol.* 27:227—236.
Roehrig, J. T., Hunt, A. R., Johnson, A. J., and Hawkes, R. A. (1989) Synthetic peptides derived from the deduced amino acid sequence of the E-glycoprotein of Murray Valley encephalitis virus elicit antiviral antibody. *Virology* 171:49—60.
Rose, G. D., Geselowitz, A. R., Lesser, G. J., Lee, R. H., and Zehfus, M. H. (1985b) Hydrophobicity of amino acid residues in globular proteins. *Science* 229:834—838.
Rose, G. D., Gierasch, L. M., and Smith, J. A. (1985a) Turns in peptides and proteins. *Adv. Protein Chem.* 37:1—109.
Sasaki, A., Mikawa, Y., Sakamoto, Y., Yamada, H., Ikeda, Y., and Ohno, T. (1988) Computer graphic analysis of antigenic sites on the insulin molecule. *Mol. Immunol.* 25:157—163.
Satterthwait, A. C., Arrhenius, T., Hagopian, R. A., Zavala, F., Nussenzweig, V., and Lerner, R. A. (1989) The conformational restriction of synthetic peptides, including a malaria peptide, for use as immunogens. *Phil. Trans. R. Soc. London B* 323:565—572.
Schaaper, M. M., Lankhof, H., Pujik, W. C., and Meloen, R. H. (1989) Manipulation of antipeptide immune response by varying the coupling of the peptide with the carrier protein. *Mol. Immunol.* 26:81—85.

Schoofs, P. G., Geysen, H. M., Jackson, D., Brown, L. E., Tang, X. L., and White, D. O. (1988) Epitopes of an influenza viral peptide recognized by antibody at single amino acid resolution. *J. Immunol.* 140:611—616.

Schulze-Gahmen, U., Klenk, H. D., and Beyreuther, K. (1986) Immunogenicity of loop-structured short synthetic peptides mimicking the antigenic site A of influenza virus hemagglutinin. *Eur. J. Biochem.* 159:283—289.

Schulze-Gahmen, U., Rini, J. M., Arevalo, J., Stura, E. A., Kenten, J. H., and Wilson, I. A. (1988) Preliminary crystallographic data, primary sequence, and binding data for an anti-peptide Fab and its complex with a synthetic peptide from influenza virus hemagglutinin. *J. Biol. Chem.* 263:17100—17105.

Scibienski, R. J. (1973) Denaturation of lysozyme by Freund's complete adjuvant. *J. Immunol.* 111:114—120.

Sheriff, S., Silverton, E. W., Padlan, E. A., Cohen, G. H., Smith-Gill, S., Finzel, B. C., and Davies, D. R. (1987) Three-dimensional structure of an antibody-antigen complex. *Proc. Natl. Acad. Sci. U.S.A.* 84:8075—8079.

Shi, P. T., Riehm, J. P., Todd, P. E. E., and Leach, S. J. (1984) The antigenicity of myoglobin-related peptides synthesised on polyacrylamide and polystyrene resin supports. *Mol. Immunol.* 21:489—496.

Smith, A. M., and Benjamin, D. C. (1991) The antigenic surface of staphylococcal nuclease. II. Analysis of the N-1 epitope by site-directed mutagenesis. *J. Immunol.* 146:1259—1264.

Smith, A. M., Woodward, M. P., Hershey, C. W., Hershey, E. D., and Benjamin, D. C. (1991) The antigenic surface of staphylococcal nuclease. I. Mapping epitopes by site-directed mutagenesis. *J. Immunol.* 146: 1254—1258.

Smyth, M. S., Hoey, E. M., Trudgett, A., Martin, S. J., and Brown, F. (1990) Chemically synthesized peptides elicit neutralizing antibody to bovine enterovirus. *J. Gen. Virol.* 71:231—234.

Soderquist, M. E., and Walton, A. G. (1980) Structural changes in proteins adsorbed on polymer surfaces *J. Colloid Interface Sci.* 75:386—397.

Stanfield, R. L., Fieser, T. M., Lerner, R. A., and Wilson, I. A. (1990) Crystal structures of an antibody to a peptide and its complex with peptide antigen at 2.8 Å. *Science* 248:712—719.

Stanley, K. K. (1983) Solubilization and immune-detection of β-galactosidase hybrid proteins carrying foreign antigenic determinants. *Nucl. Acids Res.* 11:4077—4092.

Stura, E. A., Stanfield, R. L., Fieser, T. M., Balderas, R. S., Smith, L. R., Lerner, R. A., and Wilson, I. A. (1989) Preliminary crystallographic data and primary sequence for anti-peptide Fab B13I2 and its complex with the C-helix peptide from myohemerythrin. *J. Biol. Chem.* 264:15721—15725.

Tainer, J. A., Getzoff, E. D., Paterson, Y., Olson, A. J., and Lerner, R. A. (1985) The atomic mobility component of protein antigenicity. *Annu. Rev. Immunol.* 3:501—535.

Tam, J. P. (1988) Synthetic peptide vaccine design: synthesis and properties of a high-density multiple antigenic peptide system. *Proc. Natl. Acad. Sci. U.S.A.* 85:5409—5413.

Thornton, J. M., Edwards, M. S., Taylor, W. R., and Barlow, D. J. (1986) Location of "continuous" antigenic determinants in the protruding regions of proteins. *EMBO J.* 5:409—413.

Thornton, J. M., and Sibanda, B. L. (1983) Amino and carboxy-terminal regions in globular proteins. *J. Mol. Biol.* 167:443—460.

Trifilieff, E., Dubs, M. C., and Van Regenmortel, M. H. V. (1991) Antigenic cross-reactivity potential of synthetic peptides immobilized on polyethylene rods. *Mol. Immunol.* 28:889—896.

Tulip, W. R., Varghese, J. N., Webster, R. G., Air, G. M., Laver, W. G., and Colman, P. M. (1989) Crystal structures of neuraminidase-antibody complexes. *Cold Spring Harbor Symp. Quant. Biol.* LIV:257—263.

Underwood, P. A. (1982) Mapping of antigenic changes in the haemagglutinin of Hong Kong influenza(H3N2) strains using a large panel of monoclonal antibodies. *J. Gen. Virol.* 62:153—169.

Underwood, P. A. (1985) Theoretical considerations of the ability of monoclonal antibodies to detect antigenic differences between closely related variants, with particular reference to heterospecific reactions. *J. Immunol. Meth.* 85:295—307.

Van Regenmortel, M. H. V. (1984) Molecular dissection of antigens by monoclonal antibodies. In *Hybridoma Technology in Agricultural and Veterinary Research* (N. J. Stern, H. R. Gamble, eds.), Rowman and Allanheld, Totowa, NJ, pp. 43—82.

Van Regenmortel, M. H. V. (1986) Which structural features determine protein antigenicity? *Trends Biochem. Sci.* 11:36—39.

Van Regenmortel, M. H. V. (1987) Antigenic cross-reactivity between proteins and peptides: new insights and applications. *Trends Biochem. Sci.* 12:237—240.

Van Regenmortel, M. H. V. (1989a) The concept and operational definition of protein epitopes. *Phil. Trans. R. Soc. London B* 323:451.

Van Regenmortel, M. H. V. (1989b) Structural and functional approaches to the study of protein antigenicity. *Immunol. Today* 10:266—272.

Van Regenmortel, M. H. V., Briand, J. P., Muller, S., and Plaué, S. (1988) Synthetic polypeptides as antigens. In *Laboratory Techniques in Biochemistry and Molecular Biology,* Vol. 19, Elsevier, Amsterdam, pp. 1—227.

Van Regenmortel, M. H. V., and Daney de Marcillac, G. (1988) An assessment of prediction methods for locating continuous epitopes in proteins. *Immunol. Lett.* 17:95—108.

Walter, G. (1986) Production and use of antibodies against synthetic peptides. *J. Immunol. Meth.* 88:149—161.

Welling, G. W., Weijer, W. J., Van der Zee, R., and Welling-Wester, S. (1985) Prediction of sequential antigenic regions in proteins. *FEBS Lett.* 188:215—218.

Westhof, E., Altschuh, D., Moras, D., Bloomer, A. C., Mondragon, A., Klug, A., and Van Regenmortel, M. H. V. (1984) Correlation between segmental mobility and the location of antigenic determinants in proteins. *Nature (London)* 311:123—126.

Wiley, D. C., and Skehel, J. J. (1987) The structure and function of the hemagglutinin membrane glycoprotein of influenza virus. *Annu. Rev. Biochem.* 56:365—394.

Wilson, I. A., Haft, D. H., Tainer, J. A., Getzoff, E. D., Lerner, R. A., and Brenner, S. (1985) Identical short peptide sequences in unrelated proteins can have different conformations: a testing ground for theories of immune recognition. *Proc. Natl. Acad. Sci. U.S.A.* 82:5255—5259.

Wilson, I. A., Niman, H. L., Houghten, R. A., Cherenson, A. R., Connolly, M. L., and Lerner, R. A. (1984) The structure of an antigenic determinant in a protein. *Cell* 37:767—778.

Young, R. A., and Davis, R. W. (1983) Efficient isolation of genes by using antibody probes. *Proc. Natl. Acad. Sci. U.S.A.* 80:1194—1198.

Chapter
2

Structure of Protein Epitopes Deduced from X-Ray Crystallography

Eduardo A. Padlan
Laboratory of Molecular Biology
National Institute of Diabetes and Digestive and Kidney Diseases
National Institutes of Health
Bethesda, Maryland

INTRODUCTION

The study of epitopes and of their interaction with specific antibodies is greatly aided by the availability of three-dimensional structural information. In this respect, X-ray diffraction and other techniques that provide spatial relationships between molecules can make significant contributions to the structural analysis of epitopes. Recent X-ray crystallographic studies of Fab-antigen complexes have now permitted the direct visualization of the interaction between several antibody combining sites and their epitopes. Three of these complexes involve hen egg white lysozyme (Amit et al., 1986; Padlan et al., 1989; Sheriff et al., 1987), which has been the subject of numerous immunochemical studies, and two involve the neuraminidase of influenza virus (Colman et al., 1987; Colman et al., 1989; Tulip et al., 1989). In addition, the structure of a Fab complexed to its anti-idiotypic Fab has been determined (Bentley et al., 1989), although no structural details are as yet available.

The structures of the uncomplexed lysozyme and neuraminidase are available. This permits the examination of the possible occurrence of conformational changes on the structure of the antigen upon binding to the antibody. This also permits the investigation of the possible correlation between antigenicity and the inherent flexibility of the epitope, as deduced from the crystallographic thermal factors of the uncomplexed molecule.

In the sections following, the three-dimensional structure of the antibody-antigen complexes are described which have been obtained using X-ray crystallography, the structure of protein epitopes deduced from these studies, and the possible correlation between the antigenicity of a particular region of a protein molecule and its thermal mobility, large-probe accessibility, hydrophilicity, or other structural property.

X-RAY STRUCTURE OF ANTIBODY-ANTIGEN COMPLEXES

The antibodies investigated in these X-ray crystallographic studies were murine hybridoma proteins which bind to their specific antigens with high affinity. All the complexes were between Fab fragments and intact antigens.

It must be pointed out that the structural analyses of these antibody-antigen complexes were done only at medium resolution (circa 3 to 2.5 Å), so that there is the possibility of large errors in the atomic coordinates. At resolutions such as these, average errors of about 0.5 Å can be expected for the most ordered, usually interior, parts of the molecule. Larger errors can be expected for the more exposed regions, loops, and, especially, side chains. A consequence of this is that contacts between residues cannot be described with certainty and one can only talk of potential hydrogen bonds, possible salt links, etc. Although interatomic contacts can be analyzed in terms of the errors in the atomic positions, that will not be done here; instead the molecular contacts between antibodies and their epitopes will be described here simply as they have been described by the original authors, especially since the definition of what constitutes an interatomic contact usually varies between authors.

Structure of the Complex of D1.3 Fab and Hen Egg White Lysozyme

The X-ray structure of the D1.3 Fab-lysozyme complex was determined by the method of multiple isomorphous heavy-atom replacement to 2.8-Å resolution (Amit et al., 1986). Preliminary refinement has resulted in a crystallographic R factor of 0.28 with a standard deviation of C–C bond lengths of 0.03 Å. the error in the atomic positions was estimated to be about 0.6 Å. The Fab was found to be in an almost fully extended conformation with a Fab bend (the angle between the pseudodyads in the variable and in the constant modules) of almost 180°; otherwise the D1.3 Fab was found to have the same quaternary structure as those of other known Fabs. Comparison of the structure of the lysozyme in the complex with that of an uncomplexed form of the antigen, determined at 1.6-Å resolution, gave a root-mean-square deviation of 0.64 Å for the α-carbon positions, which is statistically not significant since it is comparable to the estimated error of the D1.3 structure. Thus, no gross conformational changes in the structure of the antigen had occurred upon complexation with the antibody.

The interface between antibody D1.3 and lysozyme is extensive, with 748 Å^2 of the surface of the lysozyme and 690 Å^2 of the antibody buried upon complex formation. There is a close complementarity between the antibody-combining site surface and that of the epitope, with solvent mostly excluded from the interface. All six complementarity determining regions (CDRs) of antibody D1.3 participate in antigen binding, with 17 antibody residues making contact with 16 lysozyme residues. Two of the contact residues from the antibody are from the framework. The combining site has a cleft between the third CDRs of the light and heavy chains; the side chain of Gln^{121} of lysozyme fits snugly in this cleft. The epitope consists of residues from two stretches of polypeptide chain, residues 18 to 27 and 116 to 129 of the lysozyme.

There are twelve potential hydrogen bonds between antibody D1.3 and lysozyme and many van der Waals contacts; eight of the potential hydrogen bonds involve main-chain atoms. There are no salt bridges despite the fact that two arginines, two aspartic acids, and one histidine from the antibody and one arginine and one aspartic acid from the antigen are involved in the contact. Many aromatic residues participate in the binding, including two tryptophans, five tyrosines, one phenylalanine, and one histidine from the antibody and one tyrosine from the antigen. The contact between antibody D1.3 and its epitope (Amit et al., 1986) is summarized in Table 1.

Structure of the Complex of HyHEL-5 Fab and Hen Egg White Lysozyme

The X-ray structure of the HyHEL-5 Fab-lysozyme complex in two crystal forms was determined by the method of molecular replacement, one form to a resolution of 3.0 Å and the other to 2.5 Å (Sheriff et al., 1987). Only the results from the 2.5 Å analysis will be discussed here. The structure of the complex was refined to a crystallographic R factor of 0.245 with a root-mean-square deviation from ideal bond lengths of 0.012 Å. The estimated error of the atomic positions was 0.40 Å. The Fab bend was found to be 161°. The quaternary association of the variable domains and of the constant domains of HyHEL-5 Fab was found to be canonical, i.e., as found in other Fabs. No gross conformational changes were found to occur in the lysozyme although some movement was observed to have occurred in some parts of the antigen; for example, the α-carbon of Pro^{70} had moved by about 1.7 Å. The aromatic ring of Trp^{63} of the lysozyme was found to have rotated by 180° even though it is not involved in the contact with the antibody.

TABLE 1.
Antibody D1.3 Residues Involved in the Contact with Lysozyme

	Antibody Residues	Lysozyme Residues in Contact
Light Chain		
CDR1	His^{30}	Leu^{129}
	Tyr^{32}	Leu^{25}, Gln^{121}, Ile^{124}
FR2	Tyr^{49}	Gly^{22}
CDR2	Tyr^{50}	Asp^{18}, Asn^{19}, Leu^{25}
CDR3	Phe^{91}	Gln^{121}
	Trp^{92}	Gln^{121}, Ile^{124}
	Ser^{93}	Gln^{121}
Heavy Chain		
FR1	Thr^{30}	Lys^{116}, Gly^{117}
CDR1	Gly^{31}	Lys^{116}, Gly^{117}
	Tyr^{32}	Lys^{116}, Gly^{117}
CDR2	Trp^{52}	Gly^{117}, Thr^{118}, Asp^{119}
	Gly^{53}	Gly^{117}
	Asp^{54}	Gly^{117}
CDR3	Arg^{96}	Arg^{21}, Gly^{22}, Tyr^{23}
	Asp^{97}	Gly^{22}, Tyr^{23}, Ser^{24}, Asn^{27}
	Tyr^{98}	Thr^{118}, Asp^{119}, Val^{120}, Gln^{121}
	Arg^{99}	Asn^{19}, Gly^{22}

The surface area buried in the complex is about 750 Å^2 for both the Fab and lysozyme. The interaction between HyHEL-5 and lysozyme is very tight, and there are no solvent molecules in the interface. All six CDRs are involved in the interaction with the antigen, as well as one residue from the framework. In all, 17 residues from the HyHEL-5 are in contact with 14 residues from the lysozyme. In addition, 11 residues from the antibody and 10 from the antigen are at least partly buried by the interaction. The HyHEL-5 combining site has a groove running between the third CDRs of the light and heavy chains. At the bottom of this groove lie the carboxylates of two glutamic acid side chains from the heavy chain; two arginines from the lysozyme form a ridge that fits into this groove. The epitope consists of three oligopeptide segments: the first includes residues from the stretch 41 to 53, the second contains residues 67 to 70, and the third consists of residue 84 of the lysozyme.

There are 10 potential hydrogen bonds between HyHEL-5 and lysozyme, 74 van der Waals contacts, and 3 salt bridges. The salt bridges involve two arginines from the lysozyme and two glutamic acids from the antibody. Several aromatic side chains are involved in the interaction, including three tryptophans and two tyrosines from the antibody and one tyrosine from the lysozyme. The contact between antibody HyHEL-5 and its epitope (Sheriff et al., 1987) is summarized in Table 2.

TABLE 2.
Antibody HyHEL-5 Residues Involved in the Contact with Lysozyme

	Antibody Residues	Lysozyme Residues in Contact
Light Chain		
CDR1	Asp^{31}	Asp^{48}
	Tyr^{32}	Pro^{70}
CDR2	Asp^{50}	Pro^{70}
CDR3	Trp^{91}	Arg^{45}, Gly^{49}, Arg^{68}
	Arg^{93}	Arg^{45}, Asn^{46}, Thr^{47}
	Pro^{95}	Arg^{45}
Heavy Chain		
CDR1	Trp^{31}	Tyr^{53}, Arg^{68}
	Glu^{35}	Arg^{68}
FR2	Trp^{47}	Arg^{45}
CDR2	Glu^{50}	Arg^{45}, Arg^{68}
	Ser^{55}	Gln^{41}, Leu^{84}
	Ser^{57}	Gln^{41}, Thr^{43}
	Thr^{58}	Thr^{43}
	Asn^{59}	Thr^{43}, Asn^{44}
CDR3	Gly^{95}	Arg^{68}
	Tyr^{97}	Gly^{67}, Arg^{68}, Thr^{69}, Pro^{70}

Structure of the Complex of HyHEL-10 Fab and Hen Egg White Lysozyme

The X-ray structure of the HyHEL-10 Fab-lysozyme complex was analyzed by the method of molecular replacement of 3.0-Å resolution (Padlan et al., 1989). Crystallographic refinement resulted in an R factor of 0.24 with deviations from ideality of 0.011 Å for bond lengths. The error in atomic positions was estimated to be 0.4 Å. The Fab bend was found to be 147° and the quaternary association of the variable and of the constant domains of HyHEL-10 Fab was found to be canonical. No major changes in the structure of the lysozyme were observed, although the α-carbon of Gly^{102} was found to have moved by 2.13 Å relative to the uncomplexed lysozyme structure. The aromatic ring of Trp^{62} of the lysozyme was found to have rotated by 150°, apparently to avoid close contacts with side chains from the antibody.

The complementarity of the antibody and antigen contacting surfaces is very close and there are no cavities large enough to accommodate a water molecule. The area of the lysozyme that is in contact with the antibody is 774 Å^2, whereas 720 Å^2 of the HyHEL-10 combining site are in contact with the epitope. All six CDRs contribute to the binding, as well as one residue from the framework. In all, 19 residues from the antibody are in direct contact with the antigen and 15 residues from the lysozyme interact with the antibody. The combining site has a protuberance, consisting mainly of the side chains of two tyrosines residues; this protrusion fits into the active-site cleft of the

TABLE 3.
Antibody HyHEL-10 Residues Involved in the Contact with Lysozyme

	Antibody Residues	Lysozyme Residues in Contact
Light Chain		
CDR1	Gly^{30}	Gly^{16}
	Asn^{31}	His^{15}, Gly^{16}, Lys^{96}
	Asn^{32}	Gly^{16}, Tyr^{20}
CDR2	Tyr^{50}	Asn^{93}, Lys^{96}
	Gln^{53}	Thr^{89}, Asn^{93}
CDR3	Ser^{91}	Tyr^{20}
	Asn^{92}	Tyr^{20}, Arg^{21}
	Tyr^{96}	Arg^{21}
Heavy Chain		
FR1	Thr^{30}	Arg^{73}
CDR1	Ser^{31}	Arg^{73}, Leu^{75}
	Asp^{32}	Lys^{97}
	Tyr^{33}	Trp^{63}, Lys^{97}, Ile^{98}, Ser^{100}, Asp^{101}
CDR2	Tyr^{50}	Arg^{21}, Ser^{100}
	Ser^{52}	Asp^{101}
	Tyr^{53}	Trp^{63}, Leu^{75}, Asp^{101}
	Ser^{54}	Asp^{101}
	Ser^{56}	Asp^{101}, Gly^{102}
	Tyr^{58}	Arg^{21}, Ser^{100}, Gly^{102}
CDR3	Trp^{95}	Arg^{21}, Ser^{100}, Gly^{102}

lysozyme. The epitope is made up of four stretches of polypeptide chain; it consists of a central helix (residues 88 to 99) and some surrounding residues. The lysozyme residues that contact HyHEL-10 are residues 15, 16, 20, and 21 on one side of the helix; residues 89, 93, and 96 to 98, which constitute the exposed surface of the helix; residues 100 to 102, which are part of the loop that extends beyond the helix; residue 63, which lies in the active-site cleft; and residues 73 and 75, which are on the other side of the cleft. In addition, three other residues are partly buried by the interaction.

There are 14 potential hydrogen bonds between HyHEL-10 and the lysozyme, 1 weak salt link (the closest approach of the interacting residues is 3.6 Å and the salt bridge is exposed to the solvent), and 111 van der Waals interactions. Seven of the contacting residues from the antibody have aromatic side chains: six tyrosines and one tryptophan; one tyrosine and one tryptophan from the lysozyme are involved in the contact. The contact between antibody HyHEL-10 and its epitope (Padlan et al., 1989) is summarized in Table 3.

Structure of the Complex of NC41 Fab and Influenza Virus Neuraminidase

The X-ray structure of the NC41 Fab-neuraminidase complex was determined at 3-Å resolution by the method of multiple isomorphous heavy-atom replacement (Colman et al., 1987); it has been refined, using 2.9-Å data to a crystallographic R factor of 0.187 (Tulip et al., 1989). The root-mean-square deviation of bond lengths from ideality is 0.022 Å, and the estimated error in atomic positions is 0.3 Å. The Fab bend was found to be approximately 150°. The quaternary association of the variable domains of NC41 Fab was initially thought to differ significantly from that found in other Fab structures to make it an outlier (Colman et al., 1987); however, later results showed that the relative disposition of the variable domains in NC41 is within the observed range (Tulip et al., 1989). Possible conformational changes in the antibody or antigen could not be ascertained because the structure of the uncomplexed Fab was not known and the structure of the neuraminidase had not been fully refined.

The surface area that had become inaccessible in the formation of the complex is 878 $Å^2$ on the neuraminidase and 885 $Å^2$ on the Fab. There is a remarkable shape complementarity of the interacting surfaces and there appear to be no water molecules buried in the interface. Only five of the six CDRs are in direct contact with the antigen, with the CDR1-L of NC41 not contributing to the binding at all. In all, 20 residues from the antibody are in contact with 22 residues from the antigen. Three framework residues contribute to the paratope. The epitope is extensive, being comprised of five polypeptide segments. In addition to the 22 amino acids that are in direct contact with the antibody, five other residues are partly buried, as are atoms in five other amino acid residues from two other segments and two sugar residues from a neighboring carbohydrate (Tulip et al., 1989). No further details of the interaction are currently available.

Structure of the Complex of NC10 Fab and Influenza Virus Neuraminidase

The X-ray structure of the NC10 Fab-neuraminidase complex was determined by a combination of molecular replacement and multiple isomorphous heavy-atom replacement methods to 3-Å (0.3-mm) resolution (Colman et al., 1989). Crystallographic refinement has yielded an R factor of 0.20 (Tulip et al., 1989), but some regions of the structure are not yet fully refined. Unfortunately, these include parts of the interface so that details of the contacts, including buried surface areas, are not yet clear. The constant domains of the Fab are disordered in the crystal and are not visible. Nevertheless, it is obvious that the epitopes recognized by antibodies NC41 and NC10 are largely overlapping. However, the mode of attachment of the two antibodies is very different, so that one Fv is rotated roughly 90° relative to the other when bound. Moreover, only four of the six CDRs of NC10 are in contact with the antigen, with the second CDR of the light chain and the first CDR of the heavy chain not involved in the binding at all.

THE STRUCTURE OF PROTEIN EPITOPES

Although fine details of the lysozyme epitopes are available from the X-ray studies, the picture for the neuraminidase epitopes is far from complete. Therefore, the discussion that follows will be concerned only with the epitopes on hen egg white lysozyme for antibodies D1.3, HyHEL-5, and HyHEL-10 as revealed by X-ray crystallography.

Structure of Lysozyme

Hen egg white lysozyme is a 14.6-kDa glycosidase whose crystal structure has been determined at high resolution in various crystal forms. Its three-dimensional structure is approximately 46% helical and 16% β-pleated sheet; the structure is stabilized by four disulfide bridges. It is rugged and its crystal structure under 1000 atmospheres (101.3 megapascal) of pressure (Kundrot and Richards, 1987) differs from that observed under standard conditions by only 0.59 Å on the average for all atoms and by only 0.17 Å for the atoms in the backbone. It is bean-shaped with an extensive cleft running along the middle (Plate 1A);* this cleft can accommodate a linear hexasaccharide substrate. The total solvent-accessible area of the molecule is about 5500 Å^2.

Table 4 shows the occurrence of the various amino acid types in hen egg white lysozyme and their solvent accessibilities [computed as described elsewhere (Padlan, 1990), using atomic coordinates in the Protein Data Bank File 2LYM (Bernstein et al., 1977)]. Because lysozyme is a small protein, it is not particularly meaningful to compare its amino acid content to that of proteins in general. However, the amino acids that are usually found buried in the interior of water-soluble, globular proteins (Padlan, 1990), i.e., Cys, Ile, Leu, Met, Phe, Trp, and Val, represent 30.2% of the residues in lysozyme, nearly the same as the 28.0% for proteins in general (Klapper, 1977); the amino acids that are usually exposed to solvent, i.e., Arg, Asn, Asp, Gln, Glu, Gly, Lys, Pro, Ser, and Thr, constitute 57.4% of the total number of residues in lysozyme, essentially identical to the 56.9% for other proteins. Moreover, it is seen in Table 4 that, by and large, the exposure patterns for the various amino acid types parallel those found in other water-soluble proteins. These results imply that lysozyme is not an unusual protein so that the conclusions and generalizations made for lysozyme as an antigen are probably applicable to other protein antigens.

General Nature of the Lysozyme Epitopes

These epitopes are essentially nonoverlapping. The epitope for D1.3 is at the end of the molecule where the N- and C-termini are located (Plate 1B), the epitope for HyHEL-10 is located around the middle and includes part of

---

*Plate 1 follows page 298.

TABLE 4.
Exposures for Hen Egg White Lysozyme[a]

	Exposure[b]						Average Exposure (SD)	
	Bu	mB	pB	mE	Ex	Total	Lysozyme	Water-Soluble Proteins[c]
Ala	4	0	4	3	1	12	0.403 (0.312)	0.430 (0.381)
Arg	0	0	2	5	4	11	0.742 (0.152)	0.571 (0.235)
Asn	0	1	5	3	5	14	0.706 (0.220)	0.610 (0.281)
Asp	1	1	0	2	3	7	0.603 (0.272)	0.590 (0.315)
Cys	7	0	0	1	0	8	0.118 (0.198)	0.157 (0.206)
Gln	1	0	0	0	2	3	0.647 (0.344)	0.579 (0.275)
Glu	0	1	0	1	0	2	0.430 (0.190)	0.648 (0.255)
Gly	2	0	0	0	10	12	0.833 (0.373)	0.686 (0.464)
His	0	1	0	0	0	1	0.360 (—)	0.375 (0.287)
Ile	3	2	1	0	0	6	0.200 (0.188)	0.186 (0.233)
Leu	5	0	3	0	0	8	0.191 (0.250)	0.206 (0.255)
Lys	0	0	3	3	0	6	0.595 (0.126)	0.703 (0.204)
Met	2	0	0	0	0	2	0.000 (0.000)	0.209 (0.265)
Phe	1	1	1	0	0	3	0.277 (0.121)	0.198 (0.225)
Pro	0	0	0	0	2	2	0.915 (0.085)	0.552 (0.334)
Ser	4	1	1	2	2	10	0.406 (0.370)	0.586 (0.355)
Thr	3	0	0	3	1	7	0.471 (0.362)	0.507 (0.323)
Trp	3	1	1	1	0	6	0.313 (0.256)	0.221 (0.209)
Tyr	0	3	0	0	0	3	0.330 (0.078)	0.356 (0.249)
Val	3	1	0	0	2	6	0.340 (0.376)	0.230 (0.285)
Total	39	13	21	24	32	129	0.484 (0.356)	0.462 (0.364)

[a] Protein Data Bank File 2LYM.
[b] An amino acid whose side chain has a fractional accessibility value between 0.00 and 0.20 is designated as completely buried (Bu), between 0.20 and 0.40 as mostly buried (mB), between 0.40 and 0.60 as partly buried (pB), between 0.60 and 0.80 as mostly exposed (mE), and at least 0.80 as completely exposed (Ex). In the special case of glycine, the residue is designated as completely exposed if its α-carbon is accessible to solvent; otherwise, it is designated as completely buried.
[c] For 50 highly refined, water-soluble proteins (Padlan, 1990).

the catalytic cleft (Plate 1C), and the epitope for HyHEL-5 is at the other end, away from the termini, and includes portions of the so-called "antigenic loop" (Arnon, 1977) of the enzyme (Plate 1D). Together, these epitopes constitute more than 40% of the total solvent-accessible surface of the antigen.

The segments that constitute the three epitopes are presented in Table 5. The epitope for antibody D1.3 is made up of residues from two segments of polypeptide chain, widely separated in sequence but close together in space. Antibody HyHEL-5 is made up mainly of residues from two neighboring segments and one nearby residue, and antibody HyHEL-10 is composed of residues from four different segments of the antigen. In all three cases, the epitope is discontinuous. Considering that these epitopes each present a surface area of interaction of about 750 Å^2, it comes as no surprise that all three are discontinuous (Barlow et al., 1986).

TABLE 5.
Lysozyme Segments in the Epitopes for Antibodies D1.3, HyHEL-5, and HyHEL-10

D1.3
ASP^{18}, ASN^{19}, ARG^{21}, GLY^{22}, TYR^{23}, SER^{24}, LEU^{25}, ASN^{27}
LYS^{116}, GLY^{117}, THR^{118}, ASP^{119}, VAL^{120}, GLN^{121}, ILE^{124}, LEU^{129}
HyHEL-5
Gln^{41}, Thr^{43}, Asn^{44}, Arg^{45}, Asn^{46}, Thr^{47}, Asp^{48}, Gly^{49}, Tyr^{53}
Gly^{67}, Arg^{68}, Thr^{69}, Pro^{70}
Leu^{84}
HyHEL-10
His^{15}, Gly^{16}, Tyr^{20}, Arg^{21}
Trp^{63}
Arg^{73}, Leu^{75}
Thr^{89}, Asn^{93}, Lys^{96}, Lys^{97}, Ile^{98}, Ser^{100}, Asp^{101}, Gly^{102}

Amino Acids and Secondary Structural Elements in the Lysozyme Epitopes

The residues that form the epitope for antibody D1.3 come mainly from the segments anterior to the second helix and to the C-terminal helix of the molecule, and from those helices themselves (Plate 1B); those that form the HyHEL-10 epitope come from the exposed side of a central helix and from nearby loop regions (Plate 1C); and those in the HyHEL-5 epitope originate mainly from two antiparallel β strands and the tight turn that connects them, and from a neighboring loop structure (Plate 1D). The presence of a variety of different secondary structural elements in these epitopes suggests that the antigenicity of a region does not depend on the existence of a particular structural element in that region.

The distribution of amino acids that occur in the three lysozyme epitopes is presented in Table 6. Some amino acids are not represented in that list; specifically, there are no cysteines, methionines, or phenylalanines, which are among those usually buried in water-soluble proteins, or are there alanines, which have been found to be exposed about half the time, or glutamic acids, which are usually exposed to solvent (Padlan, 1990). Considering that this is a very limited sample, it is remarkable that most of the different amino acid types are found in one or another of these epitopes. This suggests that there is no preference for certain amino acids to be present in antigenic determinants.

It is conceivable, nevertheless, that the presence of certain amino acid types in an epitope could result in a higher immunogenic potential (Padlan, 1985) or in immunodominance. Furthermore, theoretical calculations suggest that only a few residues in epitopes contribute the major portion of the interaction energy and that the rest may simply serve to provide the necessary complementarity with the antibody-combining site (Novotny, 1990).

TABLE 6.
Amino Acid Residues in the Lysozyme Epitopes

	Antibody		
Amino acid	D1.3	HyHEL-5	HyHEL-10
Ala			
Arg	1	2	2
Asn	2	2	1
Asp	2	1	1
Cys			
Gln	1	1	
Glu			
Gly	2	2	2
His			1
Ile	1		1
Leu	2	1	1
Lys	1		2
Met			
Phe			
Pro		1	
Ser	1		1
Thr	1	3	1
Trp			1
Tyr	1	1	1
Val	1		

Mobility, Hydrophilicity, and Accessibility of the Lysozyme Epitopes

The possible correlation between antigenicity and various other structural parameters has been hypothesized. These parameters include hydrophilicity (Hopp and Woods, 1981), mobility as evidenced by high crystallographic thermal factors (Tainer et al., 1984; Westhof et al., 1984), large-probe accessibility (Novotny et al., 1986), and "protrusion index" (Thornton et al., 1986). The antigenicity of hen egg white lysozyme had been predicted on the basis of these parameters and it is clear that the predictions have been, to a certain degree, correct.

For example, the stretches in lysozyme with the highest hydrophilicities are those around residues 16, 48, and 116; these residues are contained in the epitopes for antibodies HyHEL-10, HyHEL-5, and D1.3, respectively (Table 5). From the X-ray analyses of the enzyme, the most mobile segments, i.e., those with the highest crystallographic thermal factors, are those around residues 48, 70, 102, and the C-terminus; again, these residues are part of one or another of the three epitopes discussed above. Furthermore, the regions in lysozyme with the highest "protrusion index" (Thornton et al., 1986), are the segments 38 to 54 and 64 to 80; these include most of the epitope for HyHEL-5 (Table 5). Even further, the regions that are most accessible to a spherical probe of 10-Å radius are centered around 48, 70, and 116 (Novotny et al., 1986); these, also, are in the epitopes.

However, there are many other residues that are in the epitopes for D1.3, HyHEL-5, and HyHEL-10, but which have not been predicted by these methods to be likely found in antigenic sites. These include Trp^{63}, Thr^{89}, and Asn^{93} which are not only part of the HyHEL-10 epitope but are actually near the center of the epitope (Plate 1C). Moreover, there are regions that are part of epitopes which are not particularly accessible to large probes, or are they particularly mobile (Davies et al., 1988). Indeed, there are no special physical or chemical attributes which could be ascribed to these epitopes except that they are all exposed.

Generalizations

The results from X-ray studies of the antibody-lysozyme complexes lead to the conclusion that protein epitopes are discontinuous, are made up of 15 to 20 amino acid residues, and present a surface area of interaction of 700 to 900 Å². Moreover, it would seem that antigenicity neither requires the presence of certain amino acid types, nor particular secondary structural elements, nor is the antigenicity of a given region correlated with its mobility or flexibility. It is probably safe to conclude that any part of a protein, or of any macromolecule, can be antigenic (Benjamin et al., 1984) as long as that part is accessible to the molecules which trigger the immune response. The manifestation of immunogenicity, of course, depends on the regulatory mechanisms governing the immune response of the host organism.

CONCLUSION

More complexes of antibody and protein or peptide antigens are under investigation by X-ray diffraction (Altschuh et al., 1989; Delbaere et al., 1989; Stanfield et al., 1990) and by other means, e.g., by two-dimensional NMR (Anglister and Zilber, 1990; Levy et al., 1989) so that additional three-dimensional results on protein epitopes will become available in the near future. It is doubtful that the new results will lead to different conclusions from the ones based on the currently known structures. The new results, however, should provide more clues to the understanding of the molecular events in the immune response.

REFERENCES

Altschuh, D., Kocher, H.-P., Quesniaux, V. F. J., Schmitter, D., Van Regenmortel, M. H. V., and Thierry, J.-C. (1989) Crystallization and preliminary X-ray investigation of a complex between a Fab fragment and its antigen, cyclosporin. *J. Mol. Biol.* 209:177.

Amit, A. G., Mariuzza, R. A., Phillips, S. E. V., and Poljak, R. J. (1986) Three-dimensional structure of an antigen-antibody complex at 2.8 Å resolution. *Science* 233:747.

Anglister, J., and Zilber, B. (1990) Antibodies against a peptide of cholera toxin differing in cross-reactivity with the toxin differ in their specific interactions with the peptide as observed in ^{1}H NMR spectroscopy. *Biochemistry* 29:921.

Arnon, R. (1977) Immunochemistry of lysozyme. In *Immunochemistry of Enzymes and their Antibodies* (M. R. J. Salton, ed.), Wiley, NY, pp. 1—28.

Barlow, D. J., Edwards, M. S., and Thornton, J. M. (1986) Continuous and discontinuous protein antigenic determinants. *Nature (London)* 322:747.

Benjamin, D. C., Berzofsky, J. A., East, I. J., Gurd, F. R. N., Hannum, C., Leach, S. J., Margoliash, E., Michael, J. G., Miller, A., Prager, E. M., Reichlin, M., Sercarz, E. E., Smith-Gill, S. J., Todd, P. E., and Wilson, A. C. (1984) The antigenic structure of proteins: A reappraisal. *Annu. Rev. Immunol.* 2:67.

Bentley, G. A., Bhat, T. N., Boulot, G., Fischmann, T., Navaza, J., Poljak, R. J., Riottot, M.-M., and Tello, D. (1989) Immunochemical and crystallographic studies of antibody D1.3 in its free, antigen-liganded and idiotope-bound states. *Cold Spring Harbor Symp. Quant. Biol.* 54:239.

Bernstein, F. C., Koetzle, T. F., Williams, G. J. B., Meyer, E. F., Jr., Brice, M. D., Rodgers, J. R., Kennard, O., Shimanouchi, T., and Tasumi, M. (1977) The Protein Data Bank: A computer-based archival file for macromolecular structures. *J. Mol. Biol.* 112:535.

Colman, P. M., Laver, W. G., Varghese, J. N., Baker, A. T., Tulloch, P. A., Air, G. M., and Webster, R. G. (1987) Three-dimensional structure of a complex of antibody with influenza virus neuraminidase. *Nature (London)* 326:358.

Colman, P. M., Tulip, W. R., Varghese, J. N., Tulloch, P. A., Baker, A. T., Laver, W. G., Air, G. M., and Webster, R. G. (1989) Three-dimensional structures of influenza virus neuraminidase-antibody complexes. *Phil. Trans. R. Soc. London B* 323:511.

Davies, D. R., Sheriff, S., and Padlan, E. A. (1988) Antibody-antigen complexes. *J. Biol. Chem.* 263:10541.

Delbaere, L. T. J., Vandonselaar, M., Quail, J. W., Waygood, E. B., and Lee, J. S. (1989) Crystallization of the complex of a monoclonal fab fragment with the histidine-containing protein of the phosphoenolpyruvate: Sugar phosphotransferase system of *Escherichia coli*. *J. Biol. Chem.* 264:18645.

Hopp, T. P., and Woods, K. R. (1981) Prediction of protein antigenic determinants from amino acid sequences. *Proc. Natl. Acad. Sci. U.S.A.* 78:3824.

Klapper, M. H. (1977) The independent distribution of amino acid near neighbor pairs into polypeptides. *Biochem. Biophys. Res. Commun.* 78:1018.

Kundrot, C. E., and Richards, F. M. (1987) Crystal structure of hen egg white lysozyme at a hydrostatic pressure of 1000 atmospheres. *J. Mol. Biol.* 193:157.

Levy, R., Assulin, O., Scherf, T., Levitt, M., and Anglister, J. (1989) Probing antibody diversity by 2D NMR: comparison of amino acid sequences, predicted structures, and observed antibody-antigen interactions in complexes of two antipeptide antibodies. *Biochemistry* 28:7168.

Novotny, J. (1991) Protein antigenicity: a thermodynamic approach. *Mol. Immunol.* 28:201.

Novotny, J., Handshumacher, M., Haber, E., Bruccoleri, R. E., Carlson, W. B., Fanning, D. W., Smith, J. A., and Rose, G. D. (1986) Antigenic determinants in proteins coincide with surface regions accessible to large probes (antibody domains). *Proc. Natl. Acad. Sci. U.S.A.* 83:226.

Padlan, E. A. (1985) Quantitation of the immunogenic potential of protein antigens. *Mol. Immunol.* 22:1243.

Padlan, E. A. (1990) On the nature of antibody combining sites: unusual structural features that may confer on these sites an enhanced capacity for binding ligands. *Proteins: Struct. Funct. Genet.* 7:112.

Padlan, E. A., Silverton, E. W., Sheriff, S., Cohen, G. H., Smith-Gill, S. J., and Davies, D. R. (1989) Structure of an antibody-antigen complex: crystal structure of the HyHEL-10 Fab-lysozyme complex. *Proc. Natl. Acad. Sci. U.S.A.* 86:5938.

Sheriff, S., Silverton, E. W., Padlan, E. A., Cohen, G. H., Smith-Gill, S. J., Finzel, B. C., and Davies, D. R. (1987) Three-dimensional structure of an antibody-antigen complex. *Proc. Natl. Acad. Sci. U.S.A.* 84:8075.

Stanfield, R. L., Fieser, T. M., Lerner, R. A., and Wilson, I. A. (1990) Crystal structure of an antibody to a peptide and its complex with peptide antigen at 2.8 Å. *Science* 248:712.

Tainer, J. A., Getzoff, E. D., Alexander, H., Houghten, R. A., Olson, A. J., Lerner, R. A., and Hendrickson, W. A. (1984) The reactivity of anti-peptide antibodies is a function of the atomic mobility of sites in a protein. *Nature (London)* 312:127.

Thornton, J. M., Edwards, M. S., Taylor, W. R., and Barlow, D. J. (1986) Location of 'continuous' antigenic determinants in the protruding regions of proteins. *EMBO J.* 5:409.

Tulip, W. R., Varghese, J. N., Webster, R. G., Air, G. M., Laver, W. G., and Colman, P. M. (1989) Crystal structures of neuraminidase-antibody complexes. *Cold Spring Harbor Symp. Quant. Biol.* 54:257.

Westhof, E., Altschuh, D., Moras, D., Bloomer, A. C., Mondragon, A., Klug, A., and Van Regenmortel, M. H. V. (1984) Correlation between segmental mobility and the location of antigenic determinants in proteins. *Nature (London)* 311:123.

Chapter

3

Antigen Mimicry with Synthetic Peptides

S. Vuilleumier and M. Mutter
Institut de Chimie Organique, Université de Lausanne
Lausanne, Switzerland

INTRODUCTION

The aim of this chapter is to review the attempts to design by chemical methods synthetic peptide analogs of antigenic determinants in protein antigens which mimic the conformation of these epitopes in the native antigen, and to provide a brief overview of currently available synthetic methods for stabilizing conformational features in short synthetic peptides.

The development of techniques for the synthesis of peptides by chemical methods, particularly solid-phase peptide synthesis, has had a major impact on immunology (Plaué et al., 1990). Methods have been introduced for the rapid synthesis of hundreds of peptides in sufficient quantities and purity for use in ELISA immunoassays (Geysen et al., 1987; Houghten, 1985), allowing the mapping of continuous epitopes by comparing the antigenicity of a large number of analogs of a given peptide sequence (replacement sets), in which each residue in the sequence is replaced in turn by one of the other natural amino acids. In addition, overlapping peptides covering the whole sequence of a protein can be rapidly synthesized and their antigenic properties compared with those of the corresponding proteins (see this volume, Chapters 1, 4, and 11). Antibodies to most regions of a protein can be induced by immunizing with short synthetic peptides (Lerner, 1984). In particular, site-specific antipeptide antibodies can be generated against parts of the protein structure which are not antigenic when the entire protein is used as the immunogen (see this volume, Chapter 4). This is of great interest in the characterization of gene products and in the development of diagnostic reagents specific for a given protein. Peptide sequences can be chosen for use as synthetic immunogens from the primary structure of a protein, using prediction codes for continuous antigenic determinants obtained from correlations between experimentally observed antigenic determinants in proteins of known structure with properties such as side-chain hydrophilicity, surface accessibility, and segmental mobility (see this volume, Chapter 6; Van Regenmortel and Daney de Marcillac, 1988, for a recent overview). Synthetic peptides have also proved useful in studies of interactions in T-cell receptor MHC peptide complexes (Chapter 5, this volume; Kourilsky and Claverie, 1989) and may also serve in the development of synthetic vaccines (Chapter 16; Milich, 1989). These aspects of the use of synthetic peptides in immunological research will not be discussed further here.

The importance of the conformational features of protein antigens for recognition by antibodies has been recognized early on (see this volume, Chapter 1, 4, and 11; Crumpton, 1974, for a review of classical work on protein antigenicity; Benjamin et al., 1984 for a more recent review). The reactivity of a protein to antibodies raised against the native protein is well-known to diminish upon unfolding, reduction, fragmentation, or chemical modification of the protein, and the specificity of antibodies raised against denatured antigens has been shown to differ markedly from that of antibodies against the native protein. Furthermore, proteolytic fragments of proteins were found to be poor substitutes for the native antigen in the reaction with antiprotein antibodies, and structural studies showed that such fragments were generally largely unfolded in aqueous solution (reviewed by Wetlaufer, 1981). It has recently been shown that certain peptide sequences may show regular structural features under certain conditions (for a review, see Wright et al., 1988).

Although the experimental conditions under which short peptides show cross-reactive antigenicity (and immunogenicity) with the cognate native antigen still need clarification (Dyson et al., 1988; Van Regenmortel, 1989; this volume, Chapter 4 and 11), it appears that antibodies which bind to both short peptides and the protein probably recognize small surface patches of the cognate protein dominated by short peptide sequences and including only a small number of residues. In contrast, calculations have shown most antigenic determinants on protein antigens recognized by antibodies to be unlikely to involve only local continuous stretches of amino acid residues (Barlow et al., 1986). Therefore, antipeptide antibodies cross-reactive with the protein possess, as a rule, less affinity for the cognate native protein antigen than typical antibodies raised against the native protein, because of the imperfect fit expected between antigen-binding regions of antipeptide antibodies and the partly complementary surface of a protein surface. Similarly, antibodies raised against the native protein, which cross-react with short peptides, bind peptides less tightly than the native protein. The use of longer peptides to mimic protein antigens does not necessarily lead to increased cross-reactivity, perhaps because longer peptides may adopt better defined but nonnative conformations. Therefore, it appears that methods are required to restrict the conformational space of small flexible peptides and to mimic secondary structural elements and discontinuous antigenic determinants in proteins, so that the proportion and affinity of region- and conformation-specific antibodies elicited by immunization with the peptide can be increased (Jemmerson, 1987; Jemmerson and Blankenfeld, 1989).

SYNTHETIC PEPTIDE MIMICS OF LOOPS IN PROTEINS

The use of synthetic methods to restrict the conformation of polypeptides can be traced back to the classical work on antigenicity and immunogenicity of synthetic polymers, which showed that antigenic recognition of synthetic polypeptides was not only dependent on amino acid sequence or composition but also on conformation (Sela, 1966; Sela et al., 1967; Arnon, 1974). The same authors also studied the importance of conformation for the antigenicity in natural proteins in the case of an antigenic determinant of hen egg white lysozyme, which builds a loop stabilized by a disulfide bond in the native protein structure. Antipeptide antibodies raised against the loop peptide stabilized by the disulfide bond recognized the linear form of the peptide less well than the cyclic form (Maron et al., 1971). A synthetic form of the loop coupled to a synthetic branched polypeptide yielded a fully synthetic antigen which elicited antibodies reactive with native lysozyme. This binding reaction could not be inhibited by the open-chain form of the peptide (Arnon et al., 1971). This constituted the first example of a fully synthetic construct able of eliciting the production of antibodies with specificity for a conformation-dependent determinant of a protein. Following this report, cyclized versions of synthetic peptides have often been used in order to obtain protein-specific antibodies (e.g., Dreesman et al., 1982). A selection of studies undertaken to increase the potential of short peptides for mimicking conformation-dependent features of loops in the cognate protein antigen is presented in the following.

Myoglobin peptide analogs were synthesized with nonnatural cysteines in the N- and C-termini, and the open-chain and cyclized forms of these peptides were compared in their conformational, antigenic, and immunogenic properties. Although no significant difference in the conformation of both forms of the peptide were apparent in the circular dichroism spectra of the peptides, the native protein and the linear form of the peptide were both poorly effective in binding antibodies raised against the cyclized form of the peptide (Dorow et al., 1985), suggesting that these antibodies had specificities for partially denatured forms of the protein. In another study of peptides related to the postulated "flap" region of human renin, the disulfide-bridged forms of the peptides, but not the original peptide sequences, were recognized by polyclonal antibodies raised against human renin (Fehrentz et al., 1988). Two-dimensional nuclear magnetic resonance (NMR) spectroscopy experiments indicated that ring closure of these peptides stabilizes the peptide in a β-hairpin structure consistent with the model of renin. In contrast, a comparison of the antigenicity of open-chain and cyclized forms of a loop from scorpion toxin-α studied with an antitoxin antiserum indicated that artificial cyclization of the loop sequence did not result in a good mimic of the loop conformation, since the naturally occurring linear form of the peptide was more antigenic in various different immunoassays (Fourquet et al., 1988). The circular dichroism spectra of linear and cyclic forms of the sequence were markedly different; the cyclized form showed some of the characteristics of a β-turn structure. Since the cysteines in the natural protein are close to each other, but not paired, the authors suggested that slightly less constrained versions of the loop may represent more efficient mimics of the loop structure.

In the case of the loop structure of antigenic site A from influenza virus hemagglutinin, the natural peptide sequence was modified to increase its potential for a β-hairpin conformation and cyclized through a disulfide bridge for additional stabilization of the desired conformation (Schulze-Gahmen et al., 1986). Unlike previously described attempts to obtain protein-reactive antibodies with linear peptides including this sequence, antipeptide antibodies raised against the peptide sequence analog were able to react with the cognate protein, although very weakly and with less specificity than antiprotein antibodies. However, the model peptide was not recognized by antibodies raised against the protein antigen. In a detailed study of the effect of loop size on the antigenicity of a cyclic loop peptide, peptides derived from the same hemagglutinin loop were cyclized through lactame formation between the N-terminal amino group and side-chain functional groups, using linkers of different length (Plaué, 1990). In this case, antiprotein antibodies cross-reacted with the synthetic peptide antigen analog, depending on the conformation on the loop and the form in which the peptide was presented to the antiprotein antibodies. Antibodies raised against these peptides were able to bind the virus antigen in ELISA under certain conditions. Most importantly, a high proportion of mice, for which influenza virus infection is lethal, were protected against an intranasal challenge with influenza virus (Muller et al., 1990).

SYNTHETIC PEPTIDE MIMICS OF ELEMENTS OF SECONDARY STRUCTURE IN PROTEINS

It is possible to stabilize the conformation of short, flexible peptides by carrying out chemical modifications of the original sequence. An important factor in the stabilization of conformational features in a given polypeptide chain is that of amphiphilicity (Tanford, 1980). Molecules such as proteins, which have spatially segregated hydrophobic and hydrophilic surfaces, may be regarded as amphiphilic. Secondary structural elements of globular proteins lying along the protein surface often show a more hydrophobic face directed against the protein core and a more hydrophilic face directed against the solvent. Amphiphilicity is also important for the stabilization of secondary structure in peptides and proteins which bind to apolar surfaces. Short peptides, which show hydrophilic as well as hydrophobic residues, are able to adopt conformations in aqueous medium in which hydrophobic residues are shielded against the polar solvent through intermolecular association. The periodicity of hydrophobic residues in the peptide sequence determines for a large part the secondary structure adopted (e.g., DeGrado and Lear, 1985; Mutter and Hersperger, 1990). The use of amphiphilic features for the stabilization of secondary structures in short peptides have been described for both β-sheet and α-helix structural types (for reviews, see Kaiser, 1987; DeGrado, 1988; Mutter and Vuilleumier, 1989).

As part of a strategy to assign secondary structure elements to protein primary structures with antipeptide antibodies ("conformational sequencing," Beyreuther et al., 1987), a tetrapeptide sequence with high β-turn-forming potential inserted between two short sequences of β-sheet-forming residues was used as an immunogen to induce the formation of β-turn-specific antibodies. The peptide showed conformational features indicative of a mixture of β-structure and β-turn as judged by circular dichroism (CD), and antibodies raised against this peptide appeared to recognize the model-turn peptide better than the control peptides with partial sequence similarity of same length but different conformation (Schulze-Gahmen et al., 1985). The same authors also proposed a method to mimic putative helical sequences by designing peptides which include only the relevant residues of a helix face (every fourth residue in the sequence), alternating with Ala spacer amino acids to approximate the helical pitch between residues on the same face of a helix. Antibodies against such a helix mimic peptide derived from lactose permease recognized the sodium dodecyl sulfate (SDS)-treated but not the urea-denatured cognate protein (Beyreuther et al., 1987).

Using a similar approach, it was possible to gain evidence for a helical antigenic site at the N-terminus of melittin defined by an antimelittin antiserum (Von Grünigen and Schneider, 1989). Two amphiphilic synthetic model peptides were designed; each mimics one face of the N-terminal melittin helix when they adopt a helical conformation, while omitting residues of the melittin sequence which would be situated on the other face of the helix. Whereas melittin itself inhibited the binding of the antimelittin antiserum to microtiter plates coated with either peptide in an ELISA immunoassay, the helix-face model peptides were inhibitory in the homologous situation only, as either helix-face peptide inhibited the binding of antimelittin antiserum only when the same model peptide was coated on microtiter plates.

Gras-Masse et al. (1988) also made use of amphiphilicity-driven structure formation to restore native proteinlike conformation in a peptide which alone was unorganized by elongation of the peptide with an unrelated amphiphilic sequence. Using this construct, it was possible to raise not only protein-reactive, but conformation-specific antibodies using a synthetic peptide.

Peptide mimetics (Farmer, 1980), designed to replace the peptide backbone by a nonpeptide framework, can also contribute to stabilize defined peptide backbone conformations. A number of peptide mimetics for β-turns (see Olson et al., 1990, and references therein) β-sheet, and α-helix elements (for a review, see Kemp, 1990, and references therein) have been reported. However, only few applications have so far been described in studies of antigenic recognition. Synthetic peptide sequences, thought to be important in the recognition of the malaria parasite by antibodies, have been forced into a helixlike conformation by replacing the [i − (i + 4)] H bonds of helices by hydrazone-ethane ($-NN=CHCH_2CH_2-$) links (Satterthwait et al., 1988). Antibodies against these synthetic peptides strongly cross-reacted with living *Plasmodium falciparum* sporozoites. Conformational analysis by NMR indicates a relaxed helical structure for these "shaped" peptides (Satterthwait et al., 1989). Side-chain lactame ring formation between residues (i) and (i + 4) has recently been proposed as a further possibility to achieve helixlike conformation in short peptides (Ösapay and Taylor, 1990). An immunodominant peptide of hemagglutinin, previously shown by two-dimensional NMR (Dyson et al., 1988) to partially adopt β-turn conformation in solution, was locked in that conformation using a novel spirocyclic proline mimic (Hinds et al., 1988).

Unnatural and nonproteinogenic amino acid building blocks may also be used to modulate the conformation of synthetic peptides. For example, the incorporation of α-aminoisobutyric acid in chemically synthesized model peptides has been shown to result in increased helix formation (e.g., Karle et al., 1989; Mutter et al., 1986a; O'Neil and DeGrado, 1990), because of the restricted conformational space available to this amino acid (see Karle and Balaram, 1990, for a recent review).

SYNTHETIC PEPTIDE MIMICS OF DISCONTINUOUS ANTIGENIC DETERMINANTS IN PROTEINS

As mentioned in the introduction, linear peptides, as a rule, poorly mimic the conformation of antigenic determinants on protein antigens, which consist of patches of the protein surface comprised of amino acid residues brought together by the folding of the polypeptide chain. However, methods that allow the synthesis of a large number of peptide analogs and the rapid screening of their binding to antibodies (Geysen et al., 1987) can be used to identify linear peptides which best mimic the complementary binding site of a given antibody specific for a discontinuous antigenic determinant of a protein, even when the structure of the protein or the epitope is unknown. The peptides, which can be made to include unnatural amino acids and D-configured amino acids, were termed mimotopes (Geysen et al., 1986). Unfortunately, reciprocal experiments to determine if the selected peptides are, in turn, able to elicit protein-specific antibodies against the native antigen have not been described.

In another approach using linear peptides, spatially adjacent residues, determined to constitute an antigen determinant, are directly linked via peptide bonds using glycine residues as spacers. These peptides do not exist in the native protein but attempt to mimic the specific surface patterns of the epitope (reviewed in Atassi, 1984). Such "surface-simulation" peptides (five for myoglobin and three for hen egg white lysozyme) were claimed to account for the quasitotality of the antibody response to the native protein, to elicit the formation of protein-reactive antibodies, and to stimulate the proliferation of protein-specific T cells (Atassi, 1984).

Recently, a linear synthetic peptide including two tandemly joined stretches of sequence originating from the α and β subunits of human choriogonadotropin was described. It elicited the formation of site-specific antibodies able of recognizing the protein in solution, thus mimicking a conformational epitope previously defined by a monoclonal antibody against the native protein (Bidart et al., 1990).

The question of the native conformation of the antigen was not directly addressed in these studies. No description of the conformational features of these constructs was provided. Following is a discussion of the methods currently developed in the de novo design of proteins for the step-by-step construction of tertiary structures, which may provide a more generally applicable approach in order to mimic discontinuous antigenic determinants of proteins.

USE OF THE METHODS OF PROTEIN DE NOVO DESIGN FOR THE CONSTRUCTION OF DISCONTINUOUS ANTIGENIC DETERMINANTS BY CHEMICAL METHODS

In the construction of polypeptides with tertiary structure (de novo protein design), the polypeptide sequence is considered in terms of secondary structure elements linked by turns or loops which upon folding yield the target tertiary structure. The segments representing secondary structure elements are often made amphiphilic in order to facilitate the formation of a structure with proteinlike hydrophobic core and hydrophilic surface (for reviews, see DeGrado, 1988; Mutter and Vuilleumier, 1989; Richardson and Richardson, 1989). The use of such folding units as scaffolds for the grafting of discontinuous epitopes has been proposed (Mutter et al., 1986b; Vorherr, 1987).

Using a similar approach, Kaumaya et al. (1990) synthesized model peptides, designed to adopt stable secondary and tertiary structures such as αα and four-helix bundle topologies in solution, which included residues of lactate dehydrogenase C_4, important for the antigenic recognition of the protein. The comprehensive structural characterization of these models by a number of different methods allows to determine the importance of conformational features for the antigenicity and immunogenicity of these constructs.

In the past few years, another approach has been used for the stabilization of secondary-structure elements in more complex structures (Mutter, 1988). Rather than being linked by loops to a linear polypeptide chain, secondary structure-forming peptide blocks are assembled by covalent attachment to a well-defined common synthetic carrier into a branched polypeptide, in order to facilitate the adoption by such constructs of a compact structure. The multifunctional carrier portion of the molecule is designed to favor intramolecular interactions between the covalently fixed peptide blocks and determine the packing topology of the molecule by the number, type, and spatial arrangement of its functional groups (peptide block "anchoring points"). Accordingly, these novel macromolecules were termed template-assembled synthetic proteins (TASP). The construction of TASP molecules is achieved by standard methods of peptide synthesis. Orthogonal protection techniques in combination with segment-condensation strategies allow for the chemical synthesis of TASP molecules with a variety of different proteinlike arrangements of secondary structure blocks. TASP molecules with $\beta\alpha\beta$, 4α, and $4\alpha,4\beta$-like packing arrangements with the expected conformational and physicochemical properties have been described (Ernest et al., 1990; Mutter and Vuilleumier, 1989, review; Rivier et al., 1990). The TASP approach appears well-suited for the controlled construction of synthetic peptide immunogens. The flexibility of synthetic methods allows for different epitopes to be grafted on the same carrier. Compared with the multiple-antigenic peptide (MAP) approach of Tam (e.g., Tam and Lu, 1989), conceived as an immunogenicity amplification systems for the grafting of peptides of immunological interest, the TASP approach offers the advantage of a better control of the conformational features of epitopes. Studies of the usefulness of the TASP approach in the design of better mimics of continuous and discontinuous antigenic determinants are under way.

CONCLUSION AND OUTLOOK

It is sometimes difficult to evaluate studies of antigenicity with synthetic peptides since extensive comparisons of the conformational and immunological properties of peptides and their cognate antigens are not always possible. It is to be hoped that the wide palette of methods of peptide and protein synthesis and of conformational and immunological analysis now readily available will allow future work to address the various aspects of cross-reactive antigenicity of peptides and proteins in a more integrated manner. Throughout the examples described above, two main approaches for mimicking a desired immunological effect using chemically synthesized peptides are apparent. The first, "functional" approach aims mainly at observing the desired effect using a synthetic peptide, which can then be said to mimic the functionally relevant chemical features of the antigen of interest. The second, "structural" approach first attempts to stabilize short linear peptides in the conformation thought to be important for the immunological process under study using the tools of "rational" peptide and protein design, and then confront these constructs with immunological reality. Using the latter rather than the former approach in mimicking antigens with synthetic peptides may lead to a better understanding of the importance of conformation in all stages of antigen recognition.

REFERENCES

Arnon, R. (1974) Conformation-dependent antigenic determinants in proteins and synthetic polypeptides. In *Peptides, Polypeptides and Proteins,* (E. R. Blout, P. A. Bovey, M. Goodman, and N. Lotan, eds.), Wiley, NY, pp. 538—552.

Arnon, R., Maron, E., Sela, M., and Anfinsen, C. B. (1971) Antibodies reactive with native lysozyme elicited by a completely synthetic antigen. *Proc. Natl. Acad. Sci. U.S.A.* 68:1450—1455.

Atassi, M. Z. (1984) Antigenic structures of proteins. Their determination has revealed important aspects of immune recognition and generated strategies for synthetic mimicking of protein binding sites. *Eur. J. Biochem.* 145:1—20.

Barlow, D. J., Edwards, M. S., and Thornton, J. M. (1986) Continuous and discontinuous protein antigenic determinants. *Nature (London)* 322:747—748.

Benjamin, D. C., Berzofsky, J. A., East, I. J., Gurd, F. R. N., Hannum, C., Leach, S. J., Margoliash, E., Michael, J. G., Miller, A., Prager, E. M., Reichlin, M., Sercarz, E. E., Smith-Gill, S. J., Todd, P. E., and Wilson, A. C. (1984) The antigenic structure of proteins: A reappraisal. *Annu. Rev. Immunol.* 2:67—101.

Beyreuther, K., Schulze-Gahmen, U., Bieseler, B., and Prinz, H. (1987) Towards conformational sequencing of proteins: Assignment of secondary structures by antipeptide antibodies. In *Chemical Synthesis in Molecular Biology,* (H. Blöcker, R. Frank, and H.-J. Fritz, eds.), GBF Monographs, Vol. 8, VCH Verlag, Weinheim, pp. 199—222.

Bidart, J.-M., Troalen, F., Ghillani, P., Rouas, N., Razafindratsita, A., Bohuon, C., and Bellet, D. (1990) Peptide immunogen mimicry of a protein-specific structural epitope on human choriogonadotropin. *Science* 248:736—739.

Crumpton, M. J. (1974) Protein antigens: Molecular bases of antigenicity and immunogenicity. In *The Antigens,* Vol. 2, (M. Sela, ed.), Academic Press, NY, pp. 1—78.

DeGrado, W. F. (1988) Design of peptides and proteins. *Adv. Protein Chem.* 39:51—124

DeGrado, W. F., and Lear, J. D. (1985) Induction of peptide conformation at apolar water interfaces. 1. A study with model peptides of defined hydrophobic periodicity. *J. Am. Chem. Soc.* 107:7684—7689.

Dorow, D. S., Shi, P.-T., Carbone, F. R., Minasian, E., Todd, P. E. E., and Leach, S. J. (1985) Two large immunogenic and antigenic myoglobin peptides and the effect of cyclization. *Mol. Immunol.* 22:1255—1264.

Dreesman, G. R., Sanchez, Y., Ionescu-Matiu, I., Sparrow, J. T., Six, H. R., Peterson, D. L., Hollinger, F. B., and Melnick, J. L. (1982) Antibody to hepatitis B surface antigen after a single inoculation of uncoupled synthetic HBsAg Peptides. *Nature (London)* 295:158—160.

Dyson, H. J., Lerner, R. A., and Wright, P. E. (1988) The physical basis for induction of protein-reactive antipeptide antibodies. *Annu. Rev. Biophys. Biophys. Chem.* 17:305—324.

Ernest, I., Vuilleumier, S., Fritz, H., and Mutter, M. (1990) Synthesis of a 4-helix bundle-like template-assembled protein (TASP) by condensation of a protected peptide on a conformationally constrained cyclic carrier. *Tetrahedron Lett.* 31:4015—4018.

Farmer, P. S. (1980) Bridging the gap between bioactive peptides and nonpeptides: some perspectives in design. In *Drug Design,* Vol. 10, (E. J. Ariëns, ed.), Academic Press, San Diego, pp. 119—143.

Fehrentz, J.-A., Heitz, A., Seyer, R., Fulcrand, P., Devilliers, R., Castro, B., Heitz, F., and Carelli, C. (1988) Peptides mimicking the flap of human renin: synthesis, conformation, and antibody recognition. *Biochemistry* 27:4071—4078.

Fourquet, P., Bahraoui, E., Fontecilla-Camps, J. C., Van Rietschoten, J., Rochat, H., and Granier, C. (1988) Immunochemistry of scorpion toxins. Synthesis and antigenic properties of a model of a loop region specific to α-toxins. *Int. J. Peptide Protein Res.* 32:81—88.

Geysen, H. M., Rodda, S. J., and Mason, T. J. (1986) A priori delineation of a peptide which mimics a discontinuous antigenic determinant. *Mol. Immunol.* 23:709—715.

Geysen, H. M., Rodda, S. J., Mason, T. J., Tribbick, G., and Schoofs, P. G. (1987) Strategies for epitope analysis using peptide synthesis. *J. Immunol. Methods* 102:259—274.

Gras-Masse, H., Jolivet, M., Drobecq, H., Aubert, J. P., Beachey, E. H., Audibert, F., Chedid, L., and Tartar, A. (1988) Influence of helical organization on immunogenicity and antigenicity of synthetic peptides. *Mol. Immunol.* 25:673—678.

Hinds, M. G., Richards, N. G. J., and Robinson, J. A. (1988) Design and synthesis of a novel peptide β-turn mimetic. *J. Chem. Soc., Chem. Commun.* 1447—1449.

Houghten, R. A. (1985) General method for the rapid solid-phase synthesis of a large number of peptides: Specificity of antigen-antibody interaction at the level of individual amino acids. *Proc. Natl. Acad. Sci. U.S.A.* 82:5131—5135.

Jemmerson, R. (1987) Antigenicity and native structure of globular proteins: low frequency of peptide reactive antibodies. *Proc. Natl. Acad. Sci. U.S.A.* 84:9180—9184.

Jemmerson, R., and Blankenfeld, R. (1989) Affinity considerations in the design of synthetic vaccines intended to elicit antibodies. *Mol. Immunol.* 26:301—307.

Kaiser, E. T. (1987) Design principles in the construction of biologically active peptides. *Trends Biochem. Sci.* 12:305—309.

Karle, I. L., and Balaram, P. (1990) Structural characteristics of α-helical peptide molecules containing Aib residues. *Biochemistry* 29:6747—6756.

Karle, I. L., Flippen-Anderson, J. L., Uma, K., and Balaram, P. (1989) Modular design of synthetic protein mimics. Characterization of the helical conformation of a 13-residue peptide in crystals. *Biochemistry* 28:6696—6701.

Kaumaya, P. T., Berndt, K. D., Heidorn, D. B., Trewhella, J., Kezdy, F. J., and Goldberg, E. (1990) Synthesis and biophysical characterization of engineered topographic immunogenic determinants with αα topology. *Biochemistry* 29:13—23.

Kemp, D. S. (1990) Peptidomimetics and the template approach to nucleation of β-sheets and α-helices in peptides. *Trends Biotechnol.* 8:249—255.

Kourilsky, P., and Claverie, J.-M. (1989) MHC-Antigen interaction: what does the T-Cell receptor see? *Adv. Immunol.* 45:107—193.

Lerner, R. A. (1984) Antibodies of predetermined specificity in biology and medicine. *Adv. Immunol.* 36:1—44.
Maron, E., Shiozawa, C., Arnon, R., and Sela, M. (1971) Chemical and immunological characterization of a unique antigenic region in lysozyme. *Biochemistry* 10:763—771.
Milich, D. R. (1989) Synthetic T and B cell recognition sites: implications for vaccine development. *Adv. Immunol.* 45:195—282.
Muller, S., Plaué, S., Samama, J. P., Valette, M., Briand, J.-P., and Van Regenmortel, M. H. V. (1990) Antigenic properties and protective capacity of a cyclic peptide corresponding to site A of influenza virus haemagglutin. *Vaccine* 8:308—314.
Mutter, M. (1988) Nature's rules and chemist's tools: a way for creating novel proteins. *Trends Biochem. Sci.* 13:260—265.
Mutter, M., Altmann, K.-H., Flörsheimer, A., and Herbert, J. (1986a) Sequence dependence of secondary structure formation. Helix-forming potential of amphiphilic oligopeptides containing Aib residues. *Helv. Chim. Acta* 69:786—792.
Mutter, M., Altmann, K.-H., Müller, K., Vuilleumier, S., and Vorherr, T. (1986b) Approaches to synthetic vaccines. Design of epitope-containing amphiphilic peptides matching the antigenic structure in the native protein. *Helv. Chim. Acta* 69:985—995.
Mutter M., and Hersperger, R. (1990) Peptides as conformational switch: medium-induced conformational transitions of designed peptides. *Angew Chem. Int. Ed. Engl.* 29:185—187 (*Angew. Chem.* 102:195—197).
Mutter, M., and Vuilleumier, S. (1989) A chemical approach to protein design — template-assembled synthetic proteins (TASP). *Angew. Chem. Int. Ed. Engl.* 28:535—554 (*Angew. Chem.* 101:551—571).
Ösapay, G., and Taylor, J. W. (1990) Multicyclic polypeptide model compounds. 1. Synthesis of a tricyclic amphiphilic α-helical peptide using an oxime resin, segment-condensation approach. *J. Am. Chem. Soc.* 112:6046—6051.
Olson, G. L., Voss, M. E., Hill, D. E., Kahn, M., Madison, V. S., and Cook, C. M. (1990) Design and synthesis of a protein β-turn mimetic. *J. Am. Chem. Soc.* 112:323—333.
O'Neil, K. T., and DeGrado, W. F. (1990) A thermodynamic scale for the helix-forming tendencies of the commonly occurring amino acids. *Science* 250:646—651.
Plaué, S. (1990) Synthesis of cyclic peptides on solid support. Application to analogs of hemagglutinin of influenza virus. *Int. J. Pept. Protein Res.* 35:510—517.
Plaué, S., Muller, S., Briand, J.-P., and Van Regenmortel, M. H. V. (1990) Recent advances in solid-phase peptide synthesis and preparation of antibodies to synthetic peptides. *Biologicals* 18:147—157.
Richardson, J. S., and Richardson, D. C. (1989) The de novo design of protein structures. *Trends Biochem. Sci.* 14:304—309.
Rivier, J., Miller, C., Spicer, M., Andrews, J., Porter, J., Tuchscherer, G., and Mutter, M. (1990) Total synthesis of TASP 4α molecules by solid-phase methods. In *Innovation and Perspectives in Solid-Phase Synthesis,* (R. Epton, ed.), SPCC (UK), Birmingham, pp. 39—50.
Satterthwait, A. C., Arrhenius, T., Hagopian, R. A., Zavala, F., Nussenzweig, V., and Lerner, R. A. (1988) Conformational restriction of peptidyl immunogens with covalent replacements for the hydrogen bond. *Vaccine* 6:99—103.
Satterthwait, A. C., Arrhenius, T., Hagopian, R. A., Zavala, F., Nussenzweig, V., and Lerner, R. A. (1989) The conformational restriction of synthetic peptides, including a malaria peptide, for use as immunogens. *Phil. Trans. R. Soc. London B* 323:565—572.

Schulze-Gahmen, U., Klenk, H.-D., and Beyreuther, K. (1986) Immunogenicity of loop-structured short synthetic peptides mimicking the antigenic site A of influenza virus hemagglutinin. *Eur J. Biochem.* 159:283—289.

Schulze-Gahmen, U., Prinz, H., Glatter, U., and Beyreuther, K. (1985) Towards assignment of secondary structures by anti-peptide antibodies. Specificity of the immune response to a β-turn. *EMBO J.* 4:1731-1737.

Sela, M. (1966) Immunological studies with synthetic polypeptides. *Adv. Immunol.* 5:29—129.

Tam, J. P., and Lu, Y. A. (1989) Vaccine engineering: enhancement of immunogenicity of synthetic peptide vaccines related to hepatitis in chemically defined models consisting of T- and B-cell epitopes. *Proc. Natl. Acad. Sci. U.S.A.* 86:9084—9088.

Tanford, C. (1980) *The Hydrophobic Effect: Formation of Micelles and Biological Membranes,* 2nd ed., Wiley-Interscience, NY.

Van Regenmortel, M. H. V. (1989) The concept and operational definition of protein epitopes. *Phil. Trans. R. Soc. London B* 323:451—466.

Van Regenmortel, M. H. V., and Daney de Marcillac, G. (1988) An assessment of prediction methods for locating continuous epitopes in proteins. *Immunol. Lett.* 17:95—107.

Von Grünigen, R., and Schneider, C. H. (1989) Antigenic structure of the hexacosapeptide melittin: evidence for three determinants, one with a helical conformation. *Immunology* 66:339—342.

Vorherr, T. (1987) Design, synthese und konformationsuntersuchungen von künstlichen Polypeptiden mit βαβ-Topologie. Ph. D. Thesis, Basel University, Basel.

Wetlaufer, D. B. (1981) Folding of protein fragments. *Adv. Protein Chem.* 34:61—92.

Wright, P. E., Dyson, H. J., and Lerner, R. A. (1988) Conformation of peptide fragments of proteins in aqueous solution: implications for initiation of protein folding. *Biochemistry* 27:7167-7175.

Chapter
4

Antigen Mimicry with Anti-Idiotypic Antibodies

Neil S. Greenspan
*Institute of Pathology
Case Western Reserve University
Cleveland, Ohio*

INTRODUCTION

The primary focus of this chapter is the mimicry of antigen by anti-idiotypic antibody (Ab), but we will consider aspects of molecular mimicry in general in attempting to incorporate mimicry by anti-idiotypic Ab into a broader conceptual framework. In the remainder of this introductory section, we will discuss why anti-idiotypic mimicry of antigen is of interest, and review aspects of terminology pertaining to antigens and Abs, especially anti-idiotypic Abs. Subsequent sections will focus on: (1) the nature and implications of idiotope overlap, (2) the nature of idiotopes, paratopes, epitopes, and sites of noncovalent interaction in general, (3) the types (structural, immunochemical, and functional) of molecular mimicry, and (4) the potential and limitations of anti-idiotypic mimicry. A neo-Darwinian perspective on the phenomenon of anti-idiotypic mimicry will be presented in the conclusion.

Two major sources of interest in anti-idiotypic mimicry of antigen can readily be identified. First, investigation of anti-idiotypic mimicry, and molecular mimicry in general, might be expected to reveal principles of broad biological or biochemical interest, given that: (1) a deep understanding of molecular mimicry presupposes a sophisticated understanding of molecular recognition, and (2) most important biological phenomena involve molecular recognition events. In a narrower immunological context, interest in anti-idiotypic mimicry has been based on the idea that anti-idiotypic Abs, including those able to mimic foreign antigens, play a central role in the regulation of immune responses (Jerne, 1974). This concept remains controversial (Langman and Cohn, 1986; Paul, 1989), particularly with regard to the adult immune system. It may be, however, that regulation mediated by anti-idiotypic molecules has greater relevance to the immature than to the adult immune system (Howard, 1989). Molecular mimicry may also be of importance in alloreactivity mediated by T cells (Lechler et al., 1990), T-cell repertoire development (Carbone and Bevan, 1989), and in immunopathological processes, especially autoimmune phenomena (Burdette and Schwartz, 1987; Oldstone, 1987). Second, there is great interest in exploiting anti-idiotypic mimics, as is true for molecular mimics of other origins, for research or medical purposes. Two major proposed applications for anti-idiotypic (anti-Ids) mimics are: (1) isolation of cellular receptors for ligands that are not available in sufficient quantities or that are inconvenient to work with (reviewed in Gaulton and Greene, 1986 and Kohler et al., 1989) (Sege and Peterson, 1978a,b), and (2) development of surrogate vaccines (reviewed in Eichmann et al., 1987 and Finberg and Ertl, 1987) (Nisonoff and Lamoyi, 1981; Roitt et al., 1981). Readers interested in details of the experimental systems that have employed anti-idiotypic mimicry are referred to references in the reviews just cited. Potential advantages of anti-Ids in comparison with other types of molecular mimics relate to the nature of the process for producing these Abs, important features of which include: inducibility, affinity-based selection, the ability to generate a mimic for a molecule of unknown structure that is not available in large quantities or in pure form, and accessibility to most investigators.

Let us now define, in the standard way, terms required for the subsequent discussion. Later, the detailed implications of these definitions will be scrutinized. The portion of an antigen molecule that is specifically recognized by an Ab combining site (paratope) is generally referred to as an antigenic determinant (epitope). Immunoglobulins (Igs), like most glycoprotein molecules, can be used as immunogens to elicit the production of specific anti-Ig Abs. Such Abs, once produced, can noncovalently bind to epitopes on the Ig used for immunization, which serves as an antigen in this context. Three classes of epitopes on Igs have been defined: (1) isotypic determinants, which distinguish constant domains encoded by genes at distinct loci, (2) allotypic determinants, which distinguish constant (usually) or variable (less frequently) domains encoded by allelic genes at the same locus, and (3) idiotypic determinants, which are localized to the variable domains, the domains that determine the specificity of the combining site. Idiotypic determinants can distinguish Igs even of the same isotype and allotype. The remainder of this chapter will focus primarily on idiotypic determinants and anti-idiotypic Abs.

The standard concept of an epitope also applies to recognition of a foreign molecule by a T-cell receptor (TCR), as opposed to a soluble or cell-surface Ig receptor. In this case, the recognition process is more complicated in that the TCR has specificity both for a processed form of the antigen (referred to as nominal antigen, and typically a peptide fragment derived from the antigen;

see Chapter 5) and for a particular self major histocompatibility complex (MHC) antigen. Nevertheless, it is widely accepted that the amino acid residues, derived from a nominal antigen that physically interact with the TCR, constitute an epitope for the purposes of T-cell recognition. We will consider the implications of this second form of immunological recognition for anti-idiotypic mimicry later in the discussion.

By convention, an idiotypic determinant defined by a monoclonal antibody (MAb) is referred to as an idiotope (Id). Thus, an Id is an epitope located on an antibody variable (V) module [light chain variable domain (V_L)-heavy chain variable domain (V_H) pair]. The amino acid constituents of a single Id can be derived solely from V_H, solely from V_L, or from both V_H and V_L (Davie et al., 1986; Rudikoff, 1983). It is likely that much of the surface of a V module can contribute to idiotypic determinants (Greenspan and Davie, 1985a; Novotny et al., 1986; Roux et al., 1987). A set of Ids, characterizing a particular V module, is referred to as an idiotype. In theory, the idiotype for a given Ab is the set of all Ids expressed by that Ab molecule. In practice, any given polyclonal anti-idiotypic reagent, or set of anti-Ids, is likely to detect only some of the Ids that might be expressed by a given V module so that "idiotype" refers to the set of Ids detected by a given polyclonal anti-idiotypic serum or a given collection of monoclonal anti-Ids.

The possibility of multiple cycles of anti-idiotypic response has given rise to a nomenclature whereby an Ab elicited by a specific antigen is referred to as Ab1, an anti-idiotypic Ab specific for Ab1 is referred to as Ab2, an anti-idiotypic Ab specific for Ab2 is referred to as Ab3, etc. Ab2 has been further classified by some investigators into Ab2-α, -β, and -γ (Kohler, 1984). Ab2-α refers to an anti-Id able to bind to the corresponding Id in the presence of hapten or antigen. Ab2-β refers to an anti-Id that competes with hapten or antigen for binding to Ab1 and that mimics the antigen functionally. The terms "internal image" and "homobody" are frequently used synonymously with "Ab2-β." Ab2-γ refers to hapten-inhibitable anti-Ids that fail to mimic the relevant antigen (Kohler, 1984). Other, more complicated, nomenclatures have also been proposed (Gaulton and Greene, 1986). Ambiguities inherent in such nomenclatures will be discussed below. A final point of terminology is that anti-Ids are sometimes distinguished on the basis of whether they bind to many (public) or only one or a few (private) Ab1 molecules expressing a particular antigen specificity.

Why should anti-Ids mimic epitopes of foreign molecules? Given a particular Ab1, the corresponding antigen and Ab2 share the ability to interact noncovalently with the same V module. Therefore, there is a chance that some anti-Id will interact with regions of the Ab1 V module in approximately the same manner that the antigen does. One can imagine a roughly inverse relationship between the magnitude of similarity of antigen and anti-Id, with respect to recognition by the Ab1 V module, and the probability of occurrence of such an anti-Id. This postulated relationship is reminiscent of the notion that for any given epitope there is an inverse relationship between the degree of complementarity or intrinsic affinity of Ab paratopes, with respect to a given epitope, and the frequency of occurrence of such paratopes (Inman, 1978).

The following analysis originated in our own attempts to map Ids on the surface of an Ig V module. The initial step of this analysis is based on the assumption that one can evaluate mimicry of an antigen (epitope) by an anti-Id by comparing the sites on the Ab1 with which the antigen and the anti-Id interact (operationally defined as paratope and Id, respectively). Formally, there are three potential relationships between any pair of sites (e.g., two idiotopes or an Id and a paratope) expressed by a V module, or other molecule: (1) the sites are identical, (2) the sites are completely distinct and independent, and (3) the sites are nonidentical but overlapping. The nature and degree of overlap can be further classified, yielding five Id-paratope relationships (Fig. 1). Consideration of the meaning of site overlap provided the primary stimulus for developing the ideas presented below, since defining the magnitude of overlap for two Ids, or other sites of noncovalent interaction, may be method-dependent. We will discuss our studies on Id overlap as preparation for an analysis of anti-Id mimicry of antigen (overlap of paratope and Id).

IDIOTOPE OVERLAP

Our studies were focused on the variable module of the murine MAb, HGAC 39 (Ab1), specific for the N-acetylglucosamine (GlcNAc) residues of streptococcal group A carbohydrate (GAC), a cell wall polysaccharide of *Streptococcus pyogenes* (group A streptococci). We employed a panel of xenogeneic monoclonal anti-Ids (or Ab2; derived from HGAC 39-immune rat spleen cells) in a variety of assays in an effort to determine the topographic relationships of five Ids (IdX, IdI-1, -2, -3a, and -3b). These approaches included: (1) determination of the magnitude of inhibition of binding of each anti-Id to HGAC 39 mediated by hapten (GlcNAc), antigen (GAC), or other anti-Ids, in solid-phase assays (Greenspan and Davie, 1985a; summarized schematically in Fig. 2), (2) electron microscopic analysis of negatively stained complexes of HGAC 39 IgG and anti-Id IgG or Fab fragments (Roux et al., 1989; Figs. 3 and 4), and (3) evaluation of competition between anti-Ids for binding to HGAC 39 by size-exclusion chromatography (Stevens et al., 1988). We have previously compared, in detail, the results obtained from these varied approaches, and the potential sources of artifact associated with each approach (Greenspan and Monafo, 1987; Greenspan and Roux, 1988). Of primary relevance to the current discussion is the conclusion that different techniques can suggest different degrees of overlap for the same two Ids. Thus, for example, the overlap between IdI-1 and IdI-3a appears greater on the basis of the competition assays than on the basis of the electron microscopic analysis.

The concept of overlap among Ids (or other epitopes) can also be applied

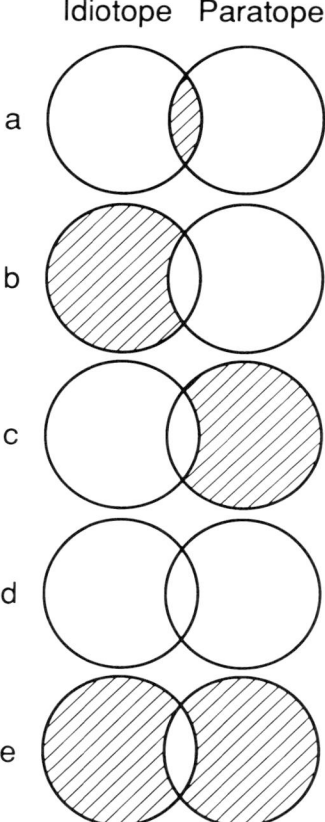

Figure 1. Schematic illustration of the possible relationships between a paratope and an idiotope on the same V module. Open areas indicate that amino acid residues (or atoms) exist in the defined subset, and shaded areas indicate that there are no amino acid residues (atoms) that correspond to that subset. Thus, the five diagrams have the following interpretations: (a) idiotope and paratope are disjoint (completely nonoverlapping); (b) all of the idiotopic residues are also paratopic residues, but there are additional paratopic residues not shared with the idiotope; (c) all of the paratopic residues are also idiotopic residues, but there are additional idiotopic residues not shared with the paratope; (d) idiotope and paratope share residues, but both idiotope and paratope contain residues not shared with the other site; and (e) the paratope and idiotope are identical in terms of component residues.

when the determinants are defined in terms of the positions in the primary structure of the Ab molecule at which amino acid substitutions affect Id expression. Such substitutions have been defined in a number of systems by comparing V domain amino acid sequences and patterns of Id expression either for independently isolated MAbs of similar antigen specificity (reviewed

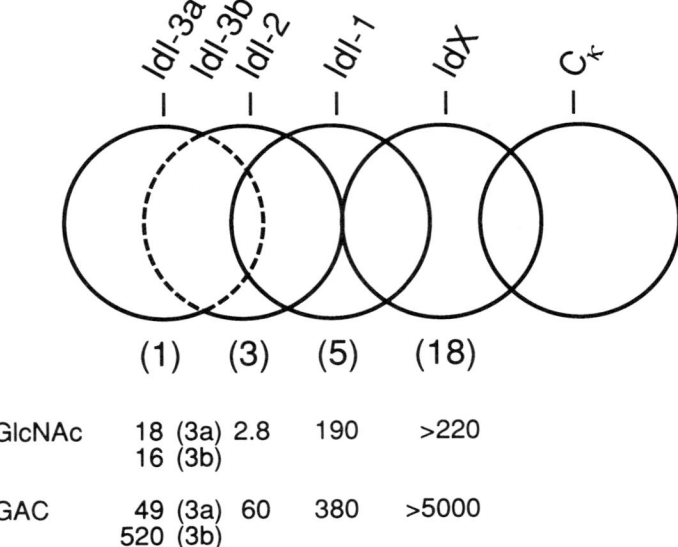

Figure 2. Schematic representation of topographic relationships among HGAC 39 Ids defined by monoclonal anti-Ids as determined from competitive binding assays (anti-Id versus anti-Id). Overlap of circles representing two sites indicates effective competition, in at least one direction, between the corresponding MAbs. Numbers in parentheses represent the number of different anti-GAC MAbs (from a total of 38 MAbs) able to displace at least 50% of radiolabeled HGAC 39 from the corresponding anti-Id, indicating a relationship between Id position (on the HGAC 39 V module) and the degree of anti-Id cross-reactivity for anti-GAC MAbs. Relative susceptibility of each anti-Id to hapten-mediated inhibition of binding to Id (HGAC 39) is indicated by the concentration of hapten (GlcNAc, mM) or antigen (GAC, μg/ml) yielding 50% inhibition. A relationship between Id position (as operationally derived from the anti-Id versus anti-Id competition assays) and the degree of hapten-mediated inhibition of the corresponding Id-anti-Id interaction is suggested. (Reproduced from Greenspan, N. S. and Davie, J. M., the *Journal of Immunology* 1985, Fig. 7 and Table II, in modified form. With permission.)

in Davie et al., 1986 and Rudikoff, 1983) (Schilling et al., 1980) or for wild-type and mutant (Id-loss variant) MAbs (Bruggemann et al., 1986; Phillips and Davie, 1990; Radbruch et al., 1985). In this context, two Ids can be considered to overlap if expression of both determinants is influenced by the same amino acid substitution(s). This definition of Id overlap could clearly accommodate a pair of Ids that are nonoverlapping in spatial extent or in terms of the competition for binding of the corresponding anti-Ids, but that are each conformationally altered by substitution of a particular (possibly distant) amino acid. Conversely, the analysis of Phillips and Davie suggests that while IdI-1 and IdI-3a overlap with respect to anti-Id competition, they may not overlap with respect to amino acid substitutions that affect Id expression.

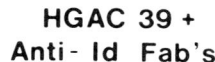

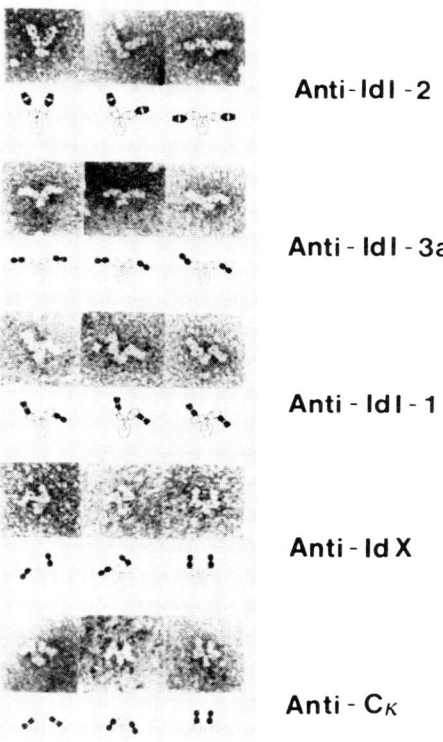

Figure 3. Electron micrographs (above; ×350,000) and interpretive diagrams (below) of HGAC 39 in complex with anti-Id MAb Fab. HGAC 39 is represented in the diagrams as an open figure and the Fab anti-Id probes are represented as solid figures. The Fab arms of the Ab targets and probes are drawn to indicate their rotational orientation as planar (oval with open center), intermediate ("bone shaped" with or without central opening), or perpendicular ("dumbbell shaped"). Ab complexes were stained with 2% uranyl formate. (Reproduced from Roux, K. H. et al., 1987, *Proc. Natl. Acad. Sci. U.S.A.*, Fig. 2. With permission.)

The solving of the three-dimensional structure of an Id(Fab)-anti-Id(Fab) complex by X-ray diffraction represents another way to define an Id (Bentley et al., 1990). This approach potentially allows the definition of an Id in terms of the amino acids (see below) that are involved in forming the noncovalent bonds between Id and anti-Id. Based on such information, one could then consider two Ids that share contact amino acids (or, more precisely, contact atoms) as overlapping. It is certainly conceivable that the magnitude of overlap in this sense would fail to be an absolutely reliable guide to the number of

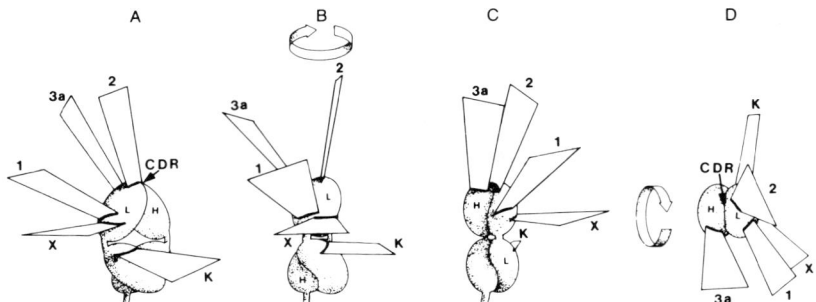

Figure 4. Three-dimensional model of HGAC 39 Fab (stippled figures), depicting approximate Id locations and planes of Id-anti-Id intersection. The paratopic region (labeled CDR, for complementarity determining regions) is indicated for orientation. A, B, and C represent the rotation of HGAC 39 Fab through 90° on the proximal-distal axis from planar (A) to intermediate (B) and perpendicular (C). D represents a 90° rotation of C to allow a "top" view of the paratope. The projections from the surface of HGAC 39 Fab represent three-dimensional depictions of rectangles corresponding to planes transecting the various anti-Id Fab probes at their widest aspects. Abbreviations: 1, IdI-1; 2, IdI-2; 3a, IdI-3a; X, IdX; K, κ constant domain epitope recognized by monoclonal antibody 187.1; L, light chain; H, heavy chain. (Reproduced from Roux, K. H. et al., 1987, *Proc. Natl. Acad. Sci.*, Fig. 4. With permission.)

amino acid substitutions affecting both Ids or to the degree of competition between the corresponding anti-Ids. As suggested above, two Ids that are spatially separate, and share no component amino acid residues (crystallographically nonoverlapping), might both be altered by the same amino acid substitution (genetically overlapping).

An example of the potential for discrepancy between the genetic and the crystallographic conceptions of a site of noncovalent interaction (a paratope in this case) is the participation of framework amino acid residues (which are classified as such because they exhibit little variation from one V module to another) as contact residues in paratope-epitope interfaces, as determined by crystallography (Amit et al., 1986; Sheriff et al., 1987). The differences between genetic and crystallographic approaches to defining Ids, or other epitopes, are also probably relevant in the case of the J558 and M104E private Ids on dextran-specific MAbs (Schilling et al., 1980). J558 and M104E are two myeloma proteins possessing identical V_L domains and nearly identical V_H domains that differ at only two amino acid positions (100 and 101). Thus, in a genetic sense, these two amino acid differences account fully for the differences in reactivity of J558 and M104E with the private anti-Ids. However, based on what is now known of paratope-protein epitope interfaces (Amit et al., 1986; Bentley et al., 1990; Colman et al., 1987; Padlan et al., 1989; Sheriff et al., 1987), it is extremely unlikely that either anti-J558 Id or anti-M104E Id, respectively, interacts with only two contact residues.

In summary, these various approaches to the study of Id expression suggest that we can specify at least four ways to define Ids and four categories of overlap for Ids, or other epitopes: (1) spatial extent, (2) physical composition in terms of contact residues, (3) amino acid sequence correlates of Id expression, and (4) competition of the corresponding anti-Ids. For the sake of brevity, we will refer to these various kinds of overlap as, respectively, spatial, compositional, genetic (or sequential), and competitive. Recent studies (Novotny et al., 1989; Paterson et al., 1990) suggest additional ways of operationally defining epitopes or paratopes and are readily accommodated into this scheme. It is conceivable, as argued above, that a pair of Ids can simultaneously exhibit different degrees of overlap in these four (or more) categories. Furthermore, it is not obvious that any one level is clearly the most important. In some contexts, the sequence correlates may be most relevant, while in other contexts competitive or compositional definitions (or overlap) may be the most useful (Greenspan and Roux, 1988). A similar perspective has been advocated for epitopes in general (Van Regenmortel, 1989).

GENERAL CONCEPTION OF IDIOTOPES, EPITOPES, AND OTHER SITES OF NONCOVALENT INTERACTION

Let us now return to the issue of formally defining the concept of Id, or, more generally, any protein epitope. A useful way to investigate the meaning of a statement (the definiens) is to determine what statement can replace the expression being defined (the definiendem) (Quine, 1987). Therefore, we can ask what expression can be used to replace, for example, "HGAC 39 expresses IdI-3a." The answer would be a statement such as "HGAC 39 binds (or is bound by) anti-IdI-3a with a particular affinity." This superficially inconsequential exchange is quite revealing, since we have replaced a phrase which tends to foster the belief that an Id (epitope) can be defined as a structure independent of the anti-Id (antibody) with an expression which makes clear that identification of an Id (epitope) is dependent on the interaction with the defining complementary structure (anti-Id in this case). Given that molecular recognition can be cooperative (the contribution of a contact residue can be influenced by the identity of noncontact residues; Chien et al., 1989; Jordan and Pabo, 1988), the above argument suggests that identification of an epitope (binding by a particular paratope with a particular affinity) carries no certain implications as to the identity of the epitope contact residues. In other words, molecular recognition can be degenerate. For example, morphine and morphine analogs can bind to the same neuronal receptors as endogenous peptides (endorphins and enkephalins), and elicit similar functional effects, despite an apparent lack of stereochemical similarity between the morphine-like compounds and the peptides (Maryanoff and Zelesko, 1978). Thus, it may be reasonable to regard an Id (or epitope) as an activity.

The above comments help us to understand why there is a lack of correspondence between the standard definition of epitope in textbooks of immunology and the usage of the term in the experimental literature. While the standard definition focuses on contact residues, the majority of studies aimed at characterizing epitopes use methods that can never identify contact residues with certainty. These methods can yield information of great value, however, as there are many reasons for attempting to characterize an epitope. In many instances (e.g., vaccine development), the central issue is to determine what primary structural differences between two molecules account for differential reactivity with a single paratope. Although differential reactivity generally involves differences in contact residues, and in some cases may solely involve differences in contact residues, it is not necessarily the case that differences in binding are solely due to differences in the identities of contact residues (due to cooperativity of recognition). Thus, mutational analysis is highly appropriate for some cases of epitope or paratope characterization, and crystallographic information is not always essential (although certainly desirable).

In the primary literature pertaining to Ids and epitopes, it is unusual to find an explicit statement as to what, in principle, would constitute a complete description of an epitope. Based on the standard definitions in textbooks, it seems likely that a complete definition of an epitope would amount to a list of contact residues (or atoms) with the corresponding spatial coordinates. It has been suggested (Laver et al., 1990) that crystallographic analysis of a complex of protein antigen and Ab Fab fragment can provide the information required for such a complete epitope characterization. If one defines a protein epitope as an undifferentiated list of contact amino acids, then crystallography is currently the only approach potentially capable of yielding a complete description, but not necessarily so. The classification of amino acid residues, on antigen or Ab, as contact or noncontact residues involves a subjective or arbitrary element (Getzoff et al., 1988; Laver et al., 1990). For example, there is no consensus on the exact interatomic distances that should be taken to indicate noncovalent interaction, nor is there a standard rule for including or excluding amino acid residues as constituents of an epitope if they contact paratopic residues only indirectly through shared hydrogen bonds to intermediary water molecules. Furthermore, it is highly likely that some contact residues are more critical to the binding energy of the paratope-epitope interaction (Novotny et al., 1989). This point is complicated, however, by the possibility that the relative importance of a particular residue, or set of residues, depends on whether one is concerned primarily with the energetics of the particular epitope-paratope interaction under consideration, or with accounting for the differences in the energies of interaction for two different epitopes with the same paratope. Thus, it is reasonable to argue that the ideal description of an epitope represents not just a list of contact residues (including spatial information), but a hierarchical list. If one allows that different hierarchies can be applied to the same epitope, depending on whether the one epitope is being analyzed in isolation or in comparison with one or more other epitopes, the likelihood that crystallography alone can provide a complete description of a protein epitope diminishes. A final limitation of crystallography relates to the flexible, dynamic nature of proteins (Karplus and McCammon, 1983), such that the range of conformations through which a given epitope oscillates is not fully captured by standard crystallographic methods.

This perspective on Ids and epitopes should, in principle, be applicable to any sites of noncovalent interaction on proteins, or even DNA or RNA. The substantial literature on the delineation of DNA sites bound by transcription regulatory factors (and the complementary sites on those DNA-binding proteins) illustrates some of the points made with respect to Ids and epitopes. Defining a DNA site as consisting only of nucleotides judged to directly contact the corresponding DNA-binding protein fails to include information relevant for understanding the sequence specificity of such interactions (Koudelka et al., 1987; Wolberger et al., 1988). Similarly, noncontact amino acid residues can play an important role, through cooperative effects on contact residues, in nucleotide sequence-specific recognition by DNA-binding proteins (Jordan and Pabo, 1988).

In conclusion, coordinated application of crystallography, or other techniques (e.g., multidimensional nuclear magnetic resonance spectroscopy) capable of providing detailed structural information, in conjunction with genetic and biochemical techniques will offer the most effective approach for characterizing Ids, epitopes, or other sites of noncovalent interaction. This process will be facilitated by improved precision in the terminology specifying sites of noncovalent interaction. It would be perfectly acceptable to continue with the term "epitope" as currently defined (contact residues). However, if this is the course to be adopted, then it would facilitate communication if investigators would explicitly recognize that many techniques can never provide a complete specification of the contact residues and only permit partial characterization of an epitope. Alternatively, a new nomenclature could be devised that would explicitly recognize the multidimensional nature of Ids, epitopes, etc.

FUNDAMENTALS OF ANTI-IDIOTYPIC MIMICRY

How do these arguments apply to an understanding of anti-idiotypic mimicry of antigen? We begin our efforts to answer this question by considering precisely what mimicry of an antigen (epitope) might mean. Once again, it is important to distinguish multiple senses of the term. One form of mimicry of one molecule by another would be structural. An ideal structural mimic would express, on some portion of its surface, the identical atoms in the identical three-dimensional distribution as are expressed by the antigen on a portion of its surface. It seems likely that this ideal would be realized infrequently and that the degree of disparity from the ideal would span a broad range. A second type of mimicry would be immunochemical — mimicry in terms of noncovalent binding. At issue in this case is whether the mimic and the object of mimicry bind to the same receptors and with the same affinities, regardless of the degree of apparent structural similarity. Several investigators have offered reasons why mimicry in an immunochemical sense does not necessarily imply the same degree of mimicry in the structural sense (Erlanger, 1985; Greenspan and Davie, 1985b; Rajewsky and Takemori, 1983; Roitt et al., 1985). At the molecular level, the potential for noncovalent bond formation or geometry (which can be shared by atoms of distinct identity) is often more relevant than atomic identity in determining the nature of a bimolecular interaction. This principle has been utilized in the design of transition state analogs for use in selecting catalytic MAbs (Pollack et al., 1986; Tramontano et al., 1986). A lack of correspondence between these two levels of mimicry could also result, for example, from the correlated expression of different sets of contact residues for anti-Id and antigen due to a restricted sample of germline variable-region gene segments or due to selective pressures. Finally, the degree of mimicry can be assessed on functional grounds, such as induction of an immune response or some other cellular response, as might be elicited by a hormone antigen. Given the complexities of most biological responses, it is easy to conceive of cases where the magnitudes of immunochemical and functional mimicry would be imperfectly correlated. In each case, mimicry is likely to behave to some extent as a continuous variable, and not as a discrete variable.

Analysis of structural similarities between antigen and anti-Id (Bruck et al., 1986; Ollier et al., 1985) is at an early stage. In most cases, assessment of anti-idiotypic mimicry of antigen has generally been confined to the immunochemical and functional (e.g., immunogenicity) levels. The first criterion generally employed in screening for putative internal image anti-Ids is whether the anti-Ids compete with antigen for binding to the Ab1 paratope. In other words, it is assumed that an Id recognized by an internal image should overlap competitively with the paratope that binds the relevant epitope. This screening strategy assumes that a useful level of functional mimicry cannot be expressed by an anti-Id that binds to a site that does not overlap competitively with the paratope, a point to which we will return below. It is worth noting in this context, that the amount of competition between anti-Id and antigen for binding to Ab1 can vary with the methods employed (Greenspan and Davie, 1985a; Greenspan et al., 1987; Stevens et al., 1986). Next, the level of functional mimicry is assessed, frequently in terms of the ability of the putative internal image to elicit Ab reactive with the antigen. If the anti-Id can induce Ab to the antigen in multiple species it is considered unlikely that mere genetic association of the Id (recognized by the putative internal image) and the paratope accounts for the functional mimicry.

Several questions are generally not addressed in such investigations. Given that the putative internal image competes with antigen for binding to the Ab1 paratope, how do the relative affinities of the two interactions compare? Thanavala et al. (1986) analyzed the binding of Ab1, specific for hepatitis B virus surface antigen (HBsAg), to Ab2 antibodies and synthetic peptides corresponding in sequence to a part of HBsAg. They found that putative internal image monoclonal anti-Ids had significantly higher affinities for Ab1 than peptide mimics of the native epitope (Thanavala et al., 1986). Interestingly, these Ab2 molecules failed to react with Ab1 molecules that could bind the peptide ligands. These results strongly support the notion that mimicry is a quantitative variable. In the GAC system as well, there appears to be a significant disparity in the affinities of Ab1 for Ab2 versus antigen or hapten (see below). Second, if immunization with Ab2 can elicit Ab reactive with the original epitope one can ask if all clones stimulated by antigen are stimulated by anti-Id and if anti-Id stimulates clones not stimulated by antigen. It is also important to know if the affinity (for antigen) and isotype distributions of Ab induced by anti-Id are comparable to those elicited by antigen. Since each experimental system may differ substantially from others in terms of immunization protocols and Ab detection procedures, merely demonstrating that anti-Id induces some Ab specific for antigen leaves unclear what magnitude of mimicry is being observed in each of the three categories defined above. In the absence of quantitative information, anti-Ids derived from unrelated systems, and labeled internal images on the basis of the typical criteria outlined above, might exhibit vastly different degrees of mimicry for their respective antigens for any of the three categories of mimicry we have discussed.

Let us now return to the perspective developed from the effort to determine Id topography. Given that anti-Id and antigen (as classes of ligands) both interact with the Ab1 paratope by noncovalent bonds, it is reasonable to consider overlap between an Id and a paratope as comparable to overlap between two Ids. Therefore, the degree of mimicry of antigen by anti-Id (particularly at the immunochemical level) can be related to the magnitude of overlap between the paratope and the Id recognized by the putative internal image. The previous arguments about the potential for disparity in the degrees of overlap exhibited for different categories of overlap now take on a new meaning. Competitive overlap between Id and paratope may not be associated with similar magnitudes of compositional, spatial, or genetic overlap, and the Id that most overlaps with the paratope in one sense may not be the Id that most overlaps in other senses. A corollary of the former point is that even if anti-Id and antigen mutually compete for binding to the Ab1 paratope, they may not interact with the same sets of contact residues and may not retain the same relative affinities when interacting with other related binding sites. Thus, the complex quantitative comparisons required to assess the relatedness of two Ids also apply to analysis of the relationship between a given Id and a paratope. Furthermore, the difficulty in inferring the relatedness of two anti-Ids by assessing the relationships of their corresponding Ids is equally applicable to inferring the relatedness of anti-Id and antigen by assessing the degrees and types of Id-paratope overlap.

Some of the potential difficulties with the current anti-Id classification system can be illustrated by considering an example. As mentioned earlier, anti-IdI-3a is a monoclonal anti-Id specific for a site on the HGAC 39 V module. The binding of anti-IdI-3a to HGAC 39 is effectively inhibited by GlcNAc or soluble GAC as well as by three other anti-Ids (anti-IdI-1, -2, and -3b). Analysis of the reactivity of anti-IdI-3a by competitive and direct binding assays revealed that this anti-Id bound more strongly than isotype-matched control Abs (not specific for GAC) to about two-thirds of the 38 GAC-specific MAbs tested (Greenspan and Davie, 1985a,b). The strength of the binding to the GAC-specific MAbs varied over a wide range. Thus, anti-IdI-3a is an immunochemical mimic of GAC in that it competes effectively with GAC or GlcNAc for binding to HGAC 39 and also binds, albeit with a wide range of functional affinities, to about two-thirds of a large set of paratopes able to bind GAC. It is, however, an imperfect mimic of GAC at the immunochemical level, as it fails to bind a significant number of anti-GAC MAbs. Furthermore, although we have not yet formally measured the relevant intrinsic affinities, a variety of binding assays suggest that anti-IdI-3a binds to HGAC 39, and other anti-GAC MAbs, with much greater intrinsic affinities than the hapten, GlcNAc, or the antigen, GAC.

This latter result can be interpreted in light of the known three-dimensional structures of protein antigen-MAb Fab fragment complexes (Amit et al., 1986; Colman et al., 1987; Padlan et al., 1989; Sheriff et al., 1987) and a single Id Fab(D1.3)-anti-Id Fab complex (Bentley et al., 1990). Lysozyme, the influenza virus neuraminidase, and the idiotypic anti-lysozyme MAb D1.3 interact with their respective Abs over large surfaces involving many noncovalent bonds. For example, in the case of the interaction between lysozyme and the antibody D1.3, 16 amino acid residues derived from the antigen interact with amino acid residues of the Ab. Although the detailed contacts are not yet fully resolved for the Id-anti-Id complex, it appears that a surface area comparable to those for the lysozyme-Fab and neuraminidase-Fab complexes are involved. It is unlikely that epitopes comparable in size to GlcNAc could form as many contacts and, therefore, larger protein epitopes would have the potential to bind much more tightly than substantially smaller epitopes. Based on the general properties of Id-anti-Id interactions it is highly likely that anti-Ids behave like other protein ligands. Since many carbohydrate and haptenic determinants are small compared to protein epitopes, such as those on lysozyme and neuraminidase, it may be common for anti-Id to bind to Ab1 with substantially greater affinity than such antigens. In addition, it has been pointed out (Glasel, 1988) that the relative contributions of the four types of noncovalent bonds are likely to differ for interactions between Abs (or other proteins) and small haptens versus interactions between Abs and macromolecular ligands. For example, small carbohydrate epitopes may not provide hydrophobic packing contributions to the energy of binding as large as those offered by protein ligands. The consequences of this relationship for the ability of the anti-Id to mimic antigen may be analyzed in terms of the overlap of the relevant Id and the paratope. Even if the set of residues determining binding to antigen is contained entirely in a larger set of residues

(Id) controlling binding to anti-Id (Fig. 1c), use of the anti-Id as an immunogen could selectively stimulate receptors on the basis of expression of those Id residues not shared with the paratope. Furthermore, it may frequently be the case that the paratope includes residues that are not involved in interacting with the anti-Id (Fig. 1b or d), increasing the probability that antigen and anti-Id will apply divergent selection pressures on the B cell repertoire. A related point is that competitive overlap between Id and paratope does not assure complete genetic overlap. For example, a single amino acid substitution in the heavy chain variable domain of a hapten-specific MAb significantly decreased expression of an Id recognized by a hapten-inhibitable anti-Id but did not affect the affinity for hapten (Radbruch et al., 1985).

Returning to our example, we have also analyzed the ability of anti-IdI-3a to serve as a functional mimic of GAC in terms of eliciting anti-GAC serum Ab. When anti-IdI-3a and two isotype-matched anti-Ids from the panel were compared as immunogens *in vivo,* anti-IdI-3a was clearly the most effective at eliciting a primary anti-GAC Ab response in C57BL/6J mice even though all three anti-Ids were comparably immunogenic (induced similar levels of serum Abs able to displace radiolabeled HGAC 39 from homologous anti-Id) (Monafo et al., 1987). While it is possible that other immunization and assay protocols would have resulted in different relative rankings of these anti-Ids in terms of their abilities to mimic GAC as immunogens, the possibility that the degree of mimicry is protocol-dependent would only add support to the contention that the term "internal image" carries no uniform implications even at the functional level. Furthermore, for the protocol used in these initial studies, anti-IdX, which does not compete with anti-IdI-3a or with antigen for binding to HGAC 39, appeared to be superior to anti-IdI-3a at priming mice for an Ab response to group A streptococci, even though this Ab was inferior at directly inducing a primary anti-GAC response (Monafo et al., 1987). These results suggest the possibility that a single anti-Id may not be the best mimic of a given epitope in all functional contexts, and that an anti-Id that fails to compete with hapten or antigen for binding to Ab1 (i.e., Ab2-α) is not necessarily devoid of the potential for functional mimicry, a point also made by others (Erlanger, 1985; Francotte and Urbain, 1984; Kohler et al., 1989; Schick et al., 1987). In conclusion, the current schemes for classifying anti-Ids are ambiguous at two levels: (1) the exact immunochemical and functional criteria for classification as an internal image are unclear, or at least variable from system to system, and (2) the structural and immunochemical implications of a given magnitude of functional mimicry are uncertain.

Another factor complicating the analysis of anti-idiotypic mimicry of antigen is the influence of structural context. Differences between antigen and anti-Id, at sites separate from those that directly interact with Ab1, can modulate the nature or the consequences of the interaction. For example, even if a portion of the surface of an anti-Id V module perfectly mimicked (structurally) a carbohydrate epitope, it is extremely unlikely that this site on the anti-Id could be presented at a density (epitopes per unit area or per unit volume) approaching that possible for bacterial polysaccharide determinants. Other differences between the antigen molecule and the anti-Id, such as net charge or flexibility, might also have consequences for the interaction of these two ligands with the Ab1 paratope. Consistent with these notions, we have found that IgG3 anti-GAC mAbs bind in a cooperative fashion to surfaces bearing multiple GlcNAc epitopes (Greenspan et al., 1987; Greenspan et al., 1988; Greenspan et al., 1989) but do not manifest this same effect, or manifest it to a much smaller extent, in binding to anti-Id (Greenspan et al., 1987). Thus, differences in the general molecular and geometric properties of antigen and anti-Id could be associated with disparities in the magnitudes of structural mimicry versus immunochemical or functional mimicry.

The use of anti-Ids to elicit humoral immune responses represents a particularly important situation where the magnitude of structural or immunochemical mimicry may not be consistent with the magnitude of functional mimicry. In vaccine development, the interest is in mimicry of both antigenic and immunogenic properties of the target molecule (Zanetti et al., 1987). Where most protein antigens are concerned, a response by a given B cell requires both an epitope recognized by the V module of the surface immunoglobulin and a sequence with two properties: (1) the ability to bind to one of the expressed class II MHC molecules, and (2) the ability to be recognized, in conjunction with a self-class II MHC molecule, by the T-cell receptor molecules of one or more helper T cells. It is possible for the B- and T-cell epitopes to be derived from distinct sets of amino acid residues in the antigen. Thus, mimicry, to any given degree, of an antigen molecule with respect to B-cell receptors does not necessarily predict the degree of mimicry for T-cell receptors, or for Ab responses which depend on T-cell help for the relevant B cells. Studies of reovirus type 3, however, indicate that a single stretch of amino acids (in the anti-Id V module) can account for mimicry with respect to both T-cell and B-cell receptors on the basis of both amino acid sequence similarity (T cell) and, presumably, similarity of secondary structure, and therefore, tertiary structure (B cell) (Williams et al., 1989a).

Mimicry at the level of T-cell receptors is of interest in and of itself, and not solely as it affects mimicry at the level of the elicitation of B-cell responses. The principles already discussed at length with respect to mimicry of antigen by anti-Id apply to recognition by TCR as well as by Ab. Thus, we would predict that attempts to define the contact residues involved in interactions with the MHC molecule (agretope) and the TCR (epitope) by comparison of the MHC binding and T-cell stimulatory properties of peptides differing by one or a few defined amino acid sequence differences (Allen et al., 1987) are unlikely to be definitive, particularly if very limited numbers of mutations are examined at each position. Evidence for cooperativity in TCR recognition of peptide, when the peptide is bound to an appropriate MHC molecule, has been obtained in studies of T-cell recognition of a class I MHC molecule-restricted murine cytomegalovirus peptide (Reddehase et al., 1989). In this study, two residues of the cytomegalovirus peptide that would have been identified as interacting with the MHC molecule, according to the scheme of Allen et al. (1987), were shown to be dispensable in a shorter peptide that retained the ability to sensitize target cells for lysis by cytotoxic T lymphocytes. Similar evidence of complexity in the structure-function relationships of peptides recognized (by TCR) in the context of class II MHC antigens has been obtained in a study of myoglobin peptides (Kurata and Berzofsky, 1990).

POTENTIAL AND LIMITATIONS OF ANTI-IDIOTYPIC MIMICRY

A likely source of possible limitations of anti-idiotypic mimicry is the nature of the anti-idiotypic molecule. As pointed out above, many ligands are quite small in comparison to an Ab V module, which has a diameter of roughly 35 to 40 Å, and are of different chemical nature. Therefore, there is potential for small ligands to bind to sites inaccessible to Ab (including anti-idiotypic) V modules. This effect has been postulated to contribute to the ability of rhinoviruses to escape from the neutralizing Ab response (Rossmann et al., 1985). A related mechanism, based on studies of the structure of foot-and-mouth disease virus, would result in functional concealment of a conserved receptor binding site on the virus by placement of the conserved residues in a context of highly variable residues (Acharya et al., 1989). In this case, the V module of an anti-Id mimic of a small cellular receptor might have a "footprint" too large to interact only with the conserved residues, and nonoptimal interactions with the variable residues would diminish the affinity of the interaction. One approach that might overcome this limitation is illustrated by a study demonstrating the ability of a peptide, derived from the amino acid sequence of an anti-Id complementary-determining region, to mimic the biological effects of the whole anti-Id on cellular receptors for the reovirus type 3 (Williams et al., 1989b). Of course, such a peptide surrogate is likely to bind to the desired target molecules with lower intrinsic affinity or diminished specificity relative to the original anti-Id.

Another factor that could potentially influence the quality of anti-idiotypic mimicry is the type of protein secondary structure associated with a given protein epitope. The related question of mimicry of nonprotein antigens was already discussed (see Section on Fundamentals of Anti-Idiotypic Mimicry). Immunoglobulin V modules are composed of two principal types of secondary structure: β-strands and loops or turns between the strands. The complementary determining regions are derived from the loops that allow the polypeptide backbone to reverse direction. Whether immunoglobulin V modules (anti-idiotypic or otherwise) can mimic structures that involve primarily other secondary structures, such as α-helices, is not known. The evidence that the same amino acid sequence in different contexts can adopt unrelated conformations (Wilson et al., 1985) suggests that if Ig V modules can mimic, to some predefined degree, a particular sequence of amino acids arranged in, for example, an α-helical conformation, then the mimicry will likely require: (1) considerable flexibility in the hypervariable loops, (2) sequences that are not predictably related to those of the mimicked ligand, or (3) both of the above.

Although it is possible to envision the production of useful anti-idiotypic vaccines, in principle, several obstacles to the implementation of such vaccines can be identified. First of all, while many anti-idiotypic Abs used for immunization in experimental systems have elicited Ab responses to the desired pathogen, these responses have often been relatively weak. This deficiency could possibly be remedied with an effective adjuvant, but immunogenic potency of anti-Ids remains a concern. Second, it is questionable whether a monoclonal or polyclonal anti-idiotypic Ab, that mimics a particular epitope, could successfully elicit a protective response to a pathogen protein or glycoprotein such as the influenza hemagglutinin, that is subject to rapid mutational drift. However, it is conceivable that some anti-Id vaccines could be useful in this context, based on the sharing of Ids by Abs specific for different epitopes on the same protein antigen (Kohno et al., 1982; Metzger et al., 1980; Moran et al., 1984). As noted earlier, anti-Ids can elicit antigen-specific Ab even if they are not immunochemical mimics for the antigen. Third, anti-idiotypic Abs able to mimic appropriate epitopes recognized by B cells might, in some cases, be required to effectively mimic epitopes recognized by $CD4^+$ and $CD8^+$ T cells in order to elicit substantial protective immunity, and as pointed out above, mimicry at the B cell level does not guarantee mimicry at the level of class I MHC antigen- or class II MHC antigen-restricted recognition. Fourth, use of an anti-idiotypic immunogen to elicit a protective response to a protein or glycoprotein target that is not subject to substantial drift, would require not just that the anti-Id elicits such a response, but that the response generated with the anti-Id was superior, overall, to the response generated by any other possible vaccine formulation. In the case of protein or glycoprotein antigens, there are many alternative approaches to the creation of subunit vaccines, some of which are likely to be more potent inducers of the desired immune response. Fifth, the immunization with anti-Id has to be free of serious side effects. One group, studying immune responses to herpes simplex virus type 2 (HSV2), reported that immunization with anti-idiotypic Abs specific for MAbs against HSV2, was correlated with shorter survival time following challenge with HSV2 (Kennedy et al., 1984). Of course, similar concerns are relevant for vaccine preparations of any origin.

In considering the relative merits of the anti-idiotypic approach to the selection of molecular mimics, it is relevant that many of the properties of anti-idiotypic mimics can be obtained by selecting antibodies in standard ways (i.e., immunization with the target molecule). For example, antireceptor MAbs, expressing agonist or antagonist activities, have been selected by immunizing with receptor, in one form or another (Clark and Ledbetter, 1986), as well as with antiligand antibody. Consequently, there are cases where the anti-idiotypic approach might work, but it might not be the most efficient approach.

The potential of the anti-idiotypic approach will concern us next. In the interval since anti-idiotypic Abs were first shown to be useful in the study of receptors (Sege and Peterson, 1978a, 1978b), anti-idiotypic Abs have been of demonstrated value in identifying, purifying, and otherwise characterizing such molecules (Gaulton and Greene, 1986). In this period, the focus has been primarily on cell-surface receptors and soluble extracellular molecules. Recently, the anti-idiotypic approach has been extended to the study of intracellular receptor molecules, such as a molecule mediating retention in the endoplasmic reticulum (Vaux et al., 1990). It appears likely that the potential of Abs, anti-idiotypic or otherwise, to identify almost any site on almost any protein molecule will be more fully exploited in the future for the analysis of intracellular phenomena.

In this context, it is interesting to consider the suggestion (Herskowitz, 1987) that it should be possible to create dominant negative mutations in diploid cells by engineering and expressing genes coding for defective gene products that interfere with the function of the corresponding wild-type gene products. This concept has been supported by recent studies (Friedman et al., 1988; Trono et al., 1989). However, this approach has significant limitations, in that it may not be obvious in many instances (particularly for proteins that function as monomers) how to engineer defective gene products with the requisite ability to interfere with the function of the wild-type gene product. A potentially more general strategy, linking the essence of Herskowitz's idea with the capabilities of the Ab response, can be imagined. The essence of the approach suggested by Herskowitz is to express a gene product that binds to a site on a target gene product that interferes with a function of that gene product by virtue of a noncovalent interaction. As we have discussed, Abs, anti-idiotypic and otherwise, are employed routinely in exactly this manner. Therefore, if Abs or appropriate Ab-derived fragments, of whatever origin, could be expressed intracellularly and targeted to the appropriate intracellular compartment, it might be possible to use Abs to create dominant negative mutations, or to mediate other alterations in cellular behavior. The feasibility of this strategy is supported by two recent studies. In the first (Carlson, 1988), a MAb specific for yeast alcohol dehydrogenase I, and capable of neutralizing enzymatic activity, was inducibly expressed in *Saccharomyces cerevisiae* with an apparent reduction in alcohol dehydrogenase I activity. A second study (Biocca et al., 1990), demonstrated that by altering the hydrophobic cores of the mu heavy chain and lambda light chain signal peptides, it is possible to express functional heavy and light chains of a hapten-specific Ab in the cytoplasm of COS cells. In addition, this latter group demonstrated the feasibility of targeting the Ab to the nucleus through attachment of the SV40 virus large T antigen nuclear localization signal.

There are at least two potential advantages of the proposed Ab-based strategy over antisense RNA. First, as pointed out by Carlson, the intracellular expression and targeting of Abs permits disruption of the interactions of molecules not directly encoded by cellular genes (nonprotein molecules).

Second, the antibody-based approach potentially offers mutations of finer resolution. Many proteins mediate a variety of functions. Shutting off the expression of the gene encoding such a multifunctional protein eliminates all functions simultaneously. An Ab binding to a site associated with one particular function might leave other functions intact, permitting evaluation of the consequences of losing that single functional activity. Of course, the above argument refers to the potential of the approach, and it is likely that there will be instances where the binding of intracellularly targeted Abs would alter several functions of a target molecule. Another limitation of this approach relates to the potential for cross-reactivity of a given V module with intracellular molecules other than the molecule targeted for inactivation (Meyer, 1990).

CONCLUSIONS

It has been established that anti-idiotypic Abs can successfully be used for the identification, purification, or characterization of cell-surface receptors and other molecules. The potential of anti-idiotypic vaccines is less certain, despite some impressive examples of mimicry of pathogen-derived molecules by anti-Id, as for example in the studies on reovirus type 3 (Gaulton and Greene, 1986). Anti-idiotypic immunogens frequently elicit relatively weak responses, and for most protein or glycoprotein target molecules alternative strategies, based on recombinant DNA techniques, appear to have greater potential at present. However, it is possible to imagine advances that would improve the results with anti-Id-based vaccines, at least with respect to the magnitudes of the elicited responses.

The perspective of anti-idiotypic mimicry of antigen developed in this chapter is readily accommodated into the modern neo-Darwinian framework. As pointed out by a noted evolutionist (Mayr, 1988), key features of the Darwinian revolution included: (1) the replacement of essentialist thinking by populational thinking, such that the emphasis shifted from the ideals and essences of biological units to the variation among units, and (2) the replacement of deterministic thinking, of the sort that dominated Newtonian physics, with probabilistic thinking. These modes of thought are most compatible with viewing anti-idiotypic mimicry as a quantitative variable. In contrast, the notion of a discrete class of anti-Ids consisting of perfect mimics of exogenous epitopes is essentialist and is not compatible with a neo-Darwinian view (or with much of the empirical evidence). As we have argued, the label "internal image" conveys no uniform message, as individual investigators utilize different criteria for classifying anti-Ids as internal images. As noted by Darwin and emphasized by Mayr, natural selection favors the best available phenotype without any requirement that the selected phenotype approach perfection. This principle applies to the artificial selection involved in identification of anti-idiotypic mimics, and is embodied in the recently described methods for generating peptide ligands for receptors of choice (Cwirla et al., 1990; Devlin et al., 1990; Scott and Smith, 1990) or RNA receptors for ligands of choice (Ellington and Szostak, 1990; Tuerk and Gold, 1990).

ACKNOWLEDGMENT

I thank Laurence J. N. Cooper for critical review of the manuscript.

REFERENCES

Acharya, R., Fry, E., Stuart, D., Fox, G., Rowlands, D., and Brown, F. (1989) The three-dimensional structure of foot-and-mouth disease virus at 2.9 Å resolution. *Nature (London)* 337:709.

Allen, P. M., Matsueda, G. R., Evans, R. J., Dunbar, J. B., Jr., Marshall, G. R., and Unanue, E. R. (1987) Identification of the T-cell and Ia contact residues of a T-cell antigenic epitope. *Nature (London)* 327:713.

Amit, A. G., Mariuzza, R. A., Phillips, S. E. V., and Poljak, R. J. (1986) Three-dimensional structure of an antigen-antibody complex at 2.8 Å resolution. *Science* 233:747.

Bentley, G. A., Boulot, G., Riottot, M.-M., and Poljak, R. J. (1990) Three-dimensional structure of an idiotope-anti-idiotope complex. *Nature (London)* 348:254.

Biocca, S., Neuberger, M. S., and Cattaneo, A. (1990) Expression and targeting of intracellular antibodies in mammalian cells. *EMBO J.* 9:101.

Bruck, C., Co, M. S., Slaoui, M., Gaulton, G. N., Smith, T., Fields, B. N., Mullins, J. I., and Greene, M. I. (1986) Nucleic acid sequence of an internal image-bearing monoclonal anti-idiotype and its comparison to the sequence of the external antigen. *Proc. Natl. Acad. Sci. U.S.A.* 83:6578

Bruggemann, M., Muller, H.-J., Burger, C., and Rajewsky, K. (1986) Idiotypic selection of an antibody mutant with changed hapten binding specificity, resulting from a point mutation in position 50 of the heavy chain. *EMBO J.* 5:1561.

Burdette, S., and Schwartz, R. S. (1987) Idiotypes and idiotypic networks. *N. Engl. J. Med.* 317:219.

Carbone, F. R., and Bevan, M. J. (1989) Major histocompatibility complex control of T cell recognition. In *Fundamental Immunology:* 2nd Ed., (W. E. Paul, ed.), Raven Press, NY, pp. 541—567.

Carlson, J. R. (1988) A new means of inducibly inactivating a cellular protein. *Mol. Cell. Biol.* 8:2638.

Chien, N. C., Roberts, V. A., Giusti, N. M., Scharff, M. D., and Getzoff, E. D. (1989) Significant structural and functional change of an antigen binding site by a distant amino acid substitution: proposal of a structural mechanism. *Proc. Natl. Acad. Sci. U.S.A.* 86:5532.

Clark, E. A., and Ledbetter, J. A. (1986) Amplification of the immune response by agonistic antibodies. *Immunol. Today* 7:267.

Colman, P. M., Laver, W. G., Varghese, J. N., Baker, A. T., Tulloch, P. A., Air, G. M., and Webster, R. G. (1987) Three-dimensional structure of a complex of antibody with influenza virus neuraminidase. *Nature (London)* 326:358.

Cwirla, S. E., Peters, E. A., Barrett, R. W., and Dower, W. J. (1990) Peptides on phage: a vast library of peptides for identifying ligands. *Proc. Natl. Acad. Sci. U.S.A.* 87:6378.

Davie, J. M., Seiden, M. V., Greenspan, N. S., Lutz, C. T., Bartholow, T. L., and Clevinger, B. L. (1986) Structural correlates of idiotopes. *Annu. Rev. Immunol.* 4:147.

Devlin, J. J., Panganiban, L. C., and Devlin, P. E. (1990) Random peptide libraries: a source of specific protein binding molecules. *Science* 249:404.

Eichmann, K., Emmrich, F., and Kaufmann, S. H. E. (1987) Idiotypic vaccinations: consideration towards a practical application. *CRC Crit. Rev. Immunol.* 7:193.

Ellington, A. D., and Szostak, J. W. (1990) In vitro selection of RNA molecules that bind specific ligands. *Nature (London)* 346:818.

Erlanger, B. F. (1985) Anti-idiotypic antibodies: what do they recognize? *Immunol. Today* 6:10.

Finberg, R. W., and Ertl, H. (1987) The use of antiidiotypic antibodies as vaccines against infectious agents. *CRC Crit. Rev. Immunol.* 7:269.

Francotte, M., and Urbain, J. (1984) Induction of anti-tobacco mosaic virus antibodies in mice by rabbit antiidiotypic antibodies. *J. Exp. Med.* 160:1485.

Friedman, A. D., Triezenberg, S. J., and McKnight, S. L. (1988) Expression of a truncated viral trans-activator selectively impedes lytic infection by its cognate virus. *Nature (London)* 335:452.

Gaulton, G. N., and Greene, M. I. (1986) Idiotypic mimicry of biological receptors. *Annu. Rev. Immunol.* 4:253.

Getzoff, E. D., Tainer, J. A., and Lerner, R. A. (1988) The chemistry and mechanism of antibody binding to protein antigens. *Adv. Immunol.* 43:1.

Glasel, J. A. (1988) Opiate receptors and molecular shapes. In *Anti-idiotypes, Receptors, and Molecular Mimicry*, D. S. Linthicum and N. R. Farid, eds., Springer-Verlag, New York, pp. 135—153.

Greenspan, N. S., Dacek, D. A., and Cooper, L. J. N. (1988) Fc region-dependence of IgG3 anti-streptococcal group A carbohydrate antibody functional affinity. I. The effect of temperature. *J. Immunol.* 141:4276.

Greenspan, N. S., Dacek, D. A., and Cooper, L. J. N. (1989) Cooperative binding of two antibodies to independent antigens by an Fc-dependent mechanism. *FASEB J.* 3:2203.

Greenspan, N. S., and Davie, J. M. (1985a) Serologic and topographic characterization of idiotopes on murine monoclonal anti-streptococcal group A carbohydrate antibodies. *J. Immunol.* 134:1065.

Greenspan, N. S., and Davie, J. M. (1985b) Analysis of idiotope variability as a function of distance from the binding site for anti-streptococcal group A carbohydrate antibodies. *J. Immunol.* 135:1914.

Greenspan, N. S., and Monafo, W. J. (1987) Topographic analysis with monoclonal anti-idiotopes: probing the functional anatomy of immunoglobulin variable domains. *Int. Rev. Immunol.* 2:391.

Greenspan, N. S., Monafo, W. J., and Davie, J. M. (1987) Interaction of IgG3 anti-streptococcal group A carbohydrate (GAC) antibody with streptococcal group A vaccine: enhancing and inhibiting effects of anti-GAC, anti-isotypic, and anti-idiotypic antibodies. *J. Immunol.* 138:285.

Greenspan, N. S., and Roux, K. H. (1988) Categories of idiotope overlap and idiotypic mimicry of antigen. In *Theoretical Immunology*, Part II, (A. S. Perelson, ed.), Addison-Wesley, Redwood City, CA, pp. 215—231.

Herskowitz, I. (1987) Functional inactivation of genes by dominant negative mutations. *Nature (London)* 329:219.

Howard, J. C. (1989) Summary: the new pragmatics of immunology. *Cold Spring Harbor Symp. Quant. Biol.* 54:947.

Inman, J. K. (1978) The antibody combining region: speculations on the hypothesis of general multispecificity. In *Theoretical Immunology*, (G. I. Bell, A. S. Perelson, and G. H. Pimbley, eds.), Dekker, NY, pp. 243—278.

Jerne, N. K. (1974) Towards a network theory of the immune system. *Ann. Immunol. (Inst. Pasteur)* 125 C:373.

Jordan, S. R., and Pabo, C. O. (1988) Structure of the lambda complex at 2.5 Å resolution: details of the repressor-operator interactions. *Science* 242:893.

Karplus, M., and McCammon, J. A. (1983) Dynamics of proteins: elements and function. *Annu. Rev. Biochem.* 53:263.

Kennedy, R. C., Adler-Storthz, K., Burns, J. W., Henkel, R. D., and Dreesman, G. R. (1984) Anti-idiotype modulation of herpes simplex virus infection leading to increased pathogenicity. *J. Virol.* 50:951.

Kohler, H. (1984) The immune network revisited. In *Idiotypy in Biology and Medicine*, (H. Kohler, J. Urbain, and P.-A. Cazenave, eds.), Academic Press, San Diego, pp. 3—14.

Kohler, H., Kaveri, S., Kieber-Emmons, T., Morrow, W. J. W., Muller, S., and Raychaudhuri, S. (1989) Idiotypic networks and nature of molecular mimicry: an overview. *Meth. Enzymol.* 178:3.

Kohno, Y., Berkower, I., Minna, J., and Berzofsky, J. A. (1982) Idiotypes of antimyoglobin antibodies. Shared idiotypes among monoclonal antibodies to distinct determinants of sperm whale myoglobin. *J. Immunol.* 128:1742.

Koudelka, G. B., Harrison, S. C., and Ptashne, M. (1987) Effect of non-contacted bases on the affinity of 434 operator for 434 repressor and Cro. *Nature (London)* 326:886.

Kurata, A., and Berzofsky, J. A. (1990) Analysis of peptide residues interacting with MHC molecule or T cell receptor: can a peptide bind in more than one way to the same MHC molecule? *J. Immunol.* 144:4526.

Langman, R. E., and Cohn, M. (1986) The "complete" idiotype network is an absurd immune system. *Immunol. Today* 7:100.

Laver, W. G., Air, G. M., Webster, R. G., and Smith-Gill, S. J. (1990) Epitopes on protein antigens: misconceptions and realities. *Cell* 61:553.

Lechler, R. I., Lombardi, G., Batchelor, J. R., Reinsmoen, N., and Bach, F. H. (1990) The molecular basis of alloreactivity. *Immunol. Today* 11:83.

Maryanoff, B. E., and Zelesko, M. J. (1978) Stereochemical considerations in structural comparisons of enkephalins and endorphins with exogenous opiate agents. *J. Pharm. Sci.* 67:590.

Mayr, E. (1988) *Toward a New Philosophy of Biology: Observations of an Evolutionist*, Belknap Press, Cambridge, MA, pp. 196—214.

Metzger, D. W., Miller, A., and Sercarz, E. E. (1980) Sharing of an idiotypic marker by monoclonal antibodies specific for distinct regions of hen lysozyme. *Nature (London)* 287:540.

Meyer, D. I. (1990) Receptor anti-idiotypes: mimics–or gimmicks? *Nature (London)* 347:424.

Monafo, W. J., Greenspan, N. S., Cebra-Thomas, J. A., and Davie, J. M. (1987) Modulation of the murine immune response to streptococcal group A carbohydrate by immunization with monoclonal anti-idiotope. *J. Immunol.* 139:2702.

Moran, T., Liu, Y.-N., Schulman, J. L., and Bona, C. A. (1984) Shared idiotopes among monoclonal antibodies specific for A/PR/8/34 (H1N1) and X-31(H3N2) influenza viruses. *Proc. Natl. Acad. Sci. U.S.A.* 81:1809.

Nisonoff, A., and Lamoyi, E. (1981) Hypothesis: implications of the presence of an internal image of the antigen in anti-idiotypic antibodies: possible application to vaccine production. *Clin. Immunol. Immunopathol.* 21:397.

Novotny, J., Bruccoleri, R. E., and Saul, F. A. (1989) On the attribution of binding energy in antigen-antibody complexes McPC 603, D1.3, and HyHEL-5. *Biochemistry* 28:4735.

Novotny, J., Handschumacher, M., and Haber, E. (1986) Location of antigenic epitopes on antibody molecules. *J. Mol. Biol.* 189:715.

Oldstone, M. B. A. (1987) Molecular mimicry and autoimmune disease. *Cell* 50:819.

Ollier, P., Rocca-Serra, J., Somme, G., Theze, J., and Fougereau, M. (1985) The idiotypic network and the internal image: possible regulation of a germ-line network by paucigene encoded Ab2 (anti-idiotypic antibodies in the GAT system). *EMBO J.* 4:3681.

Padlan, E. A., Silverton, E. W., Sheriff, S., Cohen, G. H., Smith-Gill, S. J., and Davies, D. R. (1989) Structure of an antibody-antigen complex: crystal structure of the HyHEL-10 FAb-Lysozyme complex. *Proc. Natl. Acad. Sci. U.S.A.* 86:5938.

Paterson, Y., Englander, S. W., and Roder, H. (1990) An antibody binding site on cytochrome c defined by hydrogen exchange and two-dimensional NMR. *Science* 249:755.

Paul, W. E. (1989) The immune system: an introduction. In *Fundamental Immunology:* 2nd Ed., (W. E. Paul, ed.), Raven Press, NY, pp. 3—19.

Phillips, N. J., and Davie, J. M. (1990) Idiotope structure and genetic diversity in anti-streptococcal group A carbohydrate antibodies. *J. Immunol.* 145:915.

Pollack, S. J., Jacobs, J. W., and Schultz, P. G. (1986) Selective chemical catalysis by an antibody. *Science* 234:1570.

Quine, W. V. (1987) *Quiddities: An Intermittently Philosophical Dictionary,* Belknap Press, Cambridge, MA, pp. 43—45.

Radbruch, A., Zaiss, S., Kappen, C., Bruggemann, M., Beyreuther, K., and Rajewsky, K. (1985) Drastic change in idiotypic but not antigen-binding specificity of an antibody by a single amino-acid substitution. *Nature (London)* 315:506.

Rajewsky, K., and Takemori, T. (1983) Genetics, expression, and function of idiotypes. *Annu. Rev. Immunol.* 1:569—607.

Reddehase, M. J., Rothbard, J. B., and Koszinowski, U. H. (1989) A pentapeptide as minimal antigenic determinant for MHC class I-restricted T lymphocytes. *Nature (London)* 337:651.

Roitt, I. M., Male, D. K., Guarnotta, G., de Carvalho, L. P., Cooke, A., and Ivanyi, J. (1981) Idiotypic networks and their possible exploitation for manipulation of the immune response. *Lancet* I:1041.

Roitt, I. M., Thanavala, Y. M., Male, D. K., Hay, F. C. (1985) Anti-idiotypes as surrogate antigens: structural considerations. *Immunol. Today* 6:265.

Rossmann, M. G., Arnold, E., Erickson, J. W., Frankenberger, E. A., Griffith, J. P., Hecht, H.-J., Johnson, J. E., Kamer, G., Luo, M., Mosser, A. G., Rueckert, R. R., Sherry, B., and Vriend, G. (1985) Structure of a human common cold virus and functional relationship to other picornaviruses. *Nature (London)* 317:145.

Roux, K. H., Monafo, W. J., Davie, J. M., and Greenspan, N. S. (1987) Construction of an extended three-dimensional idiotope map by electron microscopic analysis of idiotope-anti-idiotope complexes. *Proc. Natl. Acad. Sci. U.S.A.* 84:4984.

Rudikoff, S. (1983) Immunoglobulin structure-function correlates: antigen binding and idiotypes. *Contemporary Topics Mol. Immunol.* 9:169.

Schick, M. R., Dreesman, G. R., and Kennedy, R. C. (1987) Induction of an anti-hepatitis B Surface Antigen Response in mice by noninternal image (Ab2alpha) anti-idiotypic antibodies. *J. Immunol.* 138:3419.

Schilling, J., Clevinger, B., Davie, J. M., Hood, L. (1980) Amino acid sequence of homogeneous antibodies to dextran and DNA rearrangements in heavy chain V-region gene segments. *Nature (London)* 283:35.

Scott, J. K., and Smith, G. P. (1990) Searching for peptide ligands with an epitope library. *Science* 249:386.

Sege, K., and Peterson, P. A. (1978a) Anti-idiotypic antibodies against anti-vitamin A transporting protein react with prealbumin. *Nature (London)* 271:167.

Sege, K., and Peterson, P. A. (1978b) Use of anti-idiotypic antibodies as cell-surface receptor probes. *Proc. Natl. Acad. Sci. U.S.A.* 75:2443.

Sheriff, S., Silverton, E. W., Padlan, E. A., Cohen, G. H., Smith-Gill, S. J., Finzel, B. C., and Davies, D. R. (1987) Three-dimensional structure of an antibody-antigen complex. *Proc. Natl. Acad. Sci. U.S.A.* 84:8075.

Stevens, F. J., Carperos, W. E., Monafo, W. J., and Greenspan, N. S. (1988) Size-exclusion HPLC analysis of epitopes. *J. Immunol. Methods* 108:271.

Stevens, F. J., Jwo, J., Carperos, W. E., Kohler, H., and Schiffer, M. (1986) Relationships between liquid- and solid phase antibody association characteristics: implications for the use of competitive ELISA techniques to map the spatial location of idiotopes. *J. Immunol.* 137:1937.

Thanavala, Y. M., Brown, S. E., Howard, C. R., Roitt, I. M., and Steward, M. W. (1986) A surrogate hepatitis B virus antigenic epitope represented by a synthetic peptide and an internal image anti-idiotype antibody. *J. Exp. Med.* 164:227.

Tramontano, A., Janda, K. D., and Lerner, R. A. (1986) Catalytic antibodies. *Science* 234:1566.

Trono, D., Feinberg, M. B., and Baltimore, D. (1989) HIV-1 Gag mutants can dominantly interfere with the replication of the wild-type virus. *Cell* 59:113.

Tuerk, C., and Gold, L. (1990) Systematic evolution of ligands by exponential enrichment: RNA ligands to bacteriophage T4 DNA polymerase. *Science* 249:505.

Van Regenmortel, M. H. V. (1989) Structural and functional approaches to the study of protein antigenicity. *Immunol. Today* 10:266.

Vaux, D., Tooze, J., and Fuller, S. (1990) Identification by anti-idiotype antibodies of an intracellular membrane protein that recognizes a mammalian endoplasmic reticulum retention signal. *Nature (London)* 345:495.

Williams, W. V., London, S. D., Weiner, D. B., Wadsworth, S., Berzofsky, J. A., Robey, F., Rubin, D. H., and Greene, M. I. (1989a) Immune response to a molecularly defined internal image idiotype. *J. Immunol.* 142:4392.

Williams, W. V., Moss, D. A., Kieber-Emmons, T., Cohen, J. A., Myers, J. N., Weiner, D. B., and Greene, M. I. (1989b) Development of biologically active peptides based on antibody structure. *Proc. Natl. Acad. Sci. U.S.A.* 86:5537.

Wilson, I. A., Haft, D. H., Getzoff, E. D., Tainer, J. A., Lerner, R. A., and Brenner, S. (1985) Identical short peptide sequences in unrelated proteins can have different conformations: a testing ground for theories of immune recognition. *Proc. Natl. Acad. Sci. U.S.A.* 82:5255.

Wolberger, C., Dong, Y., Ptashne, M., and Harrison, S. C. (1988) Structure of a phage 434 Cro/DNA complex. *Nature (London)* 335:789.

Zanetti, M., Sercarz, E., and Salk, J. (1987) The immunology of new generation vaccines. *Immunol. Today* 8:18.

Chapter 5

Prediction of T Cell-Recognized Epitopes in Proteins

Shan Lu
Victor E. Reyes
Christopher M. Bositis
Thomas G. Goldschmidt
Valery Lam
Christopher H. Sorli
Rochelle R. Torgerson
Robert A. Lew
Robert E. Humphreys
Department of Pharmacology
University of Massachusetts Medical School
Worcester, MA

INTRODUCTION

Eventually we want to determine which peptides in foreign pathogens might structurally mimic self-proteins and lead to autoimmune responses. As a step to that goal, we need to understand in biophysical terms, why only some peptides in foreign antigens are selected for recognition by T cells. Simply put, what is the prototypic structure of a T cell-presented epitope? Our primary objective in this chapter is to present the theoretical and experimental evidence for what we think that prototypic structure is. We hypothesize that recurrent aliphatic residues in some peptides digested from a foreign antigen can stabilize helical coiling of those peptides by forming a longitudinal, hydrophobic strip (Elliott et al., 1987; Lu et al., 1990). Such coiling can lead to protection from proteolysis and/or to scavenging and transfer of the peptide to a MHC desetope (Reyes et al., 1991; Stille et al., 1987). This principle also leads to ideas about engineering of peptide vaccines to increase potency or to broaden MHC restriction of the response (Goldschmidt et al., 1990).

The epitopes on the protein antigen are of two general types of structure. Superficial, hydrophilic, haptenic epitopes are sensitive to denaturation or proteolysis and are recognized by antibodies (Geysen et al., 1987; Novotny et al., 1987). Boosting of the antibody response to the haptenic determinants depends upon T cell recognition of an epitope unique to the protein or carrier which expresses the hapten (Bluestein et al., 1971; Mozes and McDevitt, 1969). These T cell-recognized determinants can be found in proteolytic digests of antigenic proteins (Allen et al., 1984; Shimonkevitz et al., 1983). Any one T cell-recognized epitope can usually be presented by only a few MHC determinants. Thus, in any individual, although antibody responses can be directed to most determinants, only some T cell-recognized determinants are seen. In developing peptide vaccines for a population with various MHC alleles, one might then be forced to define and synthesize all T cell-presented peptides. Later, we will consider a possible method to circumvent that restriction. Furthermore, we might be able to lessen the immunogenicity of proteins used in therapy or diagnosis. Finally, we might be able to develop algorithms to look for structural homology in a helical context between segments of foreign antigens and self-proteins. Although we now deal primarily with biophysical mechanisms regulating antigen processing and presentation, the ultimate goal is clearly the application of these principles to clinical problems which require the enhancement or suppression of immunity, or the identification of homologies which might initiate autoimmune processes.

THE GENERAL THEORY

We hypothesize that selection of T cell-presented epitopes from digested fragments of an antigenic protein is governed by helical coiling of sequences in or near the T cell-presented epitope, against walls of the endosomal digestion vesicle or in a protein receptor with a hydrophobic floor (Elliott et al., 1987; Lu et al., 1990; Stille et al., 1987). Helical coiling is dictated by recurrent placement of hydrophobic amino acids only at positions which form a longitudinal hydrophobic strip along one side of the helix (Lu et al., 1990; Torgerson et al., 1991). Those residues anchor adjacent, helical coils as they hydrogen bond to each other through carbonyl-amido proton bridges along the peptidyl backbone of the helix. Hydrophobic residues not in the axial, hydrophobic strip might compete for helix formation (Lu et al., 1990). This principle also governs nucleation of helices in nascent proteins by directing the folding of helices against locally hydrophobic regions of the growing protein (Reyes et al., 1989). Thus, the sequence of structural helices in proteins and of T cell-presented epitopes (which might be part of structural helices or have a propensity to coil as a helix with an axial, hydrophobic strip after excision) can be predicted from the strip-of-helix hydrophobicity index (SOHHI) (Elliott et al., 1987; Reyes et al., 1988, 1990, 1991; Stille et al., 1987). The SOHHI is the mean hydrophobicity of residues at positions n, $n + 4$, $n + 7$, $n + 11$, $n + 15$, and $n + 18$ in a primary sequence, depending upon the number of turns or positions in a longitudinal strip for which the index is calculated. Theoretical, structural, and experimental data to support the hypothesis that cooperativity in binding of residues in such longitudinal hydrophobic strips determines helix formation in proteins and selection of T cell-presented epitopes is presented here.

BIOPHYSICS OF HELIX FORMATION

We hypothesize that recurrent hydrophobic amino acids stabilize the coiling of a peptide against a hydrophobic surface. As a second loop of an α-helix coils against the first, hydrophobic residues along one side of the helix — in a longitudinal, hydrophobic strip — anchor the growing helix. The fundamental hypothesis is that intercalation in a hydrophobic region of recurrent, hydrophobic side chains of Leu, Ile, Val, Phe, and Met, which fall in a narrow, longitudinal, hydrophobic strip when a sequence is coiled as an α-helix against that surface, stabilize hydrogen bonds or other interactions among adjacent loops of the growing helix (Fig. 1). Although interloop hydrogen bonds between amido and carbonyl functions along the peptidyl backbone of a helix stabilize that structure in solution, the helix can also be stabilized by anchoring the successively formed loops to a hydrophobic surface by hydrophobic residues found selectively in the n, $n + 4$, $n + 7$, $n + 11$, $n + 15$, etc., positions, which characterize a longitudinal strip along the helix. The occasional finding of single amino acids with nonbulky side chains (Ala, Ser) in longitudinal, hydrophobic strips of structural helices implies that another structure of the protein might be jumped over to allow the extension of a growing helix. Extension of local structure as an α-helix can also be inhibited by hydrophobic residues on the surface opposing that of the axial, hydrophobic strip (Fig. 2). Sequences with every other amino acid being hydrophobic could lead to formation of a β-pleated sheet against an organizing hydrophobic core of the nascent protein (Fig. 2).

SELECTION OF T CELL-PRESENTED SEQUENCES

The biophysical principles that appear to govern the folding of helices in nascent proteins appear to apply also to the selection of antigenic sequences for presentation by class I and class II MHC antigen-binding sites (desetopes)

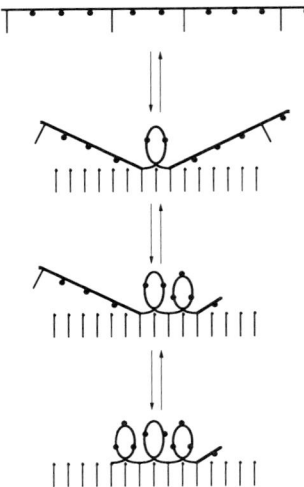

**SELECTION OF
T CELL-PPRESENTED EPITOPES**

Figure 1. Helix formation can be stabilized by recurrent hydrophobic residues which create an axial, hydrophobic strip when the helix is formed against a hydrophobic surface.

to T-lymphocyte receptors (Elliott et al., 1987; Reyes et al., 1988, 1990; Stille et al., 1987). Two types of immunogenic determinants have been described in antigenic proteins. Superficial, hydrophilic, haptenic epitopes, which are recognized by antibodies, in general require a native, intact, three-dimensional structure of the protein and are on the surface of the protein, frequently on convex areas (Geysen et al., 1987; Novotny et al., 1987). The development of a high-titered antibody response to a chemical hapten upon secondary challenge with a hapten-protein conjugate requires that the hapten be coupled to the same protein or carrier which was used in a primary immunization (Ovary and Benacerraf, 1963). Switching carriers between primary and secondary challenges with a hapten eliminates the booster effect in antihapten antibody titers arising from T cell recognition of the carrier determinant. This augmenting or helper effect from immune recognition of the same carrier molecule was found to be a function of T lymphocytes. It was also restricted by class II major histocompatibility complex (MHC) alleles in the transfer of the help from T to B cells, which would become stimulated to differentiate and proliferate as antibody-producing plasma cells. The function of class II MHC molecules is to present digested fragments of foreign antigen to T helper cells. To that end, the surface immunoglobulins of B lymphocytes bind superficial determinants of an antigenic protein. The internalized protein is digested and only some fragments are presented to T

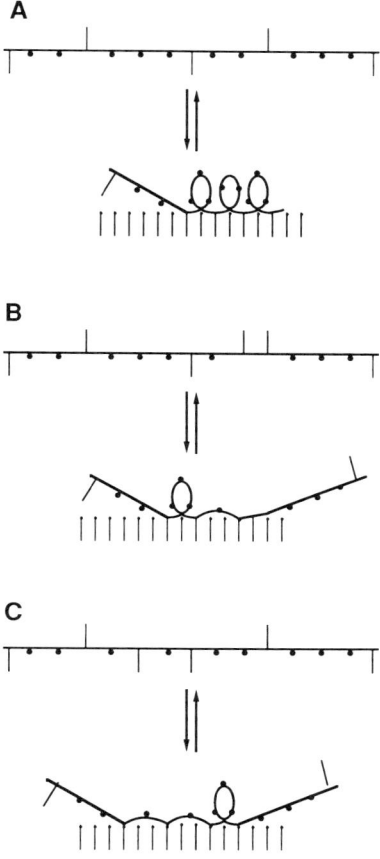

Figure 2. β-Pleated sheets might be formed when every other residue is hydrophobic and the peptide folds against a hydrophobic core.

helper cells, whose receptors are specific for both the antigen and the presenting, or restricting, MHC molecule. Through direct contact and lymphokines, the T cell prompts B cell differentiation and proliferation into antibody-producing plasma cells. The helper T cell-recognized determinants in the protein antigen are not sensitive to denaturation as are the antibody-recognized determinants and frequently remain in proteolytic digests of the antigen. Some peptides identified in such digests are capable of mediating the helper effect of the intact carrier when used in *in vitro* assays for T-B cell cooperation.

From a structural analysis of many T cell-recognized peptides, it was observed that a common feature is their general amphipathic structure (DeLisi and Berzofsky, 1985; Margalit et al., 1987). That is, when the peptides are coiled as α-helices, one axial side is hydrophobic and the other is hydrophilic. Such structures had previously been found by Kaiser and colleagues in many peptide hormones which presumably bind to receptors or membranes through their hydrophobic surface and frequently have a peptide tail which would regulate functions (Taylor and Kaiser, 1987). When the crystallographic structure of HLA-A2 class I MHC molecules was resolved, it was apparent that such amphipathic helices could fit into the putative antigen-binding trough with its hydrophobic floor (Bjorkman et al., 1987).

An alternate, not mutually exclusive hypothesis is that the amphipathic character of T cell-presented sequences of digested protein antigens reflect a step in antigen processing and selection for transfer to MHC molecules (Lu et al., 1990; Stille et al., 1987). In the course of a protein digestion, some peptides with recurrent hydrophobic residues might coil on the surface of an endosomal vesicle as helices which would be relatively resistant to digestion by proteases whose substrate-binding sites accommodate extended chains. Such helical peptides could be scavenged from the digestion sac by extrusion of the contents to a lysosome-bound vesicle or by adsorption to a transfer molecule which transports the peptide to a MHC molecule. The binding of amphipathic peptides to hydrophobic surfaces was studied by Kaiser and colleagues who found that many peptide hormones had such amphiphilic, helical character, frequently with additional uncoiled tails which interacted with regulated enzymes or other receptors (Taylor and Kaiser, 1987). We hypothesize that the principal force in stabilization, and thus selection, of such helices is derived from the quality (mean hydrophobicity and length) of the potential longitudinal, hydrophobic strip. We derived an algorithm to quantitate the SOHHI and tested both the sensitivity and efficiency of its predictions and the ability of both naturally occurring, T cell-presented and abstractly designed peptides to coil as helices in phosphate buffer in the presence of lipid vesicles (Elliott et al., 1987; Lu et al., 1990; Reyes et al., 1988, 1989; Stille et al., 1987).

ORIGIN OF THE HYPOTHESIS

In our studies of I_i, we examined the Hopp-Woods hydrophilicity plot for its primary amino acid sequence in order to make peptides to generate antisera (Elliott et al., 1987). One excellent serum was raised to the I_i sequence 183-193 (Thomas et al., 1988). Months later, upon reexamining the plot to select a second peptide, it suddenly became clear that a six-cycle oscillation in hydrophobicity at the frequency of an α-helix was present from residues I_i (146-173). Work for the next 3 years became immediately apparent. How could we test whether this sequence was just a structural helix in I_i, or if it rested in the desetope as a prototypic foreign antigen? Second, if the sequence was, in fact, a prototypic foreign antigen, could we design an algorithm based on its general structure to predict other T cell-presented peptides and could we exploit this principle in the design of peptide vaccines?

```
                    Ii  146-173
I          GLU  ARG  ASN  THR  TRP  GLU  MET  LEU
II    146       ASN  HIS  THR       LYS  SER  HIS
III   PHE  LEU  LEU  MET  ILE  VAL  TRP  HIS
IV    PRO       LYS  GLU  ASP  PHE            TRP
```

Figure 3. Sheet projection of I_i (146-173).

Looking at the primary sequence of I_i (146-173) in a sheet projection (Fig. 3), the most striking feature is its narrow, longitudinal, hydrophobic strip:

$$Phe^{146}...Leu^{150}..Leu^{153}...Met^{157}..Ile^{160}...Val^{164}$$

The primary sequence is read in the slanting coils which resemble a stripe around a barber's pole. There are salt bridges between Glu^{148} and Arg^{151}, and between Lys^{154} and Glu^{158} and other stabilizing characteristics to this helix. We focused on detection of sequences with similar longitudinal hydrophobic strips.

STRIP-OF-HELIX HYDROPHOBICITY INDEX

The strip-of-helix hydrophobicity index is the heart of several methods to look at protein structure in a helical context. The SOHHI quantitates the mean hydrophobicity of residues falling in a longitudinal, hydrophobic strip if the protein sequence is coiled as an α-helix (Fig. 4). The index for any position n in the primary sequence is the mean hydrophobicity of residues n, $n + 4, n + 7, n + 11, n + 14, n + 18$, etc., for a chosen number of turns around the helix. Turns need to be discriminated from cycles. Turns are the amino acids in any narrow axial strip along the side of the helix. A cycle represents the distance around the primary sequence from one turn up to, but not including the amino acid at the next turn. A sequence of 15 amino acids in an α-helix thus has four cycles plus 1 amino acid or five turns. The index is calculated in terms of the number of turns in a putative α-helix. Turns are analogous to landings in a spiral staircase. If one climbs three flights, one has been on four landings.

The most basic calculation and graphical display is for the SOHHI at 3, 4, 5, 6, and 7 turns through the primary sequence of a protein. Plots of SOHHI reveal two types of organized structure. In some regions, e.g., transmembranal segments, each successive value is relatively hydrophobic (SOHHI >1). One can visualize looking down the axis of the putative helix from position n: each successive residue for the number of turns analyzed is hydrophobic. Moving one's line of sight around the helix to position $n + 1$ again in the

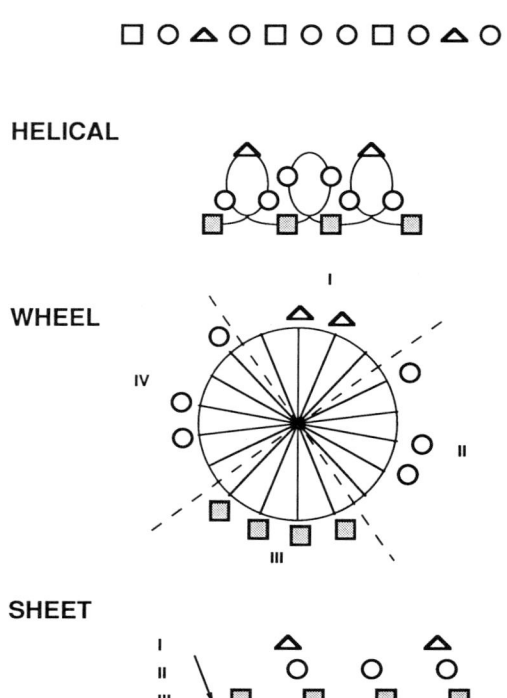

Figure 4. The strip-of-helix hydrophobicity index is the average of hydrophobicities of amino acids falling in an axial hydrophobic strip.

transmembranal segment, the axial row of residues is generally hydrophobic. This pattern repeats itself at each position around the helix. In contrast, in an amphipathic helix, the axial view from position n is hydrophobic, but looking axially from positions $n + 1$ or $n + 2$, one sees rows of generally hydrophilic amino acids. Upon returning to position $n + 4$, one is back into the line of sight from the original position n and picks up the axial, hydrophobic strip again. In the graph, the row of recurrent hydrophobic SOHHI values continues along the primary sequence of the protein, depending upon the overall length of the axial, hydrophobic strip and the number of turns used in the calculation of the SOHHI. The SOHHI was incorporated into the strip-of-helix hydrophobicity algorithm (SOHHA) at five turns to predict T cell-presented sequences because many experimentally determined T cell-presented sequences ranged from 11 to 15 amino acids. Also in preliminary surveys, five turns appeared to be the optimal length for making the selections. The SOHHI was incorporated into the structural helices algorithm (SHA) at three turns in initial measurements, but overlapping selected strips were merged. Other criteria for these two algorithms are discussed below.

SHEET PROJECTION

The sheet projection offers a simple and relatively efficient method to perform by visual inspection, in a less quantitative manner, basically the same analysis of the axial, hydrophobic strip which the computerized algorithms offer (Elliott et al., 1987; Reyes et al., 1991). This type of projection offers a superior analysis of other side-chain interactions to that of the Edmundson wheel. Graphically, the α-helix can be divided longitudinally into four quadrants with the third one being defined to be the one with the strongest axial hydrophobic strips (Fig. 4). The sheet projection represents a flat display of the surface of the helix, having cut it between quadrants one and four. The protein's sequence coils through the illustration as a stripe goes around a barber's pole. One can visualize the axial, hydrophobic strip running along quadrant III. Appearance of hydrophobic residues in other quadrants, perhaps to compete for the anchoring of successive loops during the formation of the helix, can be seen. Salt bridges between positively and negatively charged residues can be found entirely within individual axial strips or between residues which are in both adjacent strips and adjacent loops. The sheet projection is superior to the Edmundson wheel in demonstrating the axial localization of hydrophobic residues when the length of the helix exceeds three cycles. Furthermore, with the Edmundson wheel projection, one cannot identify possible salt bridges, hydrogen bonds, or other side chain interactions between cycles of the helix. Although the positions in the axial, hydrophobic strip and other intercycle interactions can be graphed with pencil and paper, it is possible, with a little practice, to evaluate these relationships by visually scanning a protein sequence.

PREDICTION OF T CELL-PRESENTED EPITOPES

A computer program was written to calculate SOHHIs at three, four, five, and six turns of a putative helix. Five-turn analyses (four cycles plus one amino acid) appeared to give the best predictions of T cell-presented peptides. In a series of well-studied antigenic proteins, all known T cell-presented sequences were found among the top predicted sequences which were ranked according to their SOHHI (Stille et al., 1987). It is possible that sequences which are predicted with the algorithm, but not experimentally reported to be T cell-presented, would be found to be so presented if additional mouse strains were tested over a range of antigen concentrations.

The sensitivity and efficiency of this predictive method were tested against the procedures of DeLisi-Berzofsky and Rothbard-Taylor (DeLisi and Ber-

**TABLE 1.
Comparisons of Methods to Predict T Cell-Presented Peptides,
Evaluated With Five Well-Studied Proteins**[a]

	Known	SOHHA α	Amphipathicity	Motifs 4	Motifs 5
Peptides	14	17	29	48	16
Sensitivity[b]					
Overlapping		0.43	0.29	0.00	0.00
Touching		0.57	0.71	0.79	0.43
Efficiency[c]					
Overlapping		0.35	0.14	0.00	0.00
Touching		0.47	0.36	0.25	0.40

[a] Chicken ovalbumin, chicken lysozyme, horse cytochrome, sperm whale myoglobin, and staphylococcal nuclease.
[b] Correct predictions per number of known T cell-presented peptides.
[c] Correct predictions per number of predictions.

zofsky, 1985; Reyes et al., 1990; Rothbard and Taylor, 1988). Sensitivity is the fraction of known T cell-presented helices that were selected. Efficiency is the fraction of the predictions that identify T cell-presented helices. It is difficult for a method to be both sensitive and efficient. The more guesses made, the more sensitive a method scores, but at some point efficiency is lost. Different levels of stringency for scoring a correct prediction were established. At our most stringent level, "overlapping" the ratio of the intersect over the union of the predicted and known segments had to be greater than or equal to 0.5. At lesser stringency, "touching" at least one common amino acid had to be identified in both predicted and known segments. At the most stringent level of comparison, the strip-of-helix hydrophobicity algorithm (SOHHA) was more sensitive and efficient than the DeLisi-Berzofsky and Rothbard-Taylor methods (Table 1). The efficiency reflected the fact that fewer predictions were made with the SOHHA than with the DeLisi-Berzofsky or the Rothbard-Taylor methods. The pattern of these results was maintained in a survey of a larger number of proteins. In summary, we now have a scheme which 35% of the time identifies a prediction that shares at least 67% of its amino acids with a peptide that is already identified to be T cell-presented. We do not know how often the predicted peptides, which overlap known determinants, have enough residues to be biologically functional. We also do not know how often predicted peptides, which do not overlap a known T cell-presented segment, will later be found to be T cell-presented, if tested in enough mouse strains or humans.

PREDICTION OF STRUCTURAL HELICES IN PROTEINS

We though that the SOHHI could be the basis for the prediction of structural helices in proteins. The biophysical principle of the axial, hydrophobic strip stabilizing a helix would presumably apply in the folding of segments of a nascent protein (Reyes et al., 1989). Such helical nucleations could fold against each other through the axial, hydrophobic strips, or through such strips against the hydrophobic β-pleated sheets or a cluster of hydrophobic residues in a "hydrophobic core" of the protein. The structural helices algorithm (SHA) predicts helices in final structures by finding eight amino acid segments, with three turns and strong axial, hydrophobic strips, and then merging overlapping segments. Because asparagine and proline are frequently found to cap N-termini, and proline and glycine to cap C-termini, those residues are used to terminate or cap predictions. The sensitivity and efficiency of this predictive method was compared at three levels of stringency against the predictive methods of Chou-Fasman and Garnier-Robson (Chou and Fasman, 1978; Garnier et al., 1978; Reyes et al., 1989). At the highest level of stringency, 34% of the SHA predictions overlapped known helices in 35 proteins by 0.5 or greater. Local binding forces might override the tendency of a segment to form a helix. In four instances, T cell-presented segments were correctly predicted with the SOHHA but were not structural helices in the crystallographic structure. Presumably, those segments, once cut from the protein during digestive processing, would be able to coil as individual peptides.

RESTRICTION OF HYDROPHOBIC RESIDUES TO A LONGITUDINAL STRIP IN HELICES

In analyses of 256 helices identified in crystallographic structures by others (Presta and Rose, 1988; Richardson and Richardson, 1988), we found that 89% of the time close approximations of helical alignment could be predicted by choosing the coiling of a sequence with the largest SOHHI (Torgerson et al., 1991). The circumferential distributions of all amino acids in the N- and C-termini, intervening segments, and entire helices, were determined in each axial quadrant. Quadrant III by definition was the axial hydrophobic strip. The standardized deviations for entire helices identified by Richardson and Richardson are shown at $p = 0.001$ stringency in Table 2. Leucine, isoleucine, valine, and phenylalanine are found in the axial strip; changed amino acids are found elsewhere. This study supports the view that the biophysical dominance of the axial hydrophobic strip regulates coiling in nascent proteins and scavenging of digested T cell-presented epitopes.

COILING OF PROTOTYPIC HELIX-1 (LYQELQKLTQTLK) ON LIPID VESICLES

We tested our theories about helical coiling of T cell-presented peptides on hydrophobic surfaces by examining the coiling of a series of peptides on

TABLE 2.
Standardized Deviations from Expected Frequencies for Amino Acids in Longitudinal Quadrants of Helices

$p = .001$	Leu	Val	Ile	Phe
I	−3.9	−2.2	−3.1	−2.4
II	−3.4	−2.9	−2.3	−2.2
III	+7.7	+6.1	+7.8	+5.9
IV	−1.1	−1.4	−2.8	−1.6
	Asp	Glu	Lys	Arg
I	+5.5	+0.7	+1.4	+0.4
II	+1.2	+1.9	+1.1	+0.6
III	−4.8	−4.4	−5.1	−3.8
IV	−1.9	+1.9	+2.9	+2.8
$p = .01$	Asn	Gln		
I	+2.5	+1.2		
II	+0.5	+1.5		
III	−3.7	−4.0		
IV	+1.1	+1.5		
$p = 0.5$	Thr	Tyr		
I	+1.9	+0.14		
II	+1.4	+1.4		
III	−2.9	−3.2		
IV	−0.1	+1.7		

lipid vesicles, as measured by circular dichroism (Lu et al., 1990). A series of 12 peptides included T cell-presented epitopes from viral proteins, some proline-containing hydrophilic peptides from I_i we had made to raise antibodies, and a prototypic helix peptide PH-1.0 which we designed (Fig. 5). This peptide had an axial, hydrophobic strip of four leucines, a lysine-aspartic acid salt bridge between the first two cycles, and favorably placed helix-stabilizing charged groups.

The circular dichroic spectra of nine peptides were determined. The differential refraction of right and left polarized light depends, in part, upon ordered arrangements of optically active centers within molecules, for example, as α-helices or β-pleated sheets. The deep trough in the spectrum extending to 222 nm is characteristic of α-helices. Measurements were made on the peptides in phosphate buffer, in trifluoroethanol which induces helix formation by enhancing backbone hydrogen bonds in a lowered dielectric medium, and in di-O-hexadecyl D,L-α-phosphatidylcholine vesicles in phosphate buffer. The I_i helix, which is hypothesized to lay in the desetope (I_i 148-164) (I_i-3), the prototypic helix (PH-1.0), and many other T cell-presented peptides without prolines were found to form helices in the presence of lipid vesicles. The degree of helicity in the various peptides was calculated from the 222-nm signal. PH-1.0, for example, was nonhelical in phosphate buffer, 58% helical in 45% trifluoroethanol, and 36% helical in phosphate buffer with lipid vesicles. In general, the degree of helicity of T cell-presented peptides without prolines in the presence of vesicles correlated with the SOHHI.

```
                    PH-1.0
        I         GLN    GLN    GLN
        II      ¹ GLU    LYS    THR
        III    \ LEU    LEU    LEU    LEU
        IV     \ TYR           THR    LYS
```

Figure 5. Sheet projection of prototypic helix peptide PH-1.0.

To test this hypothesis in a more refined way, for example, by stabilizing the peptide as a β-pleated sheet, we synthesized the analog of PH-1.0 in order to test helical coiling versus β-pleated sheet formation on lipid vesicles, as quantitated by circular dichroism (Lu et al., 1991a). We have also synthesized a series of analogs of the PH-1.0 peptides by systematically dropping out one or two of each of the residues in the axial, hydrophobic strip. At 25°C, the first members of the series coil on lipid vesicles, but the rest do not. At 4°C, coiling is extended in the series to members with three and sometimes two adjacent leucyl residues in the hydrophobic strip. In addition to testing the biophysical properties of these peptides in coiling, we would like to test their capacity to block antigen presentation.

ENGINEERING POTENCY AND RANGE OF MHC RESTRICTION

The principles of these hypotheses about scavenging and selection of peptides for presentation lead to additional ideas for the modifications of peptide vaccines to broaden the range of MHC restriction, and for therapeutic or diagnostic proteins to alter their immunogenicity (Goldschmidt et al., 1990; Lu et al., 1991b). After examining many T cell-presented peptides, it is clear that nature has almost never made the axial, hydrophobic strips perfect. They are usually broken by inclusion of a threonine, alanine, cysteine, or some other smaller residue. Perhaps, if such strips were perfect and the peptide bound to MHC desetopes but were not recognized, such peptides would compete out the presentation of other peptides that could be recognized. The imperfection of the strips allows selective presentation of a wider range of peptides by the few MHC alleles which happen to bind the peptides well. In peptide vaccine development, one is faced with the need to identify and synthesize most of the potential T cell-presented peptides in a viral protein or pathogen for universal protection. Perhaps, by engineering the potency of selected peptides, for example, by changing threonines to leucines in such axial, hydrophobic strips, one might be able to immunize persons with only low responder alleles. If enough memory T cells were generated, then upon later challenge with the wild-type peptide which occupied a low percentage of MHC desetopes, enough killing might result to afford clinical protection. This maneuver effectively circumvents the problem of MHC restriction in the development of peptide vaccines.

In addition, murine immunoglobulins or recombinant interleukins which are administered for therapeutic or diagnostic purposes might have the axial, hydrophobic strips in their putative T cell-presented peptides weakened to decrease T-cell immunogenicity. In many instances, such alterations could be made without affecting antigen-combining sites or other functional locations in the molecules.

TAKE-HOME MESSAGES

These studies can be summarized. First, the underlying biophysical hypothesis is that appropriately spaced, recurrent, hydrophobic residues V, I, L, F, and M will anchor successive cycles of an amino acid sequence coiling as an α-helix. Second, the cooperative effect of that anchoring can be quantitated by the strip-of-helix hydrophobicity index which is the mean hydrophobicity of amino acids falling in an axial strip, if the linear sequence were coiled as a helix. Third, analyses of helical structure of a series of peptides by circular dichroism shows good correlation between the strip-of-helix hydrophobicity index and helicity of peptides in the presence of lipid vesicles. Fourth, two algorithms based on the strip-of-helix hydrophobicity index, predict very well T cell-presented epitopes and structural helices in proteins. We now have a method which 35% of the time can predict 67% or more of the length of established T cell epitopes, though it is not yet clear how often those predictions will have the biological activity. It is also now possible that the propensity for amphipathicity of T cell-presented epitopes reflects their selection at a stage in processing of the antigen, rather than in actual binding in a helical form in the desetopes.

FUTURE DIRECTIONS

Given these results and theories, what are our future experiments? First, we want to test helical coiling and inhibition of antigen presentation of a systematic series of analogs of the prototypic helix-one peptide we have synthesized. Second, we would like to engineer alterations in some commonly studied antigen to increase or decrease strip-of-helix hydrophobicity indices in their known T cell-presented epitopes. We could then establish whether potency and range of MHC restriction depends upon the SOHHI. Specifically, for example, could low responders be protected from a viral challenge with an engineered peptide or an engineered vaccinia construct while the wild-type analog fails to protect. Finally, we wish to apply another algorithm, which we have developed to quantitate structural homology in a helical context, to the analysis of putative autoimmunity stimulating sequences in self- and pathogen-proteins.

SUMMARY

Leucine, isoleucine, valine, phenylalanine, and methionine, which recur in a protein or a peptide at positions that create a longitudinal, hydrophobic strip when the sequence forms an α-helix, might stabilize coiling against hydrophobic surfaces (Elliott et al., 1987; Lu et al., 1990; Reyes et al., 1989). That effect can lead to helix formation against hydrophobic cores of nascent proteins or to protease protection and scavenging of T cell-presented peptides (Reyes et al., 1989; Stille et al., 1987). Cooperativity among the residues in a longitudinal, hydrophobic strip in stabilizing helix formation is indicated by the strip-of-helix hydrophobicity index (SOHHI), which is the mean hydrophobicity of residues in such potential strips (Elliott et al., 1987; Lu et al., 1990; Reyes et al., 1990; Torgerson et al., 1991). Algorithms based on the SOHHI, with additional considerations related to length, caps, and merging, lead to sensitive and efficient predictions of structural helices and of T cell-presented epitopes (Reyes et al., 1989, 1990). The SOHHI also correlates to helical coiling of amphiphilic peptides in the presence of lipid vesicles (Lu et al., 1990). These principles might lead to techniques to alter potency and range of MHC restriction of peptide vaccines or to decrease immunogenicity of therapeutic proteins (Goldschmidt et al., 1990).

ACKNOWLEDGMENTS

This work was supported by grants CA-37645 from the National Institutes of Health and IM-582 from the American Cancer Society. Victor E. Reyes was a Fellow of N.I.H. Immunovirology Training Grant AI-07272. Thomas G. Goldschmidt and Christopher H. Sorli were Fellows of the Howard Hughes Medical Institute. Christopher M. Bositis from Dartmouth College was an Undergraduate Research Fellow of the University of Massachusetts Medical School. Valery Lam was a Fellow of N.I.H. Immunobiology Training Grant AI-07349. Rochelle R. Torgerson from Williams College was an Undergraduate Research Fellow of the Juvenile Diabetes Foundation International. We thank Ms. Marion Bonin for preparation of this manuscript.

REFERENCES

Allen, P. M., Strydom, D. J., and Unanue, E. R. (1984) Processing of lysozyme by macrophages: identification of the determinant recognized by two T-cell hybridomas. *Proc. Natl. Acad. Sci. U.S.A.* 81:2489.

Bjorkman, P. J., Saper, M. A., Samraoui, B., Bennett, W. S., Strominger, J. L., and Wiley, D. C. (1987) The foreign antigen binding site and T cell recognition regions of class I histocompatibility antigens. *Nature (London)* 329:512.

Bluestein, H. G., Green, I., and Benacerraf, B. (1971) Specific immune response genes of the guinea pig. I. Dominant genetic control of immune responsiveness to copolymers of L-glutamic acid and L-alanine and L-glutamic acid and L-tyrosine. *J. Exp. Med.* 134:458.

Chou, P. Y., and Fasman, G. D. (1978) Prediction of the secondary structure of proteins from their amino acid sequence. *Adv. Enzymol.* 47:45.

DeLisi, C., and Berzofsky, J. A. (1985) T-Cell antigenic sites tend to be amphipathic structures. *Proc. Natl. Acad. Sci. U.S.A.* 82:7048.

Elliott, W. L., Stille, C. J., Thomas, L. J., and Humphreys, R. E. (1987) An hypothesis on the binding of an amphipathic, alpha helical sequence in I_i to the desetope of class II antigens. *J. Immunol.* 138:2949.

Garnier, J., Osguthorpe, D. J., and Robson, B. (1978) Analysis of the accuracy and implications of simple methods for predicting the secondary structure of globular proteins. *J. Mol. Biol.* 120:97.

Geysen, H. M., Tainer, J. A., Rodda, S. J., Mason, T. J., Alexander, H., Getzoff, E. D., and Lerner, R. A. (1987) Chemistry of antibody binding to a protein. *Science* 235:1184.

Goldschmidt, T. G., Lu, S., Reyes, V. E., Lam, V., Torgerson, R. R., Nguyen, Q. V., Lew, R. A., and Humphreys, R. E. (1990) Toward engineering of T cell-presented epitopes. In *Vaccines*, Vol. 91, (F. Brown, R. Chanock, H. S. Ginsburg, and R. Lerner, eds.), Cold Spring Harbor Laboratory, Cold Spring Harbor, NY, p. 11.

Lu, S., Ciardelli, T., Reyes, V. E., and Humphreys, R. E. (1991a) Number and placement of hydrophobic residues in a longitudinal strip governs helix formation of peptides in the presence of lipid vesicles. *J. Biol. Chem.* 266:10054.

Lu, S., Reyes, V. E., Lew, R. A., Anderson, J., Mole, J., Humphreys, R. E., and Ciardelli, T. (1990) Role of recurrent hydrophobic residues in catalysis of helix formation by T cell-presented peptides in the presence of lipid vesicles. *J. Immunol.* 145:899.

Lu, S., Reyes, V. E., Torgerson, R. R., Lew, R. A., and Humphreys, R. E. (1991b) Common principles in protein folding and antigen presentation. *Trends in Biotechnology* 9:238.

Margalit, H., Spouge, J. L., Cornette, J. L., Cease, K. B., DeLisi, C., and Berzofsky, J. A. (1987) Prediction of immunodominant helper T cell antigenic sites from the primary sequence. *J. Immunol.* 138:2213.

Mozes, E., and McDevitt, H. O. (1969) The effect of genetic control of immune response to synthetic polypeptides on the response to homologous DNP-polypeptide conjugates. *Immunochemistry* 6:760.

Novotny, J., Handschumacher, M., and Bruccoleri, R. E. (1987) Protein antigenicity: a static surface property. *Immunol. Today* 8:26.

Ovary, Z., and Benacerraf, B. (1963) Immunological specificity of the secondary response with dinitrophenylated proteins. *Proc. Soc. Exp. Biol. Med.* 114:72.

Presta, L. G., and Rose, G. D. (1988) Helix signals in proteins. *Science* 240:1632.

Reyes, V. E., Chin, L. T., and Humphreys, R. E. (1988) Selection of class I MHC-restricted peptides with the strip-of-helix hydrophobicity algorithm. *Mol. Immunol.* 25:867.

Reyes, V. E., Fowlie, E. J., Lu, S., Phillips, L., Chin, L. T., Humphreys, R. E., and Lew, R. A. (1990) Comparison of three related methods to select T cell-presented sequences of protein antigens. *Mol. Immunol.* 27:1021.

Reyes, V. E., Lew, R. A., Lu, S., and Humphreys, R. E. (1991) Prediction of alpha helices and T cell-presented sequences in proteins with algorithms based on the strip-of-helix hydrophobicity index. In *Methods in Enzymology, Molecular Design and Modeling: Concepts and Applications,* (J. L. Langone, ed.), Academic Press, New York, 225—238.

Reyes, V. E., Phillips, L., Humphreys, R. E., and Lew, R. A. (1989) Prediction of protein helices with a derivative of the strip-of-helix hydrophobicity algorithm. *J. Biol. Chem.* 264:12854.

Richardson, J. S., and Richardson, D. C. (1988) Amino acid preferences for specific locations at the ends of α helices. *Science* 240:1648.

Rothbard, J. B., and Taylor, W. R. (1988) A sequence pattern common to T cell epitopes. *EMBO J.* 7:93.

Shimonkevitz, R., Kappler, J., Marrack, P., and Grey, H. (1983) Antigen recognition by H-2-restricted T cells. I. Cell-free antigen processing. *J. Exp. Med.* 158:303.

Stille, C. J., Thomas, L. J., Reyes, V. E., and Humphreys, R. E. (1987) Hydrophobic strip-of-helix algorithm for selection of T cell-presented peptides. *Mol. Immunol.* 24:1021.

Taylor, J. W., and Kaiser, E. T. (1987) Structure-function analysis of proteins through the design, synthesis, and study of peptide models. *Meth. Enzymol.* 154:473.

Thomas, L. J., Nguyen, Q. V., Elliott, W. L., and Humphreys, R. E. (1988) Proteolytic cleavage of I_i to p25. *J. Immunol.* 140:2670.

Torgerson, R. R., Lew, R. A., Reyes, V. E., Hardy, L., and Humphreys, R. E. (1991) Highly restricted distributions of hydrophobic and charged amino acids in longitudinal quadrants of alpha helices. *J. Biol. Chem.* 266:5521.

Chapter

6

Antigen-Antibody Reactions

Carel J. van Oss
*Department of Microbiology
State University of New York, Buffalo
School of Medicine
Buffalo, NY*

INTRODUCTION

From a chemical and even from a biochemical point of view, antigen-antibody (Ag-Ab) reactions are somewhat unusual. The bonds only involve "weak" (largely physical) interactions and are not covalent. The valencies of Abs are known quite precisely (they are either divalent or decavalent, dependent on the antibody class), but the valencies of most Ags are not as well established. In addition, different valency sites (epitopes) of an Ag often (but not always) are considerably different from each other as far as the chemical composition of the various antigenic determinants, or epitopes, is concerned. Thus plurivalency of such Ags only has meaning vis-à-vis polyclonal Abs, comprising many Ab populations, where each population has a different antibody-active site. To make matters worse, even within one population of Abs that are all directed specifically toward one given epitope, the antibody-active sites, or paratopes, while chemically fairly similar, still vary sufficiently in their amino acid composition to manifest a wide array of different affinities to that epitope.

In most cases, Ags can combine with their Abs in virtually any arbitrary proportion, so that the concept of stoichiometry becomes somewhat irrelevant to Ag-Ab reactions. Even when the binding energy of an Ag-Ab reaction is determined at the optimal binding, or "stoichiometric" ratio, that measured binding energy is still markedly proportional to the total dilution of the reagents. This phenomenon greatly complicates the experimental conditions under which meaningful Ag-Ab binding energies are to be determined, and seriously compromises the significance of most of the Ag-Ab binding constants that have been published to date. The interpretation of Ag-Ab binding affinities is often further complicated by hysteresis, i.e., the phenomenon whereby the energy of Ag-Ab *dissociation* is higher than the energy of *association,* due to the gradual formation of additional secondary Ag-Ab bonds of somewhat lesser specificity. The role of entropy in Ag-Ab reactions also is far from clear; although the formation of Ag-Ab lattices logically would seem to have to go together with an increase in order, in reality the formation of Ag-Ab complexes more often than not is accompanied by a measurable increase in entropy. Thus, the energetics of Ag-Ab reactions are fraught with difficulties that complicate the discipline of immunochemistry even more than most other fields.

NATURE OF ANTIGEN-ANTIBODY BONDS

Lifshitz-van der Waals Forces

Between all atoms that are brought closely enough together, there is a mutual attraction, caused by the interaction between the fluctuating dipole occurring in one atom, and a second dipole which the first dipole induces in a second atom. The interatomic and intermolecular forces that originate in this manner are called van der Waals-London, or dispersion forces. Via the Lifshitz approach, it can be shown that in liquids and solids van der Waals-Keesom (or dipole-dipole) and van der Waals-Debye (or dipole-induced dipole) interaction forces obey the same rules as van der Waals-London (dispersion) forces on a macroscopic scale (Chaudhury, 1984; van Oss et al., 1986a). These forces will therefore be collectively alluded to as Lifshitz-van der Waals (LW) forces.

Lifshitz-van der Waals (LW) Free Energies

LW interactions between atoms and/or molecules, when occurring in large molecules or particles, are to a significant degree additive, so that their free energy of interaction ΔG^{LW} (in the configuration of two semi-infinite flat parallel bodies) may be expressed as

$$\Delta G^{LW} = \frac{-A}{12\pi \ell^2} \quad (1)$$

where A is the Hamaker coefficient (which is linked to physical properties of the interacting materials, including those of the liquid, when the interaction takes place in a liquid medium) and l is the distance between the two parallel bodies or molecules. For a number of materials the Hamaker coefficients can be measured and/or calculated (Visser, 1972); van der Waals-London interactions can also be estimated via the Lifshitz approach (Visser, 1972), or via surface tension determinations (Israelachvili, 1974; van Oss et al., 1988). There is a direct way to determine the free energy ΔG_{132}^{LW} of the Lifshitz-van der Waals part of the interaction between two materials 1 and 2 (in a liquid medium 3), for $l = l_o$ (l_o is the minimum equilibrium distance between two parallel bodies or molecules; $l_o \approx 1.57$ Å, see van Oss et al., 1988

$$\Delta G_{132}^{LW} = \gamma_{12}^{LW} - \gamma_{13}^{LW} - \gamma_{23}^{LW} \qquad (2)$$

where γ^{LW} stands for the interfacial tensions between the materials indicated by the subscripts and where ΔG_{132}^{LW} is the same as ΔG^{LW} given in Eq. (1). Once the LW components of the surface tensions of, e.g., Ag (1), Ab (2), and of the liquid medium (3), γ_1^{LW}, γ_2^{LW}, and γ_3^{LW}, respectively, are known, the necessary elements of Eq. (2) can be obtained via Eq. (3):

$$\gamma_{ij}^{LW} = (\sqrt{\gamma_i^{LW}} - \sqrt{\gamma_j^{LW}})^2 \qquad (3)$$

Minimum Equilibrium Distance; Rate of Decay with Distance

Due to the marked increase in the Lifshitz-van der Waals attraction at short distances of interaction [see Eq. (1)], LW attractions are stronger, the better the steric fit between an epitope and its complementary paratope. The overall distance between the epitope and the paratope, as between other macromolecules and/or particles, attracted to each other via Lifshitz-van der Waals forces, can be as short as about 2Å (Israelachvili, 1974; Pressman and Grossberg, 1973) and in ideal cases is probably about 1.57Å (van Oss et al., 1988) which is of the order of magnitude of the minimum equilibrium distance ℓ_o. Up to a distance $\ell \approx 100$ Å, ΔG_{132}^{LW} decays with ℓ in proportion to $(\ell/\ell_o)^2$; [see Eq. (2)]; beyond $\ell \approx 100$ Å, the rate of decay becomes steeper, due to retardation effects in the dispersion component of the LW forces.

Attractive and Repulsive LW Forces

It should be realized that ΔG_{132}^{LW} can be negative (attractive) or positive (repulsive), depending on the value of the Hamaker constant A_{33} of the liquid medium, relative to the values of the Hamaker constant A_{11} and A_{22} of Ag and Ab. Thus, manipulation of some of the properties of the liquid medium, may turn an attractive reaction (association) into a repulsive reaction (dissociation) (Absolom and van Oss, 1986; van Oss et al., 1986a; see below). It must, however, be stressed that, while always present, LW forces are rarely the only operative ones, except in wholly apolar liquid media, such as alkanes. In aqueous media, where essentially all Ag-Ab reactions take place, LW interactions are never the only interaction forces, and usually represent less than 10% of the total interaction. The LW interaction energy is just (a usually relatively small) part of the total interaction energy, and additive to the other components.

Polar Forces

Polar forces are defined here as the forces operating in electron-acceptor/electron-donor, or Lewis acid-base interactions. Polar forces are designated by the superscript AB, for (Lewis) acid-base interactions (Fowkes, 1987; van Oss et al., 1987, 1988). (It should be stressed that in this chapter AB does *not* stand for antibody; antibody here is designated as Ab, which is not used as a superscript.) As hydrogen bonds (Brønsted acid-base interactions) are a category of polar forces, all interactions that take place in a strongly hydrogen-bonding liquid, such as water, unavoidably involve polar interactions.

"Hydrophobic" or Interfacial Interactions

Even the interaction between totally apolar (macro) molecules or particles, when immersed in water, is preponderantly (i.e., for $\approx$ 99%) polar and only for about 1% due to Lifshitz-van der Waals forces (van Oss and Good, 1988a). These interactions are familiar to most under the name of "hydrophobic" interactions, although the designation "interfacial" interactions is more appropriate (van Oss and Good, 1988a; van Oss et al., 1986a). There exist tables, portraying the degree of hydrophobicity of various amino acids (Manavalan and Ponnuswamy, 1978; Nemethy and Scheraga, 1962). These values, however, are only qualitatively linked to the Lifshitz-van der Waals constant and the available electron-acceptor (γ^+) and electron-donor (γ^-) parameters of given amino acids, and do not permit the computation of interaction energies.

Polar Free Energies

Polar energies also obey an equation analogous to Eq. (2), but the γ_{12}^{AB} term is expressed by an equation which is very different from the γ_{12}^{LW} term:

$$\gamma_{12}^{AB} = 2\left(\sqrt{\gamma_1^+ \gamma_1^-} + \sqrt{\gamma_2^+ \gamma_2^-} - \sqrt{\gamma_1^+ \gamma_2^-} - \sqrt{\gamma_1^- \gamma_2^+}\right) \quad (4)$$

where γ_i^+ and γ_i^- are the electron-acceptor and the electron-donor parameters, of the polar surface tension component γ_i^{AB} (van Oss et al., 1987), where:

$$\gamma_i^{AB} = 2\sqrt{\gamma_i^+ \gamma_i^-} \quad (5)$$

For homogeneous solids as well as for pure liquids, γ_i^{LW}, γ_i^+ and γ_i^- can be determined, e.g., via contact angle measurements* (liquid/solid) or interfacial

---

*By contact angle (θ) determinations on dry (or on hydrated) layers of proteins or peptides, with three completely characterized liquids, L (two of which liquids must be polar), the Young equation can be solved for the three unknown parameters γ_S^{LW}, γ_S^+, and γ_S^- of the solid, S (van Oss et al., 1987; 1988):

$$(1 + \cos\theta)\gamma_L = 2\left(\sqrt{\gamma_S^{LW}\gamma_L^{LW}} + \sqrt{\gamma_S^+ \gamma_L^-} + \sqrt{\gamma_S^- \gamma_L^+}\right)$$

using this equation three times, with different values for θ obtained with three different liquids, L.

tension measurements (liquid/liquid) (van Oss et al., 1987; 1988). For whole proteins, all these parameters can be measured, both for dry and for hydrated proteins (van Oss and Good, 1986b). However, a given epitope on a protein, or on a polysaccharide, is much too small for such measurements. But it is possible, in principle, to measure the characteristic γ_i parameter contributions of, for example, a given amino acid, by effecting such measurements on (dry and hydrated) layers of a homogeneous polymer of that amino acid. Once the composition of a given peptide is known, the contribution of each constituting amino acid to the total γ_i^{LW}, γ_i^+, and γ_i^- of the epitope can then be obtained from these values, derived from the corresponding poly(amino acid). The polar component of the interaction energy ΔG_{132}^{AB} can then be computed (van Oss et al., 1987; 1988). The necessary parameters of the amino acids constituting the Ab-active sites to the corresponding epitope are also known, using Eq. (6):

$$\Delta G_{132}^{AB} = 2\left[\sqrt{\gamma_3^+}\left(\sqrt{\gamma_1^-} + \sqrt{\gamma_2^-} - \sqrt{\gamma_3^-}\right) + \sqrt{\gamma_3^-}\left(\sqrt{\gamma_1^+} + \sqrt{\gamma_2^+} - \sqrt{\gamma_3^+}\right) - \sqrt{\gamma_1^-\gamma_2^-} - \sqrt{\gamma_1^-\gamma_2^+}\right] \quad (6)$$

[From the γ_i^{LW} values, ΔG_{132}^{LW}, can be determined, using Eqs. (2) and (3)].

Attractive and Repulsive AB Forces

When ΔG_{132}^{AB} has a sufficiently strongly negative value to make the total ΔG_{132}^{TOT} ($= \Delta G_{132}^{LW} + \Delta G_{132}^{AB} + \Delta G_{132}^{EL}$) value negative, a net attraction occurs. When ΔG_{132}^{TOT} has a positive value (it should be realized that ΔG_{132}^{LW}, ΔG_{132}^{AB}, and ΔG_{132}^{EL} each can be positive or negative), a repulsion prevails (van Oss et al., 1987; 1988). It is virtually always possible, by modulating the properties of the liquid medium 3, to change a negative (attractive) ΔG_{132}^{TOT} value into a positive one, thus leading to Ag-Ab dissociation (van Oss et al., 1986a).

Rate of Decay with Distance of AB Forces

Polar forces do not decay with a distance proportional to the square of that distance [as is the case with LW forces; cf. Eq (1)], but rather decrease at an exponential rate. The rate of decay with distance of ΔG^{AB} is expressed as:

$$\Delta G_\ell^{AB} = \Delta G_{\ell_o}^{AB} \exp\left[(\ell_o - \ell)/\lambda\right] \quad (7)$$

where l_o is the minimum equilibrium distance (which may be assumed to be of the same order of magnitude as for LW interactions, i.e., $l_o \approx 1.5$ Å), and where λ is the correlation length (or decay length) typical for the solvent molecules which, for liquid water, has an empirical value of the order of 2 to 10 Å for (hydration) repulsion, or even higher, i.e., of the order of 100 Å, (Christenson, 1988) for ("hydrophobic") attraction; a value for $\gamma \approx 6$Å was recently found to be a likely approximation (van Oss, 1990).

Direction Hydrogen Bonding*

Direct bonding occurring between Ag and Ab, for example, between O and C=O, NH and C=O, and NH and OH groups, has only been definitely identified in a few relatively exceptional instances, for example, in the case of *o*-substituted benzoate haptens, reacting with anti-*p*-azobenzoate antibody (Pressman and Grossberg, 1973). However, in the case of neutral hydrophilic polysaccharide Ags, such as dextrans, which are strong electron donors (van Oss et al., 1987), ruling out "hydrophobic" as well as electrostatic interactions, it is hard to conceive how they can specifically interact with Ab-active sites in any other way than in a direct closely fitting electron-donor (Ag) electron-acceptor (Ab) model. Direct hydrogen bonds between Ag and Ab may also evolve secondarily in those cases where the primary bond is between an acidic Ag and a basic Ab, e.g., with DNA-anti-DNA (high-affinity Abs), in which case the primary, electrostatic bond ultimately appears to evolve into a hydrogen bond (van Oss et al., 1985; 1986b) (see section dealing with Secondary Bonds, later in the chapter).

Electrostatic Forces

The electrostatic (EL), or Coulombic, interactions between Ag and Ab are caused by attractive forces between one or more ionized sites on the antigenic determinant and oppositely charged ions on the antibody-active site. These typically are the COO^- and the NH_2^+ groups on polar amino acids of the Ag and Ab molecules (where the Ag is a protein or a peptide). In certain hapten-Ab systems the number and position of the ionized sites have been determined (Pressman and Grossberg, 1973).

Free Energies of Electrostatic Interactions

Due to the shielding effect of the diffuse ionic double layers surrounding the charged sites, which effect varies strongly with the ambient ionic strength and with the distance between charged sites, the calculation of electrostatic interaction energies is a complicated operation. However, as a first approximation, the free energy ΔG^{EL} of attraction between a COO^- and a NH_2^+

---

*While both "hydrophobic" (interfacial) interactions and direct hydrogen bonds are caused by hydrogen bonds, the mechanisms in both cases are quite different. In "hydrophobic" (interfacial) interactions, the low energy ("hydrophobic") moieties are, in a manner of speaking, "squeezed together", through the hydrogen-bonding energy of cohesion of the surrounding water molecules. Direct hydrogen bonds, on the other hand, occur through, for example, straightforward C=O -HO binding between the opposing epitope and paratope.

group, at a distance of about 3 Å, in a medium with an ionic strength $\mu = 0.15$, is of the order of about -7 kcal/mol (Gabler, 1978) or about -12 mJ/m^2, for a charge interaction between an opposing epitope-paratope pair with a surface area of ≈ 400 Å^2. This binding energy is of the same order of magnitude as that of a fairly typical interaction between Ag and Ab (see Table 3).

Rate of Decay of EL Interactions

This is strongly a function of the (Debye) thickness of the diffuse ionic double layer $(1/\kappa)$, which is dependent on the ionic composition of the liquid medium (see Overbeek, 1952; Overbeek and Bijsterbosch, 1979; Hunter, 1981). At physiological salt concentration (i.e., 0.15 M NaCl), $1/\kappa \approx 8$ Å. The rate of decay of EL interactions with distance may be expressed as:

$$\Delta G^{EL}_\ell = \Delta G^{EL}_{\ell_o} \exp(-\kappa\ell) \tag{8}$$

It should be noted that the Debye thickness *increases* in more dilute salt solutions, e.g., the values for $1/\kappa$ are for 0.1 M NaCl: 10 Å, for 0.01 M NaCl: 100 Å, and for 10^{-5} M NaCl: 1000 Å. Thus, in more dilute salt solutions, EL interactions are measurable at much greater distances than at high ionic strengths [Eq. (8)].

As in the case of Lifshitz van der Waals and polar forces, electrostatic attractions are at a maximum at the shortest distances. Thus, here also, precision of fit and especially precise juxtaposition of oppositely charged ions on epitope and paratope favor strong electrostatic bonding.

Calcium-Bridging

As might be expected, by analogy with cell-cell interaction and cell-adhesion phenomena, purely (or mainly) electrostatic Ag-Ab interactions can occur not only through negatively charged sites on one determinant attracting positive sites on the other, but also via the binding of negatively charged epitopes to equally negatively charged paratopes by means of linkage through, for example, Ca^{2+} ions. A case in point, involving synthetic polypeptides (comprising polyglutamic acid moieties), has been described by Liberti (1975). Ag-Ab complexes of that type can be dissociated with the complexing agent ethylenediaminetetraacetic acid (EDTA). Other Ca^{2+}-dependent reactions have been observed by Kumar (unpublished observations, 1989) in certain DNA-anti-DNA interactions, and by Prickett et al. (1989), in Abs to a marker peptide used in the affinity purification of recombinant proteins.

Occurrence of Only Lifshitz-van der Waals, Only Polar, or Only Electrostatic Interactions

Exclusive Lifshitz-van der Waals Bonds

The sole occurrence of such bonds in Ag-Ab reactions are exceedingly rare, particularly if one wishes to limit such LW interactions only to those where any traces of polar (AB) reactivity may be excluded. Even the epitope polyalanine (Kabat, 1976) would only have the appearance of being entirely apolar at first sight: its side chains are, of course, apolar (as are those of polyvaline, polyleucine, polyproline), but its backbone is polar (having C=O and NH groups). More important, however, is the fact that even the interaction between totally apolar molecules, in water, turns out to be predominantly *due to polar forces** (van Oss and Good, 1988a). However, while no Ag-Ab interaction is likely to be exclusively due to LW forces (at least not when occurring in aqueous media), LW interactions can never be a priori disregarded when considering the total Ag-Ab interaction energy.

Exclusive Polar Bonds

Polar bonds alone, on the other hand, only occur quite readily in various Ag-Ab reactions. The only requirements for an Ag-Ab reaction to be exclusively polar, are that the LW *and* the EL interaction energies be zero. One clear example is the dextran-antidextran reaction. The electrostatic or ζ-potential is as close to zero as possible (van Oss et al., 1974), and, due to the strong hydration of dextran in aqueous solution, the value of ΔG^{LW}_{132} is also very low, at least as far as the primary Ag-Ab encounter is concerned. Interfacial ("hydrophobic") Ag-Ab interactions also can be just about entirely polar, i.e., when the γ^{LW} of the polar moiety is close to the γ^{LW} of water (i.e., in the case of octyl or nonyl groups), and when the ζ-potential of these apolar groups is negligible (which is often the case).

Exclusive Electrostatic Bonds

Exclusively electrostatic bonds also occur in Ag-Ab reactions. Among the better studied of these is the DNA-anti-DNA system (de Groot et al., 1980). In many protein-antiprotein systems the bonds are, at least in the *primary* Ag-Ab reaction (see below), electrostatic; a common example of this category is the bovine serum albumin (BSA)-anti-BSA system, where at pH 9.5 no precipitate occurs (at otherwise optimum ratios of Ag/Ab), but only

---

*Until the early 1980s, we tended to lump interfacial ("hydrophobic") interactions under the general category of "van der Waals bonds" (see, van Oss et al., 1980). The new, more rigorous approach to the analysis of LW and AB forces, yielded the realization that such interactions between apolar moieties, immersed in water, are largely the outcome of (Lewis) acid-base (AB) interactions, and only to a rather minor degree due to Lifshitz-van der Waals (LW) bonds [van Oss et al., 1987, 1988; see also the experimental results of Israelachvili and his colleagues (Israelachvili, 1985; Israelachvili and Pashley, 1984)].

small amounts of 10 S and 16 S complexes can be observed, although abundant precipitation takes place at pH 7.0 (van Oss et al., 1982). Another recently reported system is that of the human idiotype-anti-idiotype complex formation, which is the cause of the occurrence of 10 S IgG dimers in pooled plasma FII fractions. Almost all of these complexes dissociate at pH 4 and about one third of the complexes dissociate in 4 M NaCl, which would indicate that many if not most of the *primary* bonds are electrostatic in nature, and that about one third of the *secondary* bonds are exclusively electrostatic (Tankersley et al., 1988).

Combined Lifshitz-van der Waals, Polar, and Electrostatic Bonds

In the cases of many polysaccharide or glycoprotein Ags and of most polypeptide Ags, the Ag-Ab bond is brought about by a combination of Lifshitz-van der Waals, polar, and electrostatic interactions. Thus in these cases the "lock and key" mechanism of the Ag-Ab interaction proposed by Ehrlich in the nineteenth century, consists of the best steric fit for optimal Lifshitz-van der Waals and polar attraction, combined with the most precise juxtaposition of oppositely charged ions for maximum electrostatic attraction. Also, in preponderantly electrostatic bonding, as with BSA-anti-BSA (van Oss et al., 1982), as soon as Ag and Ab are brought closely together by electrostatic attraction (at neutral pH), in most cases, additional Lifshitz-van der Waals and polar attractions are subsequently formed between the epitope and paratope, and also between moieties of Ag and Ab immediately adjacent to the epitope and paratope. It is important to realize the complex nature of the attractive forces in all these cases when one attempts to dissociate such Ag-Ab complexes (see below).

Nonstoichiometry of Ag-Ab Reactions

As is especially apparent from the formation of soluble as well as insoluble Ag-Ab complexes (van Oss, 1984), Ags and Abs (as well as other complex-forming substances, such as cationic and anionic surfactants) can combine in a wide range of proportions. Ag-Ab reactions thus are essentially nonstoichiometric.

Valency

The nonstoichiometry of Ag-Ab reactions creates a special difficulty for the determination of the valency of Ags as well as of Abs. The valency of Ags can be determined only with complexes formed in an excess of Ab (see Table 1), while the valency of Abs can only be determined with complexes formed in an excess of Ag. Still, precipitates obtained at optimal Ag:Ab ratios (van Oss, 1984) often have close to stoichiometric Ag-Ab proportions, with perhaps a slight excess of Ag.

Valency of Antibodies

Human antibodies of the IgG, IgA, IgD, and IgE classes are divalent; antibodies of the IgM class are decavalent. It was especially important to measure the valency of antibodies of the IgM class with Ags (or haptens) with a molecular weight of not much more than 1000; with larger Ags steric hindrance effects cause a reduction in the apparent valency of IgM (Edberg et al., 1972). Secretory IgA is tetravalent.

Valency of Antigens

Most protein Ags are plurivalent only vis-à-vis a complete antiserum elicited against them, comprising antibodies against each of the epitopes. Each different valency site of protein Ags usually is an epitope with a different configuration from the other valency sites. A given monoclonal Ab can react with only one valency site of such a protein Ag. Some repeating types of biopolymer may be plurivalent, with all the epitopes being identical to each other (e.g., DNA, or tobacco mosaic virus; see Van Regenmortel, 1982), or they may have only two or three different groups of epitopes that are identical to one another within each group (DNA also can be an example of this type of Ag). On the other hand, other repeating biopolymers may be monovalent, for example, dextran in the ideal, totally unbranched form; its dominant epitope is the terminal nonreducing sugar (Kabat, 1976).

The different immunodominant epitopes of native globular proteins tend to be situated near their carboxy-terminal and at prominent places on the outer periphery of their tertiary configuration (Atassi, 1984). From known valencies of globular proteins and comparable biopolymers (e.g., viruses), it would seem that there (very roughly) is one epitope for about every 35 to 40 amino acids. As a first approximation one may thus estimate the valency N of a given globular protein to be

$$N = (M_w/5000)^{2/3} \qquad (9)$$

in which M_w is the protein's (weight-average) molecular weight (van Oss and Absolom, 1984). In Table 1 a comparison is made between the valencies N of a number of protein antigens, calculated by means of Eq. (9), and the reported values for N as measured at the extreme as well as at the near Ab excess zone with respect to the equivalence zone (see Kabat and Mayer, 1961). It can be seen that most values for N, calculated via Eq. (9), are intermediate between the two sets of reported values.

Size of Binding Sites

For polysaccharides, the size of epitopes is close to that of penta- to hexasaccharides. For proteins, the epitope size is close to that of penta- to hexapeptides, yielding a specific surface area that may vary between 250 and

TABLE 1.
Valencies of a Number of Protein Antigens

Antigen	Molecular Weight[a]	Number of Principal Epitopes (N) per Ag Molecule		
		Extreme Antibody Excess Zone[a]	Calculated According to Eq. (9)	Antibody Excess Side Equivalence Zone[a]
Bovine ribonuclease	13,400	2.8	1.9	1.55
Egg albumin	42,000	5	4.1	3
Horse serum albumin	67,000	6	5.6	4
Human γ-globulin	160,000	7	10.1	4.5
Horse apoferritin	465,000	26	20.5	14
Thyroglobulin	700,000	40	27.0	14
Viviparus hemocyanin	6,630,000	—	120.7	120
Tomato bushy stunt virus	8,000,000	90	136.8	45
Tobacco mosaic virus	40,700,000	650	404.7	130

[a] Data from Kabat and Mayer (1961).

400 Å^2 (Kabat, 1976) (see also Atassi, 1984; Cunningham, 1984), and a total surface area of contact, and thus of interaction (due to the participation of neighboring saccharide moieties or amino acids reacting secondarily), of up to 1000 Å^2 (Absolom and van Oss, 1986; see also Karush, 1976; van Oss et al., 1979, 1982).

Thermodynamics

In a general manner, the Ag-Ab interaction may be summarized as:

$$Ag + Ab = Ag\text{-}Ab + \times \text{ calories} \tag{10}$$

The equilibrium constants of that reaction are

$$K_{ass} = \frac{[Ag\text{-}Ab]}{[Ag] \cdot [Ab]} \tag{11a}$$

and

$$K_{diss} = \frac{[Ag] \cdot [Ab]}{[Ag\text{-}Ab]} \tag{11b}$$

where K_{ass} and K_{diss} stand for the association and dissociation constants, respectively, and the terms in square brackets indicate (molar) concentrations. $K_{ass} = 1/K_{diss}$ only in ideal cases. In practice one will find in many instances that the energy needed to prevent association (corresponding to K_{ass} as far as the primary interaction is concerned; see below), is less than the energy required to dissociate already existing complexes (corresponding to K_{diss}), for example, because of the continuing formation of additional secondary bonds, after the initial primary Ag-Ab complex formation (Absolom and van Oss, 1986; see also Karush, 1976; van Oss et al., 1979, 1982). This phenomenon, also called hysteresis, is discussed in more detail below. Because of the (generally) high molecular weights of Ag and Ab, and, therefore, of the relatively low molar concentrations of these reagents, molar concentrations may be used here, instead of the more accurate (but more difficult to measure) activities. Depending on the method of measurement used (see below), one obtains either K_{ass} or K_{diss}. In view of the heterogeneity and multiplicity of epitopes in most Ags, and of the heterogeneity of antibodies in antisera directed against such Ags, Eqs. (10) and (11a-b) are considerable oversimplifications. Thus K_{ass} and K_{diss} are mainly to be considered as practical constants, reflecting the average of all the subreactions involved, in all cases except the ideal situation of the reaction of a monovalent hapten with a monoclonal Ab.

Nevertheless, once the practical equilibrium constant K has been determined, the total free energy charge ΔG of the complete reaction can be derived:

$$\Delta G^{TOT} = - RT \ln K \qquad (12)$$

where R is the gas constant (1.986×10^{-3} kcal, 8.3144×10^7 ergs, or 8.3144 J, per Kelvin per mole), and T is the absolute temperature in Kelvin. It should be emphasized however that, strictly speaking, Eq. (12) is only valid for *standard conditions,* i.e., for those cases where unit molar concentrations* of both Ag and Ab were used, and is formally expressed as:

$$\Delta G^\circ = - RT \ln K^\circ \qquad (12a)$$

(where the superscripts ° indicate that standard conditions prevailed). When the binding energy between single Ag and Ab molecules is to be derived, the gas constant R must be divided by Avogadro's number, i.e., by 6.022×10^{23}, to obtain Boltzmann's constant k, so that then:

$$\Delta G^\circ = - kT \ln K^\circ \qquad (12b)$$

where k is 1.38×10^{-16} ergs per degree, or 1.38×10^{-23} J per degree. All association equilibrium constants K_{ass} (Eqs. 11a, 12, 12a,b, 13), are expressed

---

*These are the salient "standard conditions". Unless otherwise stated, ambient pressure, temperature, and pH are held to be kept constant. It should be realized that due to the high M_w of all Abs and most Ags, real unit molar concentrations are entirely unattainable in practice.

in L/mole; K_{diss} is expressed in moles/L. By measuring K at two different temperatures, the enthalpy ΔH can be calculated:

$$\frac{d \ln K}{dt} = \frac{\Delta H}{RT^2} \qquad (13)$$

which allows the determination of the entropy ΔS, by means of van't Hoff's equation:

$$\Delta G^{TOT} = \Delta H - T\Delta S \qquad (14)$$

Another way of obtaining ΔH is via microcalorimetry. If K is also determined, Eqs. (12) and (14) also yield ΔG and ΔS. ΔG, as derived from K, usually is expressed in kilocalorie per mole, but it can also be expressed in units of ergs per square centimeter (or mJ/m^2), provided that the surface area of the epitope(s) [and of the paratope(s)] is known. ΔG^{TOT} comprises ΔG^{LW} + ΔG^{AB} + ΔG^{EL}. If one measures ΔH by equilibrium determinations at different temperatures, via Eq. (13), it always is advisable to do such determinations at least at three different temperatures (van Oss et al., 1982). Contrary to general belief, the binding constant K_{ass}, as measured by the usual methods, is *not* an invariable parameter, uniquely characteristic of a given Ag-Ab reaction. For instance, at optimal Ag-Ab ratios, the K_{ass} of the BSA-anti-BSA reaction increases from 1.7×10^7 LM^{-1} to 6.5×10^{11} LM^{-1}, upon 100-fold dilution of both reagents (van Oss and Walker, 1987). While this increase is undoubtedly due, in part, to the polyclonality of the Ab (where, of course, at greater dilution the higher affinity Abs are the principal Abs that still bind), there are strong indications* that this trend must persist, even with monoclonal Abs (van Oss and Walker, 1987). Thus it must be faced that many, if not most, of the published K_{ass} values for various Ag-Ab (or Ig-receptor) interactions more closely reflect the dilution at which the measurements were done than an actual unique binding constant that might be held to be a characteristic property of the system under study. For instance, the high K_{ass} values published for the binding of IgE to Fc receptors on basophils and mast cells (e.g., Froese, 1983), would be more indicative of the very low IgE concentrations, which one is normally constrained to utilize, than of an intrinsically high K_{ass}.

The best solution for obtaining reasonably reliable K_{ass} values, notwithstanding the strong influence of the volume in which the reaction occurs, is to follow the rules given by Van Regenmortel and Hardie (1979), which include operating under constant conditions of percentage occupied binding sites (e.g., 50% binding sites occupied) and doing the measurements at a wide range of reagent concentrations.

---

*Based upon the greater ease for an Ab to bind to a site in the absence of competition or steric hindrance in the vicinity of that site, at higher dilutions.

Affinity and Avidity

Some confusion still reigns concerning the definitions of Ab affinity and Ab avidity. It is best to follow Steward (1974), and to define affinity as a thermodynamic expression of the binding energy of an antibody-active site for its homologous antigenic determinant. To quote Steward (1974): "Experimentally this term has its most precise application in monovalent hapten-anti-hapten systems" and, we should add, especially when the antibody is monoclonal. Avidity, although it is based on affinity, in addition involves factors such as Ab valency, Ag valency, Ab heterogeneity, and differences in antigenic determinants of a given Ag. Thus ΔG^{TOT} [Eqs. (12) and (14)] stands for the affinity of a monoclonal antihapten Ab toward its homologous monovalent hapten, and, in general, for the affinity of a monoclonal Ab toward a solitary nonrepeating antigenic determinant on a given Ag. However, ΔG^{TOT} can also express the avidity of a family of antibodies (one immunoglobulin class, for example, IgC) toward their homologous (plurivalent) Ag. To distinguish between these two thermodynamic expressions it may be advisable to label them ΔG^{TOT}_{AFF} and ΔG^{TOT}_{AV}, respectively; Karush (1976) calls these intrinsic affinity and functional affinity, respectively; see also Steward (1977).

Kinetics

Studies of the kinetics of the reaction

$$Ag + Ab \underset{k_{21}}{\overset{k_{12}}{\rightleftarrows}} Ag\ Ab \qquad (15)$$

which can be determined with temperature-jump relaxation and stopped-flow techniques (Froese and Sehon, 1975), have shown (in hapten-Ab systems) that the rate constants of *association* are very high (of the order of $k_{12} \approx 10^6$ to 10^8 LM^{-1}/sec) and that, in most cases, they tend to be of that order of magnitude. Binding constants appear to be determined mainly by the (much more variable and much slower) *dissociation* rate constants k_{21} (see Table 2; see also Pecht, 1982). It should be remembered that $K_{ass} = k_{12}/k_{21}$.

Orders of Magnitude of Ag-Ab Interaction Parameters

In Table 2, a number of representative thermodynamic values are given for hapten-antihapten (van Oss, 1981) and Ag-Ab interactions: for example, kinetic constants (k_{12}, k_{21}), association constants (K_{ass}), free energies of association (ΔG), enthalpy associated with formation (ΔH), and the entropy (ΔS) accompanying the formation of Ag-Ab complexes. In general, K_{ass} can vary from 10^3 to 10^{10} L/mol and ΔG from -4 to -13 kcal/mol. As most Ag-Ab reactions are exothermic, ΔH tends to be negative (usually from 0 to

TABLE 2.
Typical Kinetic Data for Some Selected Hapten-Antibody Reactions

Antibody	Hapten	k_{12} (LM^{-1} s^{-1})	k_{21} (s^{-1})	K_{ass}[a] (LM^{-1})
Rabbit anti-DNP	DNP-lysine	8.4×10^7	11[c]	7.7×10^7
Mouse anti-DNP[b]	DNP-lysine	1.1×10^7	0.5[c]	2.2×10^7
	DNP-lysine	1.3×10^8	53	2.0×10^6
Rabbit anti-DNP	DNP-glycine	1.9×10^8	1300	—
	DNP-aminocaproate	9.7×10^7	1.1[c]	9.1×10^7
	DNP-aminocaproate	8.0×10^7	8.7	—
	TNP-aminocaproate	4.0×10^7	27.0	—
	1N-3, 6S-2-DNP	8.0×10^7	1.4[c]	5.9×10^7
	1N-2, 5S-4-DNP[b]	9.5×10^6	76	1.5×10^5
	1N-2, 5S-4-DNP[c]	1.6×10^7	80	1.5×10^5
	1N-2, 5S-4-pNP	1.4×10^7	410	1.0×10^4
Rabbit anti-TNP	TNP-aminocaproate	9.0×10^7	1.6	—
	DNP-aminocaproate	7.5×10^7	6.7	—
Rabbit anti-p-nitrophenyl	DHNDS-NP	1.8×10^7	760	5.8×10^5
Rabbit anti-p-azobenzenearsonate	N-R'	2.0×10^7	50	—
	DNP-R'	1.1×10^7	1.4×10^{-3}	—
Bovine anti-ADHB[d]	ADHB	6.2×10^7	6000	—
Rabbit anti-fluorescein	Fluorescein	4.0×10^8	5.0×10^{-3}	6.5×10^{10}
Sheep anti-digoxin	Digoxin	1.7×10^7	3.4×10^{-4}	1.9×10^{10}
Rabbit anti-ouabain	Ouabain	1.3×10^7	6.4×10^{-3}	3.5×10^9
	Ouabain	8.0×10^6	1.5×10^{-3}	3.5×10^9

Note: k_{12}, forward reaction rate constant; k_{21}, reverse reaction rate constant; K_{ass} association constant. DNP, 2,4-dinitrophenyl; TNP, 2,4,6-trinitrophenyl; 1N-3,6S-2-DNP, 1-hydroxy-2-(2,4-dinitrophenylazo)-3,6-naphthalene disulfonate; 1N-2,5S-4-DNP,1-hydroxy-4-(2,4-dinitrophenylazo)-2,5-naphthalene disulfonate; 1N-2,5S-4-pNP,1-hydroxy-4-(p-nitrophenylazo)-2,5-naphthalene disulfonate; DHNDS-NP, 4,5-dihydroxy-3-(nitrophenylazo)-2,7-naphthalene disulfonate; N-R', 1-naphthol-4-[4-(4'-azobenzeneazo)phenylarsonate]; DNP-R', p(p-dimethylaminophenylazo)-benzenearsonate; ADHB, 4-(3-aminophenyl)-2,6-diphenyl-pyridinium-N-(4-hydroxyphenyl)-betaine.

[a] From $k_{21} = k_{12}/K_{ass}$.
[b] Mouse myeloma (MOPC 315) IgA with anti-DNP activity.
[c] Determined by equilibrium measurement.

Source: Absolom and van Oss (1986).

−10 kcal/mol). ΔS can vary from −40 to +80 entropy units per degree mole (or cal/degree mole); more often than not, ΔS is positive (see Table 3).

The energies of formation found in Ag-Ab interactions (and in hapten-antihapten interactions) agree well with the order of magnitude of the (relatively weak) physical bonds involved in such reactions. Covalent bonds have

TABLE 3.
Thermodynamic Values for a Number of Hapten/Antihapten[a] and Ag-Ab Interactions

Antibody	Haptens	K°_{ass} (LM^{-1} × 10^{-6})	ΔG° (kcal/mole)	ΔH° (kcal/mole)	ΔS° (e.u./mole)	Source
Anti-p-nitrophenyl	DHNDS-NP[b]	0.6[c]	−8.0	—	—	a
Anti-dinitrophenyl	N-DNP-aminocaproate	90[d]	−11.2	−9.5	—	a
Anti-dinitrophenyl	N-DNP-L-lysine	23[d]	−10.3	−19.6	−30.4	a
Anti-dinitrophenyl	2,4-Dinitroaniline	0.3[d]	−7.3	−8.7	−5.2	a
Anti-p-azobenzene arsonate	Terephtal-anilide-p-p'-diarsonate	0.3[d]	−7.3	−0.8	+22	a
Anti-D-phenyl-(p-axobenzoylamino)acetate	D-Phenyl-[p-(p-dimethylaminobenzeneazo)	0.3[c]	−7.4	−7.3	+0.7	a
Anti-p-azophenyl-β-lactoside	p-(p-Dimethylaminobenzeneazo)phenyl-β-lactoside	0.16[c]	−7.1	−9.7	−8.8	a
Anti-SU$_p$[e]	p-(p-aminobenzeneazo)-hippurate	34[c]	−10.2	−21.6	−38	a
Monoclonal anti-DNP-lysine	DNP-lysine		−8.1	−16.6	−28.3	f

Antibody	Antigens	K_{ass}°	ΔG°	ΔH°	ΔS°	Source
Rabbit antidextran (IgM)	Dextran	0.08	−6.6	—	—	g
Rabbit antidextran (IgG)	Dextran	0.1	−6.7	—	—	g
Goat antibovine serum albumin (IgG)	Bovine serum albumin	50	−10.3	−6.5	+13	h
Human anti-B (IgM)	Human B erythrocyte	100 to 140	−10.8 to −11.0	—	—	i
Human anti-A sera	Human A erythrocyte	0.2 to 0.6	−6.8 to −7.8	−0.6 to −12.5	16 to +124	j
Human anti-D	Human D(Rh$_o$) erythrocytes	300 to 1200	−10.6 to −12.3	+9.4 to +11.0	+74	k

[a] From van Oss and Grossberg (1979) and van Oss (1981), where the individual references are given. In Pecht (1982) many more rate constants can be found for various systems.
[b] DHNDS-NP, 4-5-dihydroxy-3-(p-nitrophenylazo)-2,7-naphthalene disulfonate.
[c] Measured by equilibrium dialysis.
[d] Measured by fluorescence quenching.
[e] $SU_p = -(CH_2)_4NHCOCH-SCH_2CONH--N=N--CONHOH_2COO-$
[f] Johnston et al. (1974) via equilibrium dialysis, fluorescence quenching, and flow calorimetry.
[g] Edberg et al. (1972) by $(NH_4)_2SO_4$ precipitation.
[h] van Oss et al. (1982) by precipitation at optimal ratio; figures in parentheses are obtained by affinity diffusion using the same system.
[i] Economidou et al. (1967) by equilibrium measurement.
[j] Steane (1974).
[k] Green (1982) by equilibrium measurements with protein A as indicator. This is a typical example of the exceptional endothermic behavior of the D-anti-D ("warm" antibody) reaction; this phenomenon is best explained by a phase change accompanying the reaction (e.g., "melting" of a lipid moiety), which fits in well with the apparently irreversible denaturation of the D-antigenic determinant following the D-anti-D reaction (van Oss et al., 1981).

Source: van Oss and Absolom (1984).

higher energies of formation (ΔG of the order of -10 to -1000 kcal/mol). The exothermicity of formation of the Ag-Ab reaction as manifested by a negative ΔH value is, for the most part, due to the electrostatic and the direct H-bonding complements of the interaction.

In the exceptional case where ΔH is positive (see Table 3), as in the D-anti-D reaction (Green, 1982), one must implicate the occurrence of a phase change (e.g., the "melting" of a lipid moiety), which agrees well with the apparently irreversible denaturation of the D(Rho) antigenic site following the D-anti-D reaction (van Oss et al., 1981).

In most typical Ag-Ab interactions, as the temperature increases, ΔH becomes less negative, while $T\Delta S$ proportionally increases, leaving ΔG approximately unchanged [see Eq. (14)] (Mukkur, 1984; van Oss et al., 1982). This is called an enthalpy-entropy compensation by Mukkur (1984). The fact that the entropy of the Ag-Ab complex formation often has a positive value (notwithstanding an increase in "order" involved in the Ag-Ab combination) is best explained by the expulsion (and thus the randomization) of water molecules that earlier participated in forming (organized) layers of water of hydration attached to the antigenic determinant as well as on the antibody-active site. Water of hydration is released after electrostatic as well as after polar bond formation between Ag and Ab. The increase in positive ΔS (or decrease in negative ΔS) with an increase in temperature accompanies the increase in interfacial or "hydrophobic" bond energy (van Oss et al., 1982). At higher temperatures, electrostatic bonds, as well as hydration, weaken, which also causes more of the water molecules of hydration to join the bulk water phase, which increases the entropy of the system (the Mukkur effect), while at the same time the polar interfacial ("hydrophobic") forces are strengthened. Thus, at higher temperatures, the decrease in electrostatic bond strength (accompanied by a decrease in enthalpy) tends to be compensated by an increase in polar ("hydrophobic") bond strength, leaving ΔG^{TOT} on the whole, unchanged.

It now also becomes possible to engage in computer modeling due to the X-ray diffraction work of Amit et al. (1986). An interesting example of such work was published recently by Novotny et al. (1989).

Affinity of Polyclonal and Monoclonal Antibodies

There are a number of observations that would, at first sight, seem to indicate that the affinity of monoclonal Abs (MAb) to their epitope is lower than that of polyclonal Abs to the same epitope. A lower apparent K_{ass} value of MAb to multivalent Ags (comprising several different epitopes) is, of course, plausible, due to the lack of cooperative cross-linking that would be obtainable by means of the different paratopes of polyclonal Abs. This drawback of MAb can be overcome by using mixtures of two or more MAb directed to different epitopes of the same Ag. Single MAb usually do not form immune precipitates with Ags, although immunoprecipitation becomes possible with mixtures of two or more MAb (Molinaro et al., 1984). Single MAb, however, can form immune precipitates with large Ags (e.g., plant viruses) with repeating identical epitopes (Halk et al., 1984). Bankert et al. (1981) have shown that various MAb directed against 4-azophthalate have a fairly wide array of binding constants (ranging from 4×10^4 to 4×10^7 LM^{-1}), the highest value of which compares quite well with the higher values obtained, in general, with polyclonal Abs against haptens (see Pfeiffer et al., 1987; see also Table 2, top eight values, pertaining to haptens).

FACTORS FAVORING Ag-Ab ASSOCIATION AND DISSOCIATION
Influence of Brownian Motion

It should be kept in mind that every single detached molecule, cell or particle, immersed in a liquid, is endowed with a Brownian energy ΔG^{BR}) of $+1.5$ kT (Einstein, 1907, 1955). This energy keeps it in solution or suspension, provided the energy of attraction between similar molecules or particles immersed in that liquid is less than $|-1.5 \text{ kT}|$ per pair of such molecules or particles (see also Van de Ven, 1989). For instance, a hapten molecule which can react with its specific paratope with an attractive energy of -6 mJ/m^2, and which has a contactable surface area with the paratope of ≈ 1.0 nm^2, would undergo an energy of attraction to the paratope of -1.5 kT, which, however, is then exactly counterbalanced by a repulsive Brownian energy of $+1.5$ kT, allowing the hapten to detach again (on an average) as soon as it becomes attached. It thus is imperative for small haptens to be attracted to a specific paratope with energies that are significantly larger than 6 mJ/m^2. On the other hand, large epitopes, with a contactable surface area with their paratope of ≈ 10.0 nm^2, which also undergo an attraction to their paratope of -6 mJ/m^2 (a value which is on the slightly low normal side), will be attracted to that paratope with an energy of -15 kT, which largely overrides the Brownian repulsion of $+1.5$ kT, so that it will remain attached. The latter condition of $\Delta G = -15 + 1.5 = -13.5$ kT, still gives rise to an equilibrium constant $K_a = 7.3 \times 10^5$ LM^{-1} [see Eq. (12b)]. Thus, to overcome repulsion due to Brownian motion, a small epitope needs a high binding energy to remain attached to its paratope, while a large epitope needs a much smaller binding energy per unit surface area.

It has been proposed that enhanced mobility of subunits of epitopes favors antigenicity (Getzoff et al., 1988; Van Regenmortel et al., 1988; Westhof et al., 1984) for improving the "fit". This concept is intuitively quite plausible, as Ehrlich's lock-and-key Ag-Ab binding mechanism quickly comes to mind: with such a device one does, of course, considerably facilitate the insertion of a key by applying a certain degree of vibrational motion, i.e., by wiggling the key into the lock. It is, however, somewhat dangerous to extrapolate the properties of relatively large-scale mechanical models to intramolecular interactions on the nanometer scale, as these deviate from each other at several levels. For instance, if one of the moieties of an epitope, consisting of one or two amino acids, is unusually motile, which is to say, if such a moiety is relatively independently endowed with a Brownian movement energy in one dimension of $+ \frac{1}{2}$ kT (which is the most plausible value, with one degree of freedom), then, for a contactable surface area between that motile epitopic moiety and its paratopic counterpart of 0.2 to 0.4 nm², a repulsion will be generated of the order of $\Delta G^{BR} \approx +5$ to $+10$ mJ/m². That repulsion energy is only slightly smaller than the total energy of attraction between epitope and paratope, which usually is of the order of $\Delta G^{TOT} \approx -8$ to -20 mJ/m². In other words, one invokes here a mechanism similar to "steric stabilization" (Napper, 1983) which, contrary to an enhanced attraction, serves to explain the repulsion between small particles with the help of adsorbed, but still motile, surfactant or polymer molecules. Thus, it may well be that a degree of enhanced mobility in some of the moieties of an epitope gives rise to a better "fit", but this would only work in the cases of epitopes with very high binding constants, where the sizable repulsion generated by the enhanced mobility is solidly counterbalanced by a high energy of attraction.

Hysteresis, or Differentiation between Primary and Secondary Bonds

Primary Bonds

The specificity of the bonds that arise between epitope and paratope is mainly due to the interactions that occur very early in the process of Ag-Ab binding. The primary bond is the principal cause of the early attraction between epitope and paratope while these moieties still are some distance apart. The distance at which epitope and paratope start attracting each other to a significant degree is likely to be less than 100 Å for electrostatic and polar (interfacial) interactions. Although the primary bond is mainly responsible for the specificity of Ag-Ab interactions, in many cases the primary bond energy tends to be significantly smaller than the total (primary + secondary) bond energy.

The primary bond energy can be determined by measuring the energy required to prevent the bond from forming. A few examples of primary bonds can be given. First, to prevent bovine serum albumin (BSA) from reacting with anti-BSA, it suffices to raise the pH from 7.0 to 9.5 (van Oss et al., 1982). However, to dissociate BSA-anti-BSA complexes, once formed, it is necessary to raise the pH to 9.5 and to add 9.7 M ethylene glycol (van Oss et al., 1979). In a purely polar system, to prevent the interaction between 3-azopyridine (P3), coupled to rabbit serum albumin, with rabbit anti-P3, it suffices to add 1.9 M dimethyl sulfoxide (DMSO), but the energy needed to dissociate anti-P3 from P3, requires the admixture of 6.4 M DMSO (van Oss et al., 1979). In purely electrostatic systems (e.g., the low- and medium-affinity DNA-anti-DNA systems (Smeenk et al., 1982), there is no measurable difference between the primary and the total energy of association, as shown by the equality between the energies of dissociation and of prevention of association (van Oss and Absolom, 1984).

While primary bonds of the sole Lifshitz-van der Waals variety are exceedingly rare, instances where the other bond types occur as the sole primary bond are common: (1) primary polar (interfacial or "hydrophobic") bonds: P3 (3-azopyridine)-anti-P3; (2) primary polar (direct hydrogen) bonds: dextran-antidextran; and (3) primary electrostatic bonds: BSA-anti-BSA; idiotype-anti-idiotype.

Secondary Bonds – Hysteresis

The greater energy needed for dissociating most Ag-Ab bonds than is required for the prevention of their association (hysteresis) is indicative of the existence of further secondary bonds that have formed subsequent to the formation of the initial primary Ag-Ab bonds. The difference between the energy of dissociation and the energy required to prevent association of Ag from Ab is equal to the energy of the secondary Ag-Ab bonds. Thus, the energy of the secondary bond (ΔG_{sec}) is obtained as follows (Absolom and van Oss, 1986):

$$\Delta G_{sec} = \Delta G_{diss} - \Delta G_{prev\ assoc} = \Delta G_{total} - \Delta G_{primary} \quad (16)$$

where ΔG_{diss} is $\Delta G_{dissociation}$ and $\Delta G_{prev\ assoc}$ is $\Delta G_{prevention\ of\ association}$.

Electrostatic bonds do not appear to occur often as secondary bonds. The purely electrostatic DNA-anti-DNA system has been studied from this aspect: the similarities of pH conditions, leading to dissociation and to prevention of association (lack of hysteresis), points to an absence of secondary electrostatic bonds in this system (Smeenk et al., 1982). Secondary electrostatic bonds are likely to be rare occurrences, as the statistical probability of negatively and positively charged amino acids on Ag and Ab (outside of the epitope and paratope) being situated exactly opposite each other is very slight and, in those rare cases where it might occur, such moieties would be indistinguishable from the epitope and paratope and thus simply show up as a system with somewhat larger than usual epitopes and paratopes.

Polar Bonds (interfacial forces or "hydrophobic" interactions). Interfacial ("hydrophobic") forces by nature represent the most common bonds involved in secondary Ag-Ab bonding. As soon as epitope and paratope have combined in a primary bond, various nonspecific (especially nonpolar) moieties of Ag and/or Ab in the immediate vicinity of epitope and paratope can undergo a mutual interfacial attraction, approach each other more closely, and bind to each other secondarily. Thus, both in cases where the primary bond is mainly polar (e.g., P3-anti-P3) and in the cases where the primary bond is largely electrostatic (BSA-anti-BSA), secondary bonds of the interfacial type are bound to develop. With time, a strengthening of existing (primary as well as secondary) interfacial bonds also takes place through the extrusion of interstitial solvent. This results in a shorter distance between epitope and paratope which enhances the interfacial attraction energy and results in an (at least partial) direct contact that replaces the epitope-water-paratope interactions, which gives rise to a further significant increase in the total energy of attraction (van Oss et al., 1986a,b).

Polar Bonds (direct hydrogen bonds) which can play a significant role in direct primary epitope-paratope interactions can also occur in secondary Ag-Ab bonding, e.g., in high-avidity DNA-anti-DNA systems (van Oss et al., 1985). Although precise binding studies have not yet been performed on this system, from preliminary data (i.e., from the pH needed to dissociate DNA-anti-DNA, or to prevent them from associating) it would not appear that the formation of secondary hydrogen bonds causes an increase in the total binding energy (van Oss et al., 1985; Absolom and van Oss, 1986). In this case, electrostatic bonds apparently gradually revert to direct hydrogen bonds without a significant change in energy. What points to the formation of hydrogen bonds in high-avidity DNA-anti-DNA complexes is the impossibility of dissociating them at high ionic strengths, although fairly low ionic strengths suffice to prevent them from forming at all. Chaotropic ions, however, which tend to dissociate hydrogen bonds, but not electrostatic bonds, do dissociate these high-avidity DNA-anti-DNA complexes (Absolom and van Oss, 1986).

Conditions Favoring Ag-Ab Association or Dissociation

In many cases, the conditions favoring association of Ag with Ab are qualitatively (and in some cases quantitatively) the inverse of the conditions favoring their dissociation. However, as shown above, when secondary bonds occur, dissociation usually requires more energy than the prevention of association, in which case a quantitative difference exists between the two opposing effects. In general, however, when the conditions required to effect dissociation are reversed, association is favored instead. For the sake of simplicity it therefore suffices to describe only the various conditions by which dissociation of Ag-Ab complexes can be achieved (see Table 4).

In most cases, dissociation is most readily achieved by *combining* the admixture of strong electron-donor solvent (e.g., DMSO, EG, propanol) to the liquid medium, with an increase (or in some cases with a drastic decrease) in pH. Only relatively weak, purely electrostatic systems dissociate well by only increasing the ionic strength; in systems with mainly interfacial bonding the opposite is often true. However, addition of chaotropic salts favors dissociation of both interfacial and electrostatic bonds (Absolom and van Oss, 1986), because they combine the power of increasing the ionic strength and of opening up, or of displacing, hydrogen bonds.

TABLE 4.
Factors Favoring Association (+) or Dissociation (−) of Ag-Ab Complexes

Variable parameter	Affected Energy Component		
	ΔG^{LW}	ΔG^{AB}	ΔG^{EL}
Increase or decrease in pH[a]			—[a]
Increase in ionic strength		(+)	−
Admixture of strong electron-donor solvents (DMSO; EG; propanol)[a]	−	—[a]	
Admixture pf chaotropic agents (KCNS; Guanidine, HCl)		−	−
Increase in temperature		+ or −	−
Addition of strong electron-donors and/or dehydrating agents (polyethylene glycol; $(NH_4)_2SO_4$)[b]		+ +[b]	
Increase in time		+	+ +
Addition of cospecific haptens	−	—	—

[a] These two approaches generally are best used in combination with each other.
[b] Also tends to cause aspecific protein aggregation.

Source: van Oss et al. (1986a).

Temperature Effects

The effect of an increase in temperature is often so multifaceted as to make its outcome difficult to predict, and indeed it often may have no net effect at all [van Oss et al., 1986a; see also the Mukkur effect described above (Mukkur, 1984; van Oss et al., 1982)]. Decreasing the dielectric constant of the medium also may have ambiguous effects, depending on the proportion of interfacial and electrostatic forces in the complexes. If total dissociation is desired, it is advisable to allow as little time as possible to elapse after the initial association to minimize the formation of secondary bonds. Dissociation of an Ag from Ag-Ab complexes by replacing it with the corresponding hapten is quite effective, but of course this is only feasible in those rare cases where the appropriate hapten happens to be available (see Table 4).

It should be kept in mind that, other factors remaining equal, a small decrease in $\Delta G^{TOT}/kT$, due to an increase in temperature, can result in a considerable decrease in K_a [Eq. (12b)]. For instance, an increase from 20° to 50°C, for an initial value of ΔG^{TOT} of -16 kT (which then becomes reduced to -13.4 kT), results in a 13.5-fold decrease in K_a from 8.9×10^6 LM^{-1} to 6.6×10^5 LM^{-1}. In Ag-Ab reactions in particular, other factors do not remain equal when the temperature increases. With an increase in temperature, $|\Delta G^{TOT}|$ often remains relatively unchanged, or is only slightly decreased (see the Mukkur effect, described above), so that the effect of temperature on K_a is negligible. The principal mechanism at work here, in most cases, is the progressive disappearance of water of hydration from hydrophilic moieties in the vicinity of epitopic and paratopic sites. These hydrophilic moieties then become increasingly hydrophobic and thus more and more attract each other by hydrophobic (interfacial) interactions as the temperature increases. These hydrophobic (interfacial) interactions are preponderantly polar hydrogen-bonding interactions (van Oss and Good, 1988a). The decrease in oriented water of hydration (van Oss and Good, 1988b) with an increase in temperature, correlates with the relative increase in the entropic energy component reported by Mukkur (1984).

REFERENCES

Absolom, D. R., and van Oss, C. J. (1986) The nature of the antigen-antibody bond and the factors affecting its association and dissociation. *CRC Crit. Rev. Immunol.* 6:1—46.

Amit, A. G., Mariussa, R. A., Phillips, S. E. V., and Poljak, R. J. (1986) Three dimensional structure of an antigen-antibody complex at 2.8 Å resolution. *Science* 233:747—753.

Atassi, M. Z. (1984) Immune recognition of proteins. In *Molecular Immunology.* (M. Z. Atassi, C. J. van Oss, and D. R. Absolom, eds.), Marcel Dekker, NY, 15—51.

Bankert, R. B., Mazzaferro, D., and Mayers, G. L. (1981) Hybridomas producing hemolytic plaques used to study the relationship between monoclonal antibody affinity and the efficiency of plaque inhibition with increasing concentrations of antigen. *Hybridoma* 1:47—58.

Borden, P., and Kabat, E. A. (1988) The specificities of polyclonal and monoclonal antiidiotypes to anti-α (1→6) dextrans; possible correlations of idiotype with amino acid sequence. *Mol. Immunol.* 25:251—262.

Chaudhury, M. K. (1984) Short range and long range forces in colloidal and macroscopic systems. Ph.D. Dissertation, SUNY, Buffalo, NY.

Christenson, H. K. (1988) Non-DLVO forces between surfaces–solvation, hydration and capillary effects. *J. Dispersion Sci. Technol.* 9:171—206.

Cunningham, R. K. (1984) In *Molecular Immunology.* (M. Z. Atassi, C. J. van Oss, and D. R. Absolom, eds.), Marcel Dekker, NY, 53—70.

de Groot, E. R., Lamers, M. C., Aarden, L. A., Smeenk, R. J. T., and van Oss, C. J. (1980) Dissociation of DNA/anti-DNA complexes at high pH. *Immunol. Commun.* 9:515—528.

Economidou, J., Hughes-Jones, N. C., and Gardner, B. (1967) The reactivity of subunits of IgM-Anti-B. *Immunology* 13:235—246.

Edberg, S. C., Bronson, P. M., and van Oss, C. J. (1972) The valency of IgM and IgG rabbit anti-dextran antibody as a function of the size of the dextran molecule. *Immunochemistry* 9:273—288.

Einstein, A. (1907) Theoretical observations on the Brownian motion. *Z. Elektrochem.* 13:41—42. [Reprinted in *Investigation on the Theory of the Brownian Movement.* Dover Publ., NY, 1955.]
Fowkes, F. M. (1987) Role of acid-base interfacial bonding in adhesion. *J. Adhesion Sci. Technol.* 1:7—27.
Froese, A. (1983) The immunoglobulin-binding receptors of rat mast-cells and rat basophilic leukemia cells. In *Structure and Function of Fc Receptors.* (A. Froese, and F. Paraskevas, eds.), Marcel Dekker, New York, 83—100.
Froese, A., and Sehon, A. C. (1975) Kinetics of antibody-hapten reactions. *Contemp. Topics Mol. Immunol.* 4:23—54.
Gabler, R. (1978) *Electrical Interactions in Molecular Biophysics.* Academic Press, New York, 245.
Getzoff, E. D., Tainer, J. A., and Lerner, R. A. (1988) The chemistry and mechanism of antibody-binding to protein antigens. *Adv. Immunol.* 43:1—98.
Green, F. A. (1982) Erythrocyte membrane phosphatidylcholine and Rh(D) antigen cryolatency. *Immunol. Commun.* 11:25—32.
Halk, E. L., Hsu, H. T., Aebig, J., and Franke, J. (1984) Production of monoclonal antibodies against three Ilarviruses and Alfalfa mosaic virus and their use in serotyping. *Phytopathology* 74:367—378.
Hunter, R. J. (1981) *Zeta Potential in Colloid Science.* Academic Press, New York.
Israelachvili, J. N. (1974) Van der Waals forces in biological systems. *Quart. Rev. Biophys.* 6:341—387.
Israelachvili, J. N. (1985) *Intermolecular and Surface Forces.* Academic Press, New York.
Israelachvili. J. N., and Pashley, R. M. (1984) Measurement of the hydrophobic interaction between two hydrophobic surfaces in aqueous electrolyte solutions. *J. Colloid Interface Sci.* 98:500—514.
Johnston, M. F. M., Barisas, B. G., and Sturtevant, T. M. (1974) Thermodynamics of hapten-binding to MOPC 315 and MOPC 460 mouse myeloma proteins. *Biochemistry* 13:390—396.
Kabat, E. A. (1976) *Structural Concepts on Immunology and Immunochemistry.* Holt, Rinehart & Winston, NY.
Kabat, E. A., and Mayer, M. M. (1961) *Experimental Immunochemistry.* C. C. Thomas, Springfield, IL, 26.
Karush, F. (1976) Multivalent binding and functional affinity. *Contemp. Topics Mol. Immunol.* 5:217—228.
Liberti, P. A. (1975) Incremental bonding site filling of anti-polypeptide antibodies. *Immunochemistry* 12:303—310.
Manavalan, P., and Ponnuswamy, P. K. (1978) Hydrophobic character of amino acid residues in globular proteins. *Nature (London)* 275:673—674.
Molinaro, G. A., Eby, W. C., Molinaro, C. A., Bartholemew, R. M., and David, G. (1984) Two monoclonal antibodies to two different epitopes of human growth hormone form a precipitin line when counter diffused as soluble immune complexes. *Mol. Immunol.* 21:771—774.
Mukkur, T. K. S. (1984) Thermodynamics of hapten-antibody interactions. *Brit. Rev. Biochem.* 16:133—167.
Napper, D. H. (1983) *Polymeric Stabilization of Colloidal Dispersions.* Academic Press, New York.

Nemethy, G., and Scheraga, H. A. (1962) The structure of water and hydrophobic bonding in proteins III. The thermodynamic properties of hydrophobic bonds in proteins. *J. Phys. Chem.* 66:1773—1789.

Novotny, J., Bruccoleri, R. E., and Saul, F. A. (1989) On the attribution of binding energy in antigen-antibody complexes McPC 603, DI_o3 and MyHEL-5. *Biochemistry* 28:4735—4749.

Overbeek, J. Th. G. (1952) The interaction between colloidal particles. In *Colloid Science*, Vol. I. (H. R. Kruyt, ed.), Elsevier, Amsterdam, 245—277.

Overbeek, J. Th. G., and Bijsterbosch, B. H. (1979) The electrical double layer and the theory of electrophoresis. In *Electrokinetic Separation Methods*. (P. G. Righetti, C. J. van Oss, and J. W. Vanderhoff, eds.), Elsevier, Amsterdam, 1—32.

Pecht, I. (1982) Dynamic aspects of antibody function. In *The Antigens*, Vol. 6. (M. Sela, ed.), Academic Press, New York, 1—68.

Pfeiffer, N. E., Wylie, D. E., and Schuster, S. M. (1987) Immunoaffinity chromatography utilizing monoclonal antibodies: factors which influence antigen-binding capacity. *J. Immunol. Meth.* 97:1—9.

Pressman, D., and Grossberg, A. L. (1973) *The Structural Basis of Antibody Specificity*. Benjamin, Reading, MA.

Prickett. K. S., Amberg, D. C., and Hopp, T. P. (1989) A calcium-dependent antibody for identification and purification of recombinant proteins. *Biotechniques* 7:580—589.

Smeenk, R. J. T., Aarden, L. A., and van Oss, C. J. (1982) Comparison between dissociation and inhibition of association of DNA/anti-DNA complexes. *Immunol. Commun.* 12:177—188.

Steane, E. A. (1974) Thermodynamic studies of erythrocyte antigen-antibody interaction and the modulation of this phenomenon for partial enzymatic digestion of the cell membrane. Ph.D. Dissertation. George Washington University, Washington, D.C.

Steward, M. W. (1974) *Immunochemistry* John Wiley & Sons, NY, 42—43.

Steward, M. W. (1977) Affinity of the antibody-antigen reaction and its biological significance. In *Immunochemistry*. (L. E. Glynn, and M. W. Steward, eds.), John Wiley & Sons, NY, 233—262.

Van de Ven, T. G. M. (1989) *Colloidal Hydrodynamics*. Academic Press, New York.

van Oss, C. J. (1981) The human immunoglobulins. In *Blood Banking*, Vol. II. (T. J. Greenwalt, and E. A. Steane, eds.), CRC Press, Boca Raton, FL, 181—193.

van Oss, C. J. (1984) Agglutination and precipitation. In *Molecular Immunology*. (M. Z. Atassi, C. J. van Oss, and D. R. Absolom, eds.), Marcel Dekker, NY, 361—379.

van Oss, C. J. (1990) Surface free energy contribution to cell interactions. In *Biophysics of the Cell Surface*. (R. Glaser, and D. Gingell, eds.), Berlin, NY, 131—152.

van Oss, C. J., and Absolom, D. R. (1984) Nature and thermodynamics of antigen-antibody interactions. In *Molecular Immunology*. (M. Z. Atassi, C. J. van Oss, and D. R. Absolom, eds.), Marcel Dekker, NY, 337—360.

van Oss, C. J., Absolom, D. R., and Bronson, P. M. (1982) Affinity diffusion. II. Comparison between thermodynamic data obtained by affinity diffusion and precipitation in tubes. *Immunol. Commun.* 11:139—148.

van Oss, C. J., Absolom, D. E., Grossberg, A. L., and Neumann, A. W. (1979) Repulsive van der Waals forces. I. complete dissociation of antigen-antibody complexes by means of negative van der Waals forces. *Immunol. Commun.* 8:11—29.

van Oss, C. J., Absolom, D. R., and Neumann, A. W. (1980) The antigen-antibody complex and erythrocyte destruction. In *Immunobiology of the Erythrocyte*. (S. G. Sandler, T. Nusbacher, and M. S. Schanfield, eds.), Alan R. Liss, NY, 157—169.

van Oss, C. J., Beckers, D., Engelfriet, C. P., Absolom, D. R., and Neumann, A. W. (1981) Elution of blood group antibodies from red cells. *Vox Sang.* 40:367—371.

van Oss, C. J., Chaudhury, M. K., and Good, R. J. (1987) Monopolar surfaces. *Adv. Colloid Interface Sci.* 28:35—64.

van Oss, C. J., Chaudhury, M. K., and Good, R. J. (1988) Interfacial Lifshitz-van der Waals and polar interactions in macroscopic systems. *Chem. Rev.* 88:927—941.

van Oss, C. J., Fike, R. M., Good, R. J., and Reinig, J. M. (1974) Cell microelectrophoresis simplified by the reduction and uniformization of the electroosmotic backflow. *Anal. Biochem.* 60:242—251.

van Oss, C. J., and Good, R. J. (1988a) On the mechanism of "hydrophobic" interactions. *J. Dispersion Sci. Technol.* 9:355—362.

van Oss, C. J., and Good, R. J. (1988b) Orientation of the water molecules of hydration of serum albumin. *J. Prot. Chem.* 7:179—183.

van Oss, C. J., Good, R. J., and Chaudhury, M. K. (1986a) Nature of the antigen-antibody interaction — Primary and secondary bonds: optimal conditions for association and dissociation. *J. Chromatog.* 376:111—119.

van Oss, C. J., Good, R. J., and Chaudhury, M. K. (1986b) The role of van der Waals forces and hydrogen bonds in "hydrophobic interactions" between biopolymers and low energy surfaces. *J. Colloid Interface Sci.* 111:378—390.

van Oss, C. J., Smeenk, R. J. T., and Aarden, L. A. (1985) Inhibition of association vs. dissociation of high-avidity DNA/anti-DNA complexes: possible involvement of secondary hydrogen bonds. *Immunol. Invest.* 14:245—253.

van Oss, C. J., and Walker, J. (1979) Concentration dependence of the binding constant of antibodies. *Mol. Immunol.* 24:715—717.

Van Regenmortel, M. H. V. (1982) *Serology and Immunochemistry of Plant Viruses*. Academic Press, New York, 204—205.

Van Regenmortel, M. H. V., and Hardie, G. (1979) Determination of avidity of antiviral antibodies at 50% binding of antibody. *J. Immunol. Meth.* 27:43—54.

Van Regenmortel, M. H. V., Muller, S., Quesniaux, V. F., Altschuh, D., and Briand, J. P. (1988) Operational aspects of epitope identification: structural features of proteins recognized by antibodies. In *Convocation on Immunology*, Vol. 10. (H. Kohler, and P. T. LoVerde, eds.), Longman, London, 113—122.

Visser, J. (1972) On Hamaker constants: a comparison between Hamaker constants and Lifshitz-van der Waals constants. *Adv. Colloid Interface Sci.* 3:331—363.

Westhof, E., Altschuh, D., Moras, D., Bloomer, A. C., Mondragon, A., Klug, A., and Van Regenmortel, M. H. V. (1984) Correlation between segmental mobility and the location of antigenic determinants in proteins. *Nature (London)* 311:123—126.

Chapter 7

Measurement of Antibody Affinity

Robert Karlsson
Pharmacia Biosensor AB
Uppsala, Sweden

Danièle Altschuh and Marc H. V. Van Regenmortel,
Institut de Biologie Moléculaire et Cellulaire
Strasbourg, France

INTRODUCTION

Studying the antigenicity of a protein consists, for the most part, in analyzing its ability to bind to specific antibody molecules. To extract maximum information from this analysis, it is necessary to study antibody binding in a quantitative manner. This means that the strength of this binding should be expressed in terms of the antibody affinity constant. For instance, when attempts are made to mimic protein epitopes by means of synthetic peptides, the best criterion to assess how closely the peptide matches the parent epitope is to measure the comparative binding affinity of an antibody capable of reacting both with the natural and synthetic structures. This type of quantitative information provides important guidelines to further improve the degree of mimicry achievable with synthetic peptides.

In general, changes in the affinity of the antibody can be used to detect alterations in structure or function in one of the two immunological reactants. Obvious applications are, for instance, the characterization of recombinant proteins and the control of protein purification schemes. The affinity of antibodies also determines their behavior in different types of immunoassays.

In order to predict the potential usefulness of monoclonal antibodies in a particular immunological test, it is therefore important to possess information on their relative affinities. Antibodies of higher affinity allow smaller amounts of an antigen to be detected (Stewart and Lew, 1985; Yolken, 1985). On the other hand, for the purification of antigens by affinity chromatography, it is preferable to use antibodies of moderate affinity that allow the antigen to be dissociated again after formation of the complex.

The interaction between antigen and antibody at equilibrium may be expressed as:

$$A + B \underset{k_d}{\overset{k_a}{\rightleftharpoons}} AB$$

where A represents free antigen, B free antibody, and AB the antigen-antibody complex when the rates of association, k_a, and dissociation, k_d, are equal. The equilibrium association constant may be calculated from:

$$K = k_a/k_d = \frac{[AB]}{[A][B]}$$

Although the equilibrium may also be defined from the dissociation of the complex ($K_{diss} = k_d/k_a$), the association equilibrium constant seems a simpler measure of antibody affinity since it increases in magnitude when the affinity is higher and a greater proportion of the antibody is bound.

BASIC EQUILIBRIUM EQUATIONS

Affinity is a thermodynamic expression of the primary interaction of a single epitope with a single paratope and, in principle, the concept should be used only for a monovalent antigen binding to a single Fab fragment. In the case of multivalent antigens and antibodies, the antibody-binding capacity should be expressed by the term *avidity,* which incorporates the role played by antigen and antibody valency in the observed interaction. The importance of the valency term in affinity measurements has been discussed by Underwood (1988).

A variety of symbols have been used to express the different parameters in affinity calculations. When the symbols used by Hardie and Van Regenmortel (1975) are employed, the equilibrium constant, K, of an antibody may be expressed in terms of the mass action law as follows:

$$K = \frac{sx}{(As - sx)(Bn - sx)} = \frac{ny}{(As - ny)(Bn - ny)} \quad (1)$$

where A = total antigen concentration (mol/L)
       s = antigen valence
       As = total antigen sites (mol sites/L)
       B = total antibody concentration (mol/L)
       n = antibody valence
       Bn = total antibody sites (mol sites/L)
       x = bound antigen concentration (mol/L)
       y = bound antibody concentration (mol/L)
       ny = sx = total bound sites

This equation is usually rearranged into forms suitable for the graphical representation of binding data, leading to the following expression:

$$r/c = K(n - sr) \quad (2)$$

where r = x/B = ny/sB : ratio of bound antigen to total antibody
       c = $A - x$ = free antigen concentration

and

$$f/d = K(s - nf) \quad (3)$$

where f = $y/A = \dfrac{sx}{nA}$: ratio of bound antibody to total antigen
       d = $B - y$ = free antibody concentration

Both equations can be used to construct what are commonly known as Scatchard plots (Day, 1990).

A plot of r/c vs sr gives the value of K as the slope and the value of n by extrapolation to the abscissa. When the antigen is monovalent ($s = 1$) there is no ambiguity in the extrapolated value of n. However, it is often found that a certain proportion of the antibody used in the binding test has been denatured during purification, in which case the r/c vs r plot does not extrapolate to $n = 1$ but to a lower value. In this case, it is possible to calculate the concentration of functionally active antibody B_{corr} from the relation:

$$B_{corr} = B_{total} - B_{total}(n - n_1)n$$

where n_1 is the extrapolated value found in the r/c vs r plot and n is the theoretical value. Once this corrected value of B has been obtained, the various parameters necessary for obtaining K can be recalculated.

In the case of large multivalent antigens, it is not possible to measure experimentally the quantity c (or x) since only some of the epitopes of the antigen molecule are likely to be free, while others are in the bound state. So-called "bound" antigen molecules may in fact possess between 0 and $s - 1$ free epitopes. For this reason, it is the concentration of free antibody

d that is measured experimentally after free and bound antibody have been separated by such procedures as ultrafiltration, centrifugation, or simple washing, when the multivalent antigen is immobilized in a solid-phase assay. The value of d is then used to calculate y and f.

A plot of f/d vs nf gives the value of K as the slope and the antigen valence s by extrapolation to the abscissa (Day, 1990; Hardie and Van Regenmortel, 1975). At any ratio of the reactants, the antigenic valency of a large, multivalent antigen corresponds to the maximum number of antibody molecules that can be bound simultaneously (Van Regenmortel, 1988).

When the experimental protocol consists in measuring free antibody instead of free antigen, it is nevertheless possible to represent the data by means of Eq. (2). After deriving the value of the antigen valence from a plot of Eq. (3) and since $ny = sx$, it is possible to calculate $r = ny/sB$ and to construct r/c vs sr plots (Hardie and Van Regenmortel, 1975).

In the case of bivalent antibody molecules, plots of f/d vs nf are often biphasic corresponding to regions where the antibody binds in a monovalent and bivalent manner, respectively (Van Regenmortel and Hardie, 1976). Near antibody saturation, the molecules bind monovalently and the slope of the plot gives a K value that is considerably smaller than in the region of antigen excess when the same antibody binds bivalently. When binding to virus particles or cell surfaces presenting a large number of identical epitopes, the two Fab arms of an IgG molecule bind to neighboring epitopes, a situation known as monogamous bivalent binding characterized by a high functional avidity.

Two f/d vs f plots representing binding data between tobacco mosaic virus particles and specific rabbit IgG and monovalent Fab fragments, respectively, are illustrated in Fig. 1. The binding data used to construct these plots were obtained as follows. A series of dilutions of a virus preparation (1 ml) were mixed with a constant concentration of specific antibody. After ultracentrifugation, the amount of free antibody (d) in the supernatant was determined and the amount of bound antibody was calculated from $y = B - d$. The plots obtained with different concentrations of Fab extrapolate to $s = 800$, which is the antigen valence of the virus. The plots obtained with IgG extrapolate to $s = 780$ (Fig. 1). The similarity in the two s values indicates that in antibody excess the IgG molecules bind univalently. The biphasic nature of the plot in Fig. 1A indicates that bivalent binding of IgG ($n = 2$) occurs at lower antibody-antigen ratios when $f < 400$. The higher slope in this part of the plot corresponds to the higher avidity of the antibodies when they bind in a bivalent manner (Day, 1990; Van Regenmortel, 1982). This interpretation of the biphasic plot is supported by the data shown in Fig. 2, which indicates that small successive additions of antibody to a given amount of virus results in the binding of fewer antibody molecules per virus particle than a single addition of the total amount of antibody. Adding small amounts of antibody to the virus favors bivalent binding which doubles the number of antigenic sites covered without increasing the number of antibody molecules

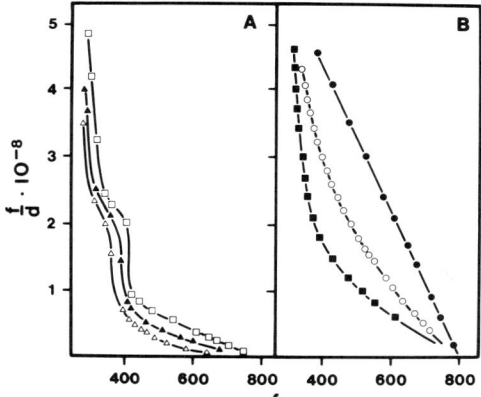

Figure 1. Determination of the avidity of tobacco mosaic virus (TMV) antibodies. (A) Plots of f/d vs f representing the interaction between TMV and specific IgG used at 6 mg/ml (□), 1.8 mg/ml (▲), and 0.6 mg/ml (△). The curves extrapolate to the antigenic valence of TMV, $s = 780$. (B) Plots of f/d vs f representing the interaction between TMV and specific Fab fragments used at 1.9 mg/ml (●), 1.18 mg/ml (○), and 0.6 mg/ml (■). The antigenic valence is $s = 800$. (From Van Regenmortel, M. H. V., *Serology and Immunochemistry of Plant Viruses*, Academic Press, New York, 1982. With permission.)

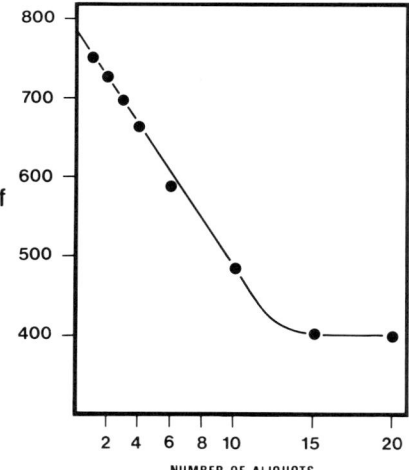

Figure 2. Variation in f observed when the same total quantity of specific IgG antibody (3.6 mg) is added to 1 mg TMV but in different aliquots. With small successive additions of IgG, the plot extrapolates to $f = 400$. Assuming monogamous bivalent binding of IgG, this corresponds to an antigenic valence of TMV of $s = 800$. When all the antibody is added at once, the antigenic valence of TMV obtained by extrapolation on the y-axis is $s = 780$. (From Van Regenmortel, M. H. V., *Serology and Immunochemistry of Plant Viruses*, Academic Press, New York, 1982. With permission.)

TABLE 1.
Calculation of Antibody Affinity Constant, K, and of Total Antigenic Sites, As, from Binding Data Obtained in Solid-Phase Immunoassay and Presented According to Eqs. (6-11)

Equation	4	5	6	7	8	9
Slope	$-K$	$-1/K$	$1/K\,As$	$K\,As$	As	$1/As$
Abscissa at origin	As	$K\,As$	$-K$	$1/As$	$1/K\,As$	$-1/K$
Ordinate at origin	$K\,As$	As	$1/As$	$-K$	$-1/K$	$1/K\,As$

Equation	10	11	12	13	14	15
Slope	$-K$	$-1/K$	$1/K\,Bn$	$K\,Bn$	Bn	$1/Bn$
Abscissa at origin	Bn	$K\,Bn$	$-K$	$1/Bn$	$1/K\,Bn$	$-1/K$
Ordinate at origin	$K\,Bn$	Bn	$1/Bn$	$-K$	$-1/K$	$1/K\,Bn$

bound. In this case, the antigen valence is obtained by multiplying the limiting value of f by 2, which again leads to $s = 800$.

When in a binding test the antigen concentration is kept constant while the antibody concentration is varied and the amount of free antibody is determined experimentally. It is possible to represent the binding data by the following transformations of the mass action relationship (Fazekas de St. Groth, 1979):

$$\frac{ny}{nd} = K\,(As - ny) \tag{4}$$

$$ny = -\frac{1}{K}\frac{ny}{nd} + As \tag{5}$$

$$\frac{1}{ny} = \frac{1}{KAs}\frac{1}{nd} + \frac{1}{As} \tag{6}$$

$$\frac{1}{nd} = KAs\frac{1}{ny} - K \tag{7}$$

$$nd = As\frac{nd}{ny} - \frac{1}{K} \tag{8}$$

$$\frac{nd}{ny} = \frac{1}{As}\,(nd) + \frac{1}{KAs} \tag{9}$$

These various representations make it possible to calculate K and As by extrapolation or from the slope of the plot as indicated in Table 1. Plots of such calculations for binding data obtained in a solid-phase immunoassay have been presented by Azimzadeh and Van Regenmortel (1990).

When in a binding test the antibody concentration is kept constant while the antigen concentration is varied and the amount of free antigen is determined experimentally. The data can be represented as follows:

$$\frac{sx}{sc} = K(Bn - sx) \tag{10}$$

$$sx = \frac{1}{K}\frac{x}{c} + Bn \tag{11}$$

$$\frac{1}{sx} = \frac{1}{KBn}\frac{1}{sc} + \frac{1}{Bn} \tag{12}$$

$$\frac{1}{sc} = KBn\frac{1}{sx} - K \tag{13}$$

$$sc = Bn\frac{sc}{sx} - \frac{1}{K} \tag{14}$$

$$\frac{sc}{sx} = \frac{1}{Bn}sc + \frac{1}{KBn} \tag{15}$$

These representations make it possible to calculate K and Bn as indicated in Table 1.

EXPERIMENTAL METHODS TO MEASURE THE EQUILIBRIUM CONSTANT

Solution-Phase Assays

In order to determine K of an antibody directed to a small monovalent antigen, it is customary to measure experimentally the concentration of free antigen c after having separated the small antigen from the larger antigen-antibody complexes, for instance, by equilibrium dialysis (Eisen, 1964; Pascual and Clem, 1988). The results are plotted according to Eq. (2).

In the case of large multivalent antigens, it is the concentration of free antibody d that is measured instead, after free and bound antibody have been separated by procedures such as ultrafiltration (Fazekas de St. Groth and Webster, 1961) or ultracentrifugation (Day, 1990). The binding data (Fig. 1) are then usually plotted according to Eq. (3).

Many procedures have been developed to separate free, labeled antigen molecules from bound complexes. Antibody can be precipitated with 50% ammonium sulfate (Kim et al., 1975), with 15% polyethylene glycol (Hetherington, 1988) or by binding to protein A (Brunda et al., 1977) or to antiimmunoglobulin antibody (Glass et al., 1973). When the antibody is biotinylated, it can be precipitated by the addition of avidin (Clark and Todd, 1982). It is also possible to remove the antigen from solution, for instance, by adsorption to charcoal (Collignon et al., 1988) or precipitation with avidin (Krüger et al., 1989).

Solid-Phase Assays

In one type of assay, a constant amount of antigen is adsorbed to the plastic surface of microtiter plates and varying amounts of antibody are added to the wells. After removing free antibody by washing, the amount of bound antibody can be measured experimentally by a variety of procedures. The binding data can be represented according to Eqs. (4) to (9). Examples of such calculations based on the experimental data of Schots et al. (1988) have been presented by Azimzadeh and Van Regenmortel (1990). The most even distribution of points and most reliable estimates of As and K were obtained from the plots of Eqs. (4) and (5), which are inverse functions of each other. Many authors use such a type of assay format in which antigen is directly adsorbed to the solid phase. Since proteins usually undergo some denaturation when they are adsorbed to plastic (Darst et al., 1988; Friguet et al., 1984; Soderquist and Walton, 1980), it is questionable whether the value of K that is measured in this way pertains to the interaction with an epitope in its native state. For this reason it is preferable to capture the antigen on the plastic by a first layer of adsorbed antibodies and to measure K by a double-antibody sandwich assay format.

Friguet et al. (1985) developed a method which uses a solid-phase assay for measuring the amount of free antibody present at equilibrium in a solution-phase antigen-antibody reaction mixture. The solution-phase mixture is incubated in antigen-coated wells, using conditions where only about 10% of the free antibody is captured. This ensures that the equilibrium is not disturbed. The proportion of free antibody is calculated from the difference in absorbance measured in the presence and absence of antigen, read from the linear portion of a calibration plot of absorbance vs antibody concentration. The method of Friguet et al. (1985) offers several advantages over other procedures. It requires no labeling of antigen or antibody and thus avoids the changes in immunoreactivity that often accompany labeling. It requires very small quantities of reagents and measures K in solution-phase equilibrium conditions. It thus avoids the ambiguities linked to measuring antibody affinity for an antigen that has been altered by adsorption to a solid phase. As pointed out by Stevens (1987), only double-liganded IgG will be scored as bound when it is assayed on the solid-phase antigen. However, at very high saturation of antibody by antigen, this type of error will be minimized (Friguet et al., 1989).

Immunoassay Using One Immobilized Reactant (BIAcore™ System)

In this type of assay, the molecules of one of the reactants are immobilized, for instance, on a dextran matrix without altering their conformation, as normally occurs when they are adsorbed on a solid phase. In one particular format of this assay, BIAcore™, a Biosensor system based on surface plasmon resonance (SPR) detection (Kretschmann and Raether, 1968), developed by Pharmacia Biosensor AB, Uppsala, has been used to monitor the reaction between antigen and antibody. SPR detects changes in refractive index close to a metal surface which allows the concentration of the reactants to be measured. One of the reactants is immobilized on a dextran matrix coupled to a thin gold film, and the other is introduced in a flow passing over the sensor surface (Löfas and Johnsson, 1990). The flow system is miniaturized to provide efficient mass transport (Eddowes, 1989). The dextran matrix extends out from the sensor surface and is easily derivatized, allowing proteins to be immobilized through amine groups. The interacting components do not need to be labeled and may be analyzed in complex samples, without prior purification. The reaction between immobilized ligand and injected analyte takes place in the hydrophilic environment defined by the dextran matrix and can be analyzed in real time. The reaction is monitored continuously and the binding curve is directly visualized on a computer screen. The integration of SPR detection, a microfluidic system, and operator-designed sensor surface into a single automated analytical system, allows the quantitative analysis of antigen-antibody interaction (Fägerstam, 1990).

The refractive index changes which are monitored continuously over time are presented in a sensorgram. The y-axis of the sensorgram corresponds to the resonance signal and is measured in resonance units (RU). The running buffer defines the baseline, and all responses are expressed relative to this level. At a given time the relative response, R, can be expressed as

$$R = R_R + R_A + R_L$$

where R_R reflects the composition of the buffer or the sample
R_A corresponds to amount of analyte bound to immobilized ligand
R_L corresponds to amount of immobilized ligand

The change in signal level with respect to time is

$$dR/dt = dR_R/dt + dR_A/dt + dR_L/dt$$

Except for the 10 to 20 s in the beginning and at the end of an injection, where running buffer is exchanged for samples and vice versa, $dR_R/dt = 0$. For covalently or biospecifically immobilized ligands, dR_L/dt is in most cases zero or close to zero and it is always measurable.

The software in the system automatically calculates R and the time derivative dR/dt, making key data for calculation of rate constants and affinity constants immediately available.

Mass Transport in BIAcore Instrument

For a reaction to occur, the analyte present in the flow stream must first be transported down into the matrix. The observed initial binding rate can be limited either by mass transport or by the intrinsic reaction rate. In a system with defined flow-cell geometry, the flow dependency of the transport of analyte down to the surface is given by (Matsuda, 1967)

$$J = kCD^{2/3}u^{1/3}$$

J = flow of analyte to the surface
C = concentration of analyte
k = a constant determined by the dimensions of the flow cell
D = diffusion coefficient
u = flow rate over the surface

The observed binding rate dx/dt can initially be limited by the transport of analyte down to the surface. As the reaction proceeds, the observed binding rate will soon reflect the intrinsic reaction rate, and finally a steady state or equilibrium binding will be reached. In order to swiftly shift the balance from mass transport to reaction rate limitation, mass transport should be as high as possible and the binding rate due to the reaction as low as possible. Mass transport can be increased using a higher flow rate but this leads to increased sample consumption and is not very practical. Instead the concentration of immobilized ligand should be kept as low as possible but still compatible with a reliably measurable response. In BIAcore™ an immobilization level of 5 to 20 × 10^{-15} mol/mm² is recommended.

Measurement of Equilibrium Constant

When used to measure the amount of free reactant present in an equilibrium mixture of antigen and antibody, the BIAcore™ instrument provides a sensorgram of the type shown in Fig. 3. This illustrates the analysis of free core protein p24 of human immunodeficiency virus (HIV) in a binding assay with immobilized monoclonal antibodies. This approach can be used only for analyzing the reaction between a monomeric protein and a monoclonal antibody binding a single site of the antigen. Blocking antibody was used to saturate the rabbit antimouse (RAMFc) surface. When the equilibrium mixture is injected, complexed antigen cannot bind since both the epitope and the RAMFc are blocked. Only free antigen can bind, and a comparison with antigen standards allows its concentration to be determined.

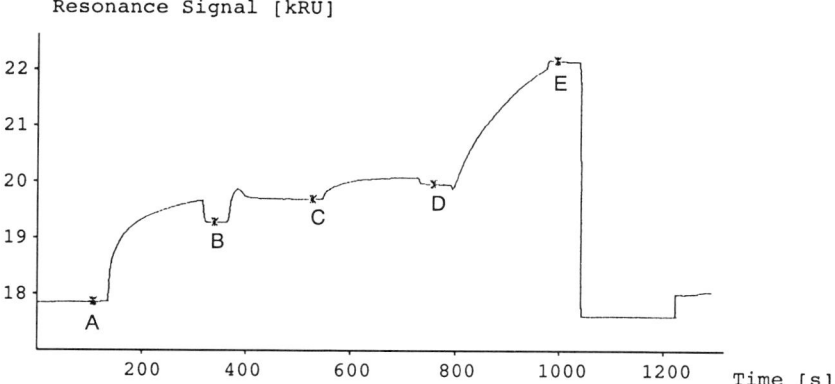

Figure 3. Determination of free antigen in BIAcore instrument. Rabbit antimouse globulin (RAMFc) is immobilized on the sensor surface and p24 antigen is determined using a sandwich assay (see text). MAb is injected (A), followed by blocking antibody (B), antigen (standard or equilibrium mixture) (C), and the secondary antibody rabbit anti-p24 serum diluted 1:300 is injected (D). The surface is then regenerated with 100 mM HCl (E).

The sensitivity of the analysis depends on the interaction time between captured antibody and antigen in solution and also on the availability of a secondary antibody which is used in the final step of the analysis. Normally concentrations as low as 50 to 100 pM can be determined in 15 min. When 15 p24 antibodies were analyzed for affinity in this way, affinities ranged from $5 \times 10^6 \, M^{-1}$ to $1 \times 10^{11} \, M^{-1}$. Values in the interval 10^6 to $10^{10} \, M^{-1}$ were obtained by analyzing the data according to Eq. (10). It is also possible to measure free antibody in analogy with the Friguet method. In this case, antigen is immobilized, the equilibrium solution is injected, and if necessary the responses amplified by the injection of rabbit antimouse antibody.

KINETIC MEASUREMENTS

Compared to the many techniques available for measuring antibody affinity at equilibrium, there are relatively few methods for measuring the kinetic rate constants of antigen-antibody interaction. Methods that detect changes in physical parameters like fluorescence (Dandliker and Levison, 1967) or absorption (Froese, 1968) in one of the reacting species can be employed for direct kinetic analysis using native molecules.

Surface-sensitive techniques can be used to continuously monitor the reaction when analyte binds to immobilized or adsorbed ligand, and potentially several of these techniques can be used for quantitative kinetic analysis. For instance, optical techniques such as ellipsometry and SPR have already been used to monitor protein-protein interactions (Cullen et al., 1987; Jönsson et al., 1985; Mayo and Hallock, 1989), and antibody- or antigen-coated piezoelectric quartz crystals have been used as transducers in a number of applications, e.g., to measure pesticides (Ngeh-Ngwaininbi et al., 1986) and microorganisms (Muramatsu, 1986). For these techniques it is important that a maximum number of immobilized ligands are active and surface chemistry becomes important.

Kinetic information can also be obtained when it is possible to quickly separate bound from free reactants (Johnstone et al., 1990; Mason and Williams, 1986; Skubitz and Smith, 1975). In this case, the antigen or antibody is often labeled with a radioactive or fluorescent probe and native molecules are no longer studied. According to a single one-step mechanism, the equilibrium association constant K should be equal to the ratio of the k_a and k_d rate constants. If a more complex molecular mechanism of antigen-antibody recognition, involving for instance conformational adaptation, is taking place, there will be a significant difference between the equilibrium constant and the ratio of the rate constants (Friguet et al., 1989).

The overall binding rate due to the reaction between matrix immobilized antibody and antigen in solution is given by:

$$\frac{dsx}{dt} = k_a (Bn - sx)(As - sx) - k_d sx \tag{16}$$

When the antigen is immobilized, the relation is:

$$\frac{dny}{dt} = k_a (As - ny)(Bn - ny) - k_d ny \tag{17}$$

Kinetic Measurements with the BIAcore System

In Eqs. (16) and (17), $(As - sx)$ and $(Bn - ny)$ are constant, because the BIAcore™ cell is continuously replenished with a constant concentration of free antigen or antibody sites. When antibody is immobilized, n is not needed since Bn is determined indirectly by the maximum number of antigen molecules that can be bound to the surface, therefore $Bn = sx_{max}$. When antibodies are monoclonal and antigens monomeric, the antigen valence will be $s = 1$. When antigen is immobilized, antibody valence must be known both for interpreting the slope value of dy/dt vs y curves and for determining the total antigen binding sites As. This is because As is determined indirectly by the maximum amount of antibody that can be bound to the surface. If y_{max} is the maximum amount of antibody that can be bound to the surface, then the total number of antigen binding sites is $As = ny_{max}$.

Since $As - sx = sc$ and $Bn - ny = nd$, Eqs. (16) and (17) can be rearranged to give:

$$\frac{dx}{dt} = k_a \, sc \, x_{max} - (k_a sc + k_d) \, x \qquad (18)$$

$$\frac{dy}{dt} = k_a \, nd \, y_{max} - (k_a nd + k_d) \, y \qquad (19)$$

When the reaction is studied at several concentrations of antigen, the slope value of each dx/dt vs x plot can be used to construct a new plot of slope values vs concentration of antigen-binding sites:

$$\text{Slope} = k_a \, sc + k_d \qquad (20)$$

or when the reaction is studied at several concentrations of antibody:

$$\text{Slope} = k_a \, nd + k_d \qquad (21)$$

From this plot, the values of k_a and k_d are readily determined.

Under equilibrium conditions, $(dsx/dt = 0$ or $dny/dt = 0)$, Eqs. (16) and (17) can be expressed in terms of Eqs. (10) and (4).

When BIAcore is used, Eq. (18) can be expressed in terms of the relative response:

$$\frac{dR}{dt} = \text{Constant} - (k_a \, c + k_d) \, (R_A) \qquad (22)$$

and Eq. (10) can be expressed as:

$$\frac{R_A}{c} = KR_{max} - KR_A \qquad (23)$$

where $R_{max} = x_{max}$

Experimental Determination of Antibody Valence

A peptide antigen (residues 110 to 135 of tobacco mosaic virus protein) was immobilized on a BIAcore™ sensor chip. The maximum amount of a monoclonal antibody or its Fab, able to bind to the surface, was determined. If antibody binding is monovalent, then the ratio of units IgG per units Fab bound should be 3 (IgG:MW = 150,000; Fab:MW = 50,000). If bivalent binding occurs, then this ratio at maximum binding should be 1.5. Figure 4 shows the relative response at steady state vs IgG or Fab concentration in the flow. When comparing the maximum amount of IgG or Fab that can be bound to the surface, the ratio of units IgG per units Fab bound is found to be 1.5. Van Regenmortel and Hardie (1976) have shown that small successive additions of antibody to a multivalent antigen like tobacco mosaic virus lead to

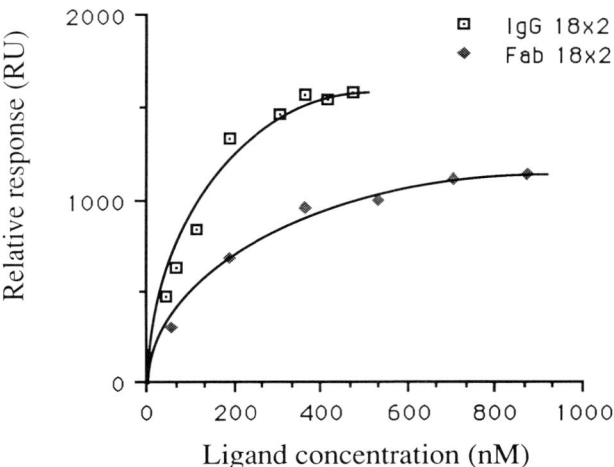

Figure 4. Comparison of the maximum amount of IgG or its corresponding Fab that can be bound to the same peptide on the sensor surface; 327 units (RU) of peptide 110 to 135 of tobacco mosaic virus proteins were immobilized. Various molar concentrations of antibody and Fab were added at a flow rate of 3 µl/min. Bound units were read after 5 min. The ratio of units IgG/Fab bounds is 1.5 (1509/1071 RU), indicating bivalent binding of IgG.

bivalent binding, whereas addition of the same amount of antibody in a single step results in monovalent binding (Fig. 2). In a kinetic experiment, the antibody is indeed added step by step in very small amounts compared to the immobilized antigen, and this explains the observed bivalent binding.

Results of Kinetic Measurements with p24 Protein

In this section, the determination of k_a and k_d of monoclonal antibodies against recombinant HIV-1 core protein p24 will be described. The BIAcore™ system (Pharmacia Biosensor AB, Uppsala, Sweden) was used for these measurements.

To aid experimental design, Eq. (18) was integrated and interaction curves were simulated. In one example, illustrated in Fig. 5, values of rate constants and x_{max} were assumed. From this figure it is clear that antigen concentrations in the interval 10 to 100 nM are suitable for kinetic analysis.

Immobilization. Immobilization of rabbit antimouse (RAM) results in sensor chips with 7000 to 8000 RU of immobilized antibody. When various hybridoma culture media were used as MAb source, the amount of bound MAb varied from 514 to 1568 RU. When the same MAb is injected repeatedly, the amount of captured MAb is reproducible within a few percent. This means that the sensor surface can be regenerated and reused without loss of antibody-binding capacity.

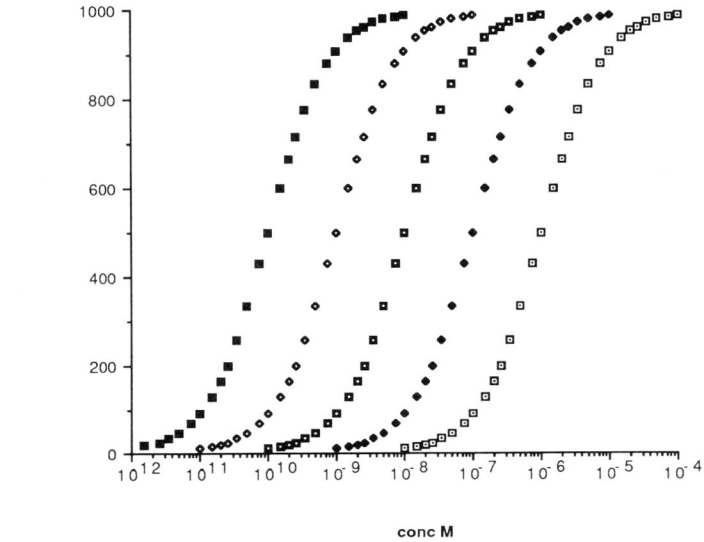
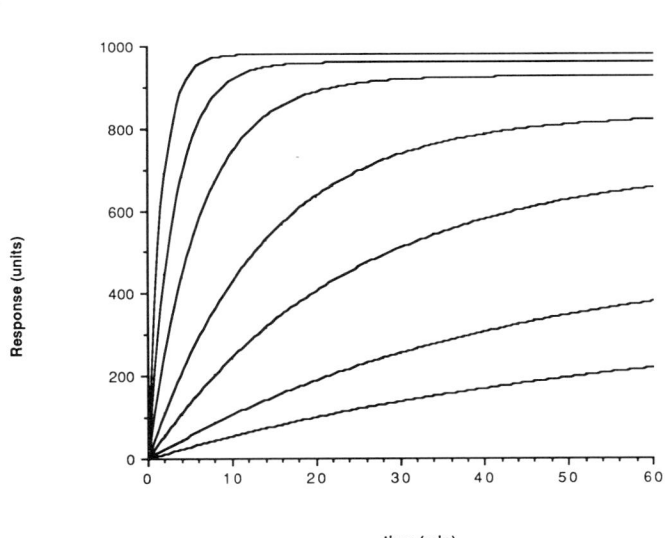

Figure 5. Simulation plots of antigen-antibody interaction on BIAcore sensor surface. In (A), steady-state values for different concentrations and affinities are illustrated; x_{max} is assumed to be 1000 units and the curves from right to left represent affinities of 10^6, 10^7, 10^8, 10^9, 10^{10} M^{-1}, respectively. In (B), calculated interaction curves, response vs time, are presented. K is assumed to be 5×10^8 M^{-1}, k_a 1×10^5 M^{-1} s^{-1} and x_{max} 1000 units. Curves from top to bottom represent antigen concentrations 100, 50, 25, 10, 5, 2, and 1 nM respectively.

Matrix Affinity and Kinetics. The experimental procedure is illustrated in Fig. 6. First anti-p24 antibody is injected and binds to covalently immobilized RAMFc; p24 is injected between report points B and C. At C the antigen injection is ended and the dissociation of bound antigen in continuous buffer flow is monitored. The interaction cycle is completed with an injection of 100 mM HCl which elutes the MAb-Ag complex and restores the RAMFc surface.

The kinetic data were evaluated as shown in Fig. 7. First, p24 at different concentrations was injected over matrix bound MAb (Fig. 7A). When each interaction curve was analyzed in a binding rate vs signal-response plot (Fig. 7B), a set of curves was obtained. Next, the slopes of these curves were plotted vs antigen concentration (Fig. 7C) and analyzed according to Eq. (20). Rate constants were evaluated from the first minutes of interaction and no correction for dissociation of MAb from RAMFc was judged necessary. (The dissociation rate of MAb was approximately 0.05 RU/s.) Values on association and dissociation rate constants were obtained as slope and intercept of the new curve. When a number of MAbs raised against p24 were analyzed in this fashion, association rate constants ranged from 3×10^4 to 7.3×10^5 $M^{-1} s^{-1}$. In many cases where the response was very stable, indicating a low value on the dissociation rate constant, the intercept obtained from Eq. (20) was negative and no meaningful value on this constant was obtained.

Steady-State Binding and Affinity. Affinity data for some anti-p24 MAbs are presented in Fig. 8. These data were obtained from an interaction time of 12 min and calculated from steady-state responses according to Eq. (23). It is clear that affinities as high as $2 \times 10^8 M^{-1}$ can be quantified in a very short time. To obtain reliable values on affinity constant concentrations leading to steady state, values ranging from 20 to 80% of the saturation response should preferably be used. For high-affinity systems, low concentrations are needed to obtain steady-state values in this region of the saturation curve and interaction times up to 1 hour or more have to be considered.

In many cases a qualitative comparison of reagents is of prime interest. Information relating to affinity and kinetics is rapidly obtained by comparing interaction curves. In Fig. 9, four anti-p24 MAbs have been bound to RAMFc and a 50 nM solution of p24 is injected. Binding curves that reach steady state can be used to compare affinity. The higher the steady-state level, the higher the affinity. Accordingly MAb 18 has higher affinity for the antigen than MAb 25 and MAb 28. Furthermore, MAb 18 reacts faster than the other MAbs, and MAb 1 shows the slowest reaction. Since all MAbs are compared using the same antigen concentration this means that MAb 1 has a lower association rate constant than MAb 18.

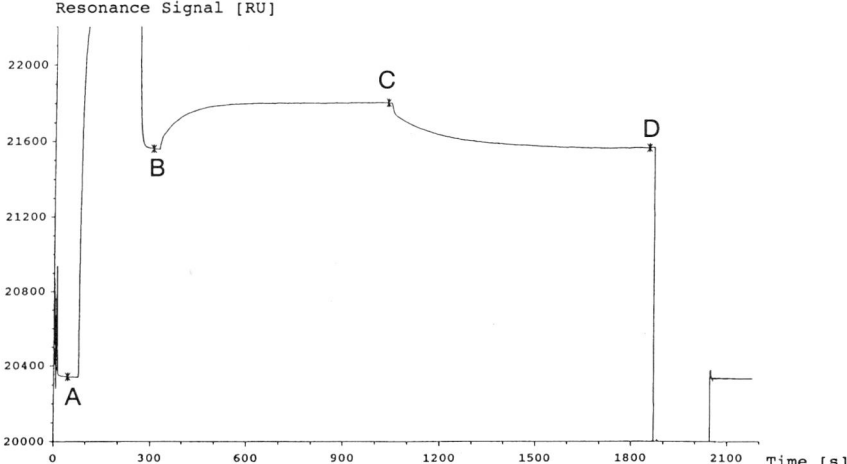

Figure 6. Kinetic analysis of p24-MAb interaction. RAMFc is immobilized on the sensor surface. At (A), MAb in culture media is injected. The refraction index of the injected MAb solution differs from the running buffer (10 mM HEPES with 0.15 M NaCl, 3.4 mM EDTA, and 0.005% Tween 20 at pH 7.4), but when the injection stops, the signal level is stabilized at a level corresponding to bound MAb. At (B), 36 µl of a 50 nM solution of p24 in running buffer is injected, and at (C), the p24 injection is terminated. Running buffer is introduced and flows over the sensor surface. At (D), 100 mM HCl is injected to regenerate the surface.

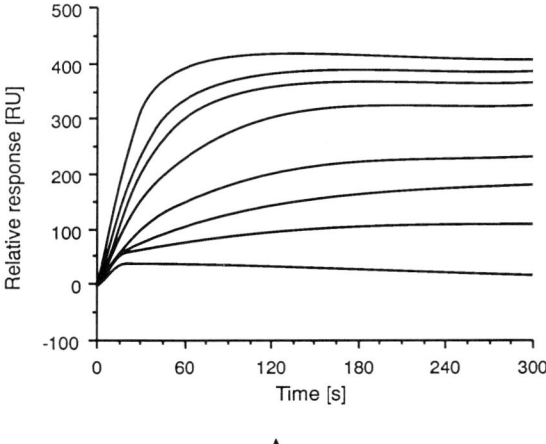

A

Figure 7. (A) Binding of p24 to matrix bound MAb 28. Curves from top to bottom correspond to injection of 300, 200, 150, 100, 50, 25, 12.5, and 0.0 nM p24 in HBS. The flow rate was 3 µl/min. (B) Evaluation of interaction curves. Plots of binding rate vs relative response. (C) Analysis of rate constants in slope value vs p24 concentration plot. From the slope of the curve, $k_{ass} = 1.4 \times 10^5$ M^{-1} s^{-1} and from the intercept with the y-axis, $K_{diss} = 7.9 \times 10^{-3}$ s^{-1}.

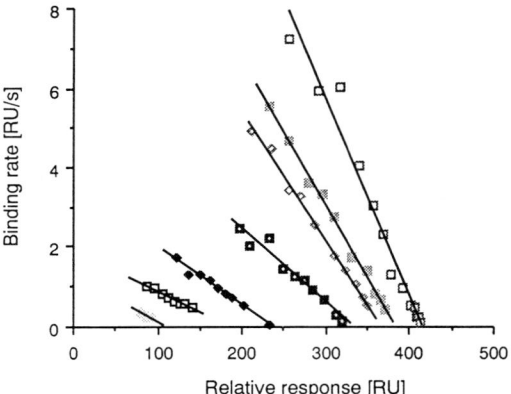

Figure 7B.

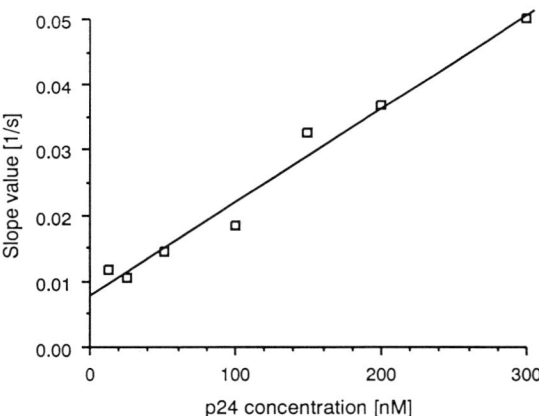

Figure 7C.

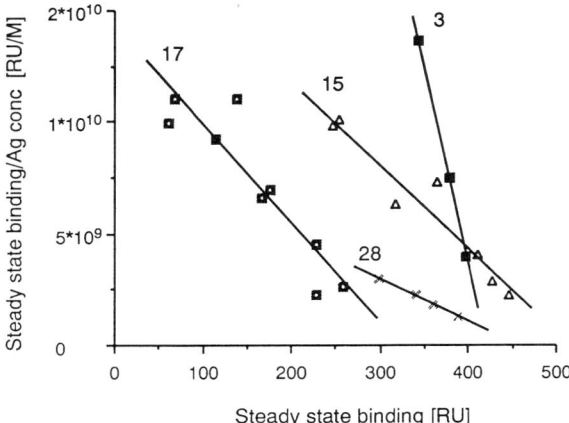

Figure 8. Plot of steady-state data R_A/C vs R_A, for determination of affinity; p24 at various concentrations were injected at 3 μl/min and allowed to interact with matrix bound MAb for 12 min. Values for K obtained from the slope of the curves are: $1.8 \times 10^8\ M^{-1}$, $4.4 \times 10^7\ M^{-1}$, $3.8 \times 10^7\ M^{-1}$, and $1.8 \times 10^7\ M^{-1}$ for MAbs 3, 17, 15, and 28, respectively.

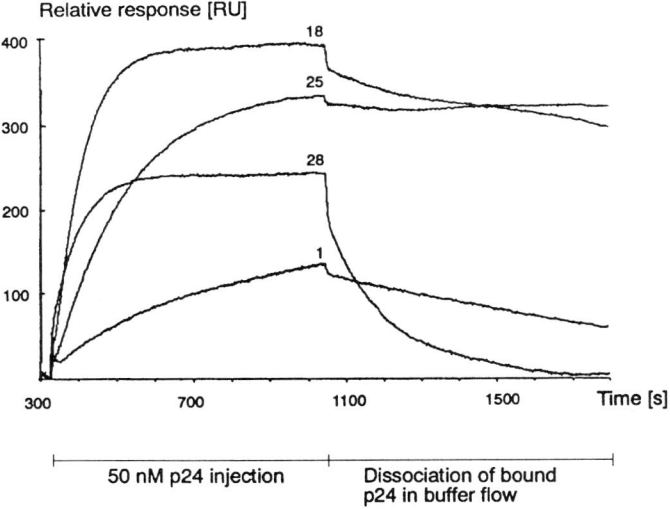

Figure 9. Comparison of interaction curves. Different MAbs are bound to RAMFc and p24 nM concentration is injected. MAbs are identified with number at the point of the interaction curves where p24 injection stops and is replaced by buffer flow.

REFERENCES

Azimzadeh, A., and Van Regenmortel, M. H. V. (1990) Antibody affinity measurements. *J. Mol. Recognition* 3:108—116.

Brunda, M. J., Minden, P., Sharpton, T. R., McClatchy, J. K., and Farr, R. S. (1977) Precipitation of radiolabelled antigen-antibody complexes with protein-A containing *Staphylococcus aureus*. *J. Immunol.* 119:193—198.

Clark, B. R., and Todd, C. W. (1982) Avidin as a precipitant for biotin-labeled antibody in a radioimmunoassay for carcinoembryonic antigen. *Anal. Biochem.* 121:257—262.

Collignon, A., Geniteau-Legendre, M., Sandre, C., Quero, A. M., and Labarre, C. (1988) Specific binding characteristics of high affinity monoclonal antidigitoxin antibodies. *Hybridoma* 7:355—366.

Cullen, D. C., Brown, R. G. W., and Lowe, C. R. (1987) Detection of immunocomplex formation via surface plasmon resonance on gold coated diffraction gratings. *Biosensors* 3:211—225.

Dandliker, W. B., and Levison, S. A. (1967) Investigation of antigen-antibody kinetics by fluorescence polarization. *Immunochemistry* 5:171—183.

Darst, S. A., Robertson, C. R., and Berzofsky, J. A. (1988) Adsorption of the protein antigen myoglobin affects the binding of conformation-specific monoclonal antibodies. *Biophys. J.* 53:533—539.

Day, E. (1990) *Advanced Immunochemistry*, 2nd ed., Wiley-Liss, NY, 693.

Eddowes, M. J. (1989) Immunosensors based upon direct measurement of surface binding: fundamental chemical limitations. *Anal. Proc.* 26:152—154.

Eisen, H. N. (1964) Equilibrium dialysis for measurement of antibody-hapten affinities. In *Methods in Medical Research*, Vol. 10 (H. N. Eisen, ed.), Year Book Med., Chicago, 106—114.

Fägerstam, L. G. (1990) A non-label technology for real time biospecific interaction analysis. In *Techniques in Protein Chemistry* (J. J. Villafranca, ed.), Academic Press, New York. in press.

Fazekas de St Groth, S. (1979) The quality of antibodies and cellular receptors. *Immunol. Meth.* 1:1—41.

Fazekas de St Groth, S., and Webster, R. G. (1961) Methods in immunochemistry of viruses. I. Equilibrium filtration. *Aust. J. Exp. Biol. Med. Sci.* 39:549—562.

Friguet, B., Djavadi-Ohaniance, L., and Goldberg, M. E. (1984) Some monoclonal antibodies raised with a native protein bind preferentially to the denatured antigen. *Mol. Immun.* 21:673—677.

Friguet, B., Chaffotte, A. F., Djavadi-Ohaniance, L., and Goldberg, M. E. (1985) Measurements of the true affinity constant in solution of antigen-antibody complexes by enzyme-linked immunosorbent assay. *J. Immunol. Meth.* 77:305—319.

Friguet, B., Djavadi-Ohaniance, L., and Goldberg, M. E. (1989) Polypeptide-antibody binding mechanism: conformational adaptation investigated by equilibrium and kinetic analysis. *Res. Immunol.* 140:355—376.

Froese, A. (1968) Kinetic and equilibrium studies on 2,4-dinitrophenol hapten-antibody systems. *Immunochemistry* 5:253—264.

Glass, D. N., Caffin, J., Maini, R. N., and Scott, J. R. (1973) Measurement of DNA antibodies by double antibody precipitation. *Ann. Rheum. Dis.* 32:342—345.

Hardie, G., and Van Regenmortel, M. H. V. (1975) Immunochemical studies of tobacco mosaic virus. I: Refutation of the alleged homogeneous binding of purified antibody fragments. *Immunochemistry* 12:903—908.

Hetherington, S. V. (1988) The intrinsic affinity constant (K) of anticapsular antibody to oligosaccharides of Haemophilus influenzae type b. *J. Immunol.* 140:3966—3970.

Jönsson, U., Malmqvist, M., Rönnberg, I., and Berghem, L. (1985) Biosensors based on surface concentration measuring devices. The concept of surface concentration. *Progr. Colloid Polymer Sci.* 70:96—100.

Johnstone, R. W., Andrew, S. M., Hogarth, M. P., Pietersz, G. A., and McKenzie, I. F. (1990) The effect of temperature on the binding kinetics and equilibrium constants of monoclonal antibodies to cell surface antigens. *Mol. Immunol.* 27:327—333.

Kim, Y. T., Kalver, S., and Siskind, G. W. (1975) A comparison of the Farr technique with equilibrium dialysis for the measurement of antibody concentration and affinity. *J. Immunol. Meth.* 6:347—354.

Kretschmann, E., and Raether, H. (1968) Radiative decay of non radiative surface plasmons excited by light. *Z. Naturforsch. A* 23:2135—2136.

Krüger, U., Wickert, L., and Wagener, C. (1989) Determination of epitope specificities and affinities of monoclonal antibodies in solution phase using biotin-labeled carcinoembryonic antigen and avidin as precipitating agent. *J. Immunol. Meth.* 117:25—32.

Löfas, S., and Johnsson, B. (1990) A novel hydrogel matrix on gold surfaces in surface plasmon resonance sensors for fast and efficient covalent immobilization of ligands. *J. Chem. Soc. Chem. Commun.* 21: 1526—1528.

Mason, D. W., and Williams, A. F. (1986) Kinetics of antibody reactions and the analysis of cell surface antigens. In *Handbook of Experimental Immunology,* Vol. 1, Immunochemistry (D. M. Weir, ed.), Blackwell, Oxford, 38.1—38.17.

Matsuda, H. (1967) Theory of the steady-state current potential curves of redox electrode reactions in hydrodynalic voltametry. II. Laminar pipe and channel flows. *J. Electroanal. Chem.* 15:325—336.

Mayo, C. S., and Hallock, R. B. (1989) Immunoassay based on surface plasmon oscillations. *J. Immunol. Meth.* 120:105—114.

Muramatsu, H. (1986) Piezoelectric immuno sensor for the detection of *Candida albicans* microbes. *Anal. Chim. Acta* 188:257—261.

Ngeh-Ngwaininbi, J., Foley, P. H., Kuan, S. S., and Guilbault, G. G. (1986) Parathion antibodies on piezoelectric crystals. *J. Am. Chem. Soc.* 108: 5444—5447.

Pascual, D., and Clem, L. W. (1988) Ligand binding by murine IgM antibodies: intramolecular heterogeneity exists in certain, but not all, cases. *Mol. Immunol.* 25:87—94.

Schots, A., Van der Leede, B. J., De Jongh, E., and Egberts, E. (1988) A method for the determination of antibody affinity using a direct ELISA. *J. Immunol. Meth.* 109:225—233.

Skubitz, K. M., and Smith, T. W. (1975) Determination of antibody-hapten association kinetics: a simplified experimental approach. *J. Immunol.* 114:1369—1374.

Soderquist, M. E., and Walton, A. G. (1980) Structural changes in proteins adsorbed on polymer surfaces. *J. Colloid Interface Sci.* 75:386—397.

Stevens, F. J. (1987) Modification of an ELISA-based procedure for affinity determination: correction necessary for use with bivalent antibody. *Mol. Immunol.* 24:1055—1060.

Steward, M. W., and Lew, A. M. (1985) The importance of antibody affinity in the performance of immunoassays for antibody. *J. Immunol. Meth.* 78:173—190.

Underwood, P. A. (1988) Measurement of the affinity of antiviral antibodies. *Adv. Virus Res.* 34:283—309.

Van Regenmortel, M. H. V. (1982) *Serology and Immunochemistry of Plant Viruses.* Academic Press, New York, 100—105.

Van Regenmortel, M. H. V. (1988) Which value of antigenic valency should be used in antibody avidity calculations with multivalent antigens? *Mol. Immunol.* 25:565—567.

Van Regenmortel, M. H. V., and Hardie, G. (1976) Immunochemical studies of tobacco mosaic virus. II. Univalent and monogamous bivalent binding of the IgG antibody. *Immunochemistry* 13:503—507.

Yolken, R. H. (1985) Solid phase immunoassays for the detection of viral diseases. In *Immunochemistry of Viruses. The Basis for Serodiagnosis and Vaccines* (M. H. V. Van Regenmortel and A. R. Neurath, eds.), Elsevier, NY, 121—138.

Chapter

8

Maturation of the Immune Response

Claudia Berek
Institute of Genetics
University of Cologne
Cologne, Germany

INTRODUCTION

Basically there are two different types of immune responses: the cell-mediated and the humoral immune response. The cellular immune response provides protection against intracellular virus infections and fungi, parasites, cancer cells, or foreign tissue. On the other hand, a humoral immune response is activated during the extracellular phase of bacterial or viral infections. In addition, the humoral immune response also plays an important role in the neutralization of toxins.

Humoral immunity is provided by immunoglobulin molecules which are antigen-specific antibodies. In a humoral immune response B lymphocytes will be activated via their immunoglobulin receptors to proliferate and to differentiate into effector cells, called plasma cells. These cells secrete large amounts of immunoglobulin molecules into the body fluids. Antigen-activated B cells may also develop into memory cells. These cells are responsible for the long-term protection of the animal. Upon a further encounter of the antigen, memory cells will be activated and provide a much faster and also stronger secondary response.

The analysis of serum antibody shows an increase in the average binding affinity of antibody for the antigen with time after immunization. Affinity measurements demonstrate that in a secondary immune response the antibody affinity is higher than in the primary response. These improvements in the antibody affinity is referred to as the maturation of the immune response (Siskind and Benacerraf, 1969).

The maturation of the immune response is unique to the humoral immune responses. No equivalent maturation in the affinity of the T-cell receptor has been observed. The requirement for the T-cell receptor to interact with both, antigen and major histocompatibility complex (MHC) and also the important role of T cells in controlling autoimmunity may place strong constraints on the degree to which the T-cell receptor can be modified.

The specificity of antibodies for the antigen is defined by the variable part of the heavy (H) and the light (L) chain. Structural analysis has demonstrated that defined parts of the variable regions determine the combining site. These complementarity determining regions (CDRs) interact strongly with the surface of the antigenic molecules.

In order to obtain antibodies of higher affinity, the structure of the antibody-binding site has to be changed. Experiments by Nussenzweig and Benacerraf (1966) indicate that there is a shift in the B cell repertoire during the response. They found that in the early response to 2,4-dinitrophenyl hapten mainly antibodies with a lambda (λ) L chain are produced, whereas mainly kappa (κ)-bearing antibodies were found to be a later response.

Weigert et al. (1970) sequenced λ L chains of myeloma proteins and found that they differed by single amino acid substitutions. These exchanges were found only in the CDRs of the variable part of the antibody molecule. From these results Weigert et al. predicted that the primary antibody structure is diversified by somatic point mutations on which antigenic selection acts sequentially.

The recent development of new techniques has allowed us to study the maturation of the immune response in more detail. The production of antigen-specific hybridoma lines (Köhler and Milstein, 1975) and the structural analysis of their antibodies produced by directly sequencing the mRNA (Hamlyn et al., 1978) has enabled us to look at the development of the antibody diversity during the course of the immune response. The detailed analysis of antibodies at various stages of the immune response has shown that both the shift in the repertoire and somatic hypermutation followed by antigenic selection leads to the increase in antibody affinity.

However, despite the knowledge accumulated in recent years, we are still far from understanding the process of the maturation of the immune response. The mechanism of hypermutation, which introduces at a high rate (10^{-3} per base pair per generation) single nucleotide exchanges specifically into the variable regions of the antibody molecules, is still not known. The high efficiency of the antigen-driven selection is also surprising. Certain substitutions that increase the affinity sometimes less than 10-fold are found in practically all mutated antibodies of a given specificity. Proceedings at the cellular level like the interaction of various cell types, such as B cells, T cells, macrophages, and follicular dendritic cells, or the importance of microenvironments for the maturation of the immune response are not really understood.

GENERATION OF THE PRIMARY ANTIBODY REPERTOIRE

The primary antibody repertoire of the mouse is extremely large. It has been estimated that up to 10^{10} different receptor molecules can be generated from the germline genes (Berek and Milstein, 1988). Thus, even a small antigenic determinant like a hapten is recognized by many different B-cell clones.

During the development of the mature B cells the variable regions of the antibodies are assembled somatically from different gene segments (Tonegawa, 1983). The variable region of the L chains are made up by two gene segments V_L and J_L; the variable part of the H chains are comprised of three gene segments, V_H, D, and J_H.

Germ-Line Diversity

There are two different types of L chains, kappa and lambda. In the mouse there are several hundred V_L genes and V_H genes, about twenty D segments and four functional J_k and J_H, and three functional $J\lambda$ gene segments.

Combinatorial Diversity

A particular V_H region may be joined to various D and J_H segments, and one V_L gene can be joined to different J_L segments. In addition, one type of L chain can form an antibody molecule with various H chains and vice versa to give rise to antibodies of different specificity.

Junctional Diversity

When the gene elements are rearranged during the development of the B cells, the various gene segments can be joined at different nucleotide positions. Thus V_H, D, and J_H regions of multiple lengths combine with each other. Furthermore, nucleotides can be inserted and deleted during the process of gene rearrangement (N-region diversity). Thus in antibodies of different specificities great differences in the length of the D and the J region have been observed. In L chains, N-region diversity has only occasionally been seen (Heller et al., 1987).

THE PRIMARY REPERTOIRE IS DETERMINED BY FREQUENCY AND AFFINITY

At the beginning of an immune response, when the antigen concentration is still high, many B-cell clones including many with low-affinity receptors are activated (Pelkonen et al., 1986). Thus, the early primary repertoire of the antigen-specific response depends on the frequency with which certain V(D)J rearrangements occur and only to some extent on the affinity of the receptor for the antigen. Thereafter, as the amount of antigen decreases, the number of antigen-specific B cells increases, and as free antibody begins to appear in the circulation, only those few B-cell clones with high-affinity receptors will further differentiate.

THE PRIMARY REPERTOIRE IS GENERATED FROM GERM-LINE SEQUENCES

The analysis of antigen-specific hybridoma lines, obtained from the fusion of spleen cells 7 days after immunization, showed that the majority of the variable regions were germ-line sequences (Clarke et al., 1990; Cumano and Rajewsky, 1985; Kaartinen et al., 1983; Malpiero et al., 1987; Wysocki et al., 1986). Only occasionally were single nucleotide substitutions observed. Suppression experiments using monoclonal antibodies specific for idiotypes of antibodies with specificity for the p-azophenylarsonate (Ars) hapten gave further evidence that prior to activation by antigen the repertoire of B cells is not diversified by somatic mutations (Manser and Gefter, 1986). Thus, hypermutation is not a mechanism to generate the primary repertoire.

ACTIVATION OF THE HYPERMUTATION MECHANISM

Only during the antigen-dependent differentiation of B cells does the hypermutation mechanism become activated. By this process single nucleotide substitutions are introduced into the variable regions of the H and the L chains. From the analysis of clonally related cells (McKean et al., 1984), and from both population kinetics (Allen et al., 1987) and the accumulation of silent mutations with time (Berek and Milstein, 1987), a rate of 10^{-3} per base pair per generation for the hypermutation process has been calculated. This is about six orders of magnitude higher than the spontaneous mutation rate in eukaryotic DNA.

Mechanistically the mutation process is not understood. The data show that the process is site-specific, changing nucleotides only in rearranged variable regions (Roes et al., 1989) and in the immediate 5'- and 3'-flanking regions (Gearhart and Bogenhagen, 1983). The idea is unlikely that the somatic diversification may be due to gene-conversion events which are comparable to processes that are responsible for the generation of V_H and V_L diversity in the chicken (Weill and Reynaud, 1987; Wysocki and Gefter, 1989).

Proliferation is not sufficient to activate the hypermutation process (Manser, 1987). Furthermore, in immune responses, which are independent of

TABLE 1.
Key Mutation in Response to Various Antigens

Hapten	Variable Region	Position	Substitution	Affinity Increase (-fold)
NP	V_H-186.2	33	Trp → Leu	10
Ars	V_H-Id^{cr}	57	Thr → Ile	3
		58	Lys → Thr	4
phOx	V_k-Ox1	34	His → Gln	8
		34	His → Asn	10

helper T cells, somatic mutations have not been observed, suggesting that the help of T cells is needed to activate the hypermutation process.

About 4 days after immunization with a T-dependent antigen, activated B cells move into the follicles of the lymphatic tissues and massive proliferation of these cells leads to the formation of germinal centers (Kroese et al., 1990). The data suggest that during the expansion of the B-cell clones in the germinal centers the hypermutation mechanism is activated (Apel and Berek, 1990).

SOMATIC MUTATIONS INCREASE THE ANTIBODY AFFINITY

Assuming that the mutation mechanism introduces nucleotide exchanges in a more or less random fashion, it is surprising to see the accumulation of somatic mutations at certain positions of the variable regions of the H and the L chain of the antibodies. An analysis of the available data suggests that there are regions within the variable parts of the antibody molecules which are more prone to the mutation process than others, so-called hot spots for somatic mutations (Berek and Milstein, 1987; Levy et al., 1988). On the other hand, the recurrence of certain mutations is due to antigenic selection. These substitutions change the amino acid sequence in such a way that the affinity for the antigen is increased. These so-called key mutations have been observed in response to various antigens (Allen et al., 1987; Berek and Milstein, 1987; Blier and Bothwell, 1987; Claflin et al., 1989; Sharon et al., 1989). Examples are given in Table 1. Whereas in the immune response to the haptens (4-hydroxy-3-nitrophenyl)acetyl (NP) and Ars haptens, mutations that increase affinity are found in the H chain, in the response to 2-phenyloxazolone (phOx), mutations were found in the L chain.

It is remarkable how efficiently the affinity-based selection operates. In the Ars response, a mere threefold increase in the affinity seems to be enough to give the B cells a proliferative advantage (Sharon et al., 1989).

A sequential increase in affinity due to increasing numbers of somatic mutations may also occur in responses to complex protein molecules. For two anti-idiotypic antibodies, which differed 15-fold in their affinity, the stepwise accumulation of somatic mutations could be demonstrated by reconstructing progenitors of clonally related somatic antibody mutants (Kocks and Rajewsky, 1988).

THE SHIFT IN THE REPERTOIRE IN THE SECONDARY RESPONSE

In immune response to haptens, as well as to influenza virus hemagglutinin, a shift in the repertoire from the primary to the secondary response was observed (Berek et al., 1985; Clarke et al., 1990; Cumano and Rajewsky, 1986; Stenzel-Poore et al., 1988). Many of the late high-affinity antibodies have V(D)J combinations which were only rarely or never observed in the primary responses. Thus the maturation of the response is due to hypermutation and selection as well as to selection of different B-cell subsets into the pool of memory cells. Why the B-cell subsets that dominate the memory response are different from those that dominate the primary response is not really understood.

MATURATION OF THE IMMUNE RESPONSE IN GERMINAL CENTERS

The germinal center may be the microenvironment where the maturation of the immune response occurs (MacLennan and Gray, 1985). In the germinal center there are mainly proliferating B cells, T-helper cells, and large numbers of follicular dendritic cells. The latter cells present antigen complexed with antibody on their surface. They are thought to be important in the selection process of the high-affinity variant B-cell clones which arise during the hypermutation phase.

The analysis of the antibody diversity of germinal center B cells has shown that by day 10 most of the cells express mutated antibodies (Apel and Berek, 1990). However, mutations that are known to increase the affinity for the antigen were not seen in these sequences. Hence the preferential expansion of the B-cell clones expressing high-affinity receptors has not yet taken place.

Hybridoma lines derived from total spleen cells 14 days after immunization (Griffith et al., 1984), as well as from separated germinal-center cells (Berek and Apel, 1990) produced antibodies that carried mutations which increase the affinity for the antigen. Thus, by the time germinal centers have started to disintegrate, the preferential expansion of high-affinity variants has occurred. Whether the expansion of these clones takes place in the germinal centers or only later is not yet clear.

The work by Coico et al. (1983) suggests that B cells in the germinal centers develop into memory cells. Affinity for antigen seems to be the determining factor as to which of the B cells differentiate further. Those B cells with reduced affinity for the antigen or which have completely lost their antigen-binding capacity seem to die in the germinal centers, whereas those with high-affinity receptors seem to develop into the memory population. An analysis of the antibody diversity of memory B cells, using the polymerase chain reaction, suggested that the memory compartment is strongly selected for high-affinity B-cell variants (Weiss and Rajewsky, 1990).

MEMORY RESPONSES

After a further injection of antigen, memory B cells are reactivated and again give rise to both plasma and memory cells. Transfer experiments (Dell et al., 1989; Siekevitz et al., 1987) showed that memory cells proliferate without the accumulation of further somatic mutations. Furthermore, the analysis of antigen-selected mutated memory cells in autoimmune mice (Shlomchick et al., 1987) suggested clonal expansion without hypermutation. On the other hand, in the immune response to phOx it was found that the number of somatic mutations increases from the early primary, to the late primary, and then to the secondary and tertiary response (Berek and Milstein, 1987). This suggests that in the memory response the hypermutation mechanism is reactivated. The accumulation of somatic mutations correlates with an increase in the affinity for the antigen (Berek, 1989). Thus an affinity maturation seems to take place not only in the primary response, but also in the memory response. Recurring rounds of mutation and selection are the basis of the maturation process.

REFERENCES

Allen, D., Cumano, A., Dildrop, R., Kocks, C., Rajewsky, K., Rajewsky, N., Roes, J., Sablitzky, F., and Siekevitz, M. (1987) Timing, genetic requirements and functional consequences of somatic hypermutation during B-cell development. *Immunol. Rev.* 96:5—22.

Apel, M., and Berek, C. (1990) Somatic mutations in antibodies expressed by germinal center B-cells early after immunisation. *Intern. Immunol.* 2:813—819.

Berek, C., (1989) Molecular dissection of an antigen-specific immune response. *J. Autoimmunity* 2:195—201.

Berek, C., and Apel, M. (1990) Maturation through hypermutation and selection. In *Molecular Evolution on Rugged Landscape,* SFI *Studies in the Sciences of Complexity,* Vol. IX (A. S. Perelson, and S. A. Kauffman, eds.), 83—91.

Berek, C., and Milstein, C. (1987) Mutation drift and repertoire shift in the maturation of the immune response. *Immunol. Rev.* 96:23—41.

Berek, C., and Milstein, C. (1988) The dynamic nature of the antibody repertoire. *Immunol. Rev.* 105:1—26.

Berek, C., Griffiths, G. M., and Milstein, C. (1985) Molecular events during maturation of the immune response to oxazolone. *Nature (London)* 316:412—418.

Blier, P. R., and Bothwell, A. (1987) A limited number of B cell lineages generates the heterogeneity of a secondary response. *J. Immunol.* 139:3996—4006.

Claflin, J. L., George, J., Dell, C., and Berry, J. (1989) Patterns of mutations and selection in antibodies to the phosphorylcholine-specific determinant in *Proteus morganii*. *J. Imunol.* 143:3054—3063.

Clarke, S. H., Staudt, L. M., Kavaler, J., Schwartz, D., Gerhard, W. U., and Weigert, M. G. (1990) V Region usage and somatic mutation in the primary and secondary responses to influenza virus hemagglutinin. *J. Immunol.* 144:2795—2801.

Coico, R. F., Bhogal, B. S., and Thorbecke, G. J. (1983) Relationship of germinal centers in lymphoid tissue to immunologic memory. *J. Immunol.* 131:2254—2257.

Cumano, A., and Rajewsky, K. (1985) Clonal recruitment and somatic mutation in the generation of immunological memory to the hapten NP. *Eur. J. Immunol.* 15:512—520.

Cumano, A., and Rajewsky, K. (1986) Structure of primary anti-(4-hydroxy-3-nitrophenyl)acetyl (NP) antibodies in normal and idiotypically suppressed C57BL mice. *EMBO J.* 5:2459—2468.

Dell, C. L., Yuanxu, L., and Claflin, J. L. (1989) Molecular analysis of clonal stability and longevity in B cell memory. *J. Immunol.* 143:3364—3370.

Gearhart, P., and Bogenhagen, D. F. (1983) Clusters of point mutations are found exclusively around rearranged V-genes. *Proc. Natl. Acad. Sci. U.S.A.* 80:3439—3442.

Griffiths, G. M., Berek, C., Kaartinen, M., and Milstein, C. (1984) Somatic mutation and the maturation of the immune response. *Nature (London)* 312:271—275.

Hamlyn, P. H., Brownlee, G. G., Cheng, C. C., Gait, M. J., and Milstein, C. (1978) Complete sequence of constant and 3' non-coding regions of an immunoglulin mRNA using the dideoxy nucleotide method of RNA sequencing. *Cell* 15:1067—1075.

Heller, M., Owens, J. D., Mushinsky, F. F., and Rudikoff, S. (1987) Amino acids at the site of V_k-J_k recombination not encoded by germ line sequences. *J. Exp. Med.* 166:637—646.

Kaartinen, M., Griffiths, G. M., Markham, A. F., and Milstein, C. (1983) mRNA Sequences define an unusually restricted IgG response to 2-phenyl-oxazolone and its early diversification. *Nature (London)* 304:320—324.

Kocks, C., and Rajewsky, K. (1988) Stepwise intraclonal maturation of antibody affinity through somatic hypermutation. *Proc. Natl. Acad. Sci. U.S.A.* 85:8206.

Köhler, G., and Milstein, C. (1975) Continuous culture of fused cells secreting antibody of predefined specificity. *Nature (London)* 256:495—497.

Kroese, F. G. M., Timens, W., and Nieuwenhuis, P. (1990) Germinal center reaction and B-lymphocytes: morphology and function. *Curr. Top. Pathol.* 84:103—148.

Levy, S., Mendel, E., Kon, S., Avnur, Z., and Levy, R. (1988) Mutational hot spots in Ig V region genes of human follicular lymphomas. *J. Exp. Med.* 168:475.

McKean, D. M., Hüppi, K., Bell, M., Staudt, L., Gerhard, W., and Weigert, M. (1984) Generation of antibody diversity in the immune response of BALB/c mice to influenza virus hemagglutinin. *Proc. Natl. Acad. Sci. U.S.A.* 81:3180—3183.

MacLennan, I. C. M., and Gray, D. (1985) Antigen driven selection of virgin and memory B-cells. *Immunol. Rev.* 91:61—85.

Malpiero, U. V., Levy, N. S., and Gearhart, P. J. (1987) Somatic mutations in antiphosphorylcholine antibodies. *Immunol. Rev.* 96:59—74.

Manser, T. (1987) Mitogen driven B-cell proliferation and differentiation are not accompanied by hypermutation of immunoglobulin variable region genes. *J. Immunol.* 139:234.

Manser, T., and Gefter, M. L. (1986) The molecular evolution of the immune response: idiotope specific suppression indicates that B cells express germ-line encoded V genes prior to antigenic stimulation. *Eur. J. Immunol.* 16:1439—1444.

Nussenzweig, V., and Benacerraf, B. (1966) Quantitative variations in L-chain types in guinea pig antihapten antibodies. *J. Exp. Med.* 124:805—818.

Pelkonen, J., Kaartinen, M., and Mäkelä, O. (1986) Quantitative representation of two germline V-genes in the early response to 2-phenyloxazolone. *Eur. J. Immunol.* 16:106.

Roes, J., Hüppi, K., Rajewsky, K., and Sablitzky, F. (1989) V Gene rearrangement is required to fully activate the hypermutation mechanism in B-cells. *J. Immunol.* 142:1022—1026.

Sharon, J., Gefter, M. L., Wysocki, L. J., and Margolies, M. N. (1989) Recurrent somatic mutations in mouse antibodies to *p*-azophenylarsonate increase affinity for hapten. *J. Immunol.* 142:596—601.

Shlomchick, M. J., Marshak-Rothstein, A., Wolfowicz, C. B., Rothstein, T. L., and Weigert, M. (1987) The role of clonal selection and somatic mutation in autoimmunity. *Nature (London)* 328:805—811.

Siskind, G. D., and Benaceraff, B. (1969) Cell selection by antigen in the immune response. *Adv. Immunol.* 10:1—50.

Siekevitz, M., Kocks, C., Rajewsky, K., and Dildrop, R. (1987) Analysis of somatic mutation and class switching in naive and memory B-cells generating adoptive primary and secondary responses. *Cell* 48:757—770.

Stenzel-Poore, M. P., Bruderer, U., and Rittenberg, M. B. (1988) The adaptive potential of the memory response: clonal recruitment and epitope recognition. *Immunol. Rev.* 105:113—136.

Tonegawa, S. (1983) Somatic generation of antibody diversity *Nature (London)* 302:575—579.

Weigert, M. (1986) The influence of somatic mutation on the immune response. *Prog. Immunol.* 6:139—144.

Weigert, M. G., Cesari, I. M., Yonkovitch, S. J., and Cohn, M. (1970) Variability in the lambda L-chain sequences of mouse antibody. *Nature (London)* 228:1045—1047.

Weill, J.-C., and Reynaud, C.-A. (1987) The chicken B cell compartment. *Science* 238:1094—1098.

Weiss, U., and Rajewsky, K. (1990) The repertoire of somatic antibody mutants accumulating in the memory compartment after primary immunization is restricted through affinity maturation and mirrors that expressed in the secondary response. *J. Exp. Med.* 172:1681—1689.

Wysocki, L., Manser, T., and Gefter, M. L. (1986) Somatic evolution of variable region structures during an immune response. *Proc. Natl. Acad. Sci. U.S.A.* 83:1847.

Wysocki, L., and Gefter, M. L. (1989) Gene conversion and the generation of antibody diversity. *Annu. Rev. Biochem.* 58:509—531.

Chapter 9

Immunoadjuvants

Arlette Adam and Vongthip Souvannavong
Institut de Biochimie
CNRS URA 1116
Université Paris-Sud
Orsay, France

INTRODUCTION

Whole microorganisms are generally immunogenic and killed or attenuated strains, when available, can provide an immunity comparable to that provided by real infections. This is not true, however, for most parasites, and the immune response elicited by viruses such as human immunodeficiency virus (HIV) does not appear to be adequate. In addition, microbial agents are difficult to prepare and their use may be accompanied by toxic reactions.

Recent developments in molecular technology and a better understanding of the immune response to an antigen have resulted in new strategies aimed at creating an ideal antigen.

It is now well-established that the elaboration of an immune response requires interactions between B cells, T cells, and antigen-presenting cells (APC). Although B cells recognize conformational determinants on the native antigen, the production of specific antibodies requires the cooperation of T-helper (Th) cells. T cells recognize only processed antigen in association with self-molecules of the major histocompatibility complex (MHC). T cells recognize epitopes processed and presented by cells bearing MHC class II molecules. Cytotoxic T lymphocytes (CTL), to destroy infected target cells, must recognize epitopes presented by cells bearing MHC class I or class II molecules. T-suppressor cells which are also stimulated by complex antigens recognize other epitopes.

Thus, the antigenicity of a complex antigen is supported by simple peptidic structures: the B- and T-cell epitopes. It was therefore reasonable to hope that synthetic peptides, which are able to mimic naturally processed antigen in antibody and T-cell recognition assays *in vitro,* might also be used as effective immunogen *in vivo.*

However, simple peptides are not by themselves immunogenic. They have to be manipulated in order to make them resemble natural immunogens. This can be achieved by coupling them with other molecules, by polymerization, or by association with oily or particulate vehicles. Efficacy of these "constructions" can be further improved by using immunostimulants. In this way, it should be possible to direct the immune response induced toward the desired type, whether humoral or cellular, as well as the isotypic profile of antibodies. The importance of such an approach for the development of new vaccines has been extensively documented (see, for example, Miller, 1989; Eppstein et al., 1990; Griffiths, 1990; Miller, 1989). In this context, we describe some representative findings in this field.

CLASSICAL ADJUVANTS

Freund's Adjuvants

The most potent adjuvant still in current use was developed in the 1930s. Previously, Ramon (1926) noticed that a local inflammation at the site of inoculation of bacterial anatoxins in horses considerably increased antibody levels. Since tuberculosis also increased the immune response of animals against unrelated antigens, inducing higher levels of antibody and delayed-type hypersensitivity (DTH), Coulaud (1935) included killed mycobacteria in paraffin oil to increase DTH to tuberculin. Finally, Freund et al. (1937) obtained high antibody levels by injecting an antigen in a water-in-oil emulsion. The antigen was suspended in saline and dispersed in mineral oil with an emulsifier such as arlacel A [Freund's incomplete adjuvant (FIA)]. The addition of killed tubercle bacilli to the oily phase [Freund's complete adjuvant (FCA)] further increased the humoral response and induced a cellular immune response. FCA has been used successfully with a variety of antigens in laboratory animals; in general it constitutes the positive control in experiments. FCA, however, cannot be used for human or veterinary vaccines because it contains a nonmetabolizable oil and its administration causes severe side effects, including granuloma and fever. That is why many investigators have tried to propose a new adjuvant formulation as efficient as FCA but acceptable for human use. N-acetylmuramyl-L-alanyl-D-isoglutamine (MDP) was identified in our laboratory as the minimal chemical structure capable of replacing mycobacteria in FCA (Ellouz et al., 1974). MDP derivatives administered with a metabolizable vehicle have been proposed. These derivatives constitute promising candidates for replacing FCA and will be described later.

Freund's complete adjuvant greatly increases the immunogenicity of poor immunogens. An example commonly used in screening experiments is provided by monoazobenzene arsonate-*N*-acetyl-L-tyrosine (ABA-Nac-L-Tyr), which is not immunogenic in FIA but induces DTH reaction when injected with FCA. It is well-established that FCA affects the isotopic pattern of synthesized immunoglobulins. More specifically, it induces the synthesis of IgG2 antibodies. Recently, a cellular basis has been provided for these biological effects of FCA. It has been shown that the administration of antigen in FCA stimulates T-helper cells of type 1 (Th1), which produce interleukin 2 (IL-2) and γ-interferon (γ-IFN), mediate inflammatory and DTH reactions, and augment IgG2a antibody responses (Grun and Maurer, 1989).

Alum

The increased immunogenic properties of diphtheria toxin after precipitation with alum were discovered in 1926 (Glenny et al.). Alum remains to this day the only adjuvant currently accepted for human use. The mineral gel adjuvant is obtained by mixing the antigen with alum, followed by the addition of NaOH which precipitates alum; alternatively, antigens can be added to preformed gels. A major disadvantage of these ionic antigen-alum complexes is their instability, since they cannot be lyophilized or frozen and must be kept in the cold; furthermore uniform preparations are difficult to obtain. The adjuvant action of alum has been attributed to a depot effect. Alum induces a granuloma at the site of injection which may increase the uptake of antigen by macrophages. *In vitro* experiments have shown that alum promotes the function of macrophages as APC and augments IL-1 release. Alum also activates the complement system, a property which is probably involved in the generation of B cell memory and enlargement of the population of potentially antigen-reactive cells in the draining lymph nodes observed in alum-treated animals (Bomford, 1986).

Studies on the isotype profile of alum-potentiated immune responses have shown the preferential elicitation of IgG1 and IgE antibodies. The latter are responsible for mediating immediate hypersensitivity reactions. Both polyclonal and antigen-specific IgE serum levels were increased in mice injected with an alum vaccine (Beck and Spiegelberg, 1989). The preferential production of IgE has been exploited to vaccinate mice against parasites (Bomford, 1986).

Recent observations by Grun and Maurer (1989) have provided a cellular basis for the modification of the isotype distribution of antibodies to antigen administered as alum complexes. They have shown that T-helper CD4+ cells of the Th2 type were elicited. The properties of these cells which produce IL-4 and IL-5, mediate hapten-carrier-linked activity, and augment IgG1 and IgE as well as IgA, are in agreement with the modifications observed in animals treated with alum.

Alum does not stimulate cell-mediated immunity and is, thus, advantageous when only humoral immunity has to be increased. The efficacy of alum in increasing humoral responses to many antigens, including toxoids and hepatitis B virus surface antigens, is well-established. Berman et al. (1990) have reported that chimpanzees immunized with recombinant HIV-1 gp120 coprecipitated with alum were protected against viral infection. For other investigators, however, alum does not appear to be suitable for use with subunits or synthetic small peptides (Sanchez-Pescador et al., 1988).

PREPARATION OF ARTIFICIAL IMMUNOGENS
Binding to a Carrier

Attachment to a carrier protein (tetanus toxoid is included among the proteins used) confers immunogenicity to most peptides. Four coupling reactions have been used: (1) glutaraldehyde which forms links between NH_2 groups; (2) carbodiimide which binds COOH to NH_2 groups; (3) bisdiazobenzidine which links tyrosine residues; and (4) maleimidobenzoyl-N-hydroxysuccinimide ester which links cysteine residues to NH_2 groups. According to peptide sequences, one or the other method is used in order to involve only one amino acid, preferably at the end of the peptide. It is also possible to add an amino acid to the natural sequence for suitable attachment to the carrier.

However, prior use of a carrier protein can inhibit the antibody response to new epitopes linked to the same protein. This phenomenon is known as epitope-specific suppression (Herzenberg and Tokuhisa, 1982). There was a possibility that a part of the carrier molecule could support the carrier effect, since a carrier protein contains B epitopes required for the antibody response to the carrier itself and distinct T epitopes recognized by T-suppressor and T-helper cells. This has been shown recently by Etlinger et al. (1990): a peptide TT73-99 corresponding to amino acid residues 73 to 99 from tetanus toxoid (TT), when linked to a B-cell epitope and injected with FCA into tetanus toxoid-primed recipients, retained its potential for carrier but not for suppressor function.

Lipids have also been used as efficient carriers. An example is provided by Brynestad et al. (1990), who used a synthetic peptide corresponding to residues 1 to 23 of glycoprotein D (gD1-23) of herpes simplex virus type 1 (HSV-1) to immunize mice against HSV-1 infection. The coupling of this peptide to palmitic acid enhanced its immunogenicity. Incorporation of the acyl peptide into liposomes further increased the immunogenicity of the peptide; inclusion of immunomodulators into the same liposome elicited the strongest response.

The polysaccharide pullulan, a linear copolymer of maltotriose, has been used to develop a new vaccine capable of inducing neutralizing antibody production without IgE synthesis. Diphtheria toxin detoxified by means of conjugation with pullulan was used as an immunogen. Subcutaneous immunization of mice with toxin-pullulan conjugate, followed by a 4-week challenge, induces a good IgG antibody response of both IgG1 and IgG2b isotypes with a diminished IgE synthesis, whereas the conventional alum-precipitated toxoid increases mainly IgE response as well as IgG1 production. In addition, the toxin-pullulan conjugate shows no detectable toxicity and is applicable to oral immunization. Therefore, the combination of toxin with pullulan represents a powerful tool for the preparation of vaccines (Yamaya et al., 1990).

Viruslike Particles

Adams et al. (1987) have described the spontaneous formation of viruslike particles (Ty-VLPs) of approximately 50 nm in diameter by fusion proteins. The latter were obtained by expression in yeast of the hybrid transposon Ty, encoding particle-forming p1 protein and the viral protein of interest. The hybrid Ty-VLPs, which are easily purified from yeast cells, express the viral proteins on their surface in a polyvalent immunogenic form. Ty-VLPs expressing, for example, the gag protein p24 and gp120 from HIV-1, have been used successfully in animal models to elicit neutralizing antibodies and even a T-cell proliferation response to p24. It must be noted that Ty-VLPs themselves are immunogenic and can elicit an immune response to yeast proteins (O'Hagan, 1990).

The capacity of hepatitis B surface antigen (HBsAg) and core (HBcAg) proteins to spontaneously assemble into 22- and 27-nm viruslike particles, respectively, has been exploited to present well-defined epitopes to the immune system. The best results were obtained with HBcAg. They were explained by the presence, on this antigen, of a number of well-defined helper T-cell epitopes (Millich et al., 1987). Chimeric particles have been expressed in yeast, as well as in bacterial cells, the coding sequences for viral epitopes replacing part of the hepatitis viral gene or being added to its C-terminal end.

Constructions with Synthetic Epitopes

Jolivet et al. (1990) presented a polyvalent construct which could confer immunogenicity to individual epitopes, provided that a strong T-cell epitope was present in the molecule. This consisted of four different synthetic peptides corresponding to antigenic sites of protein M of *S. pyogenes,* diphtheria toxin, plasmodium circumsporozoite protein, and residues 99-121 of HBsAg. The last peptide contains both B- and T-cell epitopes. The four peptides were conjugated by using glutaraldehyde and administered to guinea pigs in the presence of FCA. An antibody response to each peptide was elicited by this construct, whereas the individual antigens were not immunogenic. The presence of the viral peptide which contains a strong T-cell epitope was essential for the production of antibodies to itself and to the three other antigens.

Synthetic immunogens are now being proposed which contain both B-cell and T-cell determinants of various viral or parasitic agents; such a construct was used by Levely et al. (1990). They synthesized a peptide corresponding to residues 45 to 60 of the 1A protein of respiratory syncytial virus with T-cell stimulating activity. This peptide, which contains an antigen-binding site as well as T-cell simulating activity, was combined with a B-cell epitope derived from the viral glycoprotein, either by linear synthesis or by chemical coupling. In both cases the chimeric molecules were injected with FCA. They elicited a strong antibody response. The difference in antibody specificity elicited by the two immunogens was well explained by the difference in configuration adopted by the molecules depending on their mode of preparation, as the configuration determines the degree of accessibility of potential epitopes.

A number of T-cell epitopes, which can be recognized by CTL *in vitro* in the context of MHC class I molecules, has been identified. Until recently, however, their immunogenicity *in vivo* could not be demonstrated. Deres et al. (1989) have shown that adding a lipoprotein tail to synthetic viral peptides is a reproducible way of stimulating a primary CTL response *in vivo*. They administrated to mice a synthetic analog of the active moiety of a major lipoprotein of *E. coli*, tripalmitoyl-*S*-glycerylcysteinyl-seryl-serine (P_3CSS) coupled to peptide NP147-158 of influenza nucleoprotein (NP). In this way, CTL were primed and recognized virus-infected cells as efficiently as CTL from influenza-infected mice. Several mechanisms for this conversion to immunogenicity have been proposed: a longer half-life of the peptide, the mitogenic effect of the lipoprotein, or rather the better targeting and internalization of the peptide by APC, favored by the lipoprotein where, as in the normal pathway, it can be processed, associated with MHC class-I molecules, and presented for efficient priming of CTL.

NEW DELIVERY SYSTEMS

The physical form in which an antigen is presented to the immune system has a considerable influence on its immunogenicity. Indeed, immunization with three different forms of an isolated envelope protein from Semliki Forest virus showed that the monomeric form of the antigen is less immunogenic than the same protein presented into a defined multimeric form, such as protein micelles, or included into lipid vesicles, such as virosomes or liposomes. However, even for an antigen presented in multiple copies, an adjuvant may be necessary to obtain sufficient immunogenicity (Morein et al., 1978).

Immunostimulating Complexes (ISCOMs)

Morein et al. (1984) have recently described a novel type of immunostimulating complexes, called ISCOMs, in which antigens are presented in multiple copies and attached by hydrophobic interactions to a matrix built up by the adjuvant component Quil A combined with lipids.

The adjuvant Quil A is a saponin derived from *Quillaja saponaria molina*, with a carbohydrate moiety linked to a triterpenoid, the amphipathic quillajic acid. Quil A can now be obtained as a purified product available as a 2% sterile aqueous solution or as a lyophilized powder (Superfos Specialty Chemicals, Vedbaek, Denmark) (see Bomford, 1989; Höglund et al., 1989). With regard to its mechanism of action, it has been reported that Quil A is able to enhance markedly the murine primary antibody responses to both T-dependent antigen (TD) and T-independent antigen (TI). Thus, Quil A is interesting because most commonly used adjuvants such as alum have little or no effect on responses to TI antigens (Flebbe and Braley-Mullen, 1986). Quil A alone has been widely used as an adjuvant for a variety of vaccines in veterinary use. When used as a conventional adjuvant, however, Quil A is toxic in large doses but its effective dose can be lowered by a 100-fold when it is incorporated into ISCOMs.

ISCOMs are stable molecular structures, with a mean diameter of 35 nm, in which protein or peptide antigens are attached to a matrix produced through the interaction between Quil A and cholesterol. Cholesterol is particularly used for the construction of ISCOMs because, in a series of experiments with various lipids, it was shown that only cholesterol on its own could associate with Quil A to form the typical cagelike structure of the ISCOM matrix. Phosphatidylcholine can be used as an additional lipid to include antigens into ISCOMs. In typical ISCOMs, antigen, Quil A, and cholesterol are present in approximately equimolar proportions. When preserved by lyophilization or stored as a sterile suspension in a physiological buffer, ISCOMs have kept their morphology and immunogenicity for 3 years (Morein et al., 1984). ISCOMs can be prepared by centrifugation or the dialysis method. In both procedures, a nonionic detergent is used as a membrane-solubilizing agent to avoid a denaturing effect on the hydrophilic part of the protein, which is likely to contain epitopes. By rate zonal centrifugation in a sucrose gradient, ISCOMs sediment with a characteristic coefficient of 19 S. In the dialysis method, dialyzable nonionic detergents such as MEGA-10 (decanoyl-N-methylglucamide), are preferentially used.

Native membrane proteins used initially in ISCOMs were amphipathic proteins whose hydrophobic domains were easily integrated into ISCOMs. A model system using bovine serum albumin (BSA) was developed for studying the integration of nonamphipathic proteins into ISCOMs (Morein et al., 1990). Two methods were applied to reveal hidden hydrophobic regions of BSA: acid treatment at pH 2.5 and heating to 70°C. Both acid- and heat-treated BSA, once integrated into ISCOMs, were highly immunogenic and induced considerably higher serum antibody responses than native monomeric BSA or aggregated BSA nonintegrated into the matrix.

The efficacy of various ISCOM vaccines against viral envelope antigens has been demonstrated. These include envelope proteins from more than 20 different kinds of viruses. Such ISCOMs were at least 10 times more potent at stimulating an antibody response than micelles formed by aggregation of the membrane proteins alone (Höglund et al., 1989; Morein et al., 1984, 1987).

ISCOMs containing either a recombinant gp160 envelope glycoprotein of HIV-1 or influenza hemagglutinin have been prepared by the dialysis method using MEGA-10. In both cases, a single subcutaneous injection in mice resulted in reproducible and long-lasting priming of HIV- or influenza-specific CD8+ MHC class I-restricted CTL. The priming by ISCOM-gp160 immunization lasted at least 4 months and has been consistently successful. No such effect was induced following immunization with recombinant gp160 in conventional adjuvants such as FCA, a known potent inducer of CD4+ MHC class II-restricted CTL. Therefore, it is possible to prime antigen-specific, CD8+CD4− MHC class I-restricted CTL by immunization with exogenous intact protein using ISCOMs (Takahashi et al., 1990).

In conclusion, ISCOMs, by their important property of presenting the antigen in an accessible and multimeric form, provide an effective means to markedly enhance the immunogenicity of the included antigen. Amphipathic proteins and even nonamphipathic proteins as well as small peptides conjugated to carriers can be incorporated into ISCOMs. Once integrated, the antigen is released slowly over a prolonged period of time. ISCOMs have the same slow-release effect as conventional adjuvants but without their side effects. Both antibody response and cell-mediated immunity are induced. Of particular importance is the ability of ISCOMs to induce a MHC class I-restricted CTL response which constitutes an essential part of the immune response against viral infections.

Liposomes

The potential use of liposomes as delivery systems to increase the immunogenicity of a variety of antigens has been reported recently in a comprehensive review by Gregoriadis (1990). These vesicles are composed of one or more concentric phospholipid bilayers formed in the presence of an excess water; they were first described as adjuvants for protein antigens (Allison and Gregoriadis, 1974). Almost all water-soluble, as well as lipophilic or particulate compounds, can be incorporated in appropriate liposomes. These vesicles, which are potentially nontoxic, biodegradable, and nonimmunogenic, can be formulated with a variety of lipid compositions and structures. Liposomes of different size can be prepared. Their fluidity and stability depend on the gel-liquid crystalline transition temperature of their lipid components. Generally, the stability of liposomes is improved by increasing the liposomal cholesterol content. An optimal design does not appear to exist and, depending on individual antigens and the type of immune response which is to be elicited, fluid as well as rigid liposomes of various compositions have been used successfully (Eppstein et al., 1990, Gregoriadis, 1990).

Multilamellar vesicles can be lyophilized. A process has been described for making dehydration-rehydration vesicles (DRV) with a high yield of antigen entrapment under mild experimental conditions (Kirby and Gregoriadis, 1984).

The adjuvant activity of liposomes has been widely demonstrated by using a variety of bacterial, viral, parasitic, and tumor antigens (Gregoriadis, 1990). Moreover, incorporation within liposomes greatly reduces the amount of antigen required to induce an immune response. Interestingly enough, incorporation into liposomes has been shown to improve the immunogenicity of synthetic subunit peptides. An example, already mentioned, is provided by gD1-23 of HSV-1. It must be noted that only humoral immunity was increased by using the liposomal peptide. Cell-mediated immunity and protective immunity were only induced by the simultaneous addition of another immunomodulator (Brynestad et al., 1990). Indeed, the activity of classical adjuvants is greatly increased by their incorporation within antigen-bearing liposomes. Antigens incorporated into liposomes under well-defined conditions have also been reported to elicit increased cell-mediated responses (Gregoriadis, 1990).

Liposomes have been used as an effective delivery system for anti-idiotypic antibodies. Gastric intubation of liposomes containing anti-idiotype antibodies, specific for antibodies directed at *Streptococcus mutans,* stimulates salivary IgA response and protection. It was suggested that such a process could be exploited to augment immune responses to pathogens of mucosal surfaces (Jackson et al., 1990). It is noteworthy that liposomal antigens can be administered by a variety of routes including the oral route which leads to increased IgA immunity.

There is not, in general, a clear-cut modification of isotype distribution by incorporation into liposomes. However, it has been reported that repeated intraperitoneal injection of an allergen entrapped in liposomes can suppress the IgE response and induce an IgG response to the allergen. This could be of interest for the treatment of allergic diseases (Arora and Gangal, 1990).

In conclusion, liposomes constitute a very safe and promising means for increasing the immunogenicity of a wide variety of antigens. Their adjuvanticity can be modulated and optimized by a number of factors including lipid composition and antigen localization. Furthermore, addition of other immunomodulators and attachment of ligands at their surface to favor their interaction with a determined component of the immune system can further enhance their efficacy.

Nonionic Block Polymer Surfactants

Pluronic polyols are chemically defined nonionic block polymer surfactants. These surface-active agents are composed of hydrophobic polyoxypropylene (POP) flanked by two polymers of hydrophilic polyoxyethylene (POE). Different triblock $(POE)_a$-$(POP)_b$-$(POE)_a$ and octablock polymers, obtained by varying the size and the ratios of POP and POE, were used to define the role of the hydrophile-lipophile balance (HLB) in the biological activity (Hunter and Bennett 1984; Hunter et al., 1981). A correlation was found between the HLB of surfactants and their adjuvant activity on the immune response to BSA, following their injection in mice as an oil-in-water emulsion. All of the surfactants with strong adjuvanticity have HLB values of less than 2. This is the case of the large hydrophobic polyols such as triblocks L101 and L121 which contain 10% of POE. The large hydrophilic surfactants such as P103 and F108, containing 30 and 80%, respectively, of POE, did not stimulate antibody formation. L121 was fully adjuvant-active in stimulating antibody response, whereas L101 was more efficient in inducing granulomas. The adjuvant activity of block polymers has also been demonstrated to be correlated to their ability to promote retention of immunogens by oil droplets, which is an important component of the biologic activity of surface-active adjuvants.

Further results have been reported showing that L101, when used in an oil-in-water emulsion, is as effective as FCA or alum in increasing the production of antibodies against a synthetic peptide 9 to 21 of glycoprotein D of HSV-1 conjugated to ovalbumin. Moreover, a significant DTH reaction against purified HSV-1 virions was observed in mice immunized in the presence of L101 (Geerligs et al., 1989). Howerton et al. (1990) recently reported that the copolymer L81 in phosphate-buffered saline (PBS) induced the expression of macrophage Ia antigens *in vivo*. Indeed, L81-induced macrophages were found 10-fold more effective than normal macrophages in presenting antigen to a T-cell hybridoma. It was thus concluded that the induction of Ia expression by L81 may play a role in its immunoadjuvanticity.

A new Syntex Adjuvant Formulation (SAF), shown to be safe and efficacious when used with various antigens in several species of laboratory animals, including monkeys, was used to enhance the antibody response to influenza B virus hemagglutinin (HA). SAF consists of N-acetylmuramyl-L-threonyl-D-isoglutamine (Thr-MDP) and an emulsion of squalane, block polymer L121, and Tween 80 in PBS (Byars et al., 1990). SAF was found effective in priming mice and guinea pigs for an early and strong secondary response, following infection or a challenge with HA. This effect was obtained even in young and old animals, whose response to HA in saline was poor and inconsistent. Moreover, it was found that antibodies against human BSA injected in SAF are predominantly of the IgG2a isotype instead of the IgG1 isotype induced by the same antigen in alum.

Microparticles

Recently a number of engineered polymers have been proposed for a better delivery of drugs and antigens (Langer, 1990; O'Hagan, 1990). They consist of biodegradable microparticles of various composition from which antigen is slowly released over a prolonged period of time. In addition, polymer degradation products have been designed with adjuvant properties. An example is an L-tyrosine-based polyiminocarbonate which, upon *in vivo* degradation, releases a tyrosine ester. The immune response of mice administered with antigen incorporated in this copolymer was greatly increased (Kohn et al., 1986). Microspheres have been used successfully for parenteral as well as enteral immunizaiton, e.g., biodegradable and biocompatible poly(DL-lactide-*co*-glycolide) microspheres when administered orally with antigen in mice have been shown to induce both a systemic and a secretory IgA antibody response (Eldridge et al., 1989).

NATURAL AND BACTERIAL ADJUVANTS
Interleukins

It is difficult to call adjuvant a physiologic mediator of immune processes; we have, thus, chosen to mention only interleukin 1 (IL-1) from which a nonapeptide was identified as an active site, synthesized, and shown to have adjuvant properties.

The adjuvant activity of IL-1 *in vivo* was first demonstrated by Staruch and Wood (1983) and repeatedly observed. IL-1 has also been shown to behave as a systemic adjuvant in active immunotherapy. Mice were injected with irradiated weakly immunogenic syngeneic lung cancer tumor cells and received IL-1β locally or systemically within 10 days. Mice vaccinated with IL-1β were 70—100% tumor-free instead of 0 to 20% as control mice receiving the vaccine alone (McCune and Marquis, 1990). The early use of IL-1 as an adjuvant, however, was restricted because of its wide range of biological activities, including pyrogenicity and inflammatory effects. Later, the finding that a nonapeptide corresponding to residues 163 to 171 of IL-1β could mediate the stimulatory activity of IL-1, while being devoid of toxicity, permitted its general use. Indeed, the nonapeptide increased both primary and secondary responses to antigens (Nencioni et al., 1987) and to tumor antigens (McCune and Marquis, 1990).

Glucan

Glucan, a carbohydrate isolated from the inner cell wall of *Saccharomyces cerevisiae*, is a β-1,3-polyglucose. It has been shown to be a potent adjuvant when combined with a variety of parasite vaccines, including *Trypanosoma cruzi*, the causative agent of Chagas' disease. Results showed that glucan injected subcutaneously in conjunction with killed *T. cruzi* will exert a small but significant protection against *T. cruzi* infection over a wide challenge range (Williams et al., 1989). Glucan has also been used in combination with various antigen fractions of *L. donovani* promastigotes in an attempt to achieve complete protection of animals vaccinated against leishmaniasis. A significant increase in both humoral and cell-mediated immune responses has been observed. Moreover, a microsomal fraction has provided a significant protective immunity against infection only when combined with glucan (Obaid et al., 1989).

Bacterial Lipids

The lipopolysaccharides (LPS) isolated from the cell walls of gram-negative bacteria are potent immunomodulators. They elicit a wide range of biological effects such as activation of macrophages, polyclonal as well as specific activation of B cells, with induction of proliferation and differentiation to antibody-secreting cells. LPS, however, cause severe side effects (see Westphal et al., 1986). The adjuvant activity of bacterial LPS, first described by Johnson et al. (1956), has long been attributed to the lipid A portion of the molecule obtained by mild acid hydrolysis. The basic structure of lipid A consists of a β-1,6-linked D-glucosamine disaccharide N-acylated with (R)-3-hydroxytetradecanoyl groups and esterified by fatty acids and phosphoryl groups. This was confirmed by the total synthesis of lipid A and analogs, first described by Yasuda et al. (1982) and characterized by Ribi et al. (1982). In addition, several laboratories have successfully detoxified LPS or lipid A obtained from cell walls of various bacterial species. These retain their immunostimulatory properties but are devoid of toxicity.

Monophosphoryl lipid A (MPL) represents such a compound. Studies on the cellular and molecular basis of MPL adjuvanticity were reported. MPL has been shown to increase antibody production against sheep erythrocytes in aging mice by inducing T-helper cells to secrete γ-IFN; this lymphokine then activates macrophages to release IL-1, thereby resulting in increased responsiveness throughout the ensuing sequence of cellular and molecular events leading to antibody synthesis (Tomai and Johnson, 1989). In other studies, the antibody response to type III pneumococcal polysaccharide (SSS-III) has been shown to be increased by MPL. This adjuvant activity has been attributed to a stimulation of amplifier T cells which interact with suppressor T cells in an opposing and competitive manner to regulate the magnitude of the antibody response. MPL acts mainly to eliminate the inhibitory effects normally induced by suppressor T cells. In parallel studies, trehalose dimycolate (TDM) also increases the IgM antibody response to SSS-III, probably by a different mechanism because the effect produced by the combination of MPL with TDM was synergistic rather than additive (Baker et al., 1989). With the Ribi adjuvant system (RAS), which consists of a squalene-in-water emulsion supplemented with MPL and TDM, high antipeptide antibody response has been obtained after immunization with a synthetic peptide comprising residues 9 to 21 of glycoprotein D of HSV-1 coupled to ovalbumin. Moreover, a significant protective immunity against challenge with a lethal dose of HSV-1 has been observed (Geerligs et al., 1989).

Muramylpeptides

Natural muramylpeptides which are an ubiquitous constituent of bacterial cell walls and synthetic muramyldipeptide (MDP) can replace mycobacteria in FCA. Thus, antigens injected with MDP in FIA elicit high antibody levels and delayed hypersensitivity (Ellouz et al., 1974).

However, mineral oil or a substitute is essential for the full expression of the adjuvanticity of MDP *in vivo*. Therefore, several hundred derivatives of MDP have been synthesized in order to define the structure-activity relationship and with the goal of obtaining an analog of MDP which would be effective in the absence of mineral oil and present a reduced spectrum of biological effects (see Adam, 1985; Adam and Lederer, 1984, 1988). Indeed, some of the properties of MDP, including macrophage activation, are of potential interest for stimulating nonspecific immunity but not necessarily for augmenting the specific immune response to a given antigen (Byars and Allison, 1987); others are unacceptable for therapeutic uses. These include pyrogenicity and induction of arthritis in rats (Nagao and Tanaka, 1980) or uveitis in rabbits (Waters et al., 1986). Simple structural modifications can, however, modulate the properties of the starting molecule, and in particular suppress its pyrogenicity. We will mention only the most commonly used MDP derivatives.

Nor-MDP (*N*-acetyldesmethylmuramyl-L-alanyl-D-isoglutamine) has been used in an antifertility vaccine. It consists of a synthetic peptide corresponding to residues 109 to 145 of the β-subunit of human chorionic gonadotropin hormone, coupled to diphtheria toxin, emulsified in squalene-arlacel, and containing nor-MDP as adjuvant. This vaccine, first tested on female baboons, has been administered to human volunteers in Australia and found to be safe and effective (Jones et al., 1988).

Thr-MDP (*N*-acetylmuramyl-L-threonyl-D-isoglutamine), included in the SAF, is proposed as a promising substitute for MDP in FIA (Byars et al., 1990). Thr-MDP appears to be more effective than MDP as an adjuvant, whereas it is a 100 times less effective than MDP in pyrogenicity assays and induction of uveitis. Moreover, Thr-MDP does not affect nonspecific immunity. Similarly to MDP, it has to be included in an oily vehicle for an optimal adjuvant effect. A formulation with an efficacy comparable to that of FIA, but acceptable for clinical use, has been proposed: it consists of a stable oil-in-water emulsion of squalane (the saturated form which is a precursor of cholesterol) in pluronic polymer L121. SAF, which contains Thr-MDP, appears to be a very potent adjuvant devoid of major side effects (Byars and Allison, 1987). It increases both humoral and cellular immunity to a variety of antigens, including viral and tumoral antigens (Eppstein et al., 1990).

Murabutide (*N*-acetylmuramyl-L-alanyl-D-glutamine-*n*-butylester) has been developed by Choay Laboratories (Chedid et al., 1982) as a nonpyrogenic derivative of MDP, exhibiting most of the other properties of the parent molecule.

Another alternative to the use of FIA is the encapsulation within multilamellar vesicles. In addition, the attachment of acyl side chains to muramyl peptides makes the molecule more lipophilic, resulting in a prolonged intracellular residence time. A number of acyl derivatives, such as muroctasin (MDP-Lys-L-18), have been developed, essentially by Japanese laboratories (Azuma and Yamamura, 1989).

MTP-PE (MDP-L-alanylphosphatidylethanolamine) can be incorporated into liposomes with a high degree of efficiency. A stable reproducible preparation of liposomal MTP-PE has been produced for clinical use in humans by Ciba-Geigy Laboratories (Van Hoogevest and Frankhauser, 1989). Liposomal MTP-PE has been used in a subunit vaccine against HSV-1 infection. The antigen used was an acyl peptide containing gD1-23 of HSV-1. The presence of MTP-PE increased antibody levels and induced cellular immunity and a 70% protection of mice against lethal challenge. Adding MPL to this preparation conferred 100% protection (Brynestad et al., 1990). Sanchez-Pescador et al. (1988) have reported that MTP-PE in an oily formulation was as potent as FCA. They used as an antigen a recombinant glycoprotein D of HSV-1 termed rgD1. Several conventional adjuvants were compared for their efficacy. Optimal results were obtained when guinea pigs were injected in footpads 4 weeks before viral challenge with FCA or MTP-PE emulsified with squalene and 0.008% Tween 80. It is noteworthy that in these experiments, immunization with alum-rgD1 or with MDP covalently conjugated to rgD1 has shown little effect. This is in contrast with other findings reporting the use of MDP-antigen conjugates as effective immunogens with built-in adjuvanticity (Shapira et al., 1985).

A synthetic construct termed T1-SP10 which contains T- and B-cell epitopes from HTLV III B envelope gp120 was used to immunize rhesus monkeys. Four different adjuvants, in SAF formulation were compared: alum, poly(A:U), FIA, and Thr-MDP. Except for poly(A:U), the three adjuvants induced high levels of peptide-specific antibodies. FIA and Thr-MDP were the most effective in eliciting an HIV-specific neutralizing antibody response and a proliferative response of PBMC to the T1-SP10 and to gp120. Apparently, neither Thr-MDP nor FIA plus T1-SP10 peptide induced any toxic side effects. T1-SP10 contains epitopes recognized by neutralizing antibody, Th cells, and MHC class I and class II CTL. Hart et al. (1990) suggest that this peptide plus Thr-MDP could be a valuable HIV vaccine candidate.

The pleiotropism of muramylpeptides has been widely demonstrated and it is difficult to delineate which activities are directly responsible for the adjuvant effect. It is clear that macrophages, which play an important role in antigen processing and presentation and release a number of factors that are involved in the elaboration of an immune response, could be of importance for the mediation of the adjuvant effect. Thr-MDP, however, is a strong adjuvant and is reported as not being a macrophage activator (Eppstein et al., 1990).

It has been shown that purified B cells, cultivated in the presence of recombinant IL-2, can be stimulated by MDP to produce an optimal specific antibody response. These findings suggest that B cells could be the essential target for the adjuvant effect of muramylpeptides (Souvannavong et al., 1990). They are in agreement with recent results, showing that human tonsillar B cells could be immunized *in vitro* against various antigens in the presence of IL-2 provided MDP was added to the culture (Carroll et al., 1990). Flow cytometric analyses have shown that, although MDP was inefficient in triggering B cells to move out of the resting G_0 state, it was able to act on once-stimulated B cells, leading to an increased frequency of cells in the late G_1 (G_{1B}), S and G_2/M phases of the cell cycle (Souvannavong et al., 1990). Furthermore, MDP has been shown to markedly increase LPS-induced expression of alkaline phosphatase activity. This suggests that protein phosphorylation-dephosphorylation mechanisms could play an important role in MDP-mediated B cell activation (Souvannavong and Adam, 1990).

CONCLUSION

It is clear that with the impact of molecular technology, pure antigens and even epitopes recognized selectively by antibodies, T-helper cells, cytotoxic T cells, or T suppressor cells will be identified. Synthesis of new antigens containing chosen epitopes is now possible and a number of versatile formulations are available which provide help in focusing antigens and immunocompetent cells. New immunomodulators, apparently devoid of toxicity, are capable of further enhancing the immune response and, moreover, of orienting the type of response. It should be possible, in the near future, to design new artificial antigens that possess adequate immunogenicity.

SUMMARY

Complex antigens such as live infectious agents are often immunogenic and generally confer a protective immunity against reinfection. The challenge to investigators has been to produce a similar immune response using simple antigens from pure subunit molecules down to B-cell and T-cell epitopes. Small peptides which constitute such epitopes, however, are often poorly immunogenic by themselves or elicit the wrong type of immune response. In this chapter, we review the various approaches available for restoring and increasing an immune response to small antigens. A prerequisite is to restitute some complexity for efficient targeting to, and processing by, antigen-presenting cells. This can be achieved by coupling to a carrier or by polymerization; the use of viral vectors in order to mimic natural agents is also a valuable method. The general ways for increasing immunogenicity of a given antigen include precipitation with alum gels, inclusion into biodegradable microparticles, and association with oily vehicles such as liposomes and immunostimulating complexes (ISCOMs). Finally, the immune response can further be increased by the simultaneous use of immunomodulators such as muramylpeptides, lipopolysaccharides, and glycans. Promising results have been obtained showing that B-cell and T-cell epitopes, when appropriately manipulated, can elicit humoral as well as T-cell responses.

REFERENCES

Adam, A. (1985) Synthetic adjuvants. In *Modern Concepts in Immunology*. Vol. 1, (C. A. Bona, ed.), Wiley-Interscience, NY, 1—239.

Adam, A., and Lederer, E. (1984) Muramyl peptides: immunomodulators, sleep factors and vitamins. *Med. Res. Rev.* 4:111.

Adam, A., and Lederer, E. (1988) Muramylpeptides as immunomodulators. *ISI Atlas Sci. Immunol.* 1:205.

Adams, S. E., Dawson, K. M., Gull, K., Kingsman, S. M., and Kingsman, A. J. (1987) The expression of hybrid HIV: ty virus-like particles in yeast. *Nature (London)* 329:68.

Allison, A. C., and Gregoriadis, G. (1974) Liposomes as immunological adjuvants. *Nature (London)* 252:252.

Arora, N., and Gangal, S. V. (1990) Allergen entrapped in liposomes reduce allergenicity and induce immunogenicity on repeated injections in mice. *Int. Arch. Allergy Appl. Immunol.* 91:22.

Azuma, I., and Yamamura, Y. (1989) Immunoadjuvants for vaccine. *Adv. Immunopharmacol.* 4:149.

Baker, P. J., Fauntleroy, M. B., Stashak, P. W., Hiernaux, J. R., Cantrell, J. L., and Rudbach, J. A. (1989) Adjuvant effects of trehalose dimycolate on the antibody response to type III pneumococcal polysaccharide. *Infect. Immun.* 57:912.

Beck, L., and Spiegelberg, H. L. (1989) The polyclonal and antigen-specific IgE and IgG subclass response of mice injected with ovalbumin in alum or complete Freund's adjuvant. *Cell. Immunol.* 123:1.

Berman, P. W., Gregory, T. J., Ridle, L., Nakamura, G. R., Champe, M. A., Porter, J. P., Wurm, F. M., Hershberg, R. D., Cobb, E. K., and Eichberg, J. W. (1990) Protection of chimpanzees from infection by HIV-1 after vaccination with recombinant glycoprotein gp120 but not gp160. *Nature (London)* 345:622.

Bomford, R. (1986) Mineral gel adjuvants: why has it taken so long to find an alternative. In *Progress Towards Better Vaccines,* (R. Bell, and G. Torrigiani, eds.), Oxford. Med., NY, 177—184.

Bomford, R. (1989) Saponins as immunoadjuvants. *NATO ASI Ser.* 179:43.

Brynestad, K., Babbitt, B., Huang, L., and Rouse, B. T. (1990) Influence of peptide acylation, liposome incorporation, and synthetic immunomodulators on the immunogenicity of a 1-23 peptide of glycoprotein D of herpes simplex virus: implications for subunit vaccines. *J. Virol.* 64:680.

Byars, N. E., and Allison, A. C. (1987) Adjuvant formulation for use in vaccines to elicit both cell-mediated and humoral immunity. *Vaccine* 5:223.

Byars, N. E., Allison, A. C., Harmon, M. W., and Kendal, A. P. (1990) Enhancement of antibody responses to influenza B virus haemagglutinin by use of a new adjuvant formulation. *Vaccine* 8:49.

Carroll, K., Prosser, E., and O'Kennedy, R. (1990) Parameters involved in the *in vitro* immunization of tonsillar lymphocytes: effects of rIL-2 and muramyl dipeptide. *Hybridoma* 9:81.

Chedid, L., Parant, M. A., Audibert, F. M., Riveau, G. J., Parant, F. J., Lederer, E., Choay, J. P., and Lefrancier, P. L. (1982) Biological activity of a new synthetic muramyl dipeptide adjuvant devoid of pyrogenicity. *Infect. Immun.* 35:417.

Coulaud, E. (1935) Etat allergique durable obtenu chez les animaux de laboratoire par injection sous-cutanée de bacilles turberculeux morts enrobés dans la paraffine solide. *Rev. Tuberc.* 2:851.

Deres, K., Schild, H., Wiesmüller, K.-H., Jung, G., and Rammensee, H.-G. (1989) *In vivo* priming of virus-specific cytotoxic T lymphocytes with synthetic lipopeptide vaccine. *Nature (London)* 342:561.

Eldridge, J. H., Meulbroek, J. A., Staas, J. K., Tice, T. R., and Gilley, R. M. (1989) Vaccine-containing biodegradable microspheres specifically enter the gut-associated lymphoid tissue following oral administration and induce a disseminated mucosal immune response. *Adv. Exp. Med. Biol.* 251:191.

Ellouz, F., Adam, A., Ciorbaru, R., and Lederer, E. (1974) Minimal structural requirements for adjuvant activity of bacterial peptidoglycan derivatives. *Biochem. Biophys. Res. Commun.* 59:1317.

Eppstein, D. A., Byars, N. E., and Allison, A. C. (1990) New adjuvants for vaccines containing purified protein antigens. *Adv. Drug. Delivery Rev.* 4:233.

Etlinger, H. M., Gillessen, D., Lahm, H.-W., Matile, H., Schönfeld, H.-J., and Trzeciak, A. (1990) Use of prior vaccinations for the development of new vaccines. *Science* 249:423.

Flebbe, L. M., and Braley-Mullen, H. (1986) Immunopotentiating effects of the adjuvants SGP and Quil A. I. Antibody responses to T-dependent and T-independent antigens. *Cell. Immunol.* 99:119.

Frasca, D., Boraschi, D., Baschieri, S., Bossu, P., Tagliabue, A., Adorini, L., and Doria, G. (1988) *In vivo* restoration of T cell functions by human IL-1β or its 163-171 nonapeptide in immunodepressed mice. *J. Immunol.* 141:2651.

Freund, J., Casals, J., and Hosmer, E. P. (1937) Sensibilization and antibody formation after injection of tubercle bacilli and paraffin oil. *Proc. Soc. Exp. Biol. Med.* 37:509.

Geerligs, H. J., Weijer, W. J., Welling, G. W., and Welling-Wester, S. (1989) The influence of different adjuvants on the immune response to a synthetic peptide comprising amino acid residues 9-21 of herpes simplex virus type 1 glycoprotein D. *J. Immunol. Meth.* 124:95.

Glenny, A. T., Pope, C. G., Waddington, H., and Wallance, U. (1926) Antigenic value of toxoid precipitated by potassium alum. *J. Pathol. Bacteriol.* 29:38.

Gregoriadis, G. (1990) Immunological adjuvants: a role for liposomes. *Immunol. Today* 11:89.

Griffiths, E. (1990) Immunization. Editorial overview. *Curr. Opin. Infect. Dis.* 3:265.

Grun, J. L., and Maurer, P. H. (1989) Different T helper cell subsets elicited in mice utilizing two different adjuvant vehicles: the role endogenous interleukin 1 in proliferative responses. *Cell. Immunol.* 121:134.

Hart, M. K., Palker, T. J., Matthews, T. J., Langlois, A. J., Lerche, N. W., Martin, M. E., Scearce, R. M., McDanal, C., Bolognesi, D. P., and Haynes, B. F. (1990) Synthetic peptides containing T and B cell epitopes from human immunodeficiency virus envelope gp120 induce anti-HIV proliferative responses and high titers of neutralizing antibodies in rhesus monkeys. *J. Immunol.* 145:2677.

Herzenberg, L. A., and Tokuhisa, T. (1982) Epitope-specific regulation. I. Carrier-specific induction of suppression for IgG anti-hapten antibody responses. *J. Exp. Med.* 155:1730.

Höglund, S., Dalsgaard, K., Lövgren, K., Sundquist, B., Osterhaus, A., and Morein, B. (1989) ISCOMs and immunostimulation with viral antigens. *Subcell. Biochem.* 15:39.

Howerton, D. A., Hunter, R. L., Ziegler, H. K., and Check, I. J. (1990) Induction of macrophage Ia expression *in vivo* by a synthetic block copolymer, L81. *J. Immunol.* 144:1578.

Hunter, R., Strickland, F., and Kézdy, F. (1981) The adjuvant activity of nonionic block polymer surfactants. I. The role of hydrophile-lipophile balance. *J. Immunol.* 127:1244.

Hunter, R. L., and Bennett, B. (1984) The adjuvant activity of nonionic block polymer surfactants. II. Antibody formation and inflammation related to the structure of triblock and octablock copolymers. *J. Immunol.* 133:3167.

Jackson, S., Mestecky, J., Childers, N. K., and Michalek, S. M. (1990) Liposomes containing anti-idiotypic antibodies: an oral vaccine to induce protective secretory immune responses specific for pathogens of mucosal surfaces. *Infect. Immun.* 58:1932.

Johnson, A. G., Gaines, S., and Landy, M. (1956) Studies on the O antigen of *Salmonella typhosa*. V. Enhancement of the antibody response to protein antigens by the purified lipopolysaccharide. *J. Exp. Med.* 103:225.

Jolivet, M., Lise, L., Gras-Masse, H., Tartar, A., Audibert, F., and Chedid, L. (1990) Polyvalent synthetic vaccines: relationship between T epitopes and immunogenicity. *Vaccine* 8:35.

Jones, W. R., Bradley, J., Judd, S. J., Denholm, E. H., Ing, R. M. Y., Mueller, V. W., Powell, J., Griffin, P. D., and Stevens, V. C. (1988) Phase I clinical trial of a world health organization birth control vaccine. *Lancet* 11:1295.

Kirby, C., and Gregoriadis, G. (1984) Dehydration-rehydration vesicles: a simple method for high yield drug entrapment in liposomes. *Biotechnology* 2:979.

Kohn, J., Niemi, S. M., Albert, E. C., Murphy, J. C., Langer, R., and Fox, J. G. (1986) Single-step immunization using a controlled release, biodegradable polymer with sustained adjuvant activity. *J. Immunol. Meth.* 95:31.

Langer, R. (1990) New methods of drug delivery. *Science* 249:1527.

Levely, M. E., Mitchell, M. A., and Nicholas, J. A. (1990) Synthetic immunogens constructed from T-cell and B-cell stimulating peptides (T:B chimeras): preferential stimulation of unique T- and B-cell specificities is influenced by immunogen configuration. *Cell. Immunol.* 125:65.

McCune, C. S., and Marquis, D. M. (1990) Interleukin 1 as an adjuvant for active specific immunotherapy in a murine tumor model. *Cancer Res.* 50:1212.

Miller, J. F. A. P. (1989) Immune response. Editorial overview. *Curr. Opin. Immunol.* 2:187.

Millich, D. R., McLachlan, A., Moriarty, A., and Thornton, B. (1987) Immune response to hepatitis B core antigen (HBcAg): localization of T cell recognition sites within HBcAg/HBeAg. *J. Immunol.* 139:1223.

Morein, B., Helenius, A., Simons, K., Pettersson, R., Kääriäinen, L., and Schirrmacher, V. (1978) Effective subunit vaccines against an enveloped animal viruses. *Nature (London)* 276:715.

Morein, B., Sundquist, B., Höglund, S., Dalsgaard, K., and Osterhaus, A. (1984) Iscom, a novel structure for antigenic presentation of membrane proteins from enveloped viruses. *Nature (London)* 308:457.

Morein, B., Lövgren, K., Höglund, S., and Sundquist, B. (1987) The ISCOM: an immunostimulating complex. *Immunol. Today* 8:333.

Morein, B., Ekström, J., and Lövgren, K. (1990) Increased immunogenicity of a non-amphipathic protein (BSA) after inclusion in iscoms. *J. Immunol. Meth.* 128:177.

Nagao, S., and Tanaka, A. (1980) Muramyl dipeptide-induced adjuvant arthritis. *Infect. Immun.* 28:62.

Nencioni, L., Villa, L., Tagliabue, A., Antoni, G., Presentini, R., Perin, F., Silvestri, S., and Boraschi, D. (1987) *In vivo* immunostimulating activity of the 163-171 peptide of human IL-1β. *J. Immunol.* 139:800.

Obaid, K. A., Ahmad, S., Khan, H. M., Mahdi, A. A., and Khanna, R. (1989) Protective effect of *L. donovani* antigens using glucan as an adjuvant. *Int. J. Immunopharmacol.* 11:229.

O'Hagan, D. T. (1990) Novel nonreplicating antigen delivery systems. *Curr. Opin. Infect. Dis.* 3:393.

Ramon, G. (1926) Procédé pour accroître la production des antitoxines *Ann. Inst. Pasteur.* 40:1.

Ribi, E., Amano, K., Cantrell, J., Schwartzman, S., Parker, R., and Takayama, K. (1982) Preparation and antitumor activity of nontoxic lipid A. *Cancer Immunol. Immunother.* 12:91.

Sanchez-Pescador, L., Burke, R. L., Ott, G., and Van Nest, G. (1988) The effects of adjuvants on the efficacy of a recombinant herpes simplex virus glycoprotein vaccine. *J. Immunol.* 141:1720.

Shapira, M., Jolivet, M., and Arnon, R. (1985) A synthetic vaccine against influenza with built-in adjuvanticity. *Int. J. Immunopharmacol.* 7:719.

Souvannavong, V., and Adam, A. (1990) Increased expression of alkaline phosphatase activity in stimulated B lymphocytes by muramyl dipeptide. *Immunol. Lett.* 29:247.

Souvannavong, V., Brown, S., and Adam, A. (1990) Muramyl dipeptide (MDP) synergizes with interleukin 2 and interleukin 4 to stimulate, respectively, the differentiation and proliferation of B cells. *Cell. Immunol.* 126:106.

Staruch, M. J., and Wood, D. D. (1983) The adjuvanticity of interleukin 1 *in vivo, J. Immunol.* 130:2191.

Takahashi, H., Takeshita, T., Morein, B., Putney, S., Germain, R. N. and Berzofsky, J. A. (1990) Induction of CD8+ cytotoxic T cells by immunization with purified HIV-1 envelope protein in ISCOMs. *Nature (London)* 344:873.

Tomai, M. A., and Johnson, A. G. (1989) T cell and interferon-γ involvement in the adjuvant action of a detoxified endotoxin. *J. Biol. Response Mod.* 8:625.

Van Hoogevest, P., and Frankhauser, A. (1989) An industrial liposomal dosage form for muramyl-tripeptide-phosphatidylethanolamine (MTP-PE). In *Liposomes in the Therapy of Infectious Diseases and Cancer,* Vol. 89, (G. Lopez-Berestein, and I. J. Fidler, eds.), Alan R. Liss, NY, 117—125.

Waters, R. V., Terrell, T. G., and Jones, G. H. (1986) Uveitis induction in the rabbit by muramyl dipeptides. *Infect. Immun.* 51:816.

Westphal, O., Luderitz, O., Galanos, C., Mayer, H., and Rietschel, E. T. (1986) The story of endotoxin. *Adv. Immunopharmacol.* 3:13.

Williams, D. L., Yaeger, R. G., Pretus, H. A., Browder, I. W., McNamee, R. B., and Jones, E. L. (1989) Immunization against *Trypanosoma cruzi:* adjuvant effect of glucan. *Int. J. Immunopharmacol.* 11:403.

Yamaya, S.-I., Yamamoto, A., Komiya, T., Mizuguchi, J., and Matuhasi, T. (1990) Preparation of a diphtheria toxin-pollulan conjugate that elicits good IgG antibody production with poor IgE synthesis. *Vaccine* 8:65.

Yasuda, T., Kanegasaki, S., Tsumita, T., Takakuma, T., Homma, J. Y., Inage, M., Kusumoto, S., and Shiba, T. (1982) Biological activity of chemically synthesized analogues of Lipid A. Demonstration of adjuvant effect in hapten-sensitized liposomal system. *Eur. J. Biochem.* 124:405.

Chapter 10
Precipitation and Agglutination

Carel J. van Oss
Departments of Microbiology and Chemical Engineering
State University of New York, Buffalo
Buffalo, NY

PRECIPITATION

Solubility of Antigens, Antibodies and Their Complexes

Solubility of Biopolymers

The solubility of proteins and polysaccharides depends mainly on their polar surface properties, i.e., on their hydrophilicity. The electrical surface potential (ζ-potential) of proteins and polysaccharides contributes to their solubility only in the cases of the most highly charged proteins, such as serum albumin ($\zeta = -18$ mV). In the case of proteins and polysaccharides with a value for $\zeta \lesssim 14$ mV, the electrostatic solubility under physiological conditions of pH and ionic strength becomes negligible. For immunoglobulins the ζ-potential is of the order of only a few millivolts. Thus, in all cases of antigen-antibody (Ag-Ab) complex solubility, electrostatic forces play virtually no role, with the rare but possible exception of Ag-Ab complexes with a strong Ag- excess and an unusually high Ag ζ-potential.

Thus, the solubility of molecules of proteins, polysaccharides, Ag-Ab complexes, and other biopolymers depends largely on the interfacial (IF) free energy of interaction between biopolymer molecules, when immersed in water:

$$\Delta G_{iwi}^{IF} = -2\,\gamma_{iw} \qquad (1)$$

where γ_{iw} is the interfacial tension between the biopolymer (i) and water (w).

For solubility it is required that ΔG^{IF}_{iwi} is less negative than $-1kT$ (where k is Boltzmann's constant and T the absolute temperature: $1kT = 4 \times 10^{-14}$ ergs $= 4 \times 10^{-21}$ J), and the most pronounced solubility prevails when $\Delta G^{IF}_{iwi} > 0$ (van Oss and Good, 1989).

Mechanism of Insolubilization of Ag-Ab Complexes

Due to hydration (van Oss et al., 1986), the average ΔG^{IF}_{iwi} value for many biopolymers usually is greater than 0, thus guaranteeing complete solubility, but there usually are somewhat more hydrophobic patches on most biopolymers which makes, when such slightly hydrophobic patches approach each other, that $-1kT < \Delta G^{IF}_{iwi} < 0$. In such cases, solubility still prevails for single molecules of a biopolymer. However, when the molecular size of that biopolymer increases due to complex formation, the situation can change to $\Delta G^{IF}_{iwi} < -1kT$, which results in insolubilization because the attraction between the complexes surpasses their tendency to dissociate through Brownian motion (the free energy of which is approximately $+1$ kT per molecule or particle). For instance, if the free energy of attraction between opposing slightly hydrophobic patches on two protein molecules is $\Delta G^{IF}_{iwi} = -1.0$ mJ/m², and if each of these patches has a contactable surface area, $S_c = 1$ nm², then, in units of kT, $\Delta G^{IF}_{iwi} = -0.25$ kT, which still denotes solubility. However, when complexes arise, which can interact in such a manner that, say, eight such patches can interact, then a total contactable surface area, $S_c = 8$ nm² exists, so that then, $\Delta G^{IF}_{iwi} = -2kT$ which indicates incipient *insolubility*. This shows why, when soluble proteins with a given surface-free energy can form larger complexes (with still the same surface-free energy per unit surface area, but with a *larger surface area*), from a given size on such complexes tend to become insoluble (without the need for a change in surface properties). This has been demonstrated with IgG molecules (as antigens), complexed with similar IgG molecules (as antibodies) (van Oss et al., 1986). Thus complexes formed from perfectly soluble Ag and Ab molecules will become insoluble when they grow beyond a certain size, without the need for a change in structure, conformation, or surface properties of either Ag or Ab. In other words, for many biopolymer or biopolymer complexes, an increase in size suffices to cause insolubilization.

The solubility of biopolymers in water can be enhanced by increasing the number of exposed OH and especially O groups. Such hypersoluble biopolymers, when used as antigens, tend to become toleragenic, e.g., upon insertion of poly(ethylene oxide) groups (Sehon, 1989; Sehon et al., 1987).

Enhancement of Insolubilization of Ag-Ab Complexes

There are a number of approaches that may be used to enhance the insolubilization of biopolymers and, in particular, of soluble Ag-Ab complexes.

Flocculation through Dehydration. This procedure is often used in the guise of "salting out" (van Oss et al., 1985), usually through the admixture of fairly high concentrations of $(NH_4)_2SO_4$ [typically of the order of 1 M $(NH_4)_2SO_4$, or more]. Applied to soluble immune complexes, this approach is known as the Farr technique (Farr, 1958), and is quite effective in all cases where there is no risk of dissociation of the Ag-Ab complex at high salt concentrations. This risk exists mainly in the case of high-affinity DNA-anti-DNA complexes (de Groot et al., 1980; Smeenk and Aarden, 1980; Smeenk et al., 1982, 1983). Thus, with DNA-anti-DNA complexes it is always advisable to use precipitation by means of polyethylene glycol *in addition to salting out* (Smeenk and Aarden, 1980; see below). Precipitation by (cold) ethanol (Schultze and Heremans, 1966) is not frequently applied to Ag-Ab complexes, but the method may also be worth considering when dissociation of Ag from Ab at high salt concentrations could cause problems.

Flocculation through Phase Separation. This procedure is usually done by the admixture of ≈ 2 to 10% polyethylene glycol (PEG) (Schultze and Heremans, 1966). Usually PEG (MW ≈ 6000) concentrations of 2 to 5% are most suitable for the precipitation of soluble immune complexes, but concentrations as high as 7.5% PEG have been found preferable for very small complexes (Albini et al., 1984). For the detection of low-avidity anti-DNA Abs, e.g., in systemic lupus erythematosus, PEG precipitation is the method of choice (Smeenk and Aarden, 1980; see also the preceding section).

One drawback of both flocculation approaches is that aspecifically aggregated proteins (or nucleoproteins), or proteins which coflocculate under the influence of $(NH_4)_2SO_4$ or PEG contaminate the flocculated Ag-Ab complexes (see Albini et al., 1984).

Precipitation in Tubes

Nonstoichiometry of Ag-Ab Complex Formation

Ag-Ab complexes, like other *complex-forming* substances [e.g., aggregates of anionic and cationic surfactants (van Oss, 1984a)] are totally nonstoichiometric, i.e., Ag-Ab complexes can comprise virtually any conceivable Ag:Ab ratio (van Oss, 1984b). At large excess concentrations of either Ag or Ab, usually no precipitate is formed and only soluble Ag-Ab complexes obtain (see Fig. 1). From precipitation experiments in test tubes it became clear that only at an "equivalent" Ag:Ab ratio a maximum amount of precipitate occurs; at slight Ab *or* Ag excess, much less precipitate is obtained; at great Ab *or* Ag excess, no visible precipitate develops at all, although in the latter case the formation of soluble complexes can be detected (e.g., by analytical ultracentrifugation). However, at the "equivalence" Ag:Ab ratio no dissolved Ag *or* Ab can be detected in the supernatant by conventional methods. From Ag-Ab precipitates obtained at "equivalence" ratios, one can only obtain the valency ratios of Ag and Ab by fairly gross approximation; it is only at Ag excess that one can determine the exact valency of the Ab (Edberg et al., 1972), while the exact valency of the Ag is obtainable only at Ab excess; see also Chapter 6.

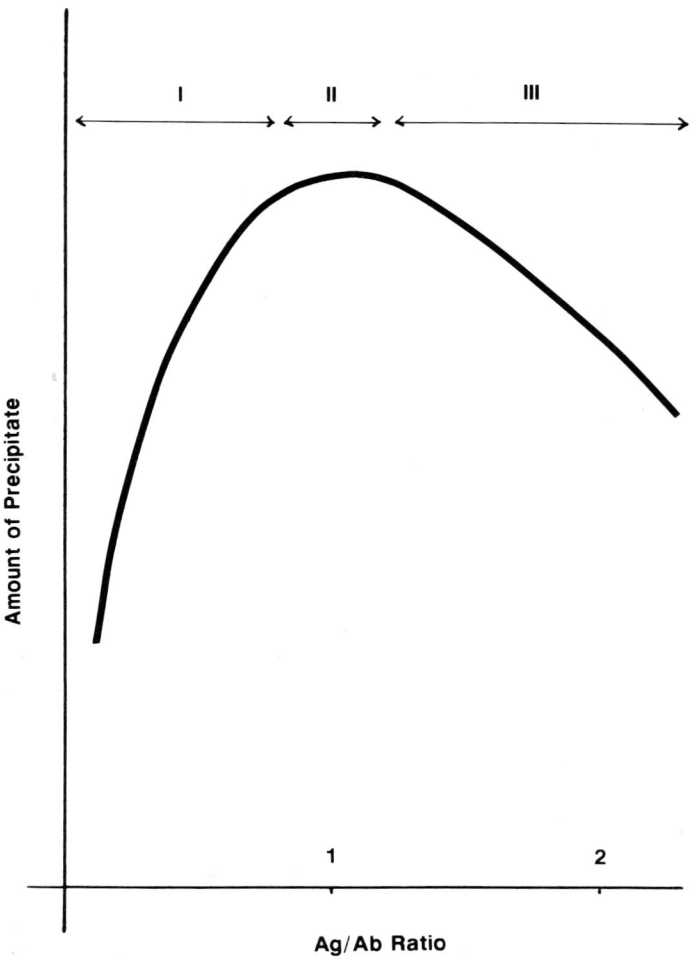

Figure 1. Plot of the amount of immune precipitate formed between a typical protein antigen and its antibody as a function of the Ag:Ab ratio. (I) Ab-excess region; (II) equivalence region; (III) Ag-excess region.

From the 1930s to the early 1960s "equivalent" (or "stoichiometric") points for a wide range of Ag:Ab ratios were obtained by determination of the amount of nitrogen found in the precipitate, measured by the Kjeldahl method; (see Kabat and Mayer, 1961). The amount of "Ab-nitrogen" could only be obtained by immune precipitation of nonproteinaceous antigens (e.g., polysaccharides). With the advent of methods of immune precipitation in gels, the use of test tubes for such procedures have become obsolete, except for a number of automated immunoassay procedures. In standardizing such automated methods, based on free-liquid immune precipitation, it should always be recalled that in all cases where precipitates are obtained that are not exactly at the "equivalence" Ag:Ab ratio, two different amounts of Ag and Ab can give rise to *the same amount of Ag-Ab precipitate* (cf. Fig. 1).

Precipitation by Double Diffusion in Gels

Properties of Precipitates Formed by Double Diffusion in Gels

Ouchterlony (1949; 1968) developed a technique in which solutions of Ag and Ab are deposited in separate wells, punched in an agar gel slab, and allowed to diffuse toward each other. At their place of encounter, a sharp, usually somewhat curved, Ag-Ab precipitate line is formed. That precipitate line actually is a precipitate membrane, or barrier, seen from above. The salient property of that precipitate membrane or barrier is its specific impermeability for both the dissolved Ag and Ab molecules situated on either side of it (van Oss and Heck, 1961). Ag and Ab molecules unrelated to the Ag and Ab that formed the precipitate can freely pass that precipitate — this is why precipitate lines formed with identical Ag-Ab systems *fuse*, whereas such lines made by two unrelated Ag-Ab systems *cross* (van Oss and Heck, 1961). The specific impermeability of the precipitate barrier formed by a given Ag-Ab system persists only as long as approximately equivalent amounts of Ag and of Ab remain present in solution, each on its own side of that barrier. This requirement also furnishes the explanation for the mechanism of specific impermeability, which is based on the fact that the barrier is *self-repairing*, that is, as soon as an accidental hole is formed, some of the soluble Ag present on one side of it will penetrate that hole, but then will immediately encounter an equivalent amount of the soluble Ab present on the other side of the barrier thus forming a precipitate, which again plugs the hole (van Oss and Heck, 1961).

One of the most important consequences of the occurrence of precipitate barriers, which are specifically impermeable only for the Ag-Ab system that formed them, and for no other Ag-Ab system, is that only Ag-Ab barriers (or lines) formed with identical systems will fuse, while barriers (or lines) formed with different systems will *cross* (see Fig. 2). This property not only has proved to be of crucial importance in the characterization of multitudinous antigens (Ouchterlony, 1968), but it also is the key to the usefulness of immunoelectrophoretic analysis (see below) as a powerful approach for detecting the presence of normal and abnormal antigens (Grabar and Burtin, 1964; Ouchterlony, 1968; van Oss and Bartholomew, 1980).

Properties of Precipitate Lines of First Formation

To understand the behavior, formation, evolution, and decay of Ag-Ab precipitate lines formed by double diffusion in gels, it is indispensable to treat the first formation of precipitate lines or barriers as a phenomenon which is separate from their subsequent evolution.

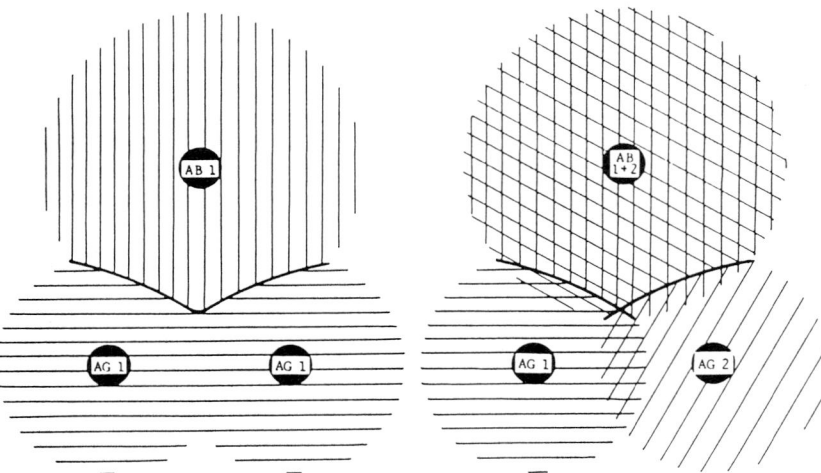

Figure 2. Diagrams of the fusing (left) and crossing (right) of precipitate lines in double immunodiffusion. (Left) When two identical Ags (AG 1), deposited in two different wells, can both precipitate with an Ab (AB 1) from the third well, fusing must occur due to the specific impermeability of the precipitate barrier formed. (Right) When two different Ags (AG 1 and AG 2), deposited in two separate wells, each precipitates with only its own Ab (AB 1 and AB 2, mixed together in the well on top), the precipitate lines cross, since each is part of a completely different system which forms its own self-repairing, specifically impermeable precipitate barrier. (From van Oss, C. J., (1984b), *Molecular Immunology*, Dekker, NY. With permission.)

Ag-Ab precipitate-forming systems, being *complex-forming systems* (see above), tend to start precipitating when their concentrations are at equivalence (E) and have reached a certain *minimum value*. (This is contrary to the precipitation of noncomplex-forming systems, which occur once a *minimum solubility product* is exceeded.) It can be proven that owing to the fact that Ag-Ab precipitation occurs when:

$$C_{Ag} = C_{Ab} = E \qquad (2)$$

the *place* where that precipitate first starts in double diffusion is largely *independent* of the starting concentrations deposited in the respective wells (van Oss, 1968). The place where the Ag-Ab precipitate first forms depends only on the distance $(a + b)$ between the wells and on the diffusion coefficients (D) of Ag and Ab, such that:

$$\frac{a}{b} = \sqrt{\frac{D_{Ag}}{D_{Ab}}} \qquad (3)$$

where a is the distance between the Ag source and the precipitate line and b the distance between the Ab source and the precipitate line. As every point

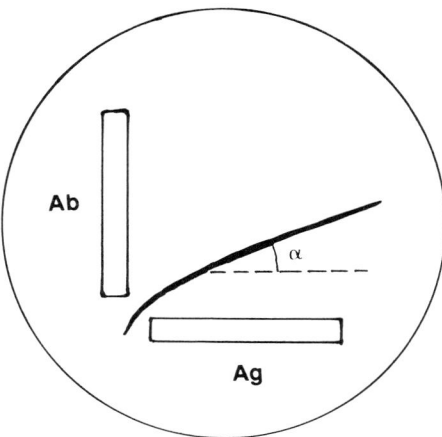

Figure 3. Double immunodiffusion of Ag vs Ab from troughs placed at right angles to one another. The precipitate line forms an angle, α, with a line parallel to the Ag trough, such that $\tan \alpha = \sqrt{D_{Ag}/D_{Ab}}$.

on the precipitate line of first formation has to obey that rule [Eq. (3)], the line of first formation, when the starting points are point-shaped (or small cylindrical) wells, must have the shape of a *circle*, with a radius R:

$$R = \frac{ab}{a - b} \qquad (4)$$

When $D_{Ag} = D_{Ab}$ (which occurs, e.g., in the case of IgG-anti-IgG systems), $a = b$ and $R = \infty$, resulting in a straight line perpendicular to the line connecting the Ag and Ab wells, exactly in the middle between the wells. A point-shaped well vs a linear trough yields parabola-shaped precipitate lines, and two linear troughs give rise to linear precipitate lines (see section on Immunoelectrophoresis below).

Equation (3) is also useful for the determination of the diffusion coefficient of a given Ag, if the diffusion coefficient of the corresponding Ab (or vice versa) is known. The best procedure for such a determination is shown in Fig. 3 in which two perpendicular rectilinear troughs are filled with Ag and Ab, respectively. The precipitate line obtained forms an angle such that (see Allison and Humphrey, 1959).

$$\frac{a}{b} = \tan \alpha = \sqrt{\frac{D_{Ag}}{D_{Ag}}} \qquad (3a)$$

This procedure has the unique possibility of determining the diffusion coefficient of an Ag without actually purifying it, provided that one has some means (e.g., by an enzymic reaction, or by an immunological reaction of identity) to identify the line formed by the Ag. In the application of this method, it is useful to know that for IgG-class antibodies, $D_{Ab} \approx 4 \times 10^{-7}$ cm²/s, at 20°C.

Evolution of Precipitate Line Geometry at Nonequivalence

If a precipitate line is formed when Ag and Ab are present at equivalent concentrations, the precipitate line will indefinitely remain in the same place where it was first formed, and it will stay thin. However, if one of the reagents (A) was present in excess in its starting well, it will ultimately be able to break down the barrier (when the other reagent begins to be exhausted), cross it, and form a new line farther down in the direction of the reagent present in lower concentration (B), with which it will react in a place closer to the starting well of B where some B is still present in solution. Thus the precipitate can do *one* of three things (van Oss and Heck, 1961):

1. It can *thicken* in the direction of the reagent (B) initially present in the lowest concentration.
2. It can form new precipitate lines in the direction of the reagent (B) initially present in the lowest concentration; then, instead of one thick line, *multiple lines* of the Liesegang variety will form.
3. Excess reagent A can dissolve the line of first formation, and form a new precipitate line closer to B; the precipitate line will then appear to *move* in the direction of the reagent (B) present in the lowest concentration.

The visible evolution with time of the place and/or thickness of the precipitate line when one of the reagents is present in excess (in contrast with the line's continuing immobility and thinness when Ag and Ab are present at equivalent concentrations), makes it possible to do a simple determination of the equivalence ratio of a given Ag-Ab system by a double-diffusion titration (Ouchterlony, 1968, p. 32; van Oss, 1968; van Oss and Heck, 1961). Here the equivalence ratio is found to correspond to the wells between which the precipitate line stays *thinnest* and does not migrate. (It is interesting to note that this equivalence ratio, found at the *thinnest line*, corresponds to the point of the curve which coincides with the greatest amount of precipitate obtained in test tubes; see Fig. 1.)

Immunoelectrophoresis

As one frequently observes with two different methods, applied in directions *perpendicular* to each other, the resolution of immunoelectrophoresis is markedly greater than that of electrophoresis alone. Immunoelectrophoresis comprises the electrophoretic separation of an antigen mixture in the first dimension, followed by the characterization of each antigen by double-diffusion precipitation in the direction perpendicular to that of the electrophoresis step (Grabar and Burtin, 1964; Ouchterlony, 1968; van Oss and Bartholomew, 1980). The property of nonidentical antigens to form crossing precipitate lines upon interaction with their corresponding antibodies (even when the antigens still partly overlap after a less than total electrophoretic separation) makes it possible to discriminate between overlapping antigens (Ouchterlony, 1968). The *shape* of the precipitate lines permits the recognition of monoclonality (a parabola-shaped line, e.g., serum albumin) or polyclonality (a fairly straight line, e.g., normal IgG) of the separated fractions (see van Oss and Bartholomew, 1980). Thus, immunoelectrophoresis is especially suited for detecting pathological monoclonal immunoglobulin abnormalities. Due to the electrophoretic dilution effect (compounded by possible electrophoretic heterogeneities of given fractions), immunoelectrophoresis is quantitatively less sensitive than ordinary double-diffusion immunoprecipitation.

Nondiffusion Transport Mechanisms Causing Ag and Ab to Converge

Counterelectrophoresis. Also called crossed-over electrophoresis, electrosyneresis, immunoelectroosmophoresis, or immunoosmophoresis, counterelectrophoresis brings Ag and Ab together by means of electrophoresis. This is only possible at a pH intermediate between the isoelectric points of Ag and Ab; in other words, Ag and Ab must have significantly different isoelectric points for this method to be applicable. The method is faster (precipitate visible in a few hours) and more sensitive (by a factor of about 3 to 4) than double-diffusion precipitation. Contrary to the implication of some of the names proposed for this method (see above), electroosmotic backflow plays *no* role in bringing Ag and Ab together.

Rheophoresis. As a method for bringing Ag and Ab together, rheophoresis or immunorheophoresis works by hydrodynamic transport engendered by the evaporation of solvent through a gap in the cover (on top of the gel chamber) situated exactly above the place (between Ag and Ab) in the gel where the precipitate is to occur. Excess solvent should be provided at both extremities of the gel to furnish liquid for capillary transport through the gel's pores. This method is also relatively fast (precipitate visible in 2 to 4 hr) and more sensitive (by a factor of 3 to 4) than double diffusion, and can be used when Ag and Ab have close or identical isoelectric points (van Oss and Bartholomew, 1980; van Oss and Bronson, 1969; van Oss et al., 1957).

In assays for hepatitis B-associated Ag (HBsAg), or Australia Ag, rheophoresis was found to be as sensitive as the complement fixation test (Jambazian and Holper, 1972).

Precipitation by Single Diffusion in Gels

Monodimensional Single Diffusion in Gels

Single diffusion of Ag solution into a gel containing a very dilute Ab solution, with an aim to producing immunological Liesegang rings (van Oss, 1984a), was first reported by Bechhold (1905). Oudin (1948) began systematic studies with this monodimensional single immunodiffusion approach, extensively reviewing this method in 1971 and in 1980 (Oudin, 1971, 1980). Outside of Oudin's laboratory at the Pasteur Institute in Paris, this approach never became popular, for a number of reasons (van Oss, 1984a):

1. In single diffusion a precipitate barrier forms virtually immediately, and then is transgressed by the more concentrated reagent in the liquid phase, to form another barrier (for a short period of time), to transgress that new barrier in its turn, etc. This makes it difficult to establish a correlation between the molecular diffusion coefficient of the progressing reagent and the rate of progression of a precipitate band (or bands) (see also section on Affinity Precipitation Methods in Gels, below).
2. The possibilities for novel qualitative and quantitative interpretations of Ab-Ag interactions with double diffusion methods are much greater.
3. The geometrical configuration of the bidimensional single-diffusion approach is much more favorable for quantitative determinations (see below).

Affinity Precipitation Methods in Gels

Affinity precipitation methods in gels, such as affinity electrophoresis (Horejsi, 1979, 1981) and affinity diffusion (van Oss et al., 1982a,b), depend on the degree to which, for example, Ag, when migrating into an Ab-containing gel, slows down as a function of Ab concentration. The dissociation constant K_d can be obtained according to

$$\frac{D_o}{D_i} = 1 + \frac{C_i}{K_d} \qquad (5)$$

where D_0 is the electrophoretic mobility (or diffusion coefficient) of Ag in the gel without Ab and D_i the electrophoretic mobility (or diffusion coefficient) of Ag in the gel at Ab concentration C_i. When D_0/D_i is plotted on the ordinate versus C_i on the abscissa, one finds $-K_d$ at the intercept of the (straight) line of the function with the abscissa, or $1/K_d$ as the slope of the line. The zero Ab concentration diffusion coefficient (D_0) of Ag is found by extrapolation to zero Ab concentration (van Oss et al., 1982a). Ideally one can obtain K_a from $1/K_d$ (see Chapter 6) only in totally homogeneous systems, with Ags with only one repeating epitope and with monoclonal Abs (in which case one would not expect precipitation to occur); however, in practice, one can obtain some useful information even in more complex systems. With heterogeneous Ag-Ab systems one finds K_a values (at least with affinity electrophoresis and diffusion methods visualized by an advancing precipitation front) that are several decimal orders of magnitude lower than those found via precipitation in tubes, because the components with the highest K_d value are measured (van Oss et al., 1982b). A further reason for the difference in the values found with affinity and equilibrium systems lies in the fact that affinity methods are kinetic systems, where one does not wait for equilibrium to set in, so that secondary (interfacial) interactions (see Chapter 6) normally have not had time to occur (van Oss, 1984b).

Affinity Electrophoresis. Affinity electrophoresis uses the degree of retardation of the electrophoretic mobility of an Ag in a gel column in which the Ab is bound to (or admixed with) the gel for obtaining equilibrium constants. Various ways of monitoring the rate of advance of Ag in the gel column can be used, including the rate of advance of an Ag-Ab precipitate, in cases where such a precipitate is formed. However, as the degree of retardation of the Ag-Ab precipitate does not necessarily accurately reflect the degree of retardation of the electrophoretic mobility of the bulk of the Ag (under precipitating as well as nonprecipitating conditions), affinity electrophoresis measured by the progression of the Ag-Ab precipitate front contains the risk of yielding erroneous equilibrium constants (van Oss et al., 1982a, b).

Affinity Diffusion. In the same manner in which one uses affinity electrophoresis to measure the equilibrium constants of Ag-Ab interaction (see Chapter 12), one may also use affinity diffusion. In the latter case, one measures the decrease in the diffusion coefficient of the Ag, in the Ab-containing gel, as a function of Ab concentrations (van Oss et al., 1982a). However, as in affinity electrophoresis (see above), if the progression of the Ag-Ab precipitate front is measured for the purpose of deriving the dissociation constant of the Ag-Ab interaction, there is a risk of obtaining erroneous results. The reason for this is that the dissociation constant of exactly those precipitate-forming reagents with the stronger propensity to dissociate (van Oss et al., 1982a,b) are measured; see section on Affinity Precipitation Methods in Gels, on the previous page.

Oudin (1971) noted that, as in molecular diffusion, the rate of progression of Ag-Ab precipitate fronts by single diffusion in Ab-containing gel tubes (with a supply of excess Ag in solution on top of the gel tubes) is proportional to the square root of time. However, the rate of progression of such Ag-Ab precipitate fronts is considerably faster than the rate corresponding to the diffusion coefficient of the Ag in free solution (see also the data given by Oudin, 1971; van Oss et al., 1982a). The explanation of this paradox is relatively simple; the molecular diffusion coefficient of, for example, albumin, as measured by visible or ultraviolet light absorption, is obtained via the progression of the inflection point of the first derivative of the absorption versus distance curve with time, i.e., one measures the rate of progression of the peak of a Gaussian curve. However, the progression of albumin in an antialbumin-containing gel, as judged by the advancing precipitate front, reflects only the diffusivity of the fastest few Ag molecules that can just attain the solubility product necessary to achieve precipitation. These few fast Ag molecules tend to be many times faster than the molecules diffusing with the Gaussian average of the bulk of the Ag (van Oss et al., 1982a).

Bidimensional Single Diffusion in Gels

Radial Immunodiffusion. In single-migration methods, only one of the components (usually the Ag) migrates or diffuses into a gel containing a homogeneous, low concentration of the other component (usually the Ab). The simplest example of this type of method is single diffusion, or radial immunodiffusion (Mancini et al., 1965), in which various concentrations of an Ag solution are deposited in small wells in the Ab-containing gel. The initial concentrations of Ag deposited in the wells must be higher than the Ab concentration of the bulk of the gel for any Ag-Ab precipitate to become visible beyond the confines of the wells (see the section on Evolution of Precipitate Line Geometry at Nonequivalence, above). After the precipitate circle around a well has reached its maximum size, the surface area of that circle (or its diameter squared) is proportional to the amount of Ag deposited in that well. Plots of Ag concentration versus precipitate circle diameter squared, therefore, yield straight lines. This method represents a reliable but slow (24 to 48 hr) method for measuring Ag concentrations (e.g., of various plasma proteins).

Electrophoretic Migration in Antibody-Containing Gels. Instead of waiting for the diffusion of an Ag into an Ag-containing gel to run its slow course, the process can be accelerated by electrophoresing the Ag into the Ab-containing gel until all growth of the rocket-shaped precipitate lines has stopped (Laurell, 1966). The final surface areas of the rockets (or their heights, as the rockets have the shape of triangles with a unit baseline) are proportional to the Ag concentrations. This method, which is somewhat more accurate than radial immunodiffusion (see above), is also about an order of magnitude faster.

Bidimensional electrophoresis in Ab-containing gels (or crossed immunoelectrophoresis) is comparable to immunoelectrophoresis in which the double immunodiffusion step has been replaced by electrophoresis (at right angles to the first electrophoresis step) into an antiserum-containing gel. With complex Ag mixtures, this gives rise to multiple rockets; the surface area under each of these is roughly proportional to the concentration of the corresponding

Ag originally present in the mixture (Laurell, 1965; see also van Oss and Bartholomew 1980).

Sensitivity and Limitations of Immunoprecipation Methods

The sensitivity of immunoprecipitation methods is not exceedingly high. One usually can determine only microgram amounts of Ab, or higher. However, there are no hard and fast rules: with IgG-class Abs, greater sensitivity can be attained than with IgM-class Abs, and with counterelectrophoresis and rheophoresis significantly higher sensitivities can be reached than with ordinary double-immunodiffusion methods. With radial immunodiffusion it is possible to determine Ag amounts in quantities as low as 10 to 20 ng, under favorable conditions.

The size of biopolymers and particles that can be used as Ags in immunoprecipitation varies from the size of small Ags (MW ≈ 10,000) and antibodies (MW ≈ 150,000 to 900,000) to the size of nanoparticles (e.g, viruses such as particles of foot-and-mouth disease virus and its sub-particles; van Oss et al., 1964), or sonicated erythrocyte stromata, which could be analyzed by double-diffusion immunoprecipitation for different blood group epitopes of the Rh family (Milgrom and Loza, 1967).

AGGLUTINATION

Mechanism of Agglutination

Agglutination is one of the oldest methods of demonstrating the occurrence of immune reactions *in vitro* — it is the destabilization of a relatively stable suspension of antigenic particles, by cross-linking them with antibodies directed to their antigenic determinants (epitopes). Because destabilization of antigenic particles can be readily detected with a rather small volume (ca. 0.1 ml of a dilute particle suspension) and because relatively few antibody molecules suffice to achieve destabilization, agglutination is an uncommonly sensitive method for detecting quite small amounts of antibody (as little as a nanogram). The sizes of antigenic particles, used in agglutination, may range from a few nanometers to about 10 μm in diameter. Antigenic particles may be cells (bacteria, red blood cells, etc.) displaying their native epitopes, or inert particles (cells as well as synthetic carriers) to which antigenic molecules have been adsorbed or covalently attached.

Visualization of Agglutination

Sedimentation Rate

According to Stokes' law, the force resisting sedimentation of a particle in a liquid medium is proportional to its radius, R, while the force inducing its sedimentation is proportional to R^3. The net force causing a particle's sedimentation is therefore proportional to R^2. Thus, when clumping causes an increase in linear particle size by a factor x, the clumps will sediment x^2 times faster than the initial monodispersed particles. For instance, single human erythrocytes, suspended in saline water, sediment at a rate of about 1 cm/hr at ambient gravity, while clumps of agglutinated erythrocytes, comprising an average of 30 cross-linked cells, sediment 1 cm in about 6 min under the same conditions. The simple visual observation of a 10-fold increase in sedimentation rate of a red cell suspension in a test tube is, therefore, indicative of significant agglutination (van Oss, 1984b). The same holds true for accelerated sedimentation in a centrifugal field, but as most cells (especially large cells such as erythrocytes) sediment rather quickly, even at relatively low g forces, the use of centrifugation in assessing agglutination focuses more on the scrutiny of the physical properties of the completely sedimented packed agglutinate than on the actual sedimentation rate (which is difficult to measure under conventional circumstances).

Aspects and Properties of Sedimented Agglutinates

Once cells (agglutinated or nonagglutinated) have been sedimented by centrifugation, there are several ways of recognizing agglutination macroscopically: by the difference in adherence to the rounded bottom of the test tube, and by the difference in dispersability that may be observed while attempting to resuspend the sedimented cells (e.g., by shaking).

Nonagglutinated, monodispersed cells or particles pack very tightly when forced to the bottom of a test tube by centrifugation; nonagglutinated cells are, therefore, deposited in a small, round, sharply delineated "button" at the bottom of the tube. Agglutinated cells, on the other hand, form large, open network structures of many cells attached to each other at a few points only; such large agglutinates cannot be packed tightly so that they tend to deposit on and adhere to the entire hemispherical inner surface of the bottom of the tube. Sedimented agglutinates thus appear as wide and thinly spread layers, often with jagged edges, covering much of the surface of the bottom of the tube. This is in sharp contrast with the small, round buttons formed by nonagglutinated cells (see Fig. 4).

For further verification or, in those cases where too few cells are available for visual inspection of the deposited clumps with the naked eye, resuspension of the cells may be attempted (e.g., by vigorous shaking of the test tubes). Nonagglutinated cells can be completely redispersed in this manner, while agglutinates are indispersable and remain present as large flocs. With large amounts of cells this phenomenon is visible with the naked eye, but when relatively few cells are present in each tube, one does well to revert to microscopic inspection of the contents of each tube.

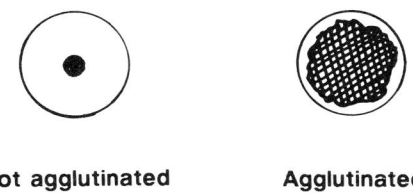

Not agglutinated   **Agglutinated**

Figure 4. Schematic drawing of the bottoms of test tubes used in hemagglutination after centrifugation. When no agglutination takes place (left), the cells sediment in a close-packed conformation and are visible as a tight little button. When agglutination has occurred (right) the cells form large flocs which, after sedimentation, adhere to most of the concave surface of the test tube bottom, usually presenting an irregular periphery.

Agglutination on Flat Surfaces

Agglutination can also be performed on flat plates (made of glass, plastic, or even cardboard). By this technique, agglutination is recognized visually by the coarse graininess of agglutinated cell or particle clumps, in contrast to the smooth aspect of monodisperse cell or particle suspensions.

Agglutination in Gels

Agglutination of very small particles (e.g., sonicated fragments of erythrocyte stromata) can even be effected in gels, by double diffusion of these very small antigenic particles against specific antisera (Milgrom and Loza, 1967). This approach is more similar to precipitation than to agglutination (see section on Sensitivity and Limitation of Immunoprecipitation Methods, p. 191).

Automated Agglutination Methods

To quantitate the results of many hemagglutination determinations in quick sequence, agglutinated cells can be separated from nonagglutinated cell suspensions. The latter may be hemolyzed and the hemolyzate conducted through a spectrophotometer which can record, via the absorptivity at 420-nm wavelength, the proportion of nonagglutinated cells, thus expressing, by difference from the total amount of cells used, a measure of the number of cells that have been agglutinated, for example, as a function of the concentration of antibody to be tested (Greenwalt and Steane, 1970).

For the quantitation of antibody (or antigen) by passive latex agglutination, the number of nonagglutinated particles (which are all close to the same size) may be automatically determined by light scattering, at such (small) forward light-scattering angles as to assure the exclusive counting of only the smallest particles (Masson et al., 1981).

Hemagglutination

Hemagglutination with IgM- and IgG-Class Antibodies

Since the early days of blood transfusion, hemagglutination, i.e., agglutination of erythrocytes with various blood group antibodies, has been the salient analytical tool in immunohematology and bloodbanking. It has long been known that with IgM-class antibodies, due to their size as well as to the availability of ten antibody sites (Edberg et al., 1972) disposed at diametrical distances of about 30 nm, hemagglutination is much more readily achieved than with antibodies of the IgG class, which have just two antibody sites, which are maximally about 12 to 14 nm apart (van Oss, 1984b). However, as IgG-class antibodies are also of considerable importance among blood group antibodies, much effort has been devoted to modifications of the environment and properties of erythrocytes to facilitate hemagglutination with IgG. With some IgG-class blood group antibodies (e.g., anti-A and anti-B), however, hemagglutination usually is readily achieved; the reasons for this are discussed below.

Intercellular Distance

Under physiological conditions of pH and ionic strength, the outer edges of the glycocalix of erythrocytes cannot approach each other to an intercellular distance, l, smaller than about 4 to 5 nm (van Oss, 1989, 1990), which, however, makes the minimum distance between the actual cell membranes of two opposing erythrocytes about 15 to 16 nm (see Fig. 5), which is slightly more than the reach of IgG-class Abs ($d \approx$ 12 to 14 nm), but quite sufficient for cross-linking by IgM-class Abs ($d \approx$ 27 to 28 nm) (van Oss, 1990).

The interactions which force erythrocytes to keep a certain minimum distance apart are threefold: (1) a Lifshitz-van der Waals (LW) attraction ($\Delta G^{LW} \approx -0.6$ mJ/m^2); an electrostatic (EL) repulsion ($\Delta G^{EL} \approx +0.5$ mJ/m^2); and (3) a polar or hydrogen-bonding [or Lewis acid-base (AB)] repulsion ($\Delta G^{AB} \approx +25$ mJ/m^2). Each of these interactions decay as a function of distance, following a different regime, resulting in a secondary minimum of attraction at a mutual distance of about 5 nm between the outer limits of the glycocalices (van Oss, 1989; 1990; see Fig. 5).

Thus, IgM-class Abs can always cross-link erythrocytes, whether the epitopes are situated on the glycocalix strands (which are, at a minimum, only about 5 nm apart), or on the cell membranes (which are at least 15 nm apart). However, IgG-class Abs can only cross-link erythrocytes if the epitopes are situated on the glycocalix edges (which is the case with ABO blood group Ags), but not if the epitopes are located on the cell membrane (which is the case with Rh blood group Ags). Therefore, to facilitate hemagglutination with anti-Rh Abs (which tend to be of the IgG-class) one of two types of measures can be taken: (1) the cells should be brought closer together, or (2) the reach of IgG-class Abs should be extended.

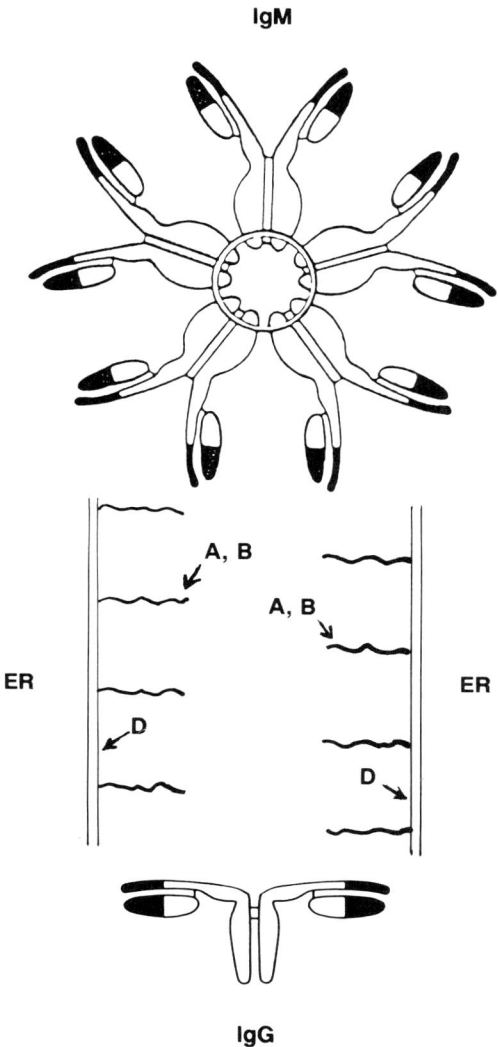

Figure 5. Schematic presentation of the opposing surfaces of two erythrocytes (ER) at their minimum equilibrium distance (about 5 nm between the tips of the glycocalix strands). Drawn approximately to scale are models of IgM and IgG molecules. IgM-class Abs clearly can specifically cross-link all erythrocytes. IgG, in its maximally open form can bridge the distance between blood group A or B epitopes, which are incorporated on the extremities of the glycocalix strands. However, IgG is too small to bridge the distance between $D(Rh_0)$ epitopes, which are situated on the cell membrane itself (drawn here as two parallel lines).

Mechanisms for Reducing the Intercellular Distance

Reduction of ℓ Through Centrifugation. This approach was first proposed by Hirszfeld and Dubiski (in van Oss, 1985), who observed that (Rh_0-positive) erythrocytes could be brought closely enough together for cross-linking with IgG-class ("incomplete") Abs at 15,000 g, but not at 3750 g (see also van Oss, 1985).

Reduction of ℓ by Decreasing the Polar Intercellular Repulsion. This approach is one of the most important ones, as the Ab repulsion between red cells under physiological conditions accounts for 98% of the total intercellular repulsive forces (see above). The electrostatic repulsion amounts to only 2% of the total repulsive forces, and the van der Waals attraction also is only about 2% of the total interaction (at closest approach).

The polar intercellular repulsion can be decreased by most methods which also cause a decrease in the cells' surface (or ζ) potential. It was long thought that the stability of cells (and other particles) in aqueous suspension was due to the balance between the van der Waals (LW) attraction and an electrostatic (EL) repulsion (see van Oss and Absolom, 1983). In the case of blood cells, including erythrocytes (as discussed above), this turns out not to be valid, as the until fairly recently neglected polar (AB) forces now can be shown to play the major role (see above). Thus earlier explanations of the destabilization of red cell suspensions through cell treatment with enzymes or by admixture of plurivalent cations [e.g., La^{3+} ions, see Lerche et al. (1979), or Al^{3+} ions, see Sachtleben and Ruhenstroth-Bauer (1961)], which were based on the decrease in ζ-potential caused by these measures (see van Oss and Absolom, 1983, 1984), have to be revised. There is no doubt that treatment of red cells with neuraminidase, bromelin or papain, as well as with plurivalent cations, causes a significant decrease in the ζ-potential of erythrocytes (van Oss and Absolom, 1984). The more important effect of either enzymic or cation treatment on erythrocytes is that they become *less* hydrophilic, thus decreasing their mutual polar (AB) repulsion, which, in turn, reduces the intercellular distance.

Papain appears to be among the most effective in decreasing the intercellular distance; it is widely used in facilitating hemagglutination with IgG-class ("incomplete") Abs. Among salts with multivalent cations, those with the highest valency are the most effective in destabilizing negatively charged particles such as erythrocytes (see Overbeek, 1952). The connection between a decrease in ζ-potential and increased hydrophobicity has been apparent since 1985 (see Holmes-Farley et al., 1985; van Oss and Good, 1988). The fact that plurivalent cations (which are electron-acceptors) cause hydrophilic electron-donating materials to become more hydrophobic (using phospholipids and Ca^{2+} as an example) was first reported by Ohki (1982), and was explained as outlined above by van Oss et al., (1988). Tannic acid treatment (which also renders erythrocytes more hydrophobic) also is effective in bringing red cells closer together and thus facilitates hemagglutination by means of IgG-class ("incomplete") Abs (Pirofsky et al., 1962).

Reduction of ℓ by Pushing Cells Closer Together by Exterior Polar (AB) Forces. This approach is the basis of the facilitation of hemagglutination by IgG-class Abs by the admixture of relatively high concentrations of serum albumin (see Race and Sanger, 1962), dextran (Gallez and Coakley, 1987; Race and Sanger, 1962; van Oss and Coakley, 1988), polyvinyl pyrrolidone (Hummel, 1963), and other water-soluble polymers (van Oss et al., 1978). When a sufficiently high concentration of water-soluble polymer is reached (e.g., of the order of 2 to 10%), a phase separation occurs between the cells and the polymers (the polymer molecules themselves may in part adsorb onto the cells, but that does not change the mechanism of the phenomenon). When the polymer concentration becomes high enough, the polar (AB) free energy of repulsion of the polymers becomes higher than the polar free energy of repulsion of the cells forcing them to occupy a smaller volume, which reduces the intercellular distance, ℓ (van Oss et al., 1990). With serum albumin, concentrations of 12 to 20% (w/v) are used to that end, while, typically, dextran concentrations between 5 and 10% serve to decrease ℓ. Higher dextran (MW $\approx$ 500,000) concentrations than 10% tend to restabilize the cells, because the concentration of adsorbed dextran then surpasses the concentration of free dextran, which reverses the roles so that in the ensuing phase separation the cells now tend to occupy a larger volume (i.e., ℓ increases) and the bulk polymers are pushed into a smaller volume by the cells (van Oss et al., 1990). This phenomenon should not be confused with the hemagglutination-facilitating effect caused by fairly low concentrations of very asymmetrical polymers of high molecular weight, or of positively charged polymers, which can cross-bind red cells and thus bring them closer together (see below).

Reduction of ℓ by Cell Cross-Binding with Polymers. This type of approach is based on a totally different mechanism from the one discussed in the preceding section. Cross-binding with polymers occurs at fairly low polymer concentrations and is done with: (1) very asymmetrical, high-molecular weight neutral or negatively charged polymers which cross-bind through adsorption and/or entanglement with two (or more) cells at a time per polymer molecule; or (2) already adsorbed biopolymer molecules which are made to precipitate with each other; or (3) positively charged polymers of low or medium molecular weight.

Cross-binding with the first class of polymers gives rise to the rouleau-formation type of hemagglutination. Red cells, which preferentially attract each other in the parallel disc conformation at an intercellular distance, ℓ, of about 7 to 9 nm (van Oss, 1990) are stabilized in that conformation by the anchoring action of cross-binding asymmetrical polymer molecules (van Oss and Absolom, 1985). Cells of a given type (e.g., human erythrocytes) attract each other in the parallel disc conformation, at the "secondary minimum" of attraction, with a very precise free energy of attraction, and slightly different cells (e.g., rabbit erythrocytes) attract each other in the same manner with a somewhat different energy of attraction (van Oss and Absolom 1985). This gives rise to the phenomenon in which rouleau formation occurring with mixtures of cells of two different species (e.g., human and rabbit erythrocytes) are totally segregated, each individual rouleau either consisting completely of human or of rabbit cells (Sewchand and Canham, 1976). This type of erythrocyte aggregation can be obtained with a variety of asymmetrical polymers: fibrinogen (Mollison, 1972), dextran (Mollison, 1972; van Oss and Coakley, 1988), nucleic acids (Ishiyama, 1963), heparin (Jan, 1979), and polymerized albumin (Jones et al., 1969). The higher the molecular weight of an asymmetrical polymer (i.e., the longer the chain length), the lower the concentration needed to obtain rouleau formation: with dextran MW $\approx$ 100,000, 1% causes rouleau formation, while with dextran MW $\approx$ 270,000, a 0.4% concentration of the polymer suffices (Mollison, 1972). The cross-binding induced by dextran can be inhibited by glucose (van Oss et al., 1978). This observation suggests the possibility that the adsorption of dextran onto erythrocyte glycocalices may be due to the presence of a lectinlike peptide with (poly)glucose specificity. This would then be comparable with the opposite of the lectin-red cell interaction (see Perera and Frumin, 1966).

Cross-binding with the second class of polymers has an entirely different mechanism. It is mediated by the aspecific adsorption of "euglobulins" (mainly of the IgM type) onto the red cells, which normally occurs under physiological conditions, but which does not, by itself, cause cross-linking. However, when the ionic strength of the suspending medium is lowered, the adsorbed euglobulins precipitate and in so doing also interact with each other intercellularly, causing cross-binding. When the red cells are washed to remove the adsorbed proteins, this type of cross-binding is no longer possible, but when the eluted euglobulins are added back to the red cell suspension, cross-binding at low ionic strength reoccurs (van Oss and Buenting, 1967). The aspect of red cells agglomerated in this manner is somewhat different from that of ordinary rouleaux; some remnants of cell stacks can still be discerned, but all clumps look as though they were painted over (probably by precipitated euglobulins), as seen by scanning electron microscopy (van Oss et al., 1978). Readdition of salt to cells agglomerated in this manner redissolves the euglobulins and causes the cells to redisperse completely. This method of erythrocyte agglomeration was formerly used as a means for removing the cryoprotectant from previously frozen, newly thawed cells, by sedimenting the agglomerates at ambient gravity, thus avoiding the need for centrifugal washing (Huggins, 1966). The elucidation of the mechanism of this class of (low ionic strength) cross-binding of erythrocytes (van Oss and Buenting, 1967), was at the origin of the development of an automated hemagglutination-enhancing method by Rosenfield et al. (1968).

Cross-binding of red cells with the third class of polymers operates through positively charged polyelectrolytes (usually of relatively low to medium molecular weight), which cross-bind erythrocytes by direct linkage (and neutralization) with the acid site of the glycocalix. Complexes of this type are most readily formed at relatively low ionic strengths and redisperse upon the addition of salt. Basic polymers of this type are: polybrene [poly(hexadimethrine bromide)] (Lalezari, 1968), protamine, and polylysine (Greenwalt and Steane, 1973; see also van Oss and Coakley, 1988). Polybrene (as well as albumin in high concentrations) induces red cells to become stomatocytic (i.e., to manifest only one dimple instead of two) (van Oss et al., 1978). It should be kept in mind that neutralization of negatively charged sites on the glycocalix also makes the cell surfaces more hydrophobic (see above), and thus more prone to agglutination.

Reduction of ℓ by Inducing Spiculation in the Red Cell Surface.
Spicules or spikes, with a small radius of curvature, undergo a much smaller repulsion than smooth parts of the cell surface. Spicules can therefore approach another cell surface much more closely than would be possible in the case of totally smooth cells. Thus, anti-blood group A or B Abs of the IgM as well as of the IgG class can cross-link red cells. Anti-A as well as anti-B blood group Abs (as well as anti-A lectins) tend to cause spiculation in red cells, but anti-Rh_0 (D) Abs do not (see also Rebuck, 1953; Salsbury and Clarke, 1967; van Oss and Mohn, 1970). Thus, hemagglutination with anti-A or anti-B blood group Abs, even of the IgG class, is never a problem. The major problems are encountered with anti-Rh_0 (D) Abs, which tend to be of the IgG class, and which leave the cells quite smooth. It should be mentioned that dextran (MW $\approx$ 40,000) also has been observed to cause spiculation (van Oss et al., 1978), which may be another reason for its usefulness in facilitating hemagglutination with "incomplete", IgG-class anti-Rh_0 (D) Abs. The reason why spiculation occurs with anti-A and anti-B Abs or lectins and not with anti-D Abs probably lies in the differences in densities of, e.g., blood group A vs blood group Rh_0 (D) epitopes per cell — the first type is of the order of 10^6 while the second is only of the order of 10^4 per cell (Steane and Greenwalt, 1980; van Oss and Mohn, 1970; see also section on Quantitative Haemagglutination, below).

Papain treatment also gives rise to surface irregularities in red cells, but the irregular processes produced by this approach tend to have a larger radius of curvature (i.e., $R \approx 0.5$ μm) than the spicules caused by, e.g., anti-A Abs ($R \approx 0.15$ μm) (van Oss and Mohn, 1970).

Methods for Extending the Reach of IgG-Class Abs

Chemical Method. The maximum distance between the two IgG paratopes can be increased by mild reduction followed by alkylation (Romans et al., 1977), which results in breaking at least some of the inter-heavy chain disulfide bonds. All inter-heavy chain disulfide bonds cannot be broken because that would result in monovalent Ab pieces, which are incapable of cross-binding. A reach of about 15 nm must be attained to achieve hemagglutination. It thus seems likely that this method mainly applies to the opening up of IgG3 with its eleven S–S bonds, and to a lesser extent to IgG2 with four S–S bonds (cf. Burton et al., 1986).

Immunochemical Method. Probably the most important method of extending the reach of IgG-class Abs (from the points of view of both blood transfusion and clinical testing) is the indirect antiglobulin, or Coombs test (Coombs et al., 1945). By this approach, red cells sensitized with ("incomplete") IgG-class Abs (which cannot themselves achieve hemagglutination) are cross-linked by means of (usually rabbit) anti-human IgG Abs. A schematic illustration of this mode of cross-linking can be found in van Oss and Absolom (1983). It is, of course, a two-step approach, but the end result is that cross-binding occurs through two human IgG molecules (one at each end), each about 12 to 14 nm long, which are cross-linked together by one (rabbit) anti-human IgG molecule with a reach of about 12 nm, resulting in an extended divalent Ab, with a total reach of $\approx$ 36 nm, i.e., slightly larger than that of IgM. For all cross-matching tests used for all blood transfusions and for all tests for Rh-Abs, the use of the indirect antiglobulin or Coombs test is still indispensable. The *direct* antiglobulin test (Coombs et al., 1946), i.e., the testing for erythrocytes already sensitized *in vivo,* by means of (rabbit) anti-human IgG Abs is and remains an indispensable test for the detection of sensitization in (suspected) cases of hemolytic disease of the newborn.

Temperature of Hemagglutination

As is usually the case with Ag-Ab interactions (which tend to be exothermic; see Chapter 11), hemagglutination generally is stronger at room temperature, or at +4°C, than at 37°C. The exception is Rh antibodies: they usually hemagglutinate better at 37°C than in the cold (i.e., they are called "warm" Abs) (Stratton and Reuton, 1958); the reasons for this lie in the unusual nature of the Rh epitope (see Table 3, Chapter 6). Thus hemagglutination, e.g., in cross-matching for blood transfusion, should be done in the cold (room temperature) as well as at 37°C.

Quantitative Hemagglutination

Titration. Titration by hemagglutination is at best, a semi-quantitative assay. It is done by making a series of increasingly dilute solutions of the antiserum in saline; the appropriate red cells are added and the serum which causes recognizable hemagglutination at the greatest dilution is considered to have the most Ab (Race and Sanger, 1962, p. 4). The Ab titer of the antiserum is then the inverse dilution of the tube containing the most dilute Ab in which hemagglutination still is observed. (For technical considerations and standardization, see Stratton and Reuton, 1958). Usually one considers that, for a given number of red cells, the amount of the Ags is reasonably constant. However, in certain cases that amount can also vary, depending, e.g., on the genetic make-up of the red cell donor; this is especially the case with the MN and Rh Ags (Race and Sanger, 1962; see below).

Other Quantitative Determinations by Hemagglutination. Quantitative hemagglutination with an excess of radioactive antibodies has been used to determine the number of antigenic determinants of a given blood group specificity per red cell. For instance, homozygous (DD, Rh_o-positive) human red cells have been shown to comprise 10,300 D epitopes, while heterozygous (Dd) red cells contain 6400 D epitopes (Masouredis, 1960; see also Greenwalt and Steane, 1973). On A-positive cells the number of antigenic determinants is much higher: $\approx$ 1,000,000 per A_1 erythrocyte. The much greater number of A than of D epitopes per erythrocyte may well be one of the major reasons why the interaction of anti-A antibodies causes spiculation in red cells, while the interaction of anti-D antibodies does not affect their smooth biconcave shape (see above).

Types of Agglutination

Active Agglutination

Apart from active hemagglutination, discussed extensively above, one of the oldest other agglutination methods is bacterial agglutination, used for the assay of antibacterial Abs in sera.

Passive Agglutination

Active hemagglutination, as discussed above, has been used in blood grouping work. Passive hemagglutination can also be done with Ags that are not an integral part of the red cells, but may be adsorbed or bound to red cells that serve solely as carrier particles. Soluble polysaccharide antigens easily adsorb directly onto the red cell surface. However, protein antigens adsorb onto red cells only after the latter have undergone treatment with, for example, 0.0056% tannic acid (10 min at 37°C) or 1.65% glutaraldehyde (several hours at room temperature). Protein antigens and haptens can also be covalently coupled to red cells by diazotization and other chemical attachment procedures, which can make passive hemagglutination and its inhibition one of the most sensitive methods for the characterization of small amounts of antibody (Adler and Adler, 1980). The method has proved especially useful for the characterization of monoclonal antibodies. With erythrocytes coupled to protein antigens or haptens, one can, of course, also characterize antibodies as well as antibody-forming cells via passive complement-mediated hemolysis (in tubes as well as in plaque assays) (Adler and Adler, 1980).

Passive agglutination with polystyrene latex and other particles has become an important tool in clinical tests, as well as in research, for the characterization of antigens as well as antibodies, either of which can be aspecifically but firmly adsorbed onto the rather hydrophobic surfaces of latex particles or covalently bound to chemically modified latices (see Masson et al., 1981). The first passive latex agglutination test was developed by Singer (1961) for the demonstration of rheumatoid factor (IgM-class autoantibody to slightly altered or aggregated IgG; see also Singer and Plotz, 1956). In that method, human IgG is aspecifically adsorbed onto the surface of polystyrene latex particles, which can then be agglutinated by sera which contain rheumatoid factor. Latex agglutination is also used to demonstrate the presence of chorionic gonadotropic hormone (usually as an inhibition of agglutination test) in pregnancy urine. It has also been used in tests for C-reactive protein, antithyroglobulin, and antistreptolysin-O antibodies, as well as in the determination of levels of circulating immune complexes, IgE, α-feto-protein, and so on (Masson et al., 1981).

Inhibition of Agglutination

Inhibition of (passive) hemagglutination can be used to measure the degree to which dissolved Ag can bind Ab, as shown by the inhibition of hemagglutination of cells coated with the same antigen. Inhibition of hemagglutination is frequently used to characterize antibodies to viruses that can agglutinate various species of erythrocytes (e.g., antibodies to measles, rubella, influenza viruses).

In a variety of (passive) latex agglutination tests, the inhibition of agglutination mode is preferred, particularly when the test is used to assay for the presence of an Ag, e.g., urinary chorionic gonadotropic hormone in pregnancy tests (see above). More recently various agglutination tests are being replaced by other types of immunoassay, such as Elisa, or blotting tests.

Agglutination with Two Different Cell Types

Mixed Agglutination. This method uses cultured cell monolayers for the characterization of antigens on the cultured cells by the intermediary of antibodies bound to these antigens. Erythrocytes, sensitized with antierythrocyte antibodies, are used as indicators of the presence of sensitized cultured cells. They are cross-linked to the monolayers with anti-immunoglobulin antibodies, much like an antiglobulin or Coombs procedure (Coombs et al., 1945; see above), and arranged as in a sandwich in two flat layers of different opposing cells.

Coagglutination. This is a method for characterizing bacteria sensitized with type-specific antibodies of the IgG class. By cross-linking them with

TABLE 1.
Leukocyte Rosetting with Erythrocytes (E)

Type of Rosetting	Type of Erythrocytes	Leukocytes Rosetted
E	Sheep E	T cells; 50% of NK cells (low-affinity E rosettes)
EAγ	E, sensitized with IgG-class Abs	B cells, some T cells, and NK cells, granulocytes, monocytes, macrophages
EAμ	E, sensitized with IgM-class Abs	Some B and T cells
EAC	E, sensitized and treated with complement; bovine erythrocytes often preferred, to avoid binding T cells with nonsensitized patches (see sheep E, above)	B cells, some non-B cells

Adapted from van Oss (1984b).

Staphylococcus aureus, strain Cowan I, which carries protein A, which binds to the Fc moieties of human IgG1, IgG2, and IgG4, the sensitized bacteria are then coagglutinated with staphylococci treated with formaldehyde and heat (Kronvall, 1973). When the type-specific antibodies are not of the IgG class, coagglutination is not possible (Hovanec et al., 1980), but in the case of IgM, direct agglutination is then practicable. Coagglutination is used for the characterization and/or typing of, for example, *Hemophilus influenzae, Neisseria meningitidis, Streptococcus pneumoniae,* and various other groups of streptococci. Coagglutination with protein A-bearing staphylococci can also be used to demonstrate sensitization with IgG-class antibodies of erythrocytes and other mammalian cells.

Rosetting. This method is closely related to coagglutination as well as to mixed agglutination. It is used primarily for the characterization of different kinds of lymphocytes. Sheep erythrocytes (E) can attach peripherally to human T lymphocytes, forming a rosette. The Rosettes are not only useful for detecting human T cells, but also for removing T cells from lymphocyte preparations, based on the fact that T lymphocytes rosetted with sheep erythrocytes (E rosettes) sediment much faster than the non-E-rosetted non-T lymphocytes. Table 1 summarizes a number of leukocyte-rosetting approaches. Protein A-bearing staphylococci, latex particles coated with IgG, and B lymphocytes have been used to characterize Rh_0 (D)-positive erythrocytes sensitized with IgG-class anti-Rh_0 (D) antibodies (EA; see Table 1) (Loren et al., 1982). There is no significant qualitative or quantitative difference between rosetting and coagglutination, except that in the former one usually employs erythrocytes, while staphylococci are more typically used in the latter.

Sensitivity of Agglutination

Due to the fact that very few Ab molecules suffice to cross-bind two cells or particles, and that the difference between freely suspended and agglutinated cells or particles is easily discernible with a very small number of particles, it is possible, under favorable conditions, to discern Ab levels as low as 1 ng to 100 pg or less. Another advantage of agglutination over, e.g., immune precipitation methods, is its short reaction time. While gel immunodiffusion methods usually require from several hours to several days to obtain the final results, the results of agglutination tests normally are available within minutes to, at most, about 1 h.

IgM-class Abs are more efficient in achieving agglutination than Abs of the IgG class, but various methods can be employed to facilitate or enhance IgG-mediated agglutination.

The size of Ags used in various agglutination methods varies from the size of small Ags (MW $\approx$ 10,000) which can be attached to cells or particles, to large cells ($\approx$ 10 μm in diameter). In passive agglutination with latex particles, the diameters of the particles used normally vary between 250 and 1000 nm.

REFERENCES

Adler, F. L., and Adler, L. T. (1980) Passive hemagglutination and hemolysis for estimation of antigens and antibodies. *Meth. Enzymol.* 70:455-466.

Albini, B., Fagundus, A. M., and Vladutiu, A. O. (1984) Circulating immune complexes. In *Molecular Immunology*, (A. Z. Atassi, C. J. van Oss, and D. R. Absolom, eds.), Dekker, NY, 381—401.

Allison, A. C., and Humphrey, J. H. (1959) Estimation of the size of antigens by gel diffusion methods. *Nature (London)* 183:1591—1592.

Bechhold, H. (1905) Strukturbildung in Gallerten. *Z. Phys. Chem.* 52:185—190.

Burton, D. R., Gregory, L., and Lefferis, R. (1986) Aspects of the molecular structure of IgG subclasses. In *Basic and Clinical Aspects of IgG Subclasses*, (F. Shakib, ed.), Karger, Basel, 7—35.

Coombs, R. R. A., Mourant, A. E., and Race, R. R. (1945) A new test for the detection of weak and "incomplete" Rh agglutinins. *Br. J. Exp. Pathol.* 26:255—266.

Coombs, R. R. A., Mourant, A. E., and Race, R. R. (1946) *In vivo* iso-sensitization of red cells in babies with haemolytic disease. *Lancet* i:264—269.

de Groot, E. R., Lamers, M. C., Aarden, L. A., Smeenk, R. J. T., and van Oss, C.J. (1980) Dissociation of DNA/anti-DNA complexes at high pH. *Immunol. Commun.* 9:515—522.

Edberg, S. C., Bronson, P. M., and van Oss, C. J. (1972) The valency of IgM and IgG rabbit anti-dextran antibody as a function of the size of the dextran molecule. *Immunochemistry* 9:273—288.

Farr, R. S. (1958) A quantitative immunochemical measure of the primary interaction between I*BSA and antibody. *J. Infect. Dis.* 103:239—262.
Gallez, D., and Coakley, W. T. (1987) Interfacial instability at cell membranes. *Prog. Biophys. Mol. Biol.* 48:155—199.
Grabar, P., and Burtin, P. (1964) *Immunoelectrophoretic Analysis*. Elsevier, NY.
Greenwalt, T. J., and Steane, E. A. (1970) Quantitative hemagglutination. II. A method for assaying red cell antigens using the Auto Analyzer. *Br. J. Haematol.* 19:691—700.
Greenwalt, T. J., and Steane, E. A. (1973) Quantitative hemagglutination. VI. Relationship of sialic acid content and aggregation by polybrene, protamine and poly-L-lysine. *Br. J. Haematol.* 25:227—237.
Holmes-Farley, S. R., Reamey, R. H., McCarthy, T. J., Deutch, J., and Whitesides, G. M. (1985) Acid-base behavior of carboxylic groups covalently attached at the surface of polyethylene: the usefulness of contact angle in following the ionization of surface functionality. *Langmuir* 1:725—740.
Horejsi, V. (1979) Some theoretical aspects of affinity electrophoresis. *J. Chromatogr.* 178:1—13.
Horejsi, V. (1981) Affinity electrophoresis. *Anal. Biochem.* 112:1—8.
Hovanec, D. L., Absolom, D. R., van Oss, C. J., and Gorzynski, E. A. (1980) Relationship to coagglutination of immunoglobulin class dissociated from *Escherichia coli*-antibody complexes. *J. Clin. Microbiol.* 12:608—609.
Huggins, C. E. (1966) Frozen blood-Clinical experience. *Surgery* 60:77—84.
Hummel, K. (1963) Quantitative Untersuchungen über die Bindung von Polyvinylpyrrolidon an die Erythrozytenoberfläche. *Blut* 9:145—164:215—237.
Ishiyama, I. (1963) Hemagglutination induced by nucleic acids. *Nature (London)* 197:912.
Jambazian, A., and Holper, J. C. (1972) Rheophoresis: a sensitive immunodiffusion method for detection of hepatitis associated antigen. *Proc. Soc. Exp. Biol. Med.* 140:560—564.
Jan, K. M. (1979) Red cell interactions in macromolecular suspension. *Biorheology* 16:137—148.
Jones, J. M., Kerwick, R. A., and Goldsmith, K. L. G. (1969) Influence of polymers on the efficacy of serum albumin as a potentiator of "incomplete" Rh agglutinins. *Nature (London)* 224:510—511.
Kabat, E. A., and Mayer, M. M. (1961) *Experimental Immunochemistry*. C. C. Thomas, Springfield, IL, 22—96.
Kronvall, G. (1973) A rapid agglutination method for typing pneumococci by means of specific antibody adsorbed to Protein A-containing *Staphylococcus*. *J. Med. Microbiol.* 6:187—190.
Lalezari, P. (1968) A new method for detection of red blood cell antibodies. *Transfusion* 8:372—380.
Laurell, C. B. (1965) Antigen-antibody crossed electrophoresis. *Anal. Biochem.* 10:358—361.
Laurell, C. B. (1966) Quantitative estimation of proteins by electrophoresis in agarose gel containing antibodies. *Anal. Biochem.* 15:45—52.
Lerche, D., Hessel, E., and Donath, E. (1979) Investigation of the La^{3+}-induced aggregation of red blood cells. *Stud. Biophys.* 78:95—106.
Loren, A. B., Matsuo, Y., Charman, D., and Yokoyama, M. M. (1982) Determination of homozygote vs. heterozygote of Rh blood group antigens via rosette assays. *Transfusion* 22:194—202.

Mancini, G., Carbonara, A. O., and Heremans, J. F. (1965) Immunochemical quantitation of antigens by single radial immunodiffusion. *Immunochemistry* 2:235—254.

Masouredis, S. P. (1960) Relationship between Rh_o (D) genotype and quantity of I^{131} anti-Rh_o (D) bound to red cells. *J. Clin. Invest.* 39:1450—1462.

Masson, P. L., Cambiaso, C. L., Collet-Cassart, D., Magnusson, C. G. M., Richards, C. B., and Sindic, C. J. M. (1981) Particle counting immunoassay. *Meth. Enzymol.* 74:106—139.

Milgrom, F., and Loza, U. (1967) Agglutination of particulate antigens in agar gel. *J. Immunol.* 98:102—109.

Mollison, P. L. (1972) *Blood Transfusion in Clinical Medicine*. Blackwell, Oxford, 150, 384.

Ohki, S. (1982) A mechanism of divalent ion-induced phosphatidylserine membrane fusion. *Biochim. Biophys. Acta* 689:1—11.

Ouchterlony, Ö. (1949) Antigen-antibody reactions in gels. *Ark. Kemi* 1:43—48; 55—59.

Ouchterlony, Ö. (1968) *Handbook of Immunodiffusion and Immunoelectrophoresis*. Ann Arbor Sci. Publ., Ann Arbor, MI.

Oudin, J. (1948) L'analyse immunochimique qualitative. Méthode par diffusion des antigènes au sein d'un immunsérum précipitant dans de la gélose. *Ann. Inst. Pasteur* 75:30—52.

Oudin, J. (1971) Simple diffusion in tubes. In *Methods in Immunology and Immunochemistry*, Vol. 3, (C. A. Williams, and M. W. Chase, eds.), Academic Press, New York, 118—138.

Oudin, J. (1980) Immunochemical analysis by antigen-antibody precipitation in gels. *Meth. Enzymol.* 70:166—198.

Overbeek, J. Th. G. (1952) Stability of hydrophobic colloids and emulsions. In *Colloid Science*, Vol. 1, (H. R. Kruyt, ed.), Elsevier, Amsterdam, 302—341.

Perera, C. B., and Frumin, A. M. (1966) Hemagglutination by Fava bean extract inhibited by simple sugars. *Science* 151:821—823.

Pirofsky, B., Cordova, M., and Imel, T. L. (1962) The function of proteolytic enzymes and tannic acid in inducing erythrocyte agglutination. *J. Immunol.* 89:767—773.

Race, R. R., and Sanger, R. (1962) *Blood Groups in Man*. Blackwell, Oxford, 341—342.

Rebuck, J. W. (1953) Structural changes in sensitized human erythrocytes observed with the electron microscope. *Anat. Rec.* 115:591—613.

Romans, D. G., Tilley, C. A., Crookston, M. C., Falk, R. E., and Dorrington, K. J. (1977) Conversion of incomplete antibodies to direct agglutinins by mild reduction: evidence for segmental flexibility within the Fc fragment of immunoglobulin G. *Proc. Natl. Acad. Sci. U.S.A.* 74:2531—2535.

Rosenfield, R. E., Spitz, C., Baz-Shany, S., Permoad, P., and Ducros, M. (1968) Low ionic concentration to augment hemagglutination for the detection and measurement of serological incompatibility. *Anal. Chem. Technicon Symp.* 1:173—175.

Sachtleben, P., and Ruhenstroth-Bauer, G. (1961) Agglutination and the electrical surface potential of red blood cells. *Nature (London)* 192:982—983.

Salsbury, A. J., and Clarke, J. A. (1967) Surface changes in red blood cells undergoing agglutination. *Rev. Fr. Etud. Clin. Biol.* 12:981—985.

Schultze, H. E., and Heremans, J. F. (1966) *Molecular Biology of Human Proteins*, Vol. 1. Elsevier, Amsterdam, 240—278.

Sehon, A. H. (1989) Modulation of antibody responses by conjugates of antigens with monomethoxypolyethylene glycol. In *Immunobiology of Proteins and Peptides, V: Vaccines*, (M. Z. Atassi, ed.), Plenum Press, NY, 341—351.

Sehon, A. H., Jackson, C. J. C., Holford-Strevens, V., Wilkinson, I., Maiti, P. K., and Lang, G. (1987) Conversion of antigens to tolerogenic derivatives by conjugation with monomethoxypolyethylene glycol. In *The Pharmacology and Toxicology of Proteins,* (J. S. Holzenberg, and J. L. Winkelhake, eds.), Alan R. Liss, NY, 205—219.

Sewchand, L. S., and Canham, P. B. (1976) Induced rouleau formation in interspecies populations of red cells. *Can. J. Physiol. Pharmacol.* 54:437—442.

Singer, J. M. (1961) The latex fixation test in rheumatic diseases. *Am. J. Med.* 31:766—779.

Singer, J. M., and Plotz, C. M. (1956) The latex fixation test. I. Application to the serologic diagnosis of rheumatoid arthritis. *Am. J. Med.* 21:888—893.

Smeenk, R. J. T., and Aarden, L. A. (1980) The use of polyethylene glycol precipitation to detect low-avidity anti-DNA antibodies in systemic lupus erythematosus. *J. Immunol. Meth.* 39:165—180.

Smeenk, R. J. T., van der Lelij, G., and Aarden, L. A. (1982) Avidity of antibodies to dsDNA. Comparison of IFT on *Crithidia luciliae,* Farr assay and PEG assay. *J. Immunol.* 128:L73—78.

Smeenk, R. J. T., Aarden, L. A., and van Oss, C. J. (1983) Comparison between dissociation and inhibition of association of DNA/anti-DNA complexes. *Immunol. Commun.* 12:177—188.

Steane, E. A., and Greenwalt, T. J. (1980) Erythrocyte agglutination. In *Immunobiology of the Erythrocyte,* (S. G. Sandler, J. Nusbacher, and M. S. Schanfield, eds.), Alan R. Liss, NY, 171—188.

Stratton, F., and Reuton, P. H. (1958) *Practical Blood Grouping.* Blackwell, Oxford, 30, 167.

van Oss, C. J. (1968) Specifically impermeable precipitate membranes formed through double diffusion in gels: behavior with complex forming and with simple systems. *J. Colloid Interface Sci.* 27:684—690.

van Oss, C. J. (1984a) Specifically impermeable precipitate membranes. *Surface Colloid Sci.* 13:115—144.

van Oss, C. J. (1984b) Agglutination and precipitation. In *Molecular Immunology,* (A. Z. Atassi, C. J. van Oss, and D. R. Absolom, eds.), Marcel Dekker, NY, 361—379.

van Oss, C. J. (1985) Stability of human red cell suspensions at 300,000 x G. *J. Dispersion Sci. Tech.* 6:139—146.

van Oss, C. J. (1989) Energetics of cell-cell and cell-biopolymer interactions. *Cell Biophys.* 14:1—16.

van Oss, C. J. (1990) Surface free energy contribution to cell interactions. In *Biophysics of the Cell Surface,* (R. Glaser, and D. Gingell, eds.), Springer-Verlag, Berlin, 131—152.

van Oss, C. J., and Absolom, D. R. (1983) Zeta potentials, van der Waals forces and hemagglutination. *Vox Sang.* 44:183—190.

van Oss, C. J., and Absolom, D. R. (1984) Hemagglutination and the closest distance of approach of normal, neuraminidase, and papain-treated erythrocytes. *Vox Sang.* 47:250—256.

van Oss, C. J., and Absolom, D. R. (1985) Influence of cell configuration and potential energy equilibria in rouleau phenomena. *J. Dispersion Sci. Tech.* 6:131—137.

van Oss, C. J., and Bartholomew, W. R. (1980) Precipitation reactions. In *Methods in Immunodiagnosis,* (N. R. Rose, and P. E. Bigazzi, eds.), John Wiley & Sons, NY, 65—90.

van Oss, C. J., and Bronson, P. M. (1969) Immunorheophoresis. *Immunochemistry* 6:775—778.

van Oss, C. J., and Buenting, S. (1967) Adsorbed euglobulins as the cause of agglomeration of erythrocytes in the Huggins blood-thawing method. *Transfusion* 7:77.

van Oss, C. J., and Coakley, W. T. (1988) Mechanisms of successive modes of erythrocyte stability and instability in the presence of various polymers. *Cell Biophys.* 13:141—150.

van Oss, C. J., and Good, R. J. (1988) Orientation of the water molecules of hydration of human serum albumin. *J. Prot. Chem.* 7:179—183.

van Oss, C. J., and Good, R. J. (1989) Surface tension and the solubility of polymers and biopolymers: the role of polar and apolar interfacial free energies. *J. Macromol. Sci. Chem.* 26:1183—1203.

van Oss, C. J., and Heck, Y. S. L. (1961) Qualitative and quantitative interpretation of double diffusion. *Z. Immun. Allergieforsch.* 122:44—57.

van Oss, C. J., and Mohn, J. F. (1970) Scanning electron mciroscopy of red cell agglutination. *Vox Sang.* 19:432—443.

van Oss, C. J., Fontaine, M., Dhennin, L., and Fontaine, M. P. (1957) Sur la mise en evidence de reactions immunologiques par zhéophorèse sur papier. *Compte Reudar Acad. Sci. Paris.* 245:407—408.

van Oss, C. J., Dhennin, L., and Dhennin, L. (1964) The antigenic connection between two different types of foot-and-mouth disease viruses and their subparticles. *Virology* 22:428—430.

van Oss, C. J., Mohn, J. F., and Cunningham, R. K. (1978) Influence of various physicochemical factors on hemagglutination. *Vox Sang.* 34:351—361.

van Oss, C. J., Bronson, P. M., and Absolom, D. R. (1982a) Affinity diffusion. I. Method for measuring dissociation constants of precipitating antibodies. *Immunol. Commun.* 11:129—138.

van Oss, C. J., Absolom, D. R., and Bronson, P. M. (1982b) Affinity diffusion. II. Comparison between thermodynamic data obtained by affinity diffusion and precipitation in tubes. *Immunol. Commun.* 11:139—148.

van Oss, C. J., Moore, L. L., Good, R. J., and Chaudhury, M. K. (1985) Surface thermodynamic properties and chromatographic and salting-out behavior of IgA and other serum proteins. *J. Prot. Chem.* 4:245—263.

van Oss, C. J., Good, R. J., and Chaudhury, M. K. (1986) Solubility of proteins. *J. Prot. Chem.* 5:385—405.

van Oss, C. J., Chaudhury, M. K., and Good, R. J. (1988) Polar interfacial interactions, hydration pressure and membrane fusion. In *Molecular Mechanisms of Membrane Fusion,* (S. Ohki, D. Doyle, T. D. Flanagan, S. N. Hui, and E. Mayhew, eds.), Plenum Press, NY, 113—122.

van Oss, C. J., Arnold, K., and Coakley, W. T. (1990) Depletion flocculation and depletion stabilization of erythrocytes. *Cell Biophys.* 17:1—16.

Chapter

11

The Behavior of Antigens and Antibodies Immobilized on a Solid Phase

John E. Butler
Department of Microbiology
University of Iowa
Iowa City, IA

INTRODUCTION

Overview

Currently employed, specific separation and assay technology in immunology and biochemistry is largely based on the principle of immobilizing one reactant on an inert, insoluble surface. This allows the immobilized reactant (receptor*) to bind (capture*) its ligand in a complex soluble mixture. Nonbound components of the mixture are then removed by washing and the bound ligand is purified by dissociation from the receptor, e.g., preparative affinity chromatography, or measured *in situ*, using a suitable detection system, as exemplified by solid-phase immunoassay (SPI). The first practical application of SPI was that of Campbell and colleagues (1961), although Landsteiner and Uhlirz demonstrated the principle of solid-phase adsorption in 1905 (Landsteiner and Uhlirz, 1905). The basic technology has now diversified into a plethora of preparative and quantitative procedures all of which share the principle of an immobilized, solid-phase reactant. This chapter briefly reviews the history of SPI, emphasizing those developments that deal

---

*The term receptor will be used throughout this chapter to indicate the immobilized, or "capture reagent"; the soluble reactant to be captured is the ligand.

with quantitative immunoassays. Although it is important for proper interpretation of SPI to understand interfacial antigen-antibody reactions on synthetic solid phases, information gained from studying such interactions may also provide useful insight into more complex reactions such as those that occur on the surfaces of cells *in vivo*.

Historical Perspective

The Emergence of Solid-phase Technology in Biochemistry and Immunochemistry

Prior to the advent of solid-phase technology, biological and medical science utilized tedious solution-phase methodologies involving separations effected by organic solvents, temperature shifts, changes in ionic strength and dielectric constants, and specific precipitating agents, as well as complicated electrophoretic and ultracentrifugational procedures. This era was also characterized by solution-phase immunoassays in which "the slowest ship in the convoy" was the separation of the bound and free reactants. Hence, the immobilization of one reactant on an inert, insoluble solid-phase greatly facilitated separation technology through affinity chromatography and simplified and accelerated immunoassays.

The practical introduction of solid-phase technology in biochemistry came through the addition of various charged, ion-exchange groups into natural polymers (Peterson and Sober, 1956). The introduction of simple chemical compounds to produce ion-exchangers paved the way for the substitution of biomolecules like enzymes, antigens, and antibodies into the same polymers. In 1968, Goldstein and Katchalski described the use of solid-phase proteases as a practical means of separating proteases from their proteolytic products.

Immunoassays Based on Solid-Phase Technology

In 1961 Campbell and associates utilized antigen immobilized on bromoacetylated cellulose to purify specific antibodies. The latter was, in fact, not dissimilar from the use of cells or bacteria as "naturally occurring solid phases" to purify antibodies specifically bound to their surfaces or merely to measure their presence *in situ* using some detection methodology. Initially the methods for measuring *in situ*-bound antibodies were indirect, secondary antibody-antigen reactions, involving such procedures as agglutination and complement-mediated lysis. Systems involving cell agglutination by cell-bound antibodies or cell lysis by complement could also be configured as inhibition assays to quantify soluble antigens by using the latter as competitive inhibitors, e.g., agglutination inhibition and complement fixation. Qualitative approaches to measuring *in situ*-bound antibodies, or detecting the presence of certain cell-surface antigens, were accomplished through the use of fluorescein-labeled antibodies.

While serology further evolved through the study of antigen-antibody reactions on natural interfaces, antigen quantitation as a tool of medical science in general, followed a different course. In 1960, Yalow and Berson described the basic principle of radioimmunoassay (RIA), whereby minute quantities of antigen in a complex biological mixture, e.g., serum, could be determined by its ability to inhibit the binding of a known amount of the same iodinated antigen to its specific antibody. RIA did not, however, involve interfacial antigen-antibody interactions, but rather tedious solution-phase immunochemistry. The time required for separation essentially determined the number of samples which could be analyzed over a given period of time, i.e., "the slowest ship in the immunoassay convoy".

A major technological advancement came about from the studies of Catt and Tregear who, in 1967, showed that proteins (antigen or antibodies) readily and stably became adsorbed on plastic surfaces. Hence, a plastic test tube, or, as currently used, a microtiter well, could be simultaneously used as a reaction vessel and as a receptor-covered solid phase, thus permitting rapid separation of bound and free analyte (ligand) by merely washing the tube or well. Adsorption of protein to synthetic polymers is largely hydrophobic (see below), and the number of useful adsorption surfaces has grown to include various plastics (polystyrene, vinyl polymers, polypropylene) and synthetic membranes, such as nitrocellulose, polyvinylidene difluoride (PVDF), and nylon. Immobilization on synthetic surfaces is not restricted to adsorption, but can also be accomplished by using functionalized synthetic surfaces which permit covalent coupling of the desired solid-phase reactant. The introduction of solid-phase technology in the field of immunoassay not only expedited and accelerated immunoassays, but also stimulated the development of such methods as immunoblotting.

Enzymes Replace Radionuclides

Until the late 1960s, enzymes as detection labels had only been used for the localization of antigens in tissues (Sternberger et al., 1970). At this time, horseradish peroxidase (HRP) and alkaline phosphatase (AP) were introduced as "signal generators" in immunoassays to quantitate antigens and antibodies (Avrameas and Guilbert, 1972; Engvall et al., 1971). The enzyme-linked immunosorbent assay (ELISA) or simply enzyme immunoassay (EIA), has gradually replaced RIA in most applications.

Apart from the safety, long shelf-life, and therefore convenience, enzymes, unlike radioisotopes (and fluors), *increase* their signal with time rather than decrease it. Hence, enzymes provide a self-amplifying system not inherent in predecessor detection systems.

The transition from radioisotopes to enzymes has proceeded so rapidly that for many new investigators and especially students, ELISA and SPI are synonymous.

ELISA: Variations on a Theme from Engvall and Perlmann

The past 20 years has witnessed the mushrooming of enzyme-mediated immunoassay into almost every area of biological and medical science. Concomitant with its widespread acceptance has been the multitude of variations in configuration and purpose; nearly all are designated ELISA after the acronym coined by Eva Engvall and Peter Perlmann in 1971. The principal modifications in the technology appear to follow several directions. First, ELISA has been modified according to purpose, either antigen or antibody quantitation. The diversity within this area is extraordinary and includes antigens ranging from synthetic peptides to whole cells and from antibody present in serum and secretions to those made *in vitro* by cultured plasma cells, e.g., "ELISPOT" technology (Czerkinsky et al., 1983a). Second, ELISAs have been modified to improve their sensitivity through the use of new enzyme substrates, through amplification involving methods to increase the enzyme:analyte ratio, or through the application of signal detection by generating fluorescent enzyme products or using chemiluminescence. Third, comparative end-point measurements have been replaced by reaction rate analyses in diagnostic laboratories where time is critical. Fourth, modifications have been so radical in certain specialized applications so as to remove ELISA altogether from the category of SPI. For example, "homogeneous" ELISAs or EIAs* depend upon the ability of an antigen-antibody interaction in solution to modify the activity of the enzyme. Finally, ELISA technology has been modified for use in so-called immunoblotting assays to detect antigens separated by electrophoresis, to determine the major antigenic proteins of a complicated mixture, and as diagnostic tools for the detection of, for example, antiviral antigens in AIDS testing.

With exception of homogeneous immunoassay, each of these variations on the original theme of Engvall and Perlmann involves the interfacial interaction of antibody and antigen and thus are appropriate for discussion in this chapter.

Hybridoma Technology and Genetic Engineering

The polyclonal nature of antibodies produced *in vivo* in animals immunized with even simple haptenic antigens has created problems when a distinction between two very similar antigens was required. Thus, the development of hybridoma technology, which culminated in the classic publication by Kohler and Milstein (1975), paved the way for the routine preparation of antibodies recognizing a single epitope; these antibodies were all derived from a single clone. Such monoclonality ensured a homogeneous response and permitted the investigator to select antibodies of the specificity needed for the task at hand. As often stated, monoclonal antibodies permit one to find

---

*Homogeneous EIA is the term used for solution phase-dependent immunoassay in contrast to "heterogeneous" EIAs in which one reactant is immobilized on a readily separable solid phase. Heterologous immunoassays are the subject of this chapter.

the needle *in* the haystack, whereas polyclonals find the needle *and* the haystack.

Monoclonal technology may also have brought with it problems which either did not exist with polyclonal antibodies or more likely, remained unrecognized. The performance of solid-phase monoclonal antibodies can vary tremendously to an extent that some may even fail to function, yet they function well in solution.

There is a great need for standardization of immunoassays in medical science. Hybridoma technology has helped fulfill this need by ensuring uniformity via the immortality of hybridoma cell lines. Recombinant DNA technology provides chimeric antibodies as standards for specific antibody immunoassay (SpAbI; Butler and Hamilton, 1991), and the field of genetic engineering will no doubt provide additional benefits to SPI. These may include engineered capture antibodies (CAb) which are highly suited for their role as solid-phase receptors, as well as engineered antigens, which reliably express the desired epitope when immobilized.

Antigen-Antibody Reactions Revisited

The interaction of antibodies with antigenic epitopes is monocovalent, and in the fluid phase follows the principles of the law of mass action. Reactions are governed by an association rate constant (k_1) and a dissociation constant (k_2), which results in equilibrium constants (K_{eq}) generally ranging from 10^5 to 10^{10} M^{-1}; higher or lower values are difficult to determine empirically using conventional methods but may be calculated after independent measurement of k_1 and k_2.

$$\text{Ag} + \text{Ab} \underset{k_2}{\overset{k_1}{\rightleftharpoons}} \text{AgAb} \qquad (1)$$

where

$$\text{where } \frac{k_1}{k_2} = K_{eq} = \frac{[\text{AgAb}]}{[\text{Ag}_f][\text{Ab}_f]}$$

[AgAb], [Ag_f], and [Ab_f] are the molar concentrations of complex, free antigen, and free antibody, respectively, at equilibrium.

First, the immobilization of one reactant would be expected to have some effect on K_{eq} when reaction kinetics for solid-phase reactions are compared to solution-phase interaction. Second, interfacial interactions involve other adjustments to the conventional wisdom of antigen-antibody reaction which is based on fluid-phase systems. For example, what is the reaction volume of an interfacial antigen-antibody reaction? Finally, the solid-phase reactant may express a different conformation than its solution-phase counterpart. This may introduce such factors as steric hindrance, epitope alteration, and changes in antibody affinity.

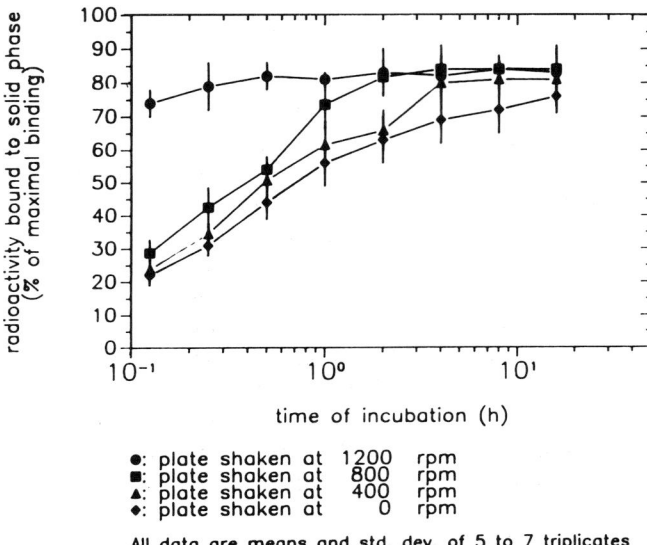

Figure 1. The diffusion dependence of solid-phase microtiter immunoassay. Data illustrate the attainment of equilibrium between an anti-pillin monoclonal and bacterial pilin adsorbed on microtiter wells incubated without agitation or vortexed at various rates indicated. Legend on figure. [From Franz, B., and Stegemann, M. (1991) *Immunochemistry of Solid-Phase Immunoassay* (J. E. Butler, ed.), CRC Press, Boca Raton, FL. With permission.]

THE CHARACTERISTICS OF INTERFACIAL ANTIGEN-ANTIBODY INTERACTIONS

The Kinetics of Interfacial Antigen-Antibody Reactions

The simplified equation below attempts to summarize the kinetics governing interfacial antigen-antibody interactions:

$$Ag_{SLD} + Ab_{SOL} \underset{k_2 D}{\overset{k_1 D}{\rightleftharpoons}} Ag_{SLD}\text{---}Ab_{SOL} \underset{k_2 R}{\overset{k_1 R}{\rightleftharpoons}} Ag_{SLD}\text{------}Ab_{SOL} \underset{k_2 A}{\overset{k_1 A}{\rightleftharpoons}} (Ag_{SLD}\text{---}Ab_{SOL})_n \quad (2)$$

Interfacial reactions kinetics include a more pronounced diffusion-dependent set of rate constants (k_1D and k_2D, constants that govern the mass transfer of reactants to the site of interaction) than do their fluid-phase counterparts. This means an overall increase in the time required for the reaction to reach equilibrium. This diffusion-dependent phase of the reaction can be largely eliminated through: (1) vigorous agitation (Fig. 1; Franz and Stegemann,

1991; Mushens and Scott, 1990), (2) confinement of the reaction volume to the liquid-solid interface, or (3) the use of colloidal microparticles capable of diffusion.

There is additional evidence that the kinetics governing the interfacial reaction of antibody and antigen (k_1R and k_2R)* also differ from those reported for solution-phase interactions. For example, the forward reaction rate (k_1) of antibody-hapten reactions are generally in the range of 10^7 m^{-1} s^{-1} (Karush, 1978; Steward, 1977; Absolom and van Oss, 1986) but may show up to a 2-log slower rate when the hapten is immobilized on a protein (Karush, 1978). The relative constancy of forward antibody-hapten reaction rates can be utilized to estimate K_{eq} values by measuring only the slower and more manageable dissociation rate constants and then calculating K_{eq} (Herron, 1984). In contrast to solution-phase reactions, the forward reaction rate constants (k_1R) for antigen-antibody reactions on synthetic surfaces has been reported to be 10^3 to 10^5 m^{-1} s^{-1} (Li, 1985; Nygren et al., 1986) and values of 10^5 to 10^6 m^{-1} s^{-1} have been reported for interfacial interactions on cell surfaces (Mason and Williams, 1980). Furthermore, increasing the concentration of solid-phase antibody decreases k_1, but does not affect dissociation rates (Fowell and Chase, 1986). Slightly higher k_1 values have been reported for divalent antibodies as compared to Fab (Mason and Williams, 1980) which may be the consequence of polyvalency (Crothers and Metzger, 1972) or surface-induced coagulation (MacRitchie, 1972; see below).

The slow rate of dissociation of antibodies from synthetic or cellular interfaces is particularly noteworthy. The k_2 values for solution-phase interactions differ considerably and may range from nearly 10^2 to 10^{-5} m^{-1} s^{-1}; essentially the off-rate determines differences in K_{eq} (Butler, 1991; Friguet et al., 1989; Froese, 1968; Steward, 1977); values of 10^{-2} m^{-1} s^{-1} or higher are most common. By contrast, k_2 rates reported for interfacial systems are in the range of 10^{-4} m^{-1} s^{-1} to 10^{-5} m^{-1} s^{-1} (Mason and Williams, 1980; Nygren et al., 1986). Of some interest is the observation that even the k_2R rates for Fab are lower than those for k_2R rates involving solution-phase interactions.

Calculation of K_{eq} for interfacial antigen-antibody reactions leads to the conclusion that solid-phase interactions, once established, are virtually irreversible within the time period over which solid-phase immunoassays are usually conducted (Berzofsky and Berkower, 1984; Nygren et al., 1985). Perhaps it is this characteristic which allows SPI to function with consistency even in the hands of the novice. Consider for a moment the multiple and often vigorous washing and reaction steps to which SPIs, especially ELISAs, are subjected. Often, incubation steps proceed 4 to 16 h in the absence of free ligand. If dissociation rates were indeed of the order of magnitude characteristic of simple antibody-hapten solution-phase systems, substantial amounts of the primary reaction would dissociate during incubation. Especially inter-

---

*The use of k_1 or k_2 without a capital suffix, e.g., k_1R, refers to cited data in which the kinetics of interfacial interaction were not subdivided into the various phases as shown in Eq. (2).

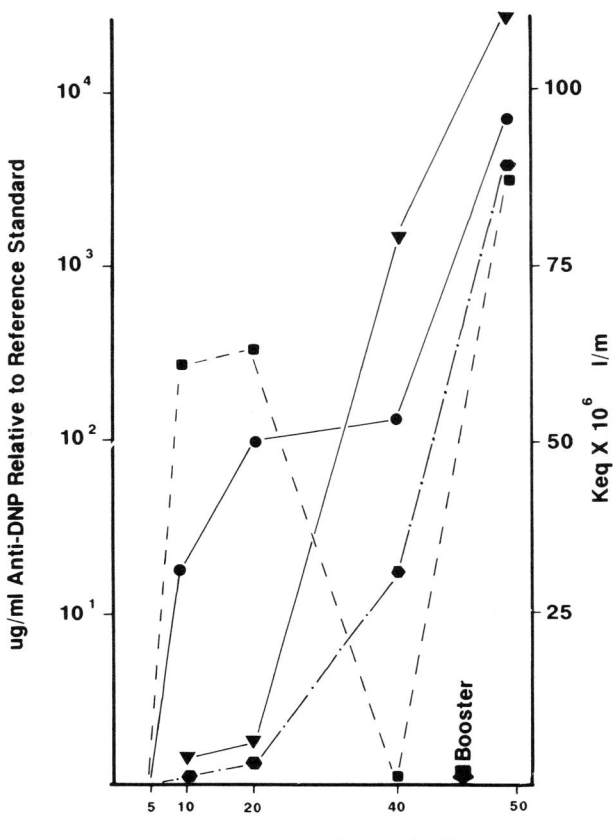

Figure 2. The affinity-dependence of solid-phase microtiter SpAbI. Data show the concentration of rat IgG anti-DNP determined by a double immunoprecipitin assay (■---■), conventional ELISA (●···●), or the amplified ELISA (●—●). The latter utilizes a multistep detection system which provides considerable opportunity for cross-linking and surface-aggregate formation. Double immunprecipitation is regarded as a reliable measure of total antibody independent of affinity. Affinity (▼—▼) determined by equilibrium dialysis. [From Butler et al. (1978b) *Immunochemistry* 15:131. With permission.]

esting are data presented in Fig. 2. While detection of rat anti-DNP (dinitrophenol) antibodies using a simple ELISA appears to be more dependent on affinity than antibody concentration, assays such as double-antibody coprecipitation or the "amplified ELISA" (a-ELISA; Bulter et al., 1978a,b) which depend on the eventual generation of large antigen-antibody complexes, appear to be less affinity dependent. Multivalency is known to cause a several log increase in the apparent K_{eq} of antibody-antigen reactions (Karush, 1970). Perhaps cross-linking of reactants within interfacial immune complexes can explain both the affinity independence of certain systems and the slow dissociation rate of interfacial antigen-antibody interactions. Fc- or C region-dependent cooperative binding of antibodies of different specificities has been described (Greenspan et al., 1989; Pearce-Pratt and Roser, 1990), raising the possibility that stability of immune complexes may not solely depend on binding-site cross-linking.

The cross-linking of antigen-antibody complexes at interfaces may also be associated with surface coagulation. It is known that passive adsorbed proteins are capable of movement; both desorption (Fenstermaker et al., 1974; Peterman, 1985) and translational diffusion along the plane on which they are immobilized (Michaeli et al., 1980). Therefore, the possibility exists for yet another kinetic phase of the interfacial interaction of antigens and antibodies, one involving the formation of aggregate clusters [see Eq. (2)]. The extent to which such cluster formation occurs would, of course, depend on the polyvalency of the antigen, the capability of the surfaced-adsorbed molecules to coagulate, and the complexity of the detection system which might promote coagulation, e.g., a-ELISA (Butler et al., 1978a). Presumably, dissociation of reactants from coagulative complexes would proceed at a slower rate than from simple antigen-antibody complexes.

The various kinetic aspects of SPI described here strongly suggest that there are numerous reasons for exercising caution before applying the kinetics of solution-phase antigen-antibody reactions to those occurring on a solid phase.

Biological Properties of Immobilized Reactants

The previous section described two characteristics of solid-phase reactants that can influence their biological activity. First, immobilized reactants are nondiffusible and are probably limited to translational surface movement and/or aggregation. Hence, any diffusion-dependent properties that characterize the same reactant in solution will be seriously affected. Second, properties which depend on the state of aggregation could be altered. Børmer (1989) reported that mouse IgG2b used as capture antibody (CAb) adsorbed to polystyrene is able to fix $C'3$ and $C1q$. These are properties normally ascribed to antibodies clustered in soluble immune complexes or on cell surfaces. Aggregation or clustering of immobilized reactants would also affect their concentrations (Fig. 3).

Figure 3 summarizes a variety of molecular changes that soluble proteins may undergo during immobilization. The model protein is depicted as expressing four functional epitopes (1 to 4), which could be antigenic determinants, enzyme catalytic sites, or a ligand receptor. Covalent attachment could lead to loss of one or more epitopes through formation of the covalent linkage or steric hindrance (Fig. 3A). Epitopes may also be sterically "buried" by passive adsorption (Fig. 3D). Passively adsorbed molecules may undergo conformational change as a consequence of unfolding to interact hydrophically

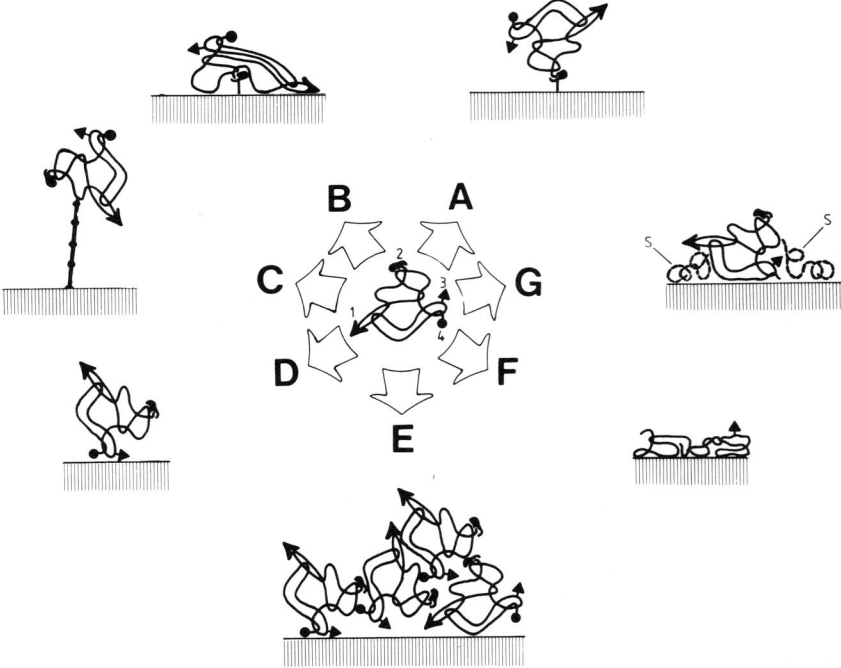

Figure 3. The conformation of solid-phase reactants. A hypothetical protein with four functional epitopes when in free solution (center, 1 to 4), is depicted after various means of immobilization on hydrophobic solid-phase (A to G). (A) Simple covalent attachment; (B) secondary hydrophobic binding of the covalently-bound protein; (C) covalent binding through a rigid "spacer"; (D) passive adsorption without conformational alteration; (E) passive adsorption accompanied by aggregation; (F) passive adsorption accompanied by severe conformational change; (G) stabilization of the protein during passive adsorption by coadsorption of a stabilizing protein(s).

with the surface (Fig. 3F). This may be so serious as to result in the loss of all epitopes or perhaps, even to permit expression of "new epitopes." The extent of adsorption-induced conformational change appears to depend on the concentration of adsorbed protein and on the nature of the molecule; rigid proteins like serum albumin appear less altered than IgG (Morrissey, 1977). Adsorbed proteins appear most distorted at low concentration and this may be overcome by coadsorption of a stabilizing protein (Fig. 3G; Dierks et al., 1986; Jitsukawa et al., 1989). While covalent immobilization may avoid adsorption-induced conformation change, this is probably only the case when attachment is to a hydrophilic, synthetic surface. Molecules covalently linked to hydrophobic surfaces, especially if incubated for long periods, can eventually bond hydrophobically as well (Fig. 3B). Immobilization methods involving the use of rigid spacers or "carrier" proteins, may prevent such secondary association with the solid phase (Fig. 3C).

All immobilization effects are not necessarily negative. Enzymes immobilized on synthetic interfaces retain their activity longer than those in solution (Schellenberger and Ulbrich, 1989), suggesting that immobilization might similarly effect antigens and antibodies. Reactive solid phases for SPI can be stored days or months prior to use with little or no deleterious effect (Voller et al., 1979). This retention of biological activity by immobilized reactants makes SPI a convenient and practical tool in biology and medicine.

Concentration and Distribution of Immobilized Reactants

One of the least understood aspects of SPI concerns the actual concentration of surface reactants and the related topic of their distribution. Unlike solution-phase reactions, the participating reactants in SPI are not uniformly distributed within the fluid of the reaction. Rather, the reaction-rate dependent interaction [k_1R; k_2R; see Eq. (2)] occurs at a fluid-solid phase interface, the actual volumetric dimensions of which are difficult to determine. Because the reaction rate-dependent kinetics are governed by reactant concentration within this volume, their magnitude remains an unknown as long as the volume remains unknown. Presumably, this could partially explain the large discrepancy between the measured K_{eq} of solid-phase CAbs and the K_{eq} of these antibodies in solution (Butler et al., 1991a; Joshi and Butler, 1991c). Some investigators have proposed that due to the confined reaction volume, the functional interfacial concentration of reactants is so high, and k_2R values so low, that interfacial reactions appear irreversible (Nygren et al., 1985). As mentioned earlier, this kinetic property of SPI may have contributed significantly to its reproducibility and success.

The issue of concentration may be strongly associated with the issue of distribution. Theoretically it is possible that interfacial reactants are (1) uniformly distributed as a monolayer of individual molecules, (2) regularly distributed as polymers (aggregates) of uniform size, and (3) randomly distributed in the form of individual molecules and polymers (aggregates) of various sizes. A more homogeneous distribution should lead to greater uniformity of reaction volume and thus more uniform reactivity over the surface. The role of distribution can be visualized in Fig. 3E, in which molecular aggregation raises the local density of epitope 1. Such aggregation could allow multivalent binding of antibodies and would, e.g., render invalid the assumption of Horeisi and Matousek (1985) that the distance between any two randomly adsorbed antigen molecules would be too great for cross-linking to bias estimates of affinity.

The nature of reactant distribution on synthetic interfaces may depend on the nature of the synthetic surface (e.g., polystyrene vs nitrocellulose), whether reactants are covalently attached or passively adsorbed, the physical chemical properties of the reactant, and the condition of immobilization. Interfacial distribution of reactants on cell membranes may depend on the state of membrane fluidity of the cell, the possibility of reactant cross-linking as in the case of lymphocyte "capping", and the nature of the cell "receptor" and its relationship to the cytoskeleton. When the various possibilities for differences in the interfacial distribution of reactants are considered, it becomes clear that few generalizations can be made and that all interfacial interactions cannot be understood by using one as a model for all others.

The Detection of Interfacial Antigen-Antibody Reactions

Our understanding of the behavior of antigens and antibodies immobilized on a solid phase depends to a large extent on their indirect detection, using immunochemical reagents coupled to some "signal generator". The primary goal of such methodology has been the development of SPI for antibody or antigen quantitation.

Modern SPI emerged in part from its historical predecessor, RIA. This is no doubt the reason why radioactive iodine was one of the initial types of "signal generators" used in SPI. By the standards of 1990, iodinated reagents have numerous disadvantages for routine diagnostics. First, health physics standards (Regulatory Guide, 1978) are more rigorously enforced than two decades earlier, in part, because of the proliferation of immunoassay throughout medical science. The widespread use of iodine in multiuse laboratories, especially those involving students where personnel changes are frequent, is potentially dangerous. Second, both ^{125}I and ^{131}I have short half-lives (57 and 9 days, respectively), necessitating the continuous generation or purchase of new signal generators. Apart from its disadvantages in routine diagnostic laboratories, radioactive iodine is still a fundamental research tool for immunochemists studying reaction kinetics and stoichiometry. In contrast to fluoresceination, biotinylation, and conjugation with enzymes, the introduction of one atom of iodine per mole of protein provides a strong detection signal typically without alteration of the biochemical or conformational properties of the protein.

Fluorescent labeling of proteins, especially antibodies, is widely used for routine SPI. The lack of any biohazards associated with fluorescence, together with advances in instrumentation that can take advantage of the subtleties of the photophysics of fluorescence, has greatly expanded its use. Chemiluminescence and time-resolve and internal reflection fluorescence are likely to receive wider application in the new generation of SPIs.

The use of enzymes covalently coupled to antibodies and antigens overcomes most of the disadvantages of radioactive labels. However, when used in heterogeneous immunoassay,* they are more cumbersome than fluorescence because of (1) the large size of the conjugate and (2) the additional enzyme-substrate reaction step required. The popularity and success of en-

---

*Homogeneous immunoassays are not SPIs and typically depend on the modification of the activity of an enzyme as a result of antibody-antigen interaction. Heterogeneous immunoassay is another term for SPI in which physical separation of bound and free reactants is required.

zymes as signal generators in SPI is due to (1) their ease and safety of use, (2) the substantial amplification of signal which they can generate, (3) their applicability to measure the reaction by rate analyses, (4) the fact that the user views a visual reaction, and (5) the generally less expensive instrumentation needed for their detection. Methods of conjugation are reviewed elsewhere (Kennedy et al., 1976).

Simple conversion of RIA to enzyme immunoassay (EIA) is often more than a simple matter of exchanging one signal generator for another. Classical RIA is a direct competitive immunoassay used to quantitate small antigens. Substituting a protein enzyme for an atom of iodine in such small molecules is sure to change their biochemical properties. Hence, the conversion of RIA to EIA often involves a switch to an indirect competitive assay* or to a homogeneous enzyme immunoassay.

Perhaps the most overrated aspects of various detection systems is their relative sensitivities. While sensitivity differences clearly exist, the claims by inventors of improved sensitivity are often the result of immunochemical adjustments rather than merely an increase in signal. "Cleaning up" the immunochemistry to reduce background "noise", or altering kinetics (Fig. 1), can alone increase the apparent sensitivity. On the other hand, improved sensitivity can be achieved through amplification using more complex indirect detection systems (Butler et al., 1978a; Guesdon et al., 1979; Nilsson, 1988), secondary enzyme activation (Self, 1985), combined EIA and RIA (Harris et al., 1979), or alternative substrates that provide fluorescent or chemiluminescent signals (Khahil, 1991).

IMMOBILIZATION OF ANTIGENS AND ANTIBODIES
Covalent Immobilization
The Chemistry of Covalent Immobilization

Simplistically speaking, synthetic surfaces that can be functionalized to allow covalent attachment of the ligand or receptor, and are either hydrophilic or hydrophobic, with some surfaces exhibiting both properties. Affinity chromatography has been generally developed using hydrophilic solid phases, e.g., dextran, agarose, and silica. To a large extent, surfaces which are logistically most practical for modern immunoassays, e.g., plastic, nylon, and nitrocellulose, have a hydrophobic character. While the energy of hydrophobic interaction is very strong, and most proteins readily adsorb to hydrophobic surfaces, this process can have a negative effect on the biological activity of the adsorbed biomolecule. Hence, there has been a justifiable effort to immobilize reactants covalently to avoid the negative consequences of hydrophobic adsorption.

---

*Indirect competitive immunoassays are those in which no modification of the antigen to be measured is required. Rather, quantitation depends on measurement of the amount of free antibody, i.e., antibody not bound by competing antigen.

Polystyrene can be treated with nitric acid to yield polynitrostyrene (Chin and Lanks, 1977; Quash et al., 1989; Rubin et al., 1980). Subsequent reduction with sodium dithionite or hydrosulfite yields polyaminostyrene which can then be coupled to protein by various means. Dimethylsuberimidate (DMS) is often employed for the coupling of proteins. Treatment with succinic anhydride results in polycarboxylstyrene which can then be coupled to protein amino groups using water-soluble carbodiimide (EDAC; Quash et al., 1989). Polycarboxylstyrene may also be modified to contain hydrazido groups with hydrazine and EDAC, resulting in polyhydrazidostyrene which can bind glycoproteins pretreated with periodate (Thomas et al., 1990). Aminystyrene is commercially available as "Covalink" from NUNC (Roskilde, DEN). Treatment of Covalink plates with N-hydroxysuccinimide and EDAC in the presence of the desired peptide or protein, results in its covalent immobilizations (Søndergard-Andersen et al., 1990). Proteins and peptides may also be coupled using suberate cross-linkers.

Coupling to polystyrene can be achieved using toluene-2,4-diisocyanate in CCl_4, which is believed to erode the surface and generate isocyanate groups capable of reacting with protein amino groups (Saito and Nagai, 1983).

Various investigators have utilized a modified form of covalent attachment in which the surface of polystyrene is at first coated with polylysine, phenylalanine-lysine, octadecylamine, or BSA, and then treated with a suitable covalent cross-linking agent such as glutaraldehyde, DMS, or EDAC, so that the ligand or protein is covalently immobilized to the adsorbed amino acid polymer or protein (Hobbs, 1989; Parsens, 1981; Papadea et al., 1985; Suter, 1982).

Radiation-sterilized polystyrene may be directly coupled to ligands in the presence of EDAC to yield covalently bound ligand (Varga et al., 1990). Irradiation is believed to cause the appearance of nucleophilic groups on the surface, a process that is increased in the presence of water and decreased in the presence of oxygen. Irradiation is deliberately utilized by NUNC to introduce such groups on the surface of their Maxisorp microtiter plates. This charge-modified surface promotes rapid hydrophilic adsorption but if incubation proceeds for a long time, adsorption will nevertheless become largely hydrophobic (Fig. 3B). Hence, all functionalized hydrophobic surfaces permit adsorption of protein if measures are not taken to prevent it. In some cases, initial adsorption may be a prerequisite for covalent bonding (Smalla et al., 1988).

Other hydrophobic surfaces have also been functionalized. A functionalized membrane, Immobilon AV, is available from Millipore. Nitrocellulose can be functionalized to express reactive aldehyde groups in "Nit-CHO" (Lauritzen et al., 1990). Conversion is via treatment with divinyl sulfone followed by ethylenediamine and finally 1% glutaraldehyde.

A great deal of information is available on covalent immobilization of reactants to hydrophilic surfaces from the work in the field of affinity chromatography (Chaiken et al., 1983; Cuatrecasas and Anfinsen, 1971). This includes a wealth of information on coupling chemistries as well as data on the nature and advantages of chemical spacers (Cuatrecasas, 1970; Inman, 1982).

Immunochemical Consequences of Covalent Immobilization

Covalent immobilization can offer several advantages: (1) immobilization of more native biomolecules (Fig. 3A), (2) generation of a surface with a higher density of biomolecules, and (3) greater stability, i.e., less desorption than occurs with passively adsorbed biomolecules. Covalent immobilization can be especially valuable for molecules that have little affinity for adsorption on synthetic surfaces, e.g., polysaccharides. While larger amounts of reactant can be immobilized covalently, a corresponding improvement in activity is not always seen. This has been demonstrated using antifluorescyl antibodies (Peterman et al., 1988). Covalent attachment may have a special advantage in solid-phase peptide immunoassay and for immobilizing membrane antigens.

Adsorption of Proteins on Plastic and Synthetic Membranes

Characteristics and Chemistry of Protein Adsorption

Proteins become adsorbed to plastic in direct linear proportion to the amount added, up to the point where it would appear that the synthetic "surface receptors" become gradually saturated (Fig. 4A). Differences in the Y intercept of the log-log linear binding plots indicate differences in affinity (avidity*) for the plastic. Differences in avidity among proteins are more apparent when data are expressed in percentage bound plots, where the binding percentage in the region of constant binding is a function of avidity (Fig. 4B). Differences in the affinity of proteins for plastic have also been observed by others (Brash and Lyman, 1969; Lee et al., 1974; Urbanek et al., 1985), as well as differences in adsorptive properties among plastics (Kenny and Dunsmoor, 1983). Above the linear-binding region, competition occurs (Cantarero et al., 1980; Kenny and Dunsmoor, 1983), and proteins with high avidity, e.g., fibrinogen, can displace previously adsorbed albumin (Fenstermaker et al., 1974). Adsorbed proteins are less stable than those covalently linked (Blanchard et al., 1990), although desorption in the presence of detergent appears only to be problematic when excessive concentrations of reactant are adsorbed (Peterman, 1985).

The data of Figure 4B are also instructive in showing that the molar concentration at which linear binding ceases, with the exception of ovalbumin, is inversely proportional to the avidity of the various proteins, and that the order of avidity, ovalbumin excluded, appears directly proportional to molecular weight. The latter suggests that avidity is probably a consequence of

---

*It is reasonable to assume that the strength of noncovalent bonding in passive adsorption is due to multisite binding which significantly decreases the dissociate rate of the complete molecule. Hence, the term avidity is more correct than affinity.

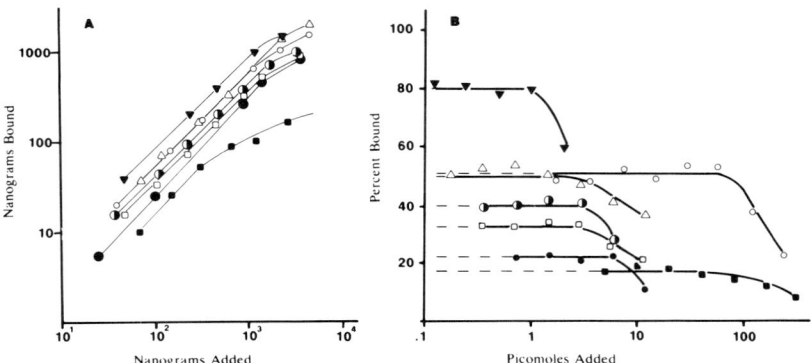

Figure 4. The characteristics of passive adsorption on polystyrene. (A) The adsorptive behavior of seven different proteins in a log-log saturation plot. ▼ Bovine IgM, 1000 kDa; △ bovine SIgA, 420 kDa; ○ ovalbumin, 44 kDa; ○ bovine IgG1, 158 kDa; □ bovine IgG2a, 152 kDa; ○ bovine serum albumin, 69 kDa; ■ bovine α-lactalbumin, 14 kDa. (B) The adsorptive behavior of the same proteins expressed in a molar percentage bound plot. Dashed lines are extrapolations in the region of constant percentage binding for which empirical data were not reported. Same symbols as in A. (From Cantarero et al., 1980.)

the surface area of the molecule which can contact the plastic. Superficially these relationships also suggest that a finite area is available for the protein to adsorb and that once protein is passively adsorbed to form a monolayer, the surface is saturated and the nature of the binding plot changes. However, neither surface-area mathematics, scanning electron microscopy (SEM) studies, or the behavior of ovalbumin, support this conclusion. At the apparent point of "receptor saturation" of polystyrene for rabbit IgG, the available surface area is covered assuming that one IgG molecule occupies an area of ca. 70 nM^2. SEM studies, using either colloidal gold particles or by direct visualization of carbon-coated protein, indicate non-uniform distribution of IgG (Butler et al., 1992b) although the chemistry of polystyrene is uniform (Rasmussen, 1990) and its surface smooth. Hence, the apparent saturation phenomenon illustrated in Fig. 4 appears consistent with the mathematical calculations but inconsistent with the formation of non-random clusters. Nevertheless, optimal capture antibody (CAb) activity is achieved at the highest coating concentration which would produce a monolayer assuming uniform distribution. This corresponds to the addition of 200 μl of CAb at 5 μg/ml (Butler et al., 1991; Joshi et al., 1992).

The passive adsorption of protein on synthetic surfaces such as polystyrene, vinyl polymers, polypropylene, nylon, and nitrocellulose (NC) is generally agreed to result from the formation of strong hydrophobic bonds. Adsorption can be inhibited by detergents and other agents capable of interfering with hydrophobic bond formation (Gardas and Lewartowska, 1988; Gripenberg and Kuruki, 1986; Kenny and Dunsmoor, 1983; Newman et al., 1981; Palfree and Elliot, 1982) and are generally facilitated by moderate salt concentrations which drive the hydrophobic interaction (Smalla et al., 1988). The pH dependence of adsorption is somewhat controversial. Generally, there is little or no pH effect, although somewhat greater adsorption seems to occur near the Ip of proteins (see below). The pH dependence may be much more important for heavily glycosylated protein and polysaccharides (Elkins et al., 1990).

As early as 1956, Bull presented data to suggest that protein adsorbed on glass underwent conformational change in the process. These data are in agreement with the thermodynamic findings of Nyilas et al. (1974) and Lyklema and Norde (1973) and the spectrophotometric studies of Burghardt and Axelrod (1983). These findings are further supported by numerous immunochemical studies. It is believed that such conformational changes allow hydrophobic groups to gain access to the hydrophobic synthetic surface. Increased adsorption of acid-treated antibodies appears to result from greater exposure of hydrophobic groups (Conradie et al., 1983).

The adsorptive process is most likely complex; it appears to be biphasic with differences in binding constants associated with each phase (Oreskes and Singer, 1961; Pesce et al., 1977). Proteins adsorbed at low concentrations may undergo the greatest conformational change (Kochwa et al., 1967; Nyilas et al., 1974). A parallel increase in the loss of antigenicity at low concentration is also supported by immunochemical studies (Fig. 5; Dierks et al., 1986; Jitsukawa et al., 1989).

A number of interesting, but puzzling, features of studies on protein adsorption are worthy of comment. First, the kinetic and thermodynamic studies of Oreskes and Singer (1961) suggest that adsorbed proteins may exist in different allosteric conformations which appear to be related to the "coating concentration" used and the nature of the protein. At very low concentrations, IgG adsorbed on polystyrene latex behaves like heat-denatured globulin (Kochwa et al., 1967). The bi- or multiphase nature of protein adsorption may be due in part to the ability of adsorbed protein to move along the plane of adsorption, i.e., "translation diffusion" (Michaeli et al., 1980). There may be some connection between observations that hydrophobic adsorption is maximal near the Ip of the protein (Bull, 1956; Elkins et al., 1990; Morressey and Stromberg, 1974; Oreskes and Singer, 1961) and evidence that passively adsorbed proteins exist in the form of clusters (Børmer, 1989; Brash and Lyman, 1969; Butler et al., 1992; Greenspan et al, 1989; Nygren, 1988). It is interesting to speculate from these diverse observations that hydrophobic surface adsorption is essentially the adsorption of aggregates that form with greatest propensity at optimal salt concentration, at the Ip of the protein, and under conditions in which the ratio of hydrophobic surface to protein is at a maximum. Increasing the concentration of added protein restores a condition unfavorable to destabilization of soluble protein. Hence, the apparent "receptor saturation" observed in adsorption plots (Fig. 4A) represents the point at which the destabilization effects of the polystyrene surface are overcome by the stabilizing effects of increasing protein concentration.

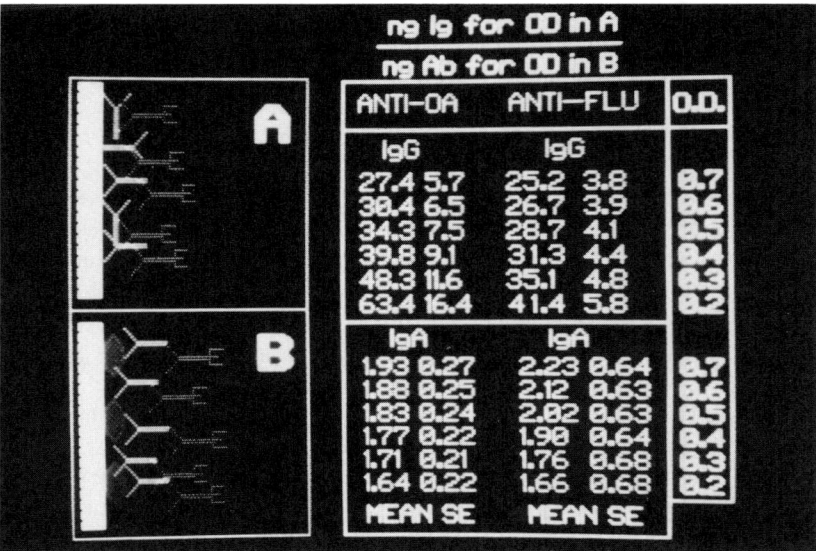

Figure 5. The comparative antigenicity of rabbit IgG and IgA directly adsorbed on plastics versus when bound to solid-phase antigens. The diagram on the left illustrates the two configurations, (A) and (B), which were employed for antibodies of both isotypes. (A) Passive adsorption; (B) immobilization via binding to antigen. The tabled values are the ratio of detectability measured as the ratios of the ng of passively adsorbed Ig* to ng of antibody bound to antigen which gave equivalent ELISA activity. For example, to produce the same OD405, approximate twice as much IgA must be passively adsorbed as compared to the amount bound to antigen. Data are presented for iodinated IgG and IgA anti-ovalbumin (OA) and anti-fluorescein (FLU). Specific enzyme-conjugated, anti-γ and anti-α secondary antibodies were employed for detection. The column on the right indicates the OD406 (enzyme activity) at which comparisons were made, i.e., the relative concentration over which comparisons were made. Note that the ratio is concentration-dependent for IgG but independent of concentration for IgA. [Modified from Dierks et al. (1986) *Mol. Immunol.* 23:403.]

Hydrophobic forces are also believed to play a major role in adsorption on NC (Bers and Garfin, 1985; Gershoni and Palade, 1982; Towbin and Gordon, 1984). Binding to NC is increased in high ionic strength buffers and reduced or inhibited by detergents. The pH is known to influence adsorption on NC; maximal binding occurs close to the pI of the protein (Nyholm and Ramlau, 1988). The pH dependence of adsorption to plastic seems less pronounced (Dierks, 1985; van Oss and Singer, 1966). By contrast, pH plays no significant role in binding or release from charge-modified nylon (Gershoni and Palade, 1982; Ramlau, 1988) although electrostatic interactions are important on this medium. The higher binding capacity of unmodified nylon compared to NC, is in part due to intrinsic charge groups on this medium. While methanol can increase binding to NC, it has little effect on nylon (Brown et al., 1991). The PVDF membranes (e.g., Immobilon-P) have the highest retention of adsorbed protein which is bound exclusively by hydro-

---

*Adsorbed Ig was affinity-purified specific antibody.

phobic bonds. Synthetic membranes show considerable heterogeneity in their binding properties and different proteins show greater variability in their affinity for any one membrane than they do for polystyrene (Brown et al., 1991). The apparent >500-fold higher capacity of membranes for adsorption is probably a result of their large internal surface area which has been estimated to be 100- to 1000-fold their planar area (Nyholm and Ramlau, 1988).

Finally, precoating with substances like glutaraldehyde and polylysine has been described as a means of facilitating stable passive adsorption (Gabrilovac et al., 1979; Pachmann and Leibold, 1976; Suter, 1982) although their value is controversial and can produce troublesome background effects (Herrmann et al., 1979).

Properties of Adsorbed Proteins

There is a substantial body of evidence to indicate that proteins in general undergo conformational change when adsorbed to synthetic surfaces. The evidence obtained from physical chemical studies (Bull, 1956; Lyklema and Norde, 1973; Morrissey and Fenstermaker, 1976; Nyilas et al., 1974; Soderquist and Walton, 1980) is strongly supported by immunochemical studies in which changes in the immunoreactivity of adsorbed vs nonadsorbed antigen is taken as evidence for a conformational change in epitopes. Kochwa et al. (1967) reported that adsorbed IgG behaved antigenically like heat-denatured material. Kennel (1982), Djavadi-Ohaniance et al. (1984), Hollander and Katchalski-Katzir (1986), and Stevens et al. (1986) all observed that monoclonal antibodies recognized adsorbed antigens differently than in solution. Friguet et al. (1984) demonstrated that monoclonals which associated only slowly with the β_2-subunit of *E. coli* tryptophan synthase, as opposed to those which bound rapidly, preferentially bound to denatured forms of the protein. Five out of a total of twelve monoclonals raised to this protein were of this class and bound easily to the adsorbed enzyme. A similar phenomenon was seen with polyclonal antibodies specific for rabbit IgG and IgA (Fig. 5). Rabbit IgA antibodies bound to their antigen on a solid phase were recognized twice as well as when merely adsorbed on plastic. By contrast, adsorbed IgG was recognized only 1/25 to 1/60 as well as IgG bound to its antigen. The ratio of detectability for IgG depended on the concentration of adsorbed IgG, lower amounts of adsorbed IgG being least detectable (Fig. 5). Loss of antigenic detectability at low concentration could be overcome by coadsorption of small amounts of albumin (Dierks, 1986). The stabilizing effect of coadsorbed proteins has now been demonstrated for a number of antigens (Jitsukawa et al., 1989) (see Figure 3F and 3G).

The changes in immunochemical reactivity of adsorbed proteins have alternative explanations. Prominent among these is steric hindrance of epitopes (Fig. 3D and 3E). Countering the argument of mere steric hindrance, is the evidence that "new epitopes" appear after adsorption (Dunn et al., 1985; Friguet et al., 1984; Mierendorf and Dimond, 1983; Stevens et al., 1986; Vaidya et al., 1985). While identifying the actual mechanism may be difficult, the consequences of using such antigens for detecting specific antibodies in patient or animal sera have the same dangerous effect.

Adsorption-induced protein changes also effect capture antibodies; monoclonal antibodies especially undergo loss of affinity and functional antibody-binding sites.

Since the description of immunoblotting (Towbin et al., 1979), NC and a number of membrane filters have been widely used as solid phases for immunoassay. In contrast to polystyrene, there have been very few attempts to investigate the characteristics of the adsorbed proteins. The most common use of NC is as the solid phase onto which proteins, first separated in polyacrylamide gel, are subsequently transferred. Hence, changes in immunoreactivity could result from the electrophoretic process, the reduction of interchain disulfide bonds, the transfer process itself, or conformational changes resulting from adsorption. For example, the failure of four out of five monoclonals specific for human IgG γ-chains to recognize IgG on immunoblots, has been ascribed to the loss of conformational epitopes due to cleavage of H and L chain disulfide bonds (Thorpe et al., 1984). Because the bond forces involved in adsorption on NC are similar to those bonding protein to plastic, similar conformational changes can be anticipated.

Noncovalent, Nonadsorptive Immobilization of Antigens

Immunochemical Immobilization

Awareness of the potential loss of antigenic or antibody activity due to passive adsorption or even through covalent bonding has prompted various investigators to devise systems which involve neither. The simplest procedure is the use of a primary capture antibody or capture antigen. For example, Fig. 5 illustrates how the antigen (ovalbumin) is used to capture either rabbit IgG or IgA on the solid-phase without adsorption (note: capture of the second reactant is done in the presence of nonionic detergent which prevents hydrophobic adsorption of the antibody directly to the plastic). The data in Fig. 5 also illustrate the positive effect of preserving immunoreactivity through the use of a nonadsorptive method of immobilization; this is most pronounced in the case of rabbit IgG.

Variations on the above theme are described throughout the literature. The use of a first-level polyclonal CAb, e.g., goat antimouse, to immobilize a second-level mouse monoclonal for use in two-site or "sandwich" ELISAs or in certain specific antibody immunoassays (SpAbI), is a common example of this type of immobilization (Hirano et al., 1989; Nustad et al., 1984; Zeiss et al., 1973). While this method may indeed yield a solid-phase monoclonal CAb which may function better than when adsorbed, a number of factors should be considered before selecting the method. First, it is predictable and has been shown empirically (Joshi and Butler, unpublished) that significantly smaller amounts of the monoclonal will be bound to the solid phase than via direct adsorption. The same is true for immunochemically immobilized antigen (Herrmann et al., 1979). The number of secondarily immobilized macromolecules will always be less than the number of adsorbed primary macromolecules. If 50% of an adsorbed monoclonal antibody (MAb) loses its activity, and immunochemical immobilization results in 50% less MAb, the end result is the same. Second, the primary CAb must be of high avidity in order to bind 50% of the secondary MAb; the first CAb may have to be affinity purified to increase antibody abundance.* Third, if the intention is to develop a sandwich assay, caution is necessary so that the detection antibody used does not recognize the first-level CAb; otherwise unacceptable background "noise" will be present (Butler, 1988).

Immunochemical immobilization of antigen (McCullough et al., 1985; Trent et al., 1976; Zigterman et al., 1988) faces the same potential problem with background as described above for antibody immobilization, but there is an additional concern. The antigen must be multivalent so that it can be both captured and still express determinants to be recognized by other antibodies (McCullough et al., 1985). If the capture monoclonal is specific for an irrelevant epitope on the antigen, this generally increases the probability that the epitopes of interest will still be available for reaction. Immunochemical immobilization of antigen can be especially useful for multivalent antigens like polysaccharides and heavy glycosylated proteins which have very low affinity for direct adsorption (Barrett et al., 1980; Carlson et al., 1982; Katz and Schiffman, 1985; Voller et al., 1976; Zigterman et al., 1988); this technique has also been shown to improve the antigenicity of immobilized antigen (Brennand et al., 1986).

Other Noncovalent Methods of Immobilization

The high affinity of avidin and streptavidin (SA) for biotin (Green, 1963; Piran and Riordan, 1990) qualifies it as an excellent first-level capture system. Unfortunately, SA has a very low affinity for polystyrene, and must be immobilized using the protein-avidin-biotin-capture (PABC) system (Fig. 6A; Suter and Butler, 1986) or through covalent attachment (Peterman et al., 1988; Nardelli et al., 1989).

The PABC system depends on the multivalency of SA which allows it to bridge CAb or Ag to an irrelevant, adsorbed, and biotinylated protein (Fig. 6A). The usefulness of the PABC is demonstrated in Fig. 6C in which the antigen-capture capacity (AgCC) of a biotinylated monoclonal is shown to increase fivefold when immobilized via the PABC vs adsorbed directly on plastic. Similarly, biotinylated monoclonals immobilized using covalently bound streptavidin also have higher AgCC than when the same monoclonals are immobilized covalently (Peterman et al., 1988).

---

*Antibody abundance refers to the percentage of an antibody preparation which is specific antibody; globulin fractions of serum or IgG fractioning purified using protein A have lower antibody abundance than affinity-purified antibody.

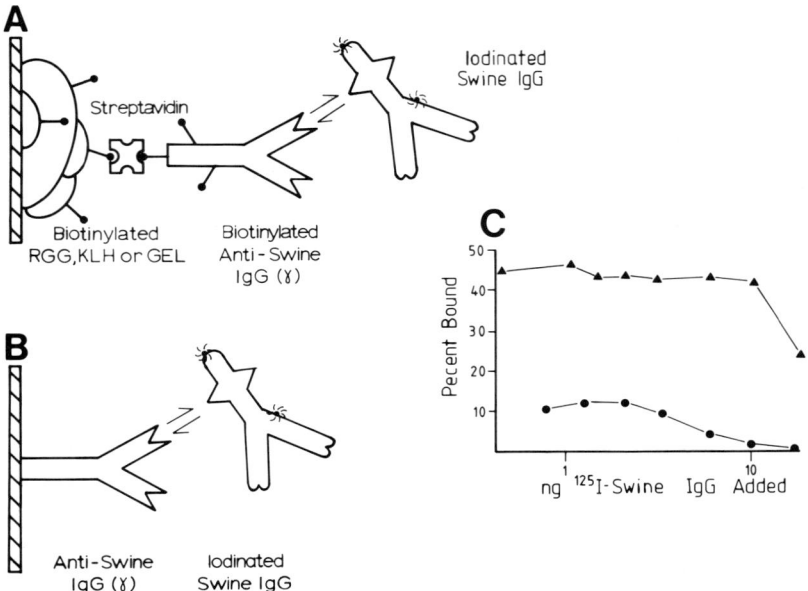

Figure 6. The antigen-capture capacity (AgCC) of a monoclonal capture antibody immobilized by a nonadsorptive, noncovalent method involving a streptavidin bridge (A) versus by direct passive adsorption (B). The percentage bound plot (C) shows the AgCC of the same monoclonal antibody after being immobilized by the two methods (▲, method A; ●, method B).

Apart from the system using covalently bound streptavidin, the original PABC system shares with immunochemical immobilization of CAbs the property that only 50% as much CAb can be immobilized as compared to direct adsorption. Furthermore, care must be used during biotinylation to avoid alteration of antibody activity, a possibility that has caused some investigators to restrict substitution to the carbohydrate moiety (O'Shannessy et al., 1984). The stoichiometry of the PABC system, including data on the effect of various degrees of biotinylation, is presented elsewhere (Suter et al., 1989).

In addition to the use of the avidin-biotin system, several other more specialized forms of noncovalent immobilization have been described. These include the use of the bacterial IgG-binding protein, protein A. The latter are restricted to IgG CAbs, which have affinity for protein A, i.e., certain subclasses or species IgG (Goudswaard et al., 1978). Perhaps the major disadvantage is the potential for high background because IgGs in the test sample or in the detection conjugate can also bind the immobilized protein A.

Lectins provide another form of noncovalent immobilization. Concanavalin A adsorbed to microtiter wells has proven to be a convenient method for immobilizing glycoprotein antigen, such as gp120 of HIV (Robinson et al., 1990). gp120 immobilized in this manner appears to be antigenically more active than adsorbed gp120.

Immobilization of Cells and Microorganisms

Viruses, Bacteria, and Cells

Virus particles can be directly adsorbed on polystyrene in the manner of proteins (Butler, unpublished data; Herrmann et al., 1979; McCullough et al., 1985; Mufson and Belshe, 1980). Our experience using adsorbed transmissible gastrointestinal virus to measure IgA, IgG, and IgM responses in swine, and adsorbed parvovirus to measure IgG2a, IgG2b, and IgG1 responses in cattle, revealed several difficulties with the procedure. First, preparations must be free of tissue culture protein or other substances which can competitively inhibit adsorption (Herrmann et al., 1979; Kenny and Dunsmoor, 1983). Second, preparations must be free of any antigens (normally of media origin) that may have been present in the vaccine preparation, since the immunized animal will also have made antibodies to these antigens. To overcome these difficulties, viruses have been immobilized immunochemically using adsorbed capture antibodies specific to the virus (Herrmann et al., 1979; McCullough et al., 1985; Trent et al., 1976; Yolken et al., 1980). Less virus is immobilized than by direct adsorption (Herrmann et al., 1979), and internalized epitopes are not exposed as they are in the case of adsorbed virus (McCullough et al., 1985).

Intact cells and bacteria have been used as antigens in SPI. Their hydrophilic properties lead to unstable adsorption unless cells or surfaces are first modified. Adsorption to poly-L-lysine-coated surfaces (Franci et al., 1985; Mazia et al., 1975; Suter et al., 1980), to surfaces pretreated with glutaraldehyde (C. Severson and G.A. Bishop, pers. commun., 1985 and 1990), or in the presence of the polyaldehyde methyl glyoxal (Czerkinsky et al., 1983b) have all been reported. Probably each of these actually results in the formation of some types of covalent bond to the accessory coating agent.

Membrane Antigens of Cells and Microorganisms

The use of whole-cell antigens theoretically exposes plasma membrane or surface antigens. An alternative procedure is immobilization of isolated cell membrane antigens. This can present a special challenge because membrane proteins are almost always isolated in the presence of nonionic detergent. Hence, passive adsorption to synthetic surfaces would be inhibited by the detergent, especially adsorption on plastic (Gardas and Lewartowska, 1988; Kenny and Dunsmoor, 1983; Newman et al., 1981). Palfree and Elliott (1982) showed that adsorption to NC in the presence of detergent was possible when concentrations were in the range of 0.01 to 0.05%. Triton, Tween, and SDS were most inhibitory, while deoxycholate and octylglucoside were least inhibitory. Detergents were much more inhibitory to adsorption on nylon (Genescreen®). It appears that both the choice of the synthetic surface and the detergent (Gardas and Lewartowska, 1988) significantly influence the adsorption of protein from detergent-containing solutions.

If the detergent-containing membrane preparation cannot be adequately diluted to permit adsorption of constituent protein on NC, two alternatives have been described. First, membrane protein preparations may be covalently linked to NC (Newman et al., 1981) or plastic (Evan, 1984). Second, SM-2 Bio-Beads can be used to remove the detergent prior to adsorption on either plastic or NC, provided the antigens of interest have a mass of 20 kDa or more (Drexler et al., 1986; Van Kreveld and Van der Hoed, 1973). The second procedure does not require 100% removal of the detergent, and this might be undesirable in any case, as hydrophobic aggregates may form. Used carefully, this method appears to be superior to glutaraldehyde-mediated immobilization.

Peptides in Solid-Phase Immunoassay

Application

A fundamental objective in all immunoassays is the quest for specificity. It has become generally recognized that antibodies recognize conformational determinants (Getzoff et al., 1988; Berzofsky, 1985; Paterson, 1989) which may occur at a frequency of one for each 2000 to 5000 Da of protein size (Absolom and van Oss, 1986; Crumpton, 1974). Being able to make subtle distinctions between epitopes on pathogens, e.g., HIV, is important both in immunodiagnostics and in vaccine development (Arnon, 1987; Javaherian et al., 1989; van Regenmortel et al., 1988). The development of automated protein sequencers that require only small amounts of protein, e.g., Applied Biosystems Sequencer, and the advent of DNA technology that allows protein sequences to be deduced from gene sequences, has permitted focus on the epitope structure of proteins to be sharpened. The advent of solid-phase peptide synthesis (Merrifield, 1963) has made it possible to synthesize specific peptides which comprise the structure of proteins. These synthetic peptides have made it possible to identify and/or map the proteins' antigenic epitopes (Atassi and Atassi, 1986; Geysen et al., 1984; Gnann et al., 1987; Neurath et al., 1990). Peptides have sometimes been employed as competitive inhibitors in immunoassay, using antibodies raised to the intact native protein (Atassi et al., 1976). In other situations, peptides have themselves been used as solid-phase antigens (see below).

Immobilization of Solid-Phase Peptides

Three general methods have been employed to immobilize peptides for SPI: conjugation with a carrier protein which is then adsorbed on a hydrophobic synthetic surface, direct adsorption of the peptide to the synthetic surface, and covalent immobilization.

Direct adsorption has been employed by a surprisingly large number of investigators (Atassi and Atassi, 1986; Geerligs et al., 1988; Lacroix et al., 1991; Neurath et al., 1990). There have been at least indirect studies on the affinity of various peptides for plastic (Neurath et al., 1990) as well as of the adsorption conditions that are most favorable for preserving antigenic activity (Geerligs et al., 1988). The latter group of investigators observed a pronounced effect of pH and a need for circa, 0.6 M NaCl during adsorption to obtain maximum antigenic activity. It is not known whether these conditions promote greater adsorption or adsorption of the peptide in a form more easily recognized by antibody. Peptides adsorbed in cyclized form appear more active (Lacroix et al., 1991). Direct synthesis of peptide on polyethylene rods circumvents the need for a separate immobilization step (Geysen et al., 1984).

Coating concentrations ranging from 0.5 to 20 µg/ml have been reported, although no data which parallel those described for protein (see Fig. 4) are available. Some have argued that the amount adsorbed is such that any two peptides could be bridged by an IgG antibody (Lacroix et al., 1991). These calculations are, of course, based on the uniform distribution of the adsorbed peptide. Whether adsorbed peptides show the same clustering properties of adsorbed protein remains to be determined.

The simplest alternative to direct adsorption is conjugation to, and subsequent adsorption of, an irrelevant carrier protein (Shirahama and Suzawa, 1985). In addition to requiring a time-consuming extra step, this method could result in loss of a functional epitope by virtue of its involvement in the covalent linkage to the carrier protein. However, such criticism is applicable to every method of immobilization.

Covalent attachment to NC has been described by Lauritzen et al. (1990) as has the covalent attachment to functionalized microtiter wells (Sødergard-Andersen et al., 1990). Immobilization involves coupling through N-hydroxysuccimide in the presence of EDAC. Angiotensin I and II are five- to tenfold more detectable by antibody when covalently coupled than when absorbed on NC. Similar improvements have been obtained with peptides on plastic, although substantial amounts of peptide are simultaneously adsorbed passively during covalent immobilization (Sødergard-Andersson et al., 1990).

There appears to be a general absence of studies which systematically compare the retention of antigenicity of the various immobilized peptides in relationship to the amount of each immobilized and in comparison to the antigenic activity of the same peptide when not immobilized on a solid phase. Judged by the results of the differential antigenicity of adsorbed vs nonadsorbed protein antigens, there is room for concern that data obtained using solid-phase peptides may not be representative of the antigenicity of these peptides in solution.

APPLICATIONS OF SOLID-PHASE ANTIBODIES AND ANTIGENS

Antigens and Antibodies in Affinity Chromatography

Applications

Affinity chromatography has been an invaluable preparative tool in biomedical science and is the focus of numerous reviews (Chaiken et al., 1983; Cuatrecasas and Anfinson, 1971). Unlike most solid-phase immunoassays that utilize hydrophobic supports and passive adsorption of the solid-phase reactant, affinity chromatography features the use of hydrophilic supports to which the solid-phase reactant is covalently bound. Affinity chromatography is not restricted to antigens and antibodies, but is employed for enzymes, membrane receptors, bacterial immunoglobulin-binding receptors, and even cells with affinity for lectins (Edelman and Rutishauer, 1974). Although applicable to nearly any molecular separation dependent on noncovalent receptor-ligand interaction, discussion of this technology is confined here to antigen-antibody interactions.

There are two major applications of affinity chromatography in immunology: the affinity purification of a substance (ligand) from a mixture which becomes bound to the solid-phase receptor (see earlier footnote), and the removal of unwanted substances from a mixture. Although these superficially represent opposite sides of the same argument, the technical considerations regarding the solid phase are often quite different. On one hand, the second application does not require that the bound ligand be dissociated or dissociated in a purified form. Hence, there are generally less stringent considerations in the choice of matrix and chemical linkage. When the ligand is to be purified by elution, the immobilizing covalent linkage must be able to tolerate the changes in pH, ionic strength, etc., encountered during elution. In addition, affinity supports constructed for purification must minimize the nonspecific adsorption of substances which might also be eluted with the "purified" ligand, and must utilize a concentration and configuration of receptors which facilitates ligand dissociation under moderate dissociation conditions that will not damage ligand, receptor, or matrix.

Supports and Methods of Immobilization

The most commonly used supports for solid-phase reactants in affinity chromatography are porous matrices with good flow rates and easily modifiable chemical groups that were initially developed for liquid chromatography (Cuatrecasas and Anfinson, 1971). Most popular have been cross-linked agaroses like CL-Sepharose 4B activated with CNBr (Axen et al., 1967). Agarose-acrylamide polymers, acrylamide, derivatized cellulose, and porous glass (Weetall, 1970) have also been used. These media have been typically packed into simple columns, e.g., modified syringe barrels, and the various buffer solutions allowed to flow through them by gravity.

Prior to the application of column chromatographic materials as supports, insoluble "natural" supports such as bacterial aggregates and red blood cells were used (Gough et al., 1966). In 1969, Avrameas and Ternynck described the use of insolubilized protein aggregates, prepared with glutaraldehyde, as immunosorbents. These cellular or protein aggregates were employed in test tubes and separation was effected by centrifugation. These immunoadsorbents were gradually replaced by the column-support matrices described above.

In recent years, low-pressure column methods have been replaced by high-pressure techniques, using functionalized silica as the column-support matrix. These offer the advantage of shorter time and large sample processing as well as kinetic analyses.

Selection of the matrix and the chemistry of coupling can be dependent on the applications. The popularity of CNBr-activated Sepharose is due to its high capacity for immobilized reactants; at least 9 mg of protein can be immobilized per milliliter of gel. By contrast, linkage via oxirane groups (Sundberg and Porath, 1974), hydrazido groups (Lamed et al., 1973), diazotization (Campbell et al., 1961), and succinimide esters (Frost et al., 1981) produce lower yields. However, because of the relative instability of the isourea and carbamate linkages formed during coupling with CNBr, pH changes during elution result in protonation of the double bonds and subsequent "leaching" of the solid-phase reactant (Hagen and Strejan, 1987). Although CNBr-activated supports are a good choice when depletion of an unwanted substance is desired, they are a poor choice for recovery of the bound ligand. One exception to this "rule" is competitive affinity elution, e.g., PC-chloride used to elute anti-PC, without the need to make changes in buffer pH.

Affinity purification is best accomplished using matrices with low nonspecific binding of unwanted materials (Nardella and Mannik, 1978), and utilizing single carbon–nitrogen bonds that resist cleavage during elution with buffers of different pH and ionic strength. It is, of course, desirable to use matrices of relatively high capacity. The two coupling procedures which we have found to meet these criteria employ 2-fluoro-1-methylpyridium toluene-4-sulfonate (FMP; Ngo, 1986) and active aldehydes in the presence of sodium cyanoborohydride.

The focus of this chapter is on the behavior of solid-phase antigens and antibodies. Unlike the immobilization of proteins on the usual hydrophobic surfaces used in immunoassay, there are few data and/or evidence for conformational alterations of immobilized reactants in affinity chromatography, although epitopes may be lost in coupling chemistry (Fig. 3C). Steric hindrance can be a major problem which has been the chief argument used to explain the better performance of reactants immobilized with "spacer" linkages (Cuatrecasas, 1970). However, care must be taken to avoid the use of highly hydrophobic aliphatic spacers which contribute to nonspecific adsorption.

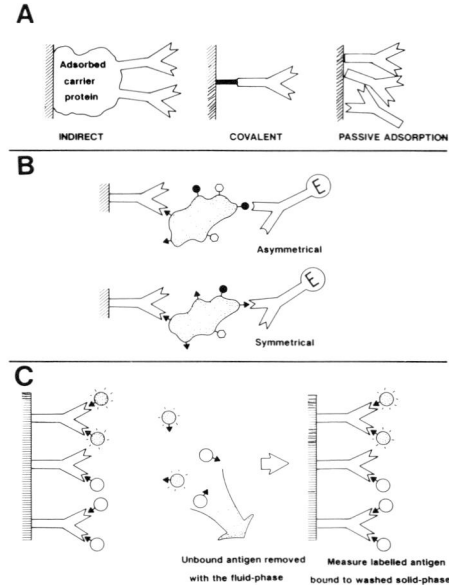

Figure 7. Solid-phase antibodies in immunoassay. (A) The most common forms of immobilization are illustrated. Indirect immobilization includes the use of streptavidin, protein A, and a primary antiglobulin. (B) Asymmetrical vs symmetrical configuration in sandwich immunoassays. E, Enzyme-labeled detection antibody. (C) Solid-phase CAb in competitive immunoassay. Burst effect and stipples are used to illustrate the labeled, competitive antigen.

Solid-Phase Antibodies in Immunoassay

Capture Antibodies in Sandwich or "Two-Site" Immunoassays

Sandwich immunoassays provide a convenient and uncomplicated method for the quantitation of multivalent antigens; the antigen is captured by one epitope and detected using a signal-generating antibody which binds to another epitope (Fig. 7B). Configurations may be either symmetric, in which both antibodies have the same specificity, or asymmetric in which the antibodies recognize different determinants (Fig. 7B). The latter configuration is especially convenient for immunoglobulin (Ig) quantitation in which specificity resides in the capture antibody and detection is done using pan-specific anti-L chain reagents that can recognize all classes and subclasses of Ig in the species under study (Butler, 1988; Butler et al., 1986). Steric hindrance is encountered with the symmetrical configuration, especially in situations in which a large signal-generating antibody conjugates is used (Butler et al., 1986). Furthermore, competition will be encountered using the asymmetrical configuration if the CAb is not totally specific (Fig. 7B; Butler, 1988; Francois-Gerard et al., 1988).

Solid-Phase Antibodies in Direct Competitive Immunoassay

The configuration illustrated in Fig. 7C is that of conventional radioimmunoassay (Yalow and Berson, 1960), in which labeled antigen directly competes with unlabeled antigen of known quantity in a reference standard or with an unknown amount of unlabeled antigen in the sample to be tested. Using a fixed amount of solid-phase antibody and a constant amount of labeled antigen in a series of reaction vessels, the system is titrated by adding increasing amounts of unlabeled antigen to different vessels, incubating the reactions for a prescribed period, removing the unbound soluble components, and measuring the amount of label bound to the solid-phase antibody. This generates a standard inhibition curve to which tested unknown specimens can be compared simultaneously.

Competitive immunoassay is necessary when the antigen to be measured is small and univalent so that it cannot be detected in a two-site sandwich assay (Fig. 7C). Labeling of antigen in direct competitive immunoassay was historically done by iodination. When done with care to avoid damage due to oxidative or reductive processes, most small antigens could be successfully labeled without loss of antigenicity. In cases where labeling difficulties are encountered or when enzyme of fluorescent markers seriously alter antigenicity, and indirect competitive SPI can be used.

Performance Criteria for Solid-Phase Antibodies

Immobilized antibodies are stable but may perform differently than their fluid-phase counterparts and may display differential activity depending on the method of their immobilization. Figure 7A depicts three general ways in which solid-phase antibodies can be immobilized. The protein carrier method includes the various nonadsorptive, noncovalent methods reviewed earlier.

The difficulty of determining concentration in solid-phase immunoassay requires the use of performance parameters which do not require absolute concentration data. Figures 4B and 6C express the activity of the solid phase and solid-phase reactant, respectively, in terms of the percentage of ligand bound when the receptor is present in excess. In Fig. 4A, the avidity of IgM for polystyrene is much higher than the avidity of serum albumin for polystyrene. In Fig. 6C, monoclonal anti-swine CAb immobilized via an SA linkage binds a higher percentage of IgG than when the same CAb is directly adsorbed on plastic. Differences in the percentage bound reflect avidity and for CAb performance, we have termed this antigen-capture capacity (AgCC; Butler et al., 1986). This term is independent of the need to know absolute solid-phase concentrations. Using the same percentage bound plots, the degree to which the percentage of captured antigen remains constant is a function of its functional CAb concentration. These two parameters have proven to be convenient and practical in evaluating the performance of capture antibodies immobilized by different methods or prepared from serum, ascites fluid, or tissue culture by different methods (Butler et al., 1986; Joshi and Butler, 1992; Suter and Butler, 1986).

The performance of CAb can also be assessed by more conventional procedures, albeit with difficulty owing to the need for absolute values of concentration. As described earlier (Suter et al., 1989), many adsorbed monoclonal antibodies appear to have a greater propensity to undergo loss of activity than do adsorbed polyclonals. This is seen in Fig. 8 in percentage bound (A) plots as well as in more traditional double-reciprocal (B) and Scatchard (C) plots.

Although Langmuir isotherm and Scatchard equations applied to SPI yield performance plots with reasonable shapes, they generate unusual values for functional antibody concentration $[Ab_t]$ or K_{eq}. Specifically, $[Ab_t]$ is seriously overestimated and K_{eq} is underestimated (Joshi and Butler, 1992; Butler et al., 1991). It would seem that these errors are due to a failure to know the true interfacial reaction volume and to assume that unbound ligand is randomly distributed in the liquid phase.

Apart from the sometimes dramatic effect seen when the performance of adsorbed monoclonal CAb is compared to the same monoclonal immobilized using the PABC system (Suter and Butler, 1986; Fig. 6C), we have observed only trivial differences in performance when CAb were immobilized covalently (Peterman et al., 1988; Butler et al., 1991) or via a primary antiglobulin CAb (unpublished data). However, covalent immobilization should not be used generically. Studies by Mize et al. (1991) have shown that when the proper covalent linkage is employed, a definite improvement in the behavior of covalently immobilized CAbs can be observed. The CAbs with high AgCC and functional CAb concentration produce immunoassays with the greatest dynamic range and greatest sensitivity.

Solid-Phase Antigens in Immunoassay

Use in Indirect Competitive Immunoassay

The problem of antigenic alteration and steric hindrance occurs when especially small antigens are labeled with enzymes or fluors. This can be overcome using an indirect competitive system (Fig. 9B). This method avoids the need to label the antigen, thus providing a practical means for the quantitation of small, univalent antigens. Essentially, the labeled antibody is present in limited amount so that a high concentration of the ligand in the sample will consume all antibody and inhibit its binding to solid-phase antigen. Standard curves, etc., are constructed in much the same manner as for direct competitive immunoassays. A variety of configurations for indirect competitive immunoassays, involving various degrees of amplification, e.g., competitive enzyme-linked immunosorbent assay (CELIA) (Yorde et al., 1976) have been described, although the basic principle is the same for all.

Solid-Phase Antigens in Specific Antibody Immunoassay (SpAbI)

One of the most important applications of SPI is in the study of antibody responses to infectious agents and experimental antigen. Specific antibody

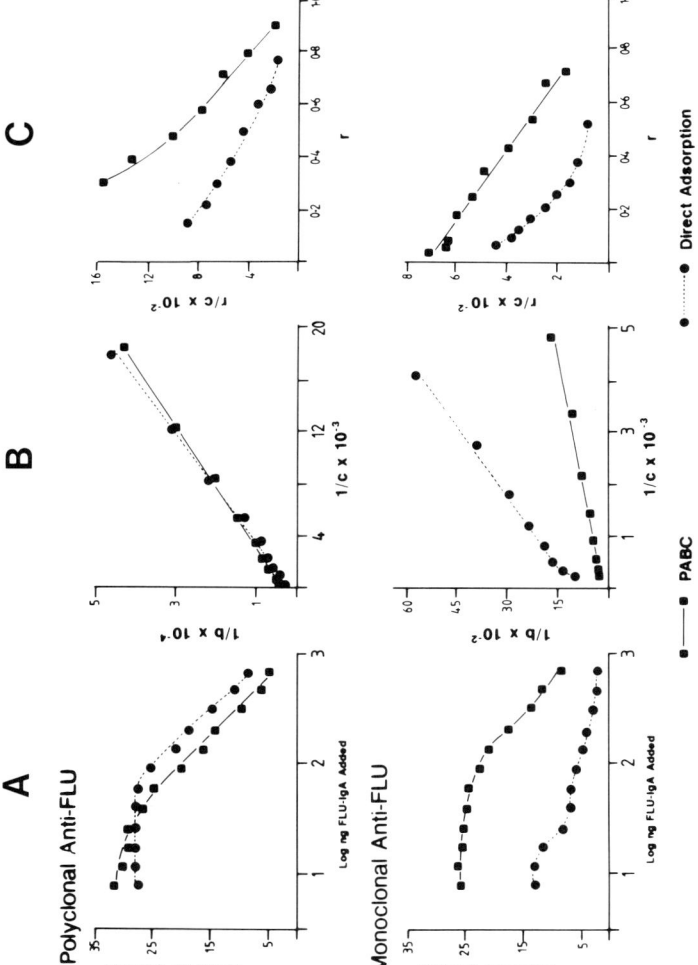

Figure 8. The comparative behavior of polyclonal and monoclonal anti-fluorescein (FLU) of equal affinity when directly adsorbed on Immulon 2 (●--●) or immobilized using the noncovalent, nonadsorptive PABC method illustrated in Fig. 6 (■—■). (A) Percentage binding plots; (B) Steward-Petty plots; (C) Scatchard analyses. ^{125}I-labeled FLU_{18}-IgA (MW = 160,000) was used as the antigen.

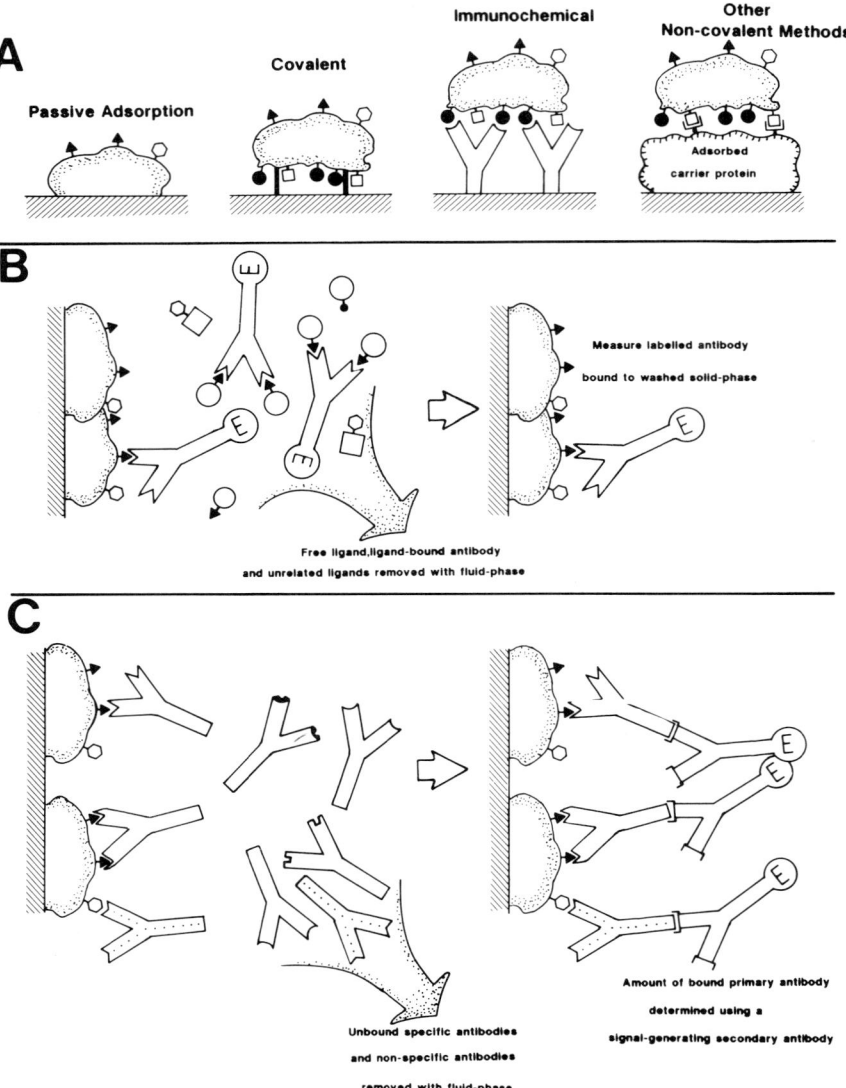

Figure 9. Solid-phase antigens in immunoassay. (A) Four general methods for the immobilization of antigen on a solid phase are illustrated. (B) The use of solid-phase antigen in an indirect competitive immunoassay. The concentration of antigen in the specimen (circle with single triangular epitope on left) is determined by measuring the amount of bound, labeled antibody that is not inhibited by free ligand in the specimen from binding the solid-phase antigen (right). (C) Solid-phase antigen in SpAbI. The amount of antibody in the specimen that becomes bound to the solid-phase antigen is determined using a secondary, signal-generating antibody which recognizes the first bound antibody.

immunoassay (SpAbI) is also subject to considerable technical difficulty. Among the list of problems encountered with SpAbI are the following:

1. The immobilized antigen may not express epitopes that are representative of the antigen *in vivo*.
2. Antigen concentration limitations and steric hindrance may permit the detection of certain antibodies at the expense of others.
3. Serum globulin may bind nonspecifically to immobilized antigens, and remedies to prevent this may limit assay sensitivity.
4. Results may be interpreted to imply that bound antibody represents the total antibody in the sample, leading the investigator to report his data in absolute units of serum concentration and therefore misrepresent immunobiological reality.

Solid-phase SpAbI is done by immobilizing the antigen of interest on a suitable synthetic surface (Fig. 9C); Fig. 9A summarizes the various methods that were discussed earlier. The specimen to be tested for antibodies is applied in a buffer containing at least nonionic detergent (to prevent adsorption of protein in the specimen to the solid phase) and often additional protein to prevent nonspecific adsorption of nonantibody globulin to the immobilized antigen. Incubation of the reaction may range from less than 1 h or until equilibrium is reached. Depending on the nature of the solid-phase, e.g., microparticles vs microtiter wells, or the degree to which agitation is supplied, equilibrium may require up to 40 h (Fig. 1). Thereafter, unbound protein and antibodies are removed, the solid phase is washed, and a suitable detection system is added (Fig. 9C). Enzyme-labeled detection systems are currently most popular, with horseradish peroxidase (HRP) and alkaline phosphatase (AP) most often used. Detection systems were discussed earlier and elsewhere (Butler, 1991; Khalil, 1991; Ngo, 1986).

Special Consideration in Performing and Interpreting SpAbI

The importance of the potential problems associated with SpAbI should not be underestimated. SpAbI can be only as good as the solid-phase antigen being used. Although sensitivity and reliability are largely technical logistic issues, the question of whether an SpAbI measures what it claims touches the issue of specificity, perhaps the most fundamental concept in specific immunity.

The stability of solid-phase antigen appears to depend on its concentration and the chemistry of the antigen in relationship to the solid phase. Most protein antigens adsorb avidity to synthetic surfaces (Fig. 4A) and do so in a linear log-log fashion until, e.g., approximately 5 µg have been added to polystyrene surface of 150 mm^2. Within the concentration range spanned by this log-linear binding region, adsorbed proteins are extremely stable. Above this range, unstable binding occurs (Blanchard et al., 1990; Cantarero et al., 1980; Herrmann et al., 1979; Peterman, 1985). Desorption of unstable antigen during SpAbI can cause "prozoning" in which desorbed antigen acts as a competitive inhibitor for the antibody being measured (Engvall, 1980; Peterman, 1985).

Hydrophilic antigens, especially polysaccharides, appear to adsorb less well to synthetic surfaces (Elkins et al., 1990; Gardas and Lewartowska, 1988) which has prompted the use of alternative methods such as capture antibodies (Barrett et al., 1980; Carlson et al., 1982; Voller et al., 1976) or precoating with poly-L-lysine (Messimer et al., 1985) or by capturing the antigen with lectins (Robinson et al., 1989). Desorption of antigens immobilized noncovalently in this manner (Barrett et al., 1980; Blanchard et al., 1990; Herrmann et al., 1979) suggests that greater stability could be obtained through covalent immobilization (Rubin et al., 1980). The various possibilities are summarized in Fig. 9A.

The problem of instability encountered when high concentrations of antigen are immobilized noncovalently as well as a reduction in activity* (Barrett et al., 1980; Carlson et al., 1982; Elkins et al., 1990) has "standardized" coating concentration in the 1 to 10 μg/ml range (Butler et al., 1978a; Engvall, 1980). The immobilization of only 400 to 700 ng per well (typical for many antigens when 200 μl is added at 5 μg/ml) is responsible for several other phenomenona which characterize solid-phase SpAbI conducted on microtiter wells. First, such "antigen limitation" means that, assuming equal affinity, minor subclasses and classes of antibodies in serum will be inhibited from binding by the more abundant IgG antibodies specific for the same determinants. This is reflected in the titration plot (Fig. 10D) and has been observed for IgA and IgE (Butler et al., 1980, 1985, 1990; Haba and Nisonoff, 1985). The erroneous data generated by such competition, led Zeiss et al. (1973) to develop a system for measuring allergen-specific IgE which circumvented the problem by at first capturing only the serum IgE before testing its activity. A similar system was used by Hirano et al. (1989), and Duermeyer et al. (1979) have applied this approach to measurement of IgM anti-hepatitis A.

The antigen-limiting nature of SpAbI, as seen among isotypes, also occurs among antibodies of the same isotype which differ in affinity. Thus, the "affinity-dependence" of SpAbI on microtiter wells (Ahlstedt et al., 1974; Butler et al., 1978b; Lehtonen and Eerola, 1982; Nimmo et al., 1984; Fig. 2) is a predictable consequence of such a configuration.

The antigenic integrity of immobilized antigen was discussed earlier; immobilization-induced changes in antigen can produce all of the following effects:

1. A reduction in functional epitope concentration making a solid-phase SpAbI even more affinity dependent or isotype biased than that which results from a low antigen concentration.

---

*It is probably that the lower activity observed at high concentrations of antigen is due to desorption, although this has been more often theorized than proven.

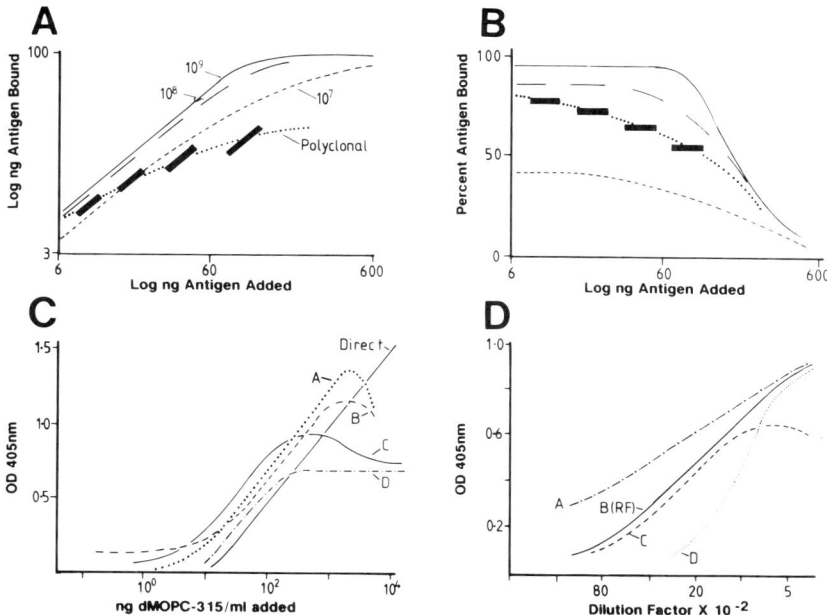

Figure 10. The nature of titration plots obtained in solid-phase SpAbI. (A) and (B): The effect of antibody affinity and heterogeneity in log-log saturation plots (A) or percentage bound plots (B). Theoretical data are given for three monoclonals of different affinities and one polyclonal. The values on the plots are the K_{eq} in m^{-1}. The darkened rectangles depict subpopulations of progressively lower affinity antibodies (left to right) which comprise the polyclonal preparation. (Data for the monoclonals are from Peterman, J.H., 1985, Ph.D. thesis, University of Iowa, Iowa City, IA. With permission.) (C) The relationship between the amount of ^{125}I-labeled IgA anti-DNP antibody (MOPC 315) bound to an adsorbed DNP-carrier antigen and its detection with antibody-enzyme conjugates of increasing size A → D. Conjugate A is the Fab fragment of the antibody conjugated 1 + 1 with alkaline phosphatase. The solid line labeled "direct", depicts the amount of radioactive antibody bound by direct counting (exact units omitted). (Data from Koertge and Butler, 1985. With permission.) (D) Parallelism in titration plots of SpAbI. Plot B (RF) is that of the reference standard used in the assay. Plot A illustrates nonparallelism due to excessively nonspecific binding. Plot C illustrates nonparallelism at low dilution caused by inhibition of binding of an isotype (e.g., IgE) being measured by high levels of another isotype not being measured, e.g., IgG. Plot D depicts nonparallelism caused by excessive background correction.

2. A loss or masking of certain eptiopes such that the solid-phase antigen is no longer representative of the antigen "seen" by antibodies *in vivo*.
3. The generation of new epitopes that are recognized by antibodies which are of no serological and diagnostic importance.
4. Clustering in the case of adsorbed antigen which could accentuate competition through steric hindrance.

Antigenic integrity in SpAbI should be a matter of considerable concern to immunobiological and microbiological investigations which depend on SpAbI for evaluating immune responses and vaccines.

There are several noteworthy aspects of SpAbI data expression and analyses. Figure 10C illustrates an important aspect of ELISA-type SpAbI. The titration of a radioactive antibody (MOPC 315) is shown in relationship to its detection, using enzyme conjugates of increasing complexity and amplification. The lower two titrations were generated using the types of indirect or secondary antibody-enzyme conjugates often used. These plots collectively illustrate that no direct stoichiometric relationship exists between enzyme signal and primary antibody bound, and that the apparent "saturation" curve of the antigen at high antibody concentration is not due to saturation of the antigen, but rather the result of steric hindrance by the detection system.

Figure 10A is a theoretical, log-log plot generated for antibodies of different affinities. These data show that the slope of the titration plot is not a function of affinity (as some have inaccurately claimed) but rather its Y intercept. Differences in the slope of a log-log plot reflect heterogeneity of affinity, typically the response seen with polyclonal antiserum. Figure 10B depicts the behavior of antibodies of differing affinities in a percentage bound plot of a SpAbI. Relevant to discussion here is that only in situations where the affinity of the antibody is very high, is 100% of the antibody bound in the region of excess antigen (the log-log linear region in Fig. 10B). Hence, caution must be exercised when reporting antibody responses in absolute units (μg/ml of serum) because it cannot be assumed that all of the antibody in the sample is antigen bound. The topic of absolute quantitation of antibodies using SpAbI is treated in detail elsewhere (Butler and Hamilton, 1991).

Figure 10D reviews the method of expressing antibody responses as titer, e.g., "end point" or "mid point." These are valid for comparing responses among different samples, provided that the titrations leading to either of these endpoints are parallel. Parallelism is a fundamental principle in the proper use of all immunoassay (Butler and Hamilton, 1991; Perlstein, 1979; Peterman and Butler, 1989). Various factors contribute to nonparallelism; the effects of nonspecific binding are most pronounced at high dilution and cause flattening of the slope, whereas competitive inhibition (curve C) is most obvious at high antibody concentration. Excessive background correction can lead to artificially steep slopes (Fig. 10D).

Parallelism can only be controlled when complete titrations with multipoint analyses are performed (Peterman and Butler, 1989). Hence, so-called "single-point" determinations, i.e., the dilution required to achieve a certain magnitude of reaction, can be dangerous to the extent that nonparallelism could go undiscovered.

IMMUNOLOGY, IMMUNODIAGNOSTICS, AND INTERFACIAL ANTIGEN-ANTIBODY INTERACTIONS

Reliability, Sensitivity, and Specificity in SPI

Sensitivity and Specificity

Sensitivity describes the minimum detectable quantity (antigen or antibody), which depends on the signal-to-noise ratio and the precision at zero dose. Mere amplification of a signal does not increase sensitivity unless it preferentially amplifies the signal and not the noise; few if any of the systems for amplifying SPI possess this property. Therefore, background reduction must be part of any scheme designed to improve sensitivity. Background "noise" in SPI originates from two major sources: the binding of components of the detection system, or nonligand compounds which are recognizable by the detection system*, directly to the synthetic solid phase, and the nonspecific binding of the same components to the protein receptor on the solid phase. In SPI, the former is generally prevented by the use of nonionic detergents which prevents hydrophobic interaction of protein with the solid phase, while the latter is prevented by the addition of a "blocking protein solution" or use of buffer conditions which discourage nonspecific protein-protein interaction. It has been shown that detergent alone does not block protein-protein interactions on NC (Bird et al., 1988) or in SpAbI when certain fluorescyl-protein antigen are used (Butler and Brown 1992). Unfortunately, increasing the concentration of the "blocking protein" can also inhibit specific interactions (Butler and Brown, 1992; Dierks, 1985; Hobbs, 1989) or cause desorption (Joshi, K. S., pers. commun.), i.e., signal and noise are both decreased. When the signal obtained in ELISA from control wells that receive all reagents but serum is used as a background correction, the genuine signal can often be overcorrected because of increased nonspecific binding of the detection system in the control well which had received no serum; this produces an artificially steep slope (curve D, Fig. 10D). In some situations, immunochemical "short-circuits" (Butler, 1988) may occur when the detection system recognizes a part of the coating antigen or vice versa. This is common in systems utilizing protein A or when CAbs recognize determinants on alkaline phosphatase (St. Laurent et al., 1990).

Background problems are exacerbated when measuring immunochemical interaction of low affinity because it means that the reactants must be used at very high concentration to drive the interaction (Graves, 1988). This raises the potential for nonspecific interaction or even nonspecific inhibition of the desired reaction. Hence, increasing the affinity of the interaction or "site occupancy" (Ekins, 1991) would be the ideal means of increasing the signal-to-noise ratio. When this is not an option, such as in SpAbI, other methods of "noise control" may be used (Graves, 1988).

---

*If in an asymmetrical sandwich ELISA for Igs, a pan-specific detection is used, it could also detect Ig not bound to the specific CAb but adsorbed anywhere on the synthetic solid phase.

Specificity describes the ability of an immunoassay to detect only the desired substance as opposed to a similar substance or even background "noise". Therefore, to obtain both high sensitivity and specificity, a high-affinity antibody which does not cross-react should be the optimum. Such an objective is most often paradoxical because antibodies with the highest affinity are those most likely to recognize other substances, albeit with lower affinity. In situations where specificity is more important than sensitivity, monoclonal antibodies are the best choice.

Antibody Activity Versus Antigen Quantitation

Reversing the role of antigen and antibody in the design of an immunoassay does not result in simple reversal of data interpretation. An antigen to be quantified has little or no heterogeneity, i.e., all antigen molecules in the test specimen, and those in the reference standard, are identical and all combine with their antibody equally well. Hence, SPI can be used to quantitate antigen in absolute units, e.g., micrograms per milliliter. When the object is to measure the amount of antibody, the same assumption of homogeneity does not apply to antibody unless a contrived system is used. For example, measurement of a given monoclonal antibody in tissue culture media or ascites can be done in absolute units in the same manner as antigen. However, serum antibodies to antigens of interest in infectious disease or in experimental studies of the immune response are not homogeneous. As illustrated in Fig. 10B, antibodies of different affinities will be bound to antigen to different degrees and also each to a different degree than the antibodies used as the reference standard; this renders invalid the expression of data in absolute units. Results are preferentially influenced by high-affinity antibody and thus are more correctly expressed as units of activity, i.e., titer (Butler and Hamilton, 1991). Titer may be more relevant to the *in vivo* situation and for evaluating the effectiveness of vaccines (Keren, 1979).

Assay Reliability

The simplest measure of assay reliability is the variation among replicates. This can be expressed as standard deviation or more often, in terms of coefficient of variation (CV) which is independent of the mean; CVs of <10% are generally considered acceptable. Variability due to temperature and other "daily variants" is usually controlled by including the standard on each daily test. The reliability of single-point determinations is not an adequate measure of reliability, unless it includes a control for parallelism. Multipoint analyses provide the simplest approach for control of parallelism (Butler and Hamilton, 1991; Peterman and Butler, 1989).

Serological SPI attempts to obtain data from *in vitro* tests which reflect events *in vivo*. The spectrum of antigenic determinants displayed by an immobilized antigen should be representative of those displayed by the same antigen *in vivo*. Although difficult, it is possible to test such a hypothesis by allowing the test antigen to first bind antibody in solution before its immobilization and subsequent detection of the bound antibody (McCullough et al., 1985). Virulence antigens have been recognized in many pathogens and protective immunity can often be correlated with antibody titers to these antigen. Developing SPIs capable of monitoring the immune response to such antigen is a criterion of reliability. An analogous situation is the correlation between the titer of IgE antibodies to an allergen measured by SPI and the magnitude of the wheal and flare obtained in clinical skin tests with the same allergen.

Another aspect of reliability concerns the specificity of the reagents for SPI. Unlike pharmaceuticals, there is no national or international standard for the specificity of immunological reagents, e.g., antibodies. Specificity is controlled only by the producer and the user. Hence, it is the responsibility of the user to prove the specificity of the reagents used in the immunoassay: "Vertrauen ist gut aber Kontrolle ist besser." It is important that the reagents be tested for specificity in the very same assay in which they will be used, because the suppliers do not know in what type of assay a consumer will use their reagent. In short, the investigator bears an important responsibility in the reliability of SPI.

Are *In Vitro* Solid-Phase Antigen-Antibody Reactions Models for Interfacial Membrane Interactions *In Vivo*?

There are more than a few similarities between the potential immunochemical behavior of surface-bound reactants *in vivo* and those attached to a solid phase *in vitro*. Beyond the fact that reactants are no longer diffusible, the reaction volume is also confined to an interface. Molecules concentrated in a small volume, such as in lymphocyte capping, should, according to the mass law, promote ligand binding. As reviewed earlier, there are data showing that the kinetics of cell surface antibody interactions are similar to those of antibodies binding solid-phase antigen (Mason and Williams, 1980). However, a simple comparison of *in vivo* receptor-ligand interaction with solid-phase receptor-ligand interactions overlooks many significant differences. Living membranes are dynamic, not chemically fixed as is presumed to be the case with synthetic solid phases. Furthermore, synthetic solid phases are hydrophobic, whereas the solvent-exposed surfaces of cell membranes are hydrophilic. Because of the dynamic fluidity of living membranes, such interfacial reaction can be proteolytically altered, endocytosed, or processed in some other manner.

Despite the differences identified above, certain principles learned from studies of antigen-antibody reactions on synthetic interfaces *in vitro* could be instructive in understanding interfacial interaction *in vivo*.

SUMMARY

It is important for immunologists and users of immunological methods to understand that a great deal of what is presented on the subject of antigen-antibody interaction in elementary textbooks of immunology is probably not applicable to interfacial antigen-antibody reactions without some modification. An effort has been made in this chapter to highlight those issues concerning solid-phase systems which deviate from conventional wisdom about fluid-phase antigen-antibody reactions. Of special concern are the issues of interfacial concentrations, the integrity of immobilized reactants, and the kinetics of interfacial interactions.

The importance of the method of immobilization cannot be overemphasized, especially with regard to the antigenic properties of antigens used, especially in SpAbI. Unfortunately, no simple generalization is possible because each antigen is different. This places the burden of assay validity on the inventor and user; following a generalized protocol is not an excuse for omitting specificity and validity tests. Unfortunately, the "publish or perish" pressures in biomedical science often do not encourage such careful evaluation.

Solid-phase immunoassay is likely to be the major *in vitro* testing system used for some time to come. Hence, investigators should make an effort to thoroughly familiarize themselves not only with the configurational possibilities provided by this system, but also with what would appear to be its unique immunochemistry as well.

REFERENCES

Absolom, D. R., and van Oss, C. J. (1986) The nature of the antigen-antibody bond and the factors affecting its association and dissociation. *CRC Crit. Rev. Immunol.* 6:1.

Ahlstedt, S., Holmgren, J., and Hanson, L. A. (1974) Protective capacity of antibodies against *E. coli* O antigen with special reference to avidity, *Int. Arch. Allergy Appl. Immunol.* 46:470.

Aron, R., (ed.) (1987) *Synthetic Vaccines,* Vols. I and II, CRC Press, Boca Raton, FL.

Atassi, H., and Atassi, M. Z. (1986) Antibody recognition of ragweed allergen Ra3: localization of the full profile of the continuous antigenic sites by synthetic overlapping peptides representing the entire chain. *Eur. J. Immunol.* 16:229—235.

Atassi, M. Z., Koketsu, J., and Habeeb, A. F. S. A. (1976) Enzymatic and immunochemical properties of lysozyme. XIII. Accurate delineation of the reaction site around the disulfide 6—127 by immunochemical study of β-propiolactone lysozyme derivative and of synthetic disulfide peptides. *Biochim. Biophys. Acta* 420:358.

Avrameas, S., and Guilbert, B. (1972) Enzyme-immunoassay for the measurement of antigen using peroxidase conjugates. *Biochimie* 54:837.

Avrameas, S., and Ternynck, T. (1969) The cross-linking of proteins with glutaraldehyde and its use for the preparation of immunosorbents. *Immunochemistry* 6:53.

Axen, R., Porath, J., and Ernback, S. (1967) Chemical coupling of peptides and proteins to polysaccharides by means of cyanogen halides. *Nature (London)* 214:1302.

Barrett, D. J., Amman, A. J., Stenmark, S., and Wara, D. W. (1980) Immunoglobulin G and M antibodies to pneumococcal polysaccharide detected by enzyme-linked immunosorbent assay. *Infect. Immunol.* 27:411.

Bers, G., and Garfin, P. (1985) Protein and nucleic acid blotting and immunobiological detection, *Biotechniques* 3:276.

Berzofsky, J. A. (1985) Instrinsic and extrinsic factors in protein antigen structure. *Science* 229:932.

Berzofsky, J. A., and Berkower, I. J. (1984) Antigen-antibody interaction. In *Fundamental Immunology* (W. E. Paul, ed.), Raven Press, NY, 595—645.

Bird, C. R., Andrew, J. H. G., and Thorpe, R. (1988) The use of Tween 20 alone as a blocking agent for immunoblotting can cause artifactual results. *J. Immunol. Meth.* 106:175.

Blanchard, G. C., Taylor, C. G., Busey, B. R., and Williamson, M. L. (1990) Regeneration of immunosorbent surfaces used in clinical, industrial and environmental biosensors. Role of covalent and non-covalent interactions. *J. Immunol. Meth.* 130:263.

Børmer, O. P. (1989) Interference of complement with the binding of carcinoembryonic antigen to solid-phase monoclonal antibodies. *J. Immunol.* 121:85.

Brash, J. L., and Lyman, D. J. (1969) Adsorption of plasma proteins in solution to uncharged hydrophobic polymer surfaces. *J. Biomed. Mater. Res.* 3:175.

Brennand, D. M., Danson, M. J., and Hough, D. W. (1986) A comparison of ELISA screening methods for the production of monoclonal antibodies against soluble protein antigens. *J. Immunol. Meth.* 93:9.

Brown, W. R., Dierks, S. E., Butler, J. E., and Gershoni, J. M. (1991) Immunoblotting: membrane filters as the solid-phase for immunoassays. In *Immunochemistry of Solid-Phase Immunoassay,* (J. E. Butler, ed.), CRC Press, Boca Raton, FL, 151—172.

Burghardt, T. P., and Axelrod, D. (1983) Total internal reflection fluorescence study of energy transfer in surface-adsorbed and dissolved bovine serum albumin. *Biochemistry* 22:979.

Butler, J. E. (1988) The immunochemistry of sandwich ELISAs. Principles and applications for the quantitative determination of immunoglobulins. In *Practical Aspects of ELISA and Other Solid-Phase Immunoassays,* (D. M. Kemeny, and S. J. Challacombe, eds.), John Wiley & Sons, New York, 155—180.

Butler, J. E. (1991) Perspectives, configuration and principles. In *Immunochemistry of Solid-Phase Immunoassay* (J. E. Butler, ed.), CRC Press, Boca Raton, FL, 1—24.

Butler, J. E., Heo, Y., Adams, P., and Richerson, H. B. (1990) The antigen-limited nature of microtiter ELISAs requires partial depletion of IgG to permit reliable determination of rabbit serum IgA antibody activity. *Molec. Immunol.* 27:319—325.

Butler, J. E., McGivern, P. L., Peterson, L., and Cantarero, L. A. (1980) Application of the amplified enzyme-linked immunosorbent assay (a-ELISA). II. Comparative quantitation of bovine serum IgG1, IgG2, IgA and IgM antibodies using the a-ELISA. *Amer. J. Vet. Res.* 41:1479—1491.

Butler, J. E., Peterman, J. H., and Koertge, T. E. (1985) The amplified enzyme-linked immunosorbent assay (a-ELISA). In *Enzyme-Mediated Immunoassay,* (T. T. Ngo, and H. M. Lenhoff, eds.), Plenum Press, NY, 241—276.

Butler, J. E., Spradling, J. E., Dierks, S. E., Heyermann, H., Peterman, J. H., and Suter, M. (1986) The immunochemistry of sandwich ELISAs. I. The binding characteristics of immunoglobulins to monoclonal and polyclonal capture antibodies adsorbed on plastic and their detection by symmetrical and asymmetrical antibody-enzyme conjugates. *Mol. Immunol.* 23:971.

Butler, J. E. and Brown, W. R. (1992) The immunochemistry of sandwich ELISAs. VII. Reaction buffers containing blocking proteins do not cause desorption of capture antibody but can interfere with specific antibody-antigen interactions. *J. Immunol. Meth.* (submitted).

Butler, J. E., and Hamilton, R. G. (1991) Quantitation of specific antibodies: methods of expression, standards, solid-phase considerations and specific applications. In *Immunochemistry of Solid-Phase Immunoassay,* (J. E. Butler, ed.), CRC Press, Boca Raton, FL, 173—198.

Butler, J. E., McGivern, P. L., and Swanson, P. (1978a) Amplification of the enzyme-linked immunosorbent assay (ELISA) for the detection of antibodies. *J. Immunol. Meth.* 20:365.

Butler, J. E., Feldbush, T. L., McGivern, P. L., and Stewart, N. (1978b) The enzyme-linked immunosorbent assay (ELISA): a measure of antibody concentration of affinity. *Immunochemistry* 15:131.

Butler, J. E., Joshi, K. S., Rosenberg, B., and Nessler, R. (1992) The immunochemistry of sandwich ELISAs. VI. The monoclonal behavior of adsorbed polyclonal capture antibodies to multivalent antigens can result from the clustering of interfacial immune complexes. (submitted).

Butler, J. E., Joshi, K. S., and Brown, W. R. (1991) The application of traditional immunochemical methods to evaluate the performance of capture antibodies immobilized on microtiter wells. In *Immunochemistry of Solid-Phase Immunoassay,* (J. E. Butler, ed.), CRC Press, Boca Raton, FL, 221—231.

Bull, H. B. (1956) Adsorption of bovine serum albumin on glass. *Biochim. Biophys. Acta* 19:464.

Campbell, D. H., Leuscher, E., and Lerman, L. S. (1961) Immunologic adsorbents. I. Isolation of antibody by means of cellulose-protein antigen. *Proc. Natl. Acad. Sci. U.S.A.* 37:575.

Cantarero, L. A., Butler, J. E., and Osborne, J. W. (1990) The binding characteristics of various proteins to polystyrene and their significance in solid-phase immunoassay. *Analyt. Biochem.* 105:375—382.

Carlson, B. A., Giebink, G. S., Spika, J. S., and Gray, E. D. (1982) Measurement of immunoglobulin G and M antibodies to type 3 pneumococcal capsular polysaccharide by enzyme-linked immunosorbent assay. *J. Clin. Microbiol.* 16:63.

Catt, K., and Tregear, G. W. (1967) Solid-phase immunoassay in antibody-coated tubes. *Science* 158:1570.

Chaiken, I. M., Wilchek, M., and Parikh, I. (eds.) (1983) *Affinity Chromatography and Biological Recognition,* Academic Press, New York, 515 pp.

Chin, N. W., and Lanks, K. W. (1977) Covalent attachment of lactoperoxidase to polystyrene tissue culture flasks. *Anal. Biochem.* 83:709.

Conradie, J. D., Govender, M., and Visser, L. (1983) ELISA solid phase: partial denaturation of coating antibody yields a more efficient solid phase. *J. Immunol. Meth.* 59:289.

Crothers, D. M., and Metzger, H. (1972) The influence of polyvalency on the binding properties of antibodies. *Immunochemistry* 9:341.

Crumpton, M. J. (1974) In *The Antigens,* Vol. II (M. Sela, ed.), Academic Press, New York, 1—78.

Cuatrecasas, P. (1970) Preparation and characterization of antigen and antibody adsorbents covalently coupled to an inorganic carrier. *Biochem. J.* 117:257.

Cuatrecasas, P., and Anfinson, C. B. (1971) Affinity chromatography. *Annu. Rev. Biochem.* 40:295.

Czerkinsky, C. C., Nilsson, L.-A., Ouchterlony, O., and Tarkowski, A. (1983a) A solid-phase enzyme-linked immunospot (ELISPOT) assay for enumeration of specific antibody-secreting cells. *J. Immunol. Meth.* 58:109.

Czerkinsky, C., Rees, A. S., Bergmeir, L. A., and Challacombe, S. J. (1983b) The detection and specificity of class specific antibodies to whole bacterial cells using a solid-phase immunoassay. *Clin. Exp. Immunol.* 53:192.

Dierks, S. E. (1985) Differential recognition of solid phase immunoglobulin and antibody bound to solid phase antigen: a method of antibody quantitation. M. S. Thesis, University of Iowa, Iowa City.

Dierks, S. E., Butler, J. E., and Richerson, H. B. (1986) Altered recognition of surface-adsorbed compared to antigen bound antibodies in the ELISA. *Mol. Immunol.* 23:403.

Djavadi-Ohaniance, L., Friguet, B., and Goldberg, M. E. (1984) Structural and functional influence of enzyme-antibody interactions: effect of eight different monoclonal antibodies on the enzyme activity of *Escherichia coli* tryptophan synthase. *Biochemistry* 23:97.

Drexler, G., Eichinger, A., Wolf, C., and Sieghart, W. (1986) A rapid and simple method for efficient coating of microtiter plates using low amounts of antigen in the presence of detergent. *J. Immunol. Meth.* 95:117.

Duermeyer, W., Wielaard, F., and van der Veen, J. (1979) A new principle for the detection of specific IgM antibodies applied in an ELISA for hepatitis A. *J. Med. Virol.* 4:25.

Dunn, S. D., Tozer, R. G., Antezak, D. F., and Hoppel, L. A. (1985) Monoclonal antibodies to *Escherichia coli* F_1-ATPase. *J. Biol. Chem.* 260:10418.

Edelman, G. M., and Rutishauser, U. (1974) Specific fractionation and manipulation of cells with chemically derivatized fibers and surfaces. *Meth. Enzymol.* 34:195.

Ekins, R. P. (1991) Competitive, non-competitive and multianalyte immunoassays. In *Immunochemistry of Solid-Phase Immunoassay,* (J. E. Butler, ed.), CRC Press, Boca Raton, FL, 105—138.

Elkins, K. L., Stashak, P. W., and Baker, P. J. (1990) Analysis of the optimal conditions for the adsorption of type III pneumococcal polysaccharide to plastic for use in solid-phase ELISA. *J. Immunol. Meth.* 130:123.

Engvall, E. (1980) Enzyme immunoassay ELISA and EMIT. *Meth. Enzymol.* 70:419.

Engvall, E., Jonsson, K., and Perlmann, P. (1971) Enzyme-linked immunosorbent assay. II. Quantitative assay of protein antigen in antibody coated tubes. *Biochim. Biophys. Acta* 251:427.

Engvall, E., and Perlmann, P. (1971) Enzyme-linked immunosorbent assay (ELISA). Quantitative assay of immunoglobulin G. *Immunochemistry* 8:871—874.

Evan, G. I. (1984) A simple and rapid solid phase enzyme-linked immunoabsorbance assay for screening monoclonal antibodies to poorly soluble proteins. *J. Immunol. Meth.* 73:427.

Fenstermaker, C. A., Grant, W. H., Morrissey, B. W., Smith, L. E., and Stromberg, R. R. (1974) Interaction of plasma proteins with surfaces. Cited in Morrisey, B. W. (1977) *Ann. N.Y. Acad. Sci.* 283:50.

Fowell, S. L., and Chase, H. A. (1986) Variation of immunosorbent performance with the amount of immobilized antibody. *J. Biotechnol.* 4:1.

Franci, C., and Vidal, J. (1988) Coupling redox and enzymic reactions improves the sensitivity of the ELISA-spot assay. *J. Immunol. Meth.* 107:239.

Francois-Gerard, C., Gerard, P., and Rentier, B. (1988) Elucidation of non-parallel EIA curves. *J. Immunol. Meth.* 111:59.

Franz, B., and Stegemann, M. (1991) The kinetics of solid-phase immunoassay. In *Immunochemistry of Solid-Phase Immunoassay* (J. E. Butler, ed.), CRC Press, Boca Raton, FL, chap. 18, 272—284.

Friguet, B., Djavadi-Ohaniance, L., and Goldberg, M. E. (1984) Some monoclonal antibodies raised with a native protein bind preferentially to the denatured antigen. *Mol. Immunol.* 21:673.

Friguet, B., Djavadi-Ohaniance, L., and Goldberg, M. E. (1989) Polypeptide-antibody binding mechanism: conformational adaptation investigated by equilibrium and kinetic analyses. *Res. Immunol.* 140:355.

Froese, A. (1968) Kinetic and equilibrium studies on 2,4-dinitrophenyl hapten-antibody systems. *Immunochemistry* 5:253.

Frost, R. G., Monthony, J. F., Englehorn, S. C., and Siebert, C. J. (1981) Covalent immobilization of proteins to N-hydroxylsuccinimide ester derivatives. Effect of protein charge on immobilization. *Biochim. Biophys. Acta* 670:163.

Gabrilovac, J., Packmann, D., Rodt, H., Jäger, G., and Theirfelder, S. (1979) Particle-labeled antibodies. I. Anti-T-cell antibodies attached to plastic beads by poly-L-lysine. *J. Immunol. Meth.* 30:161.

Gardas, A., and Lewartowska, A. (1988) Coating of proteins to polystyrene ELISA plates in the presence of detergent. *J. Immunol. Meth.* 106:251.

Geerligs, H. J., Weijer, W. J., Bloemhoff, W., Welling, G. W., and Welling-Wester, S. (1988) The influence of pH and ionic strength on the coating of peptides of herpes simplex virus type 1 in an enzyme-linked immunosorbent assay. *J. Immunol. Meth.* 106:239.

Gershoni, J. M., and Palade, G. E. (1982) Electrophoretic transfer of proteins from dodecyl sulfate-polyacrylamide gels to a positively charged membrane filter. *Anal. Biochem.* 124:396.

Getzoff, E. D., Tainer, J. A., Lerner, R. A., and Geysen, H. M. (1988) The chemistry and mechanism of antibody binding to protein antigens. *Adv. Immunol.* 43:1.

Geysen, M. H., Meloen, R. H., and Barteling, S. J. (1984) Use of peptide synthesis to probe viral antigens for epitopes to a resolution of a single amino acid. *Proc. Natl. Acad. Sci. U.S.A.* 81:3998.

Gnann, J. W., Jr., McCormick, J. B., Mitchell, S., Nelson, J. A., and Oldstone, M. B. A. (1987) Synthetic peptide immunoassay distinguishes HIV type 1 and HIV type 2 infections. *Science* 237:1346.

Goldstein, L., and Katchalski, E. (1968) Use of water-insoluble enzyme derivatives in biochemical analyses and separation. *Z. Anal. Chem.* 243:375.

Goudswaard, J., van der Donk, J. A., van Dam, R., and Vaerman, J.-P. (1978) Protein-A reactivity of various mammalian immunoglobulins. *Scand. J. Immunol.* 8:21.

Gough, P. M., Jenness, R., and Anderson, R. K. (1966) Characterization of bovine immunoglobulins. *J. Dairy Sci.* 49:718.

Graves, H. C. B. (1988) Noise control in solid-phase immunoassays by use of a matrix coat. *J. Immunol. Meth.* 111:167.
Green, N. M. (1963) Avidin 1. The use of ^{14}C-biotin for kinetic studies and for assay. *Biochem. J.* 89:585.
Greenspan, N. S., Dacek, D. A., and Cooper, L. J. N. (1989) Cooperative binding of two antibodies to independent antigens by an Fc-dependent mechanism. *FASEB J.* 3:2203.
Gripenberg, M., and Kuruki, P. (1986) Demonstration of human autoantibodies by quantitative enzyme immunoassay. *J. Immunol. Meth.* 92:145.
Guesdon, J.-L., Ternynck, T., and Avrameas, S. (1979) The use of avidin-biotin interaction in immunoenzymatic techniques. *J. Histochem. Cytochem.* 27:1131.
Hagen, M., and Strejam, G. H. J. (1987) Antigen linkage from immunosorbents. Implications for the detection of site-directed auto-anti-idiotypic antibodies. *J. Immunol. Meth.* 100:47.
Harris, C. C., Yolken, R. H., Krohan, H., and Hsu, I. C. (1979) Ultrasensitive enzymatic radioimmune assay for detection of cholera toxin and rotovirus. *Proc. Natl. Acad. Sci. U.S.A.* 76:5336.
Herrmann, J. E., Hendry, R. M., and Collins, M. F. (1979) Factors involved in enzyme-linked immunoassay of viruses and evaluation of the method for identification of enteroviruses. *J. Clin. Microbiol.* 10:210.
Herron, J. A. (1984) Equilibrium and kinetic methodology for the measurement of binding properties in monoclonal and polyclonal populations of anti-fluorescyl-IgG antibodies. In *Fluorescein Hapten: An Immunological Probe* (E. W. Voss, Jr., ed.), CRC Press, Boca Raton, FL, 49—76.
Hirano, T., Yamakawa, N., Miyajima, H., Maeda, K., Takai, S., Ueda, A., Taniguchi, O., Hashimoto, H., Hirose, S., Okumura, K., and Ovary, Z. (1989) An improved method for the detection of IgE antibody of defined specificity by ELISA using rat monoclonal anti-IgE antibody. *J. Immunol. Meth.* 119:145.
Hobbs, R. N. (1989) Solid-phase immunoassay of serum antibodies to peptides. Covalent antigen binding to adsorbed phenylalanine-lysine copolymers. *J. Immunol. Meth.* 117:257.
Holland, Z., and Katchalski-Katzir, E. (1986) Use of monoclonal antibodies to detect conformational alterations in lactate dehydrogenase isoenzyme 5 on heat denaturation and on adsorption to polystyrene plates. *Mol. Immunol.* 23:927.
Horejsi, V., and Matousek, V. (1985) Equilibrium in the protein-immobilized-ligand-soluble-ligand system: estimation of dissociation constants of protein-soluble ligand complexes from binding-inhibition data. *Mol. Immunol.* 22:125.
Howell, E. E., Nasser, J., and Schrau, K. H. (1981) Coated tube immunoassay: factors affecting sensitivity and effects of reversible protein binding to polystyrene. *J. Immunoassay* 2:205.
Inman, J. K. (1982) Covalent attachment of ligands to support using heterobifunctional reagents. In *Affinity Chromatography and Related Techniques* (T. C., Gribaan, J. Visser, and R. J. F. Nivard, eds.), Elsevier, Amsterdam, 217—233.
Javaherian, K., Kanglois, A. J., McDanal, C., Ross, K. L., Eckler, L. I., Jellis, C. L., Profy, A. T., Rusche, J. R., Bolognesi, D. P., Putney, S. D., and Matthews, T. J. (1989) Principal neutralizing domain of the human immunodeficiency virus type I envelope protein. *Proc. Natl. Acad. Sci. U.S.A.* 86:6768.
Jitsukawa, T., Nakajima, S., Sugawara, I., and Watanabe, H. (1989) Increased coating efficiency of antigens and preservation of original antigenic structure after coating with ELISA. *J. Immunol. Meth.* 116:251.

Joshi, K. S., Hoffmann, L. G., and Butler, J. E. (1992) The immunochemistry of sandwich ELISAs. V. The capture antibody performance of polyclonal antibody-enriched fraction prepared by various method. *Mol. Immunol.* (in press).

Karush, F. (1978) The affinity of antibody: range, variability and the role of multivalence. In *Immunoglobulins*, (G. W. Litmann, and R. A. Good, eds.), Plenum Press, NY, 85—115.

Karush, F. (1970) Affinity and the immune process. *Ann. N.Y. Acad. Sci.* 169:56.

Katz, M. A., and Schiffman, G. (1985) Comparison of an enzyme-linked immunosorbent assay with radioimmunoassay for the measurement of pneumococcal capsular polysaccharide antibodies. *Mol. Immunol.* 22:313.

Kennedy, J. H., Kricka, L. J., and Wilding, P. (1976) Protein-protein coupling reactions and the application of protein conjugates. *Clin. Chim. Acta* 70:1.

Kennel, S. (1982) Binding of monoclonal antibody in fluid phase and bound to solid supports. *J. Immunol. Meth.* 55:1.

Kenny, G. E., and Dunsmoor, C. L. (1983) Principles, problems and strategies in the use of antigenic mixtures for the enzyme-linked immunosorbent assay. *J. Clin. Microbiol.* 17:655—665.

Keren, D. (1979) Enzyme-linked immunosorbent assay for immunoglobulin G and immunoglobulin A antibodies to *Shigella flexneri* antigen. *Infect. Immunol.* 24:441.

Khalil, O. S. (1991) Photophysics of heterogeneous immunoassay. In *Immunochemistry of Solid-Phase Immunoassay*, (J. E. Butler, ed.), C.R.C. Press, Boca Raton, FL, 67—83.

Kochwa, S., Brownell, M., Rosenfield, R. E., and Wasserman, L. R. (1967) Adsorption of proteins by polystyrene particles. I. Molecular unfolding and acquired immunogenicity of IgG. *J. Immunol.* 99:981.

Kohler, G., and Milstein, C. (1975) Continuous culture of fused cells secreting specific antibody. *Nature (London)* 256:495.

LaCroix, M., Dionne, G., Zrein, M., Dwyer, R. J., and Chalifour, R. J. (1991) The use of synthetic peptides as solid-phase antigens. In *Immunochemistry of Solid-Phase Immunoassay*, (J. E. Butler, ed.), Boca Raton, FL, 261—268.

Lamed, R., Levin, Y., and Wilchek, M. (1973) Covalent coupling of nucleotides to agarose for affinity chromatography. *Biochim. Biophys. Acta* 304:231.

Landsteiner, K., and Uhlirz, R. (1905) Über der Absorption von Eiweisskorper. Zentlblatt fur Bacterologie u. Prasiten Kunde Bd XL H Z, *Abth 1* 40:265.

Lauritzen, E., Masson, M., Ruben, I., and Holm, A. (1990) Dot immunoblotting and immunoblotting of picrogram and nanogram quantities of small peptides on activated nitrocellulose. *J. Immunol. Meth.* 131:257.

Lee, R. G., Adamson, C., and Kim, S. W. (1974) Competitive adsorption of plasma proteins onto polymer surfaces. *Thromb. Res.* 4:485.

Lehtonen, O.-P., and Eerola, E. (1982) The effect of different antibody affinities on ELISA absorbance and titer. *J. Immunol. Meth.* 54:233.

Li, C. K. N. (1985) ELISA-based determination of immunological binding constants. *Mol. Immunol.* 22:321.

Lyklema, J., and Norde, W. (1973) Biopolymer adsorption with special reference to the serum albumin-polystyrene latex system. *Croat. Chem. Acta* 45:67.

McCullough, K. C., Crowther, J. R., and Butcher, R. N. (1985) Alteration of antibody reactivity with foot and mouth disease virus (FMV) 146S antigen before and after binding to a solid phase or complexing with specific antibody. *J. Immunol.* 82:91.

MacRitchie, F. (1972) The adsorption of protein at the solid/liquid interface. *J. Colloid Interface Sci.* 38:484.

Mason, D. W., and Williams, A. F. (1980) The kinetics of antibody binding to membrane antigens in solution and at the cell surface. *Biochem. J.* 187:1.
Mazia, D., Schatten, G., and Windfield, S. (1975) Adhesion of cells to surfaces coated with polylysine. Application to electron microscopy. *J. Cell Biol.* 66:198.
Merrifield, R. B. (1963) Solid-phase peptide synthesis. I. The synthesis of a tetrapeptide. *J. Am. Chem. Soc.* 85:2149.
Messina, J. P., Hickox, P. G., Lepow, M. L., Pollara, B., and Venezia, R. A. (1985) Modification of a direct enzyme-linked immunosorbent assay for the detection of immunoglobulin G and M antibodies to pneumococcal polysaccharide. *J. Clin. Microbiol.* 21:390.
Michaeli, I., Absolom, D. R., and van Oss, C. J. (1980) Diffusion of adsorbed protein within the plane of adsorption. *J. Colloid Interface Sci.* 77:586.
Mierendorf, R. C., Jr., and Diamond, R. L. (1983) Functional heterogeneity of monoclonal antibodies obtained using different screening assay. *Anal. Biochem.* 135:221.
Mize, P. D., Naqui, A., O'Connell, C. M., Waller, J. N., Fesler, M., Myatich, R. G., and Keating, W. E. (1991) Studies on the covalent attachment of antibodies to controlled surfaces. In *Immunochemistry of Solid-Phase Immunoassay*, (J. E. Butler, ed.), CRC Press, Boca Raton, FL, 207—219.
Morrissey, B. W. (1977) The adsorption and conformation of plasma proteins: a physical approach. *Ann. N.Y. Acad. Sci.* 283:50.
Morrissey, B. W., and Fenstermaker, C. A. (1976) Conformation of adsorbed γ-globulin and β-lactoglobulin. Effect of surface concentration. *Trans. Am. Soc. Artif. Intern. Organs* 22:278.
Morrissey, B. W., and Stromberg, R. R. (1974) The conformation of adsorbed blood proteins by infrared bound fraction measurements. *J. Colloid Interface Sci.* 46:152.
Mushens, R. E., and Scott, M. L. (1990) A fast and efficient method for quantification of monoclonal antibodies in an ELISA using a novel incubation system. *J. Immunol. Meth.* 131:83.
Nardella, F. A., and Mannik, M. (1978) Non-immunospecific protein-protein interaction of IgG: studies of the binding of IgG to IgG immunosorbents. *J. Immunol.* 120:739.
Nardelli, B., McHugh, L., and Mage, M. (1989) Polyacrylamide-streptavidin: a novel reagent for simplified construction of soluble multivalent macromolecular conjugates. *J. Immunol. Meth.* 120:233.
Neurath, A. R., Strick, N., and Lee, E. S. Y. (1990) B cell epitope mapping of human immunodeficiency virus envelope glycoproteins with long (19- to 36-residue) synthetic peptides. *J. Gen. Virol.* 71:85.
Newman, P. J., Kahn, R. A., and Hines, A. (1981) Detection and characterization of monoclonal antibodies to platelet proteins *J. Cell Biol.* 90:249.
Ngo, T. T. (1986) Facile activation of Sepharose hydroxyl groups by 2-fluoro-1-methylpyridinium toluene-4-sulfonate: preparation of affinity and covalent chromatography. *BioTechnology* 4:134.
Ngo, T. T. (1991) Enzyme systems and enzyme conjugates for solid-phase ELISA. In *Immunochemistry of Solid-Phase Immunoassay*, (J. E. Butler, ed.), CRC Press, Boca Raton, FL, 85—102.
Nimmo, G. R., Lew, A. M., Stanley, C. M., and Steward, M. W. (1984) Influence of antibody affinity on the performance of different antibody assay. *J. Immunol.* 72:177.

Nustad, K., Johansen, L., Ugelstad, J., Ellingsen, T., and Berge, A. (1984) Hydrophobic monodisperse particles as solid-phase material in immunoassays: comparison of shell and core particles with compact particles. *Eur. Surg. Res.* 16(Suppl. 2):80.

Nygren, H., Czerkinsky, C., and Stenberg, M. (1985) Dissociation of antibodies bound to surface-immobilized antigen. *J. Immunol. Meth.* 85:87.

Nygren, H., Kaartinen, M., and Stenberg, M. (1986) Determination by ellipsometry of the affinity of monoclonal antibodies. *J. Immunol. Meth.* 92:219.

Nyholm, L., and Ramlau, J. (1988) Nitrocellulose membranes as solid phase in immunoblotting. In *Handbook of Immunoblotting of Proteins,* Vol. I, (O. J. Bjerrum and N. H. H. Heegaard, eds.), CRC Press, Boca Raton, FL, 101.

Nyilas, E., Chiu, T.-H., and Herzlinger, G. A. (1974) Thermodynamics of native protein/foreign surface interactions. I. Colorimetry of the human γ-globulin/glass system. *Trans. Am. Soc. Artif. Intern. Organs* 20:480.

Oreskes, I., and Singer, J. M. (1961) The mechanism of particulate carrier reactions. Adsorption of human γ-globulin to polystyrene latex particles. *J. Immunol.* 86:338.

O'Shannessy, D., Dobersen, M. J., and Quarles, R. H. (1984) A novel procedure for labeling immunoglobulins by conjugation to oligosaccharide moieties. *Immunol. Lett.* 8:273.

Pachman, K., and Leibold, W. (1976) Insolubilization of protein antigens on polyacrylic plastic beads using polystyrene. *J. Immunol. Meth.* 12:81.

Palfree, R. G. W., and Elliott, B. E. (1982) An enzyme linked immunosorbent assay (ELISA) for detergent-solubilized Ia glycoproteins using nitrocellulose membrane discs. *J. Immunol. Meth.* 52:395.

Papadea, C., Check, I. J., and Reimer, C. B. (1985) Monoclonal antibody-based-solid-phase immunoenzymometric assays for quantifying human immunoglobulin G and its subclasses in serum. *Clin. Chem.* 31:1940.

Parsens, G. H. (1981) Antibody-coated plastic tubes in radioimmunoassay. *Meth. Enzymol.* 73:224.

Paterson, Y. (1989) Structural aspects of the immune recognition of a model protein antigen; Cytochrome C. In *The Immune Response to Structurally Defined Proteins: The Lysozyme Model.* (S. Smith Gill, and E. Sercarz, eds.), Academic Press, New York, 177—189.

Perlstein, M. T. (1979) Evaluation of commercial RIA kits. 2. Parallelism effects of protein matrices and mathematical treatment of data in evaluating an assay. *Ligand Quart.* 2:6.

Pearce-Pratt, R., and Roser, B. (1990) False-positive signals in enzyme immunoassay (EIA) interactions between rodent IgG subclasses. *J. Immunol. Meth.* 130:65.

Pesce, A. J., Ford, D. J., Gaizutis, M., and Pollak, V. W. (1977) Binding of protein to polystyrene in solid-phase immunoassay. *Biochim. Biophys. Acta* 492:399.

Peterman, J. H. (1986) The influence of antibody affinity, valency and heterogeneity on the binding behavior of anti-fluorescein antibodies in solid-phase micro-ELISA systems. Ph.D. Thesis, University of Iowa, Iowa City, IA.

Peterman, J. H., and Butler, J. E. (1989) Application of theoretical considerations to the analysis of ELISA data. *BioTechniques* 7:608.

Peterman, J. H., Tarcha, P. J., Chu, V. P., and Butler, J. E. (1988) The immunochemistry of sandwich ELISAs. IV. A comparison of the antigen capture capacity of antibody adsorbed or covalently attached to polystyrene. *J. Immunol. Meth.* 111:271.

Peterson, E. A., and Sober, H. A. (1956) Chromatography of proteins. I. Cellular ion-exchange adsorbents. *J. Am. Chem. Soc.* 78:751.

Piran, U., and Riordan, W. J. (1990) Dissociation rate constant of the biotin-streptavidin complex. *J. Immunol. Meth.* 133:141.

Quash, G. A., Thomas, V., Ogier, G., El Alaoui, S., Delcros, J. G., Ripollo, H., Roch, A. M., Legastelois, S., Gibert, R., and Ripoll, J. P. (1989) Diagnostic and therapeutic procedures with haptens and glycoproteins (antigens and antibodies) coupled covalently by specific sites to insoluble supports. In *Covalently Modified Antigens and Antibodies in Diagnosis and Therapy*. Marcel Dekker, NY, 155—186.

Ramlau, J. (1988) Protein binding to charge derivatized membranes in blotting procedures — a critical study. In *Handbook of Immunoblotting of Proteins*, Vol. I (O. J. Bjerrum, and N. H. H. Heegaard, eds.), CRC Press, Boca Raton, FL, 109.

Regulatory Guide 8.20 (1978) U.S. Nuclear Regulatory Commission, Washington, April 1978.

Robinson, J. E., Holton, Liu, J., McMurdo, H., Muciano, A. and Gohd, R. (1990) A novel enzyme-linked immunosorbent assay (ELISA) for the detection of antibodies to HIV-1 envelope glycoproteins based on immobilization of viral glycoproteins in microtiter wells coated with Con-A. *J. Immunol. Meth.* 132:63.

Rubin, R. L., Hardtke, M. A., and Carr, R. I. (1980) The effect of high antigen density on solid-phase readioimmunoassays for antibody regardless of immunoglobulin class. *J. Immunol. Meth.* 33:277.

St. Laurent, M., Martel, F., Verrette, S., and Lemieux, R. (1990) Non-specific reactivity of monoclonal antibodies in ELISA due to the presence of an antigen-like structure on the alkaline phosphatase molecule. *J. Immunol. Meth.* 133:145.

Saito, T., and Nagai, F. (1983) Immobilization of antibody to a plastic surface by toluene 2,4-diisocyanate and its application to radioimmunoassay. *Clin. Chim. Acta* 133:301.

Schellenberger, A., and Ulbrich, R. (1989) Protein stabilization by blocking the native unfolding nucleus. *Biomed. Biochim. Acta* 48:63.

Self, C. H. (1985) Enzyme amplification — A general method applied to provide an immunoassociated assay for placental alkaline phosphatase. *Immunol. Meth.* 76:389.

Shirahama, H., and Suzawa, T. (1985) Adsorption of bovine serum albumin onto styrene/acrylic acid copolymer latex. *Colloid Polymer Sci.* 263:141.

Smalla, K., Turkova, J., Coupek, J., and Hermann, P. (1988) Influence of salts on the covalent immobilization of proteins to modified copolymers of 2-hydroxyethyl methacrylate with ethylene dimethacrylate. *Biotechnol. Appl. Biochem.* 10:21.

Soderquist, M. E., and Walton, A. G. (1980) Structural changes in protein adsorbed on polymer surfaces. *J. Colloid Interface Sci.* 75:386.

Sødergard-Andersen, J., Lauritzen, E., Lind, L., and Holm, A. (1990) Covalently linked peptides for enzyme-linked immunosorbent assay. *J. Immunol. Meth.* 131:99.

Sternberger, L. A., Hardy, P. H., Jr., Coculis, J. J., and Meyer, H. G. (1970) The unlabeled enzyme method of immunohistochemistry; preparation of antigen-antibody complex (perosidase-anti-peroxidase) in identification of spirochetes. *J. Histochem. Cytochem.* 18:315.

Stevens, F. J., Jwo, O., Carperons, W., Kohler, H., and Schiffler, M. (1986) Relationship between liquid- and solid-liquid antibody association characteristics: implications for the use of competitive ELISA techniques to map the spatial location of idiotypes. *J. Immunol.* 137:1937.

Steward, M. W. (1977) Affinity of the antibody-antigen reaction and its biological significance. In *Immunochemistry: An Advanced Textbook* (L. E. Glynn, and M. W. Steward, eds.), John Wiley & Sons, London, 233—262.

Sundberg, L., and Porath, J. (1974) Preparation of adsorbents for biospecific affinity chromatography. I. Attachment of group-containing ligands to insoluble polymers by means of bifunctional oxiranes. *J. Chromat.* 90:87.

Suter, L., Bruggen, J., and Sorg, C. (1980) Use of an enzyme-linked immunosorbent assay (ELISA) for screening of hybridoma antibodies against cell surface antigens. *J. Immunol. Meth.* 39:407.

Suter, M. (1982) A modified ELISA technique for anti-hapten antibodies. *J. Immunol. Meth.* 53:103.

Suter, M., and Butler, J. E. (1986) The immunochemistry of sandwich ELISAs. II. A novel system prevents denaturation of capture antibodies. *Immunol. Lett.* 13:313.

Suter, M., Butler, J. E., and Peterman, J. H. (1989) The immunochemistry of sandwich ELISAs. III. The stoichiometry and efficacy of the protein-avidin-biotin capture (PABC) system. *Mol. Immunol.* 26:221.

Thomas, V., El Alaoui, S., Roch, A. M., and Quash, G. (1990) A novel covalent enzyme-linked immunoassay (ELISA) for simultaneously measuring free and immune complex bound antibodies with a defined specificity. II. Application to immune complexes containing viral antigens in human sera. *J. Immunol. Meth.* 133:13.

Thorpe, R., Bird, C. R., and Spitz, M. (1984) Immunoblotting with monoclonal antibodies: loss of immunoreactivity with human immunoglobulins arises from polypeptide chain separation. *J. Immunol. Meth.* 73:259.

Towbin, H., and Gordon, J. (1984) Immunoblotting and dot immunobinding — current status and outlook. *J. Immunol. Meth.* 72:313.

Towbin, H., Staehelin, T., and Gordon, J. (1979) Electrophoretic transfer of protein from polyacrylamide gels to nitrocellulose sheets: procedure and applications. *Proc. Natl. Acad. Sci. U.S.A.* 76:4350.

Trent, D. W., Jarvey, C. L., Qureshi, A., and LeStourgeon, D. (1976) Solid-phase radioimmunoassay for antibodies to flavivirus structural and nonstructural proteins. *Infect. Immunol.* 13:1325.

Urbanek, R., Kemeny, D. M., and Samuel, D. (1985) Use of enzyme-linked immunosorbent assay for measurement of allergen-specific antibodies. *J. Immunol. Meth.* 79:123.

Vaidya, H. C., Dietzler, D. N., and Ladenson, J. H. (1985) Inadequacy of traditional ELISA for screening hybridoma supernatants for murine monoclonal antibodies. *Hybridoma* 4:271.

Van Kreveld, M. E., and Van den Hoed, N. (1973) Mechanism of gel permeation chromatography: distribution coefficient. *J. Chromatogr.* 83:111.

van Oss, C. J., and Singer, J. M. (1966) The binding of immune globulins and other proteins by polystyrene latex particles. *J. Reticuloendothel. Soc.* 3:29.

van Regenmortel, M. H. V., Briand, J. P., Muller, S., and Plaue, S. (1988) Synthetic polypeptides as antigens. In *Laboratory Techniques in Biochemistry and Molecular Biology,* Vol. 19 (R. H. Burdon, and P. H. van Knippenberg, eds.), Elsevier, Amsterdam, 1—227.

Varga, J. M., Klein, G. F., and Fritsch, P. (1990) Binding of a mouse monoclonal IgE (anti-IgE) antibody to radio-derivatized polystyrene-DNP complexes. *FASEB J.* 4:2678.

Voller, A., Bidwell, D. E., and Bartlett, A. (1976) Microplate enzyme immunoassay for the immunodiagnosis of virus infections. In *Manual of Clinical Immunology* (N. R. Rose, and H. Friedman, eds.), Am. Soc. Microbiology, Washington, 506—512.

Voller, A., Bidwell, D. E., and Bartlett, A. (1979) *The Enzyme Linked Immunosorbent Assay (ELISA)*. Dynatech Laboratories Tech. Bull., Alexandria, VA.

Weetall, H. H. (1970) Preparation and characterization of antigen and antibody covalently coupled to an inorganic carrier. *Biochem. J.* 117:257.

Yalow, R. S., and Berson, S. A. (1960) Immunoassay of endogeneous plasma insulin in man. *J. Clin. Invest.* 39:1157.

Yolken, R. H., Stopa, P. J., and Harris, C. C. (1980) Enzyme immunoassay for the detection of rotovirus antigen and antibody. In *Manual of Clinical Immunology* (N. R. Rose, and H. Friedman, eds.), Am. Soc. Microbiology, Washington, 692—699.

Yorde, D. E., Sasse, E. A., Wang, T. Y., Hussa, R. O., and Garancis, J. C. (1976) Competitive enzyme-linked immunosorbent assay with use of soluble immune complexes for labeling. I. Measurement of human choriogronadotropin. *Clin. Chem.* 22:1372.

Zeiss, C. R., Pruzansky, J. J., Patterson, R., and Roberts, M. (1973) A solid-phase radioimmunoassay for the quantitation of human reagenic antibody against ragweed E. *J. Immunol.* 110:414.

Zigterman, G. J. W. J., Verhuel, A. F. M., Ernste, E. B. H. W., Rombouts, R. F. M., DeReuver, M. J., Jansze, M., Snippe, H., and Willers, J. M. N. (1988) Measurement of the humoral immune response against *Streptococcus pneumoniae* type 3 capsular polysaccharide and oligosaccharide containing antigens by ELISA and ELISPOT techniques. *J. Immunol. Meth.* 106:101.

Chapter 12

Drugs as Antigens

Johan Hoebeke
Laboratoire des Protides des Liquides Biologiques C.N.R.S.
Faculté de Médecine, Université François Rabelais
Tours Cédex, France
and
A. Donny Strosberg
Laboratoire d'Immunopharmacologie Moléculaire, C.N.R.S. and
Université Paris VII
Institut Cochin de Génétique Moléculaire
Paris, France

INTRODUCTION

Immunology and pharmacology are two disciplines which were fathered by Paul Ehrlich who was the first to postulate the existence in blood of distinct entities that could specifically neutralize invading bacteria (Ehrlich, 1990). He thus predicted the existence of antibodies 50 years before they were structurally defined as immunoglobulins.

Ehrlich attempted to mimic these hypothetic entities by chemical synthesis of molecules which would be specifically targeted toward the bacterial intruder without interference with the host organism. He thus became the father of modern chemotherapy through the invention of the first wholly synthetic antibacterial agent, "Salvarsan."

The "receptor" concept, postulated by Ehrlich, was introduced as a fruitful pharmacological hypothesis by Langley (1906). This concept postulated that the discriminatory response to stimulatory or inhibitory agents in various tissues is due to the existence of molecular structures able to specifically recognize one or a few of these agents. While this pharmacological concept remains at the basis of modern molecular pharmacology, it took many decades before these hypothetic structures could be identified as membrane proteins and, only since the cloning of the cDNA of the acetylcholine receptor of the electroplax of the torpedo fish (Noda et al., 1982), could an attempt be made to relate the primary structures of these proteins to their recognition functions.

An understanding of the molecular basis of immune recognition showed that receptorlike molecules were also involved in the immune response. The identification of the antibody function using the γ-globulin protein fraction in serum (Tiselius and Kabat, 1939) and the first primary sequence analyses of the antibodies helped to relate the antigen specificity of an antibody to the existence of variable domains in the chains of the protein (Hilschman and Craig, 1965), and, more precisely, to the hypervariable regions of these domains (Wu and Kabat, 1970). The first successful attempt to unravel the three-dimensional structure of a myeloma protein, which happened to bind vitamin K (Amzel et al., 1974), confirmed that the antigen-combining site is limited to the variable domains of the heavy and light chains and that the hapten specificity mainly resides in interactions with the hypervariable regions (Fig. 1).

From the first studies of antibodies induced against steroid molecules, the hypothesis was derived that the steroid hapten-antibody interaction could be a possible model for hormone binding by target tissue receptors (Zimmering et al., 1967). Apart from the practical use of antidrug antibodies to perform pharmacokinetic measurements by radioimmunoassays or enzyme immunoassays, the value of antidrug antibodies as analogs of receptors has been a constant topic of research in molecular immunology and pharmacology (Cook and Drayer, 1988). Moreover, the finding that anti-idiotypic antibodies against antidrug antibodies can interact with receptors (Sege and Peterson, 1978) has prompted many pharmacologists to use the anti-idiotypic approach to study membrane receptors (Langone, 1989). This chapter focuses on the use of antidrug antibodies as tools for the understanding of the corresponding receptors.

ANTIBODIES AGAINST CARDIAC GLYCOSIDES

It is not fortuitous that the first drug used as a hapten to induce antidrug antibodies has been the cardiac glycoside digitoxin (Oliver et al., 1966). Indeed, cardiac glycosides (Fig. 2) are used in patients with congestive heart failure to increase the output of the failing heart. By their inhibitory activity on the potassium influx into cells, the cardiac glycosides may, however, cause life-threatening hyperkalemia (Hoffman and Bigger, 1985). Since there are large individual variations in the dosage required to produce a beneficial therapeutic effect and in the sensitivity toward the toxic effects. careful monitoring of drug pharmacokinetics at very low serum concentrations is required. Antidigitoxin and antidigoxin antibodies (Smith et al. 1970) of high affinity

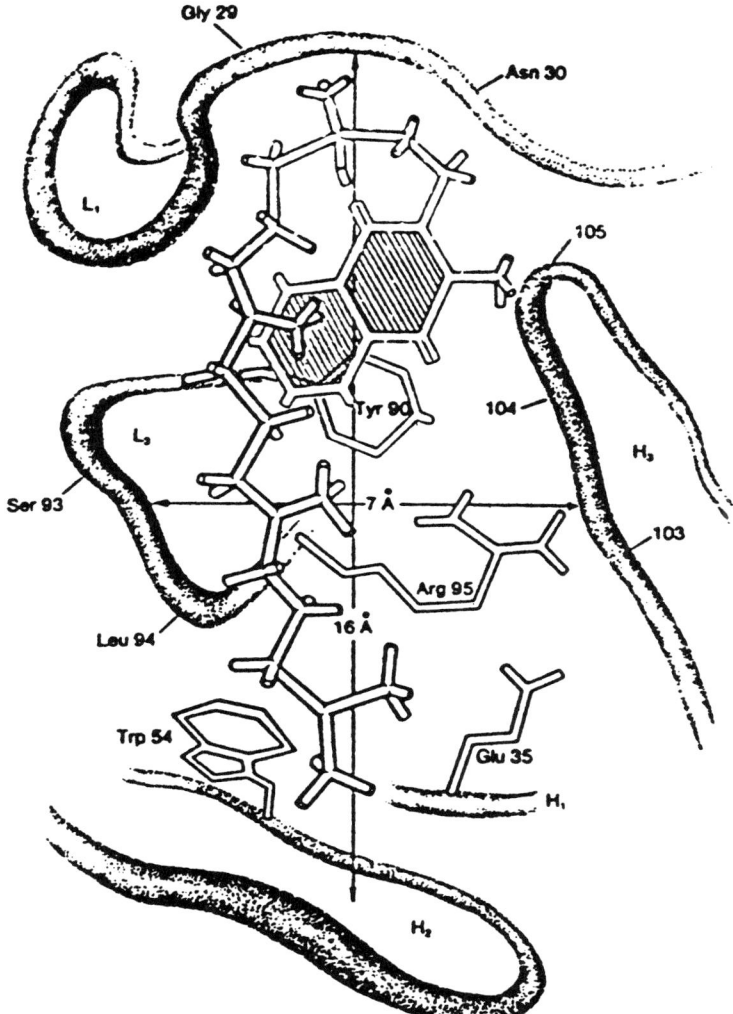

Figure 1. Complex of vitamin K and the Fab fragment of immunoglobulin NEW. L₂ and L₂ are the hypervariable regions of the light chain; H₁, H₂, and H₃ are the hypervariable regions of the heavy chain. The amino acid residues involved in vitamin K recognition are indicated. [After Amzel, L. M. et al. (1974) *Proc. Natl. Acad. Sci. U.S.A.* 71:1427—1430. With permission.]

were thus a welcome tool for the development of sensitive radioimmunoassays. The availability of polyclonal antibodies with high affinity for a hapten, such as digoxin, also induced a spate of studies to better understand the molecular basis of hapten-antibody interactions. Kinetic experiments showed that the high-affinity constant was the result of a diffusion-controlled asso-

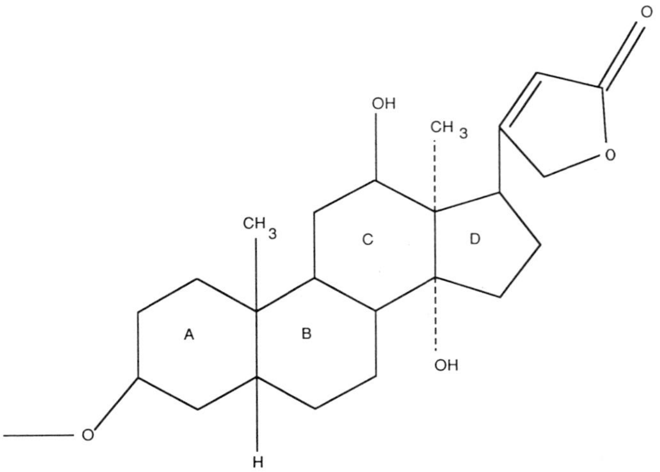

Figure 2. Structural formula of digoxigenin, the aglycon moiety of digoxin. The trisaccharide is linked to the oxygen on cycle A. The junctions of cycles A and B and cycles C and D are *cis* while cycles B and C are joined in *trans*. All antidigoxin antibodies recognize this aglycon moiety.

ciation rate and a very low dissociation rate, suggesting that the hapten-antibody interaction did occur without conformational changes and was stabilized by multiple atomic interactions between digoxin and the antibody-combining site (Smith and Skubitz, 1975). The dimensions of digoxin (30 × 9 × 9 Å) (Go et al., 1980), corresponding to the postulated antibody-combining site (Kabat, 1966) could explain the perfect fit of this hapten in its binding site. Although crystals of the Fab fragment of a monoclonal antidigoxin antibody and its complex with digoxin have been obtained (Rose et al., 1982), no three-dimensional structure analysis is yet available to support this hypothesis.

The production of high-affinity monoclonal antibodies (Köhler and Milstein, 1975) to digoxin (Mudgett-Hunter et al., 1982; Pincus et al., 1984) and digitoxin (Collignon et al., 1988) led to the analysis of the possible relationship between the primary structure of their light and heavy chains and the specificity of hapten recognition. Five monoclonal antidigoxin antibodies, sharing identical heavy and light chains according to the N-terminal sequences, displayed differences in hapten specificity (Table 1) (Mudgett-Hunter et al., 1985). Complete amino acid analysis of these chains indicated that the degree of sequence homology among the five antibodies correlated with their rank order of hapten and idiotype specificity (Panka and Margolies, 1987). Mutation of a residue outside of the hypervariable regions affected hapten specificity (Panka et al., 1988) but this could be explained by a computer analysis of the secondary structure which suggested that the involved residue could enter into hydrogen binding with amino acids of the combining site which might account for the affinity changes (Novotny et al., 1990).

TABLE 1.
Kinetic Parameters of Alprenolol Binding to an Antibody and a Receptor

	Antibody			Receptor		
t°C	k_{on} 10^6 $M^{-1}s^{-1}$	k_{off} 10^{-3} s^{-1}	K_a 10^9 M^{-1}	k_{on} 10^6 M^{-1} s^{-1}	k_{off} 10^{-3} s^{-1}	K_a 10^9 M^{-1}
25	—	—	—	2.7	1.7	1.5
27	0.025	2.1	0.012	—	—	—
37	0.054	3.5	0.015	8.5	8.7	1.0

Note: Kinetic parameters for the antibody from Hoebeke et al. (1987) and for the receptor from Affolter et al. (1985).

Genetic engineering was used to prepare single-chain Fv (sFv) fragments of antidigoxin antibodies, i.e., variable-region fragments consisting of V_H and V_L domains linked together to form a single polypeptide chain via a (Gly-Gly-Gly-Gly-Ser)$_3$ linker. The association constant of this engineered antibody-binding site was only six times lower than that of the original Fab (Huston et al., 1988). The gene of this sFv was fused to the gene of the Fc-binding fragment B of staphylococcal protein A to yield a bifunctional fusion protein (Tai et al., 1990).

Another application of the antidigoxin antibodies was to use the detoxifying properties of the Fab fragments allowing the renal elimination of the complexed drug (Lechat et al., 1984; Smith et al. 1982). The availability of the smaller sFv digoxin-binding fragments will certainly improve the immunological detoxification of digitalis compounds.

Another application of antidrug antibodies was also exemplified with the antidigoxin antibodies. Beginning with the hypothesis that antidrug antibodies could be useful tools in the study of endogenous druglike substances (Gintzler et al., 1976), the existence of humoral agents acting as digitalis glycosides on the Na$^+$ K$^+$-ATPase, and postulated by Haddy and Overbeck (1976), was confirmed by extraction of substances cross-reacting with antidigoxin antibodies in plasma from volume-expanded dogs (Gruber et al., 1980) and by inhibiting the action of these substances by *in vivo* treatment with antidigoxin antibodies (Kojima et al., 1982). Mammalian ligands which cross-react with antidigoxin antibodies and display digitalis-like activities could be the endogenous substances which had been described 10 years earlier (Fagoo et al., 1986).

ANTIBODIES AGAINST MORPHINELIKE SUBSTANCES

Morphine was a good candidate to develop a radioimmunoassay to monitor dose-therapeutic effect relationships and to study the prevalence of drug abuse for medico-legal and epidemiological studies (Spector, 1982). The first radioimmunoassay for morphine was described in 1970 (Spector and Parker, 1970).

Antimorphine antibodies were used as tools for the detection of endogenous ligands for the morphine receptor. Morphine immunoreactivity (ir-morphine) was found in rabbit and cat brain (Gintzler et al., 1976). These results were confirmed by several groups during the next decade (Blume et al., 1977; Gintzler et al., 1978; Killian et al., 1981; Shore et al., 1978) but only in 1985 would the structure of one of the ir-morphines, extracted from toad skin (Oka et al., 1985) and from beef brain and adrenal (Goldstein et al., 1985) unambiguously be determined as being morphine. Both groups who identified ir-morphines as morphine used polyclonal or monoclonal antimorphine antibodies with different fine specificities as a first approach toward unraveling their structure.

The first antimorphine monoclonal antibodies were reported in 1983 (Glasel et al., 1983). As was already observed for the polyclonal antimorphine antisera, none of these monoclonal antibodies nor the more recently reported ones (Sawada et al., 1988) were able to recognize endorphins, the peptide ligands of the morphine receptor. It had been previously suggested that the hapten-antibody binding in the opiate system could provide a macromolecular binding site model for opiate-receptor studies in view of the large array of opiate structural analogs available, of the fine specifity of the monoclonal antimorphine antibodies, and of the few degrees of conformational freedom of the planar polycyclic structures of morphine and analogs (Fig. 3) (Glasel, 1989). The rigid structure of morphine allowed, for the first time, the study of the interaction of a drug with its antibody by means of nuclear magnetic resonance using transferred ^{1}H nuclear Overhauser enhancements (TRNOE) (Glasel, 1989; Glasel and Borer, 1986). The results obtained indicated that the conformation of nalorphine, a morphine analog, has a different antibody-binding site than that found in solution or in crystals and suggested that at least one aromatic amino acid residue was closely involved in the binding of the ligand. This hypothesis was strengthened by the inhibitory activity on hapten binding of the alkylating agent, phenoxybenzamine, and by the effect of iodination on hapten binding, which pointed toward the existence of an essential tyrosine residue. From sequence comparisons of the light and heavy chains of four monoclonal antimorphine antibodies, it was suggested that this tyrosine is at position 59 in the second hypervariable region of the heavy chains (Miller and Glasel, 1989).

In view of the difficulty in purifying the morphine receptor and the availability of high-affinity polyclonal and monoclonal antimorphine antibodies, the latter were used to study the receptor by the anti-idiotypic route (Sege and Peterson, 1978). Anti-idiotypic antiserum against polyclonal antimorphine antibodies was first reported to inhibit binding of the tritiated antagonist naloxone to brain membrane preparations by noncompetitive inhibition and to inhibit contraction of electrically stimulated tissue suggesting a morphine agonistlike effect of the anti-idiotypic antibodies (Ng and Isom,

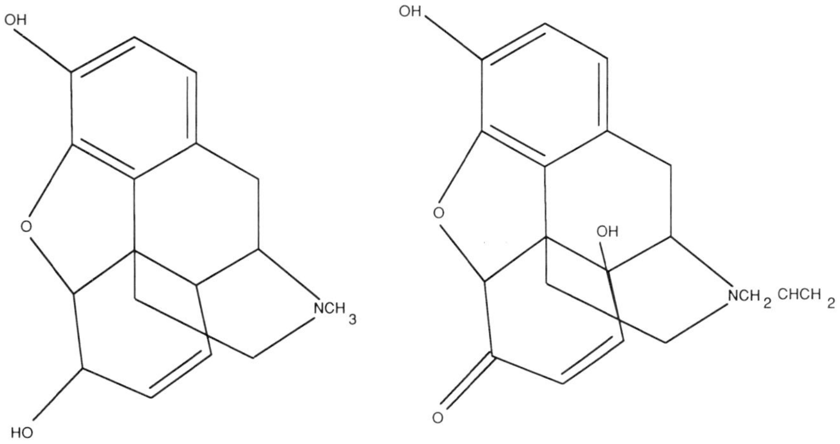

Figure 3. Structural formulas of morphine (A) and its antagonist naloxone (B).

1984; 1985). A more fundamental approach was taken using Fab fragments of monoclonal antimorphine antibodies as the idiotype and affinity-purified anti-idiotypic antibodies, characterized as competitive inhibitors of the hapten-antibody interaction (Glasel and Pelosi, 1986). One of these anti-idiotypic antimorphine antibodies displayed a subclass receptor specificity (mu > delta > kappa) which corresponded to the rank order of recognition by the anti-morphine antibody chosen as the anti-idiotypic antigen (Myers and Glasel, 1986).

As already mentioned, none of the polyclonal or monoclonal antimorphine antibodies could recognize opioid peptides, such as enkephalins and endorphins. Reciprocally, monoclonal antibodies, raised against the human β-endorphin recognized neither etorphine nor naloxone (Herz et al., 1982). These results were even more remarkable because the monoclonal described was reported to specifically recognize the tetrapeptide Tyr-Gly-Gly-Phe, a sequence present in all opioid peptides able to bind to the morphine receptor (Meo et al., 1983). Interestingly, this antibody could be used to induce monoclonal anti-idiotypic antibodies against the morphine receptor but, instead of having an agonistic physiological effect on the receptor, as did the polyclonal antimorphine and anti-β-endorphin anti-idiotypic antibodies (Ng and Isom, 1985; Schulz and Gramsch, 1985), this anti-β-endorphin anti-idiotypic antibodies had an antagonistic effect (Gramsch et al., 1988). The isolation of a monoclonal antienkephalin antibody with a higher affinity for the antagonist naloxone than for the agonist morphine (Deguchi and Yokoyama, 1985) suggests that the antimorphine antibodies mimic the agonist-binding site of the opiate receptor while the antienkephalin antibodies mimic the antagonist-binding site.

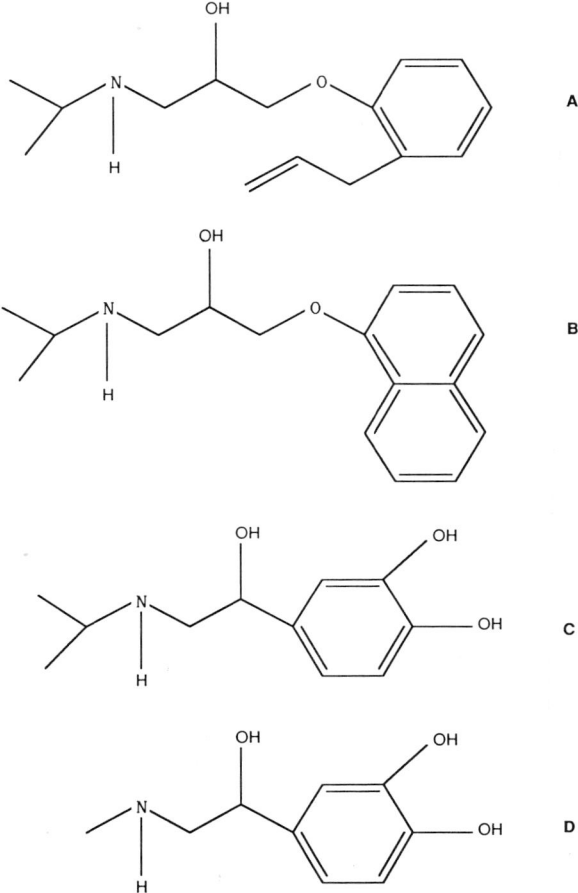

Figure 4. Structural formula of ligands of the β-adrenergic receptor: antagonist alprenolol (A), which was used for haptenization, the antagonist propranolol (B), synthetic agonist isoproterenol (C), and the natural hormone adrenaline (D).

ANTIBODIES AGAINST β-ADRENERGIC DRUGS

In contrast to the two drugs described in previous paragraphs for which the initial stimulus to raise antibodies was the development of a sensitive assay, antibodies against β-adrenergic antagonists were induced specifically to "compete with the β-adrenergic receptors." For this reason, care was taken to haptenize the drug under such conditions that the coupling did not interfere with the groups essential for recognition by the receptor. As shown in Fig. 4, the general β-adrenergic blocker, alprenolol was used because it contained a vinyl group on the phenyl ring which, by means of bromohydration, resulted in a bromohydrin with high reactivity for the thiol groups of reduced carrier protein (Hoebeke et al., 1978). The polyclonal antibodies raised in rabbits against this hapten not only recognized different β-adrenergic antagonists but also recognized the natural β-adrenergic agonists epinephrine and norepinephrine and the synthetic analog, isoproterenol (Hoebeke et al., 1978; Schreiber et al., 1980). Interestingly, a fraction of the rabbit polyclonal antibodies raised against the haptenic enantiomer ($\pm$)-alprenolol could be fractionated by stereospecific elution with ($-$)-propranolol to yield antibodies with a high affinity for the active ($-$)-stereoisomer (Rockson et al., 1980).

Two approaches were followed to raise monoclonal antialprenolol antibodies with binding properties similar to those of the β-adrenergic receptor. Hybridomas were prepared from mice immunized either with the mixed enantiomers or with the stereospecific ($-$)-alprenolol as a hapten. Both methods resulted in monoclonal antibodies sharing at least some properties with the β-adrenergic receptor (Chamat et al., 1984; Sawutz et al., 1985). Together with a stereospecific preference for the pharmacologically active ($-$)-stereoisomers, one of the monoclonal antibodies obtained in each approach was also able to recognize the agonists isoproterenol, epinephrine, and norepinephrine. This was not the case for a monoclonal antibody raised against the β-adrenergic antagonist propranolol which was haptenized by coupling the drug to bovine serum albumin (BSA) by means of the modified secondary amino group (Fig. 4) (Wang et al., 1986).

The monoclonal antibody 37A4, which showed the binding properties mentioned above, was an excellent tool to study the physicochemical characteristics of the hapten-antibody interactions and to compare the results with what is known about the ligand-receptor interactions. Indeed, the intrinsic fluorescence of this antibody was increased upon hapten binding and the increase could be used for equilibrium and kinetic studies (Hoebeke et al., 1987). Association kinetics measured by stopped-flow showed association rate constants in the $10^{-4} M^{-1} s^{-1}$ range, suggesting a conformational change upon binding of the hapten to the ligand. The nonlinearity of the observed pseudo-first-order association rate constant as a function of the hapten concentration confirmed the existence of a low-affinity binding step which, after conformational changes of the antibody-combining sites, led to formation of a high-affinity complex. In contrast, the association rate constants of ($-$)-alprenolol for the receptor were hundred times faster and were compatible with a diffusion-limited process (Table 2) (Affolter et al., 1985; Contreras et al., 1986). When the dissociation rate constants of the hapten-antibody complex are, however, compared to those of the receptor-ligand complex, the similarity is striking (Table 2). Due to the small dimensions of the hapten, the antibody-combining site may have to undergo a conformational change before it can mimic the receptor-combining site. Several pieces of evidence support this interpretation. Studies of the anti-idiotypic response against the monoclonal antialprenolol antibodies showed that the IgG fraction of one of

TABLE 2.
Synopsis of Drugs as Antigens

Drug	Receptor	Endogenous Ligand	Antibody			
			Anti-Idiotype	Sequences	Modelization	Crystals
Digitoxin	Na^+, K^+-ATPase	Yes	No	Yes	Yes	Yes
Morphine	Morphine	Yes	Yes	Yes	Yes	No
Alprenolol	β-Adrenergic		Yes	Yes	No	No
Haloperidol	Dopamine 2		Yes	Yes	Yes	No
Diazepam	GABA	Yes	No	No	No	No
Clonidine	Imidazoline	Yes	No	No	No	No
Nortriptyline	Muscarinic		No	No	No	No
SK&F 94481	Histaminic		No	No	No	No
Nifendipine	Ca^{2+}-channel		No	No	No	No
Cyclosporin	Cyclophilin		No	Yes	No	Yes

the anti-idiotypic antibodies enhanced hapten binding to the monoclonal idiotypic antibody (Chamat et al., 1986). A similar effect was shown by an antiidiotypic antibody against another antialprenolol antibody and physicochemical studies indicated that the enhancement was due to an increase in affinity for the hapten of the monoclonal idiotypic antibody. This increase could be ascribed to the 100-fold decrease of the dissociation rate of the antibody-hapten complex (Sawutz et al., 1987) (Table 1). The anti-idiotypic antibodies could induce the conformational changes leading to the high-affinity complex formation and also maintain the hapten in the antibody-combining site.

Sequencing of the different monoclonal antialprenolol antibodies shed more light on the structural basis of hapten recognition (Nahmias et al., 1988). The comparison between the V_H from antialprenolol antibodies and antibodies with a different specificity using the same V_H genes, indicated that the antialprenolol antibodies had a CDR3 region more acidic than any other described antibody. The acidic residues could serve as counterions for the positively charged haptens in the same way as the Asp residues in the transmembrane regions of the adrenergic receptors appear to be essential for binding of catecholamines (Strader et al., 1989). The comparison between the V_H of the 37A4 antibody and the other antialprenolol monoclonal antibodies suggested that tryptophan residue H103 was responsible for the intrinsic fluorescence enhancement upon hapten binding possibly because of the shortened CDR3 region of antibody 37A4.

To probe this region, a peptide was synthesized corresponding to positions H92 to 106 of monoclonal antibody 37A4 and antibodies were raised against this peptide as tools for studying the localization of the sequence into the antibody-combining site. The antipeptide antibodies specifically recognized the monoclonal antibody in an enzyme immunoassay and by Western blot of the reduced and nonreduced immunoglobulin but, surprisingly, this recognition was not inhibited by the native antibody (Cazaubon et al., 1988). By stepwise denaturation of the antibody by SDS, it appeared as if the accessibility of the peptide in the protein for the antipeptide antibodies correlated with the disappearance of the hapten-binding capacity. These results suggest that the CDR3 region of the heavy chain of 37A4 is part of a region of the antibody-combining site which is exquisitely sensitive to environmental changes, such as adsorption of the native antibody to plastic or denaturation at low SDS concentrations. These properties are compatible with conformational changes induced by the hapten. Studies by nuclear magnetic resonance of the structure of the HV3 peptide in different solvents and in the presence or absence of the hapten suggests that the conformation of the peptide is altered by the presence of alprenolol (E. Lebrun et al., in press).

As in the case of the antimorphine antibodies, the anti-idiotypic response against polyclonal or monoclonal antialprenolol antibodies yielded antibodies able to recognize the receptor but with different functional properties. Polyclonal or monoclonal anti-idiotypic antibodies activated the receptor in the same way as did agonists (Guillet et al., 1985; Schreiber et al., 1980) or inhibited agonist activation as did antagonists (Homcy et al., 1982). Although a radioimmunoassay for the β-adrenergic agonist salbutamol has been described (Loo et al., 1987), the antisalbutamol antibodies have not been characterized for their similarity to the receptor or for the properties of their anti-idiotypic antibodies.

ANTINEUROLEPTIC DRUG ANTIBODIES

Neuroleptic drugs are widely used in the treatment of psychoses. Neuroleptics of the butyrophenone and diphenylbutamine series (Fig. 5) have been used for many years before a sensitive radioimmunoassay made it possible to measure therapeutic plasma levels of these drugs in man (Michiels et al., 1975). The identification of the target of these series of drugs as a dopaminergic receptor led to a new interest in antibutyrophenone antibodies as proteins mimicking the dopamine D2 receptor-binding site or as antigens to induce anti-idiotypic antibodies able to recognize this receptor.

The first butyrophenone derivative used to induce such antibodies was spiroperidol (Schreiber et al., 1983). The antispiroperidol antibodies not only showed a high affinity for the hapten spiroperidol but also for other neuroleptic drugs of the same series and even, though very weakly, for the structurally unrelated neuroleptics of the phenothiazine series. A more complete study was undertaken to analyze the dopamine D2 receptorlike properties of antispiroperidol antibodies induced using a different method of haptenization (Luedtke et al., 1988). In rabbits it was shown that spiroperidol induced subpopulations of defined antibodies with higher affinity for the unrelated dopamine D2 antagonists iodobenzamide and domperidone (Fig. 5) than for the hapten spiroperidol. In mice no such "heteroclitic" antibodies could be shown to be induced for iodobenzamide, although antibodies heteroclitic for domperidone were obtained. Out of 36 hybridomas, no monoclonal antibody was found that could bind iodobenzamide or domperidone better than spiroperidol. Only two monoclonal antibodies showed a low affinity for these structurally unrelated dopamine-2 antagonists (Luedtke et al., 1990). Studies of the primary structure of the monoclonal antispiroperidol antibodies may shed light on the structural requirements for the recognition of the different dopamine D2 antagonists and enable a three-dimensional prediction of the antibody-combining sites.

This has been done for monoclonal antibodies directed against the neuroleptic haloperidol. Out of 13 fusions, 17 hybridomas secreted antihaloperidol antibodies (Bolger et al., 1985) of which 5 were selected for a detailed study of their binding specificities. Two of the antibodies showed a higher affinity for the folded conformation of the hapten while three others recognized the extended form. This is the energetically most favored conformation of the molecule and is probably the conformation recognized by the dopamine D2 receptor. Although the three monoclonal antibodies recognizing the ex-

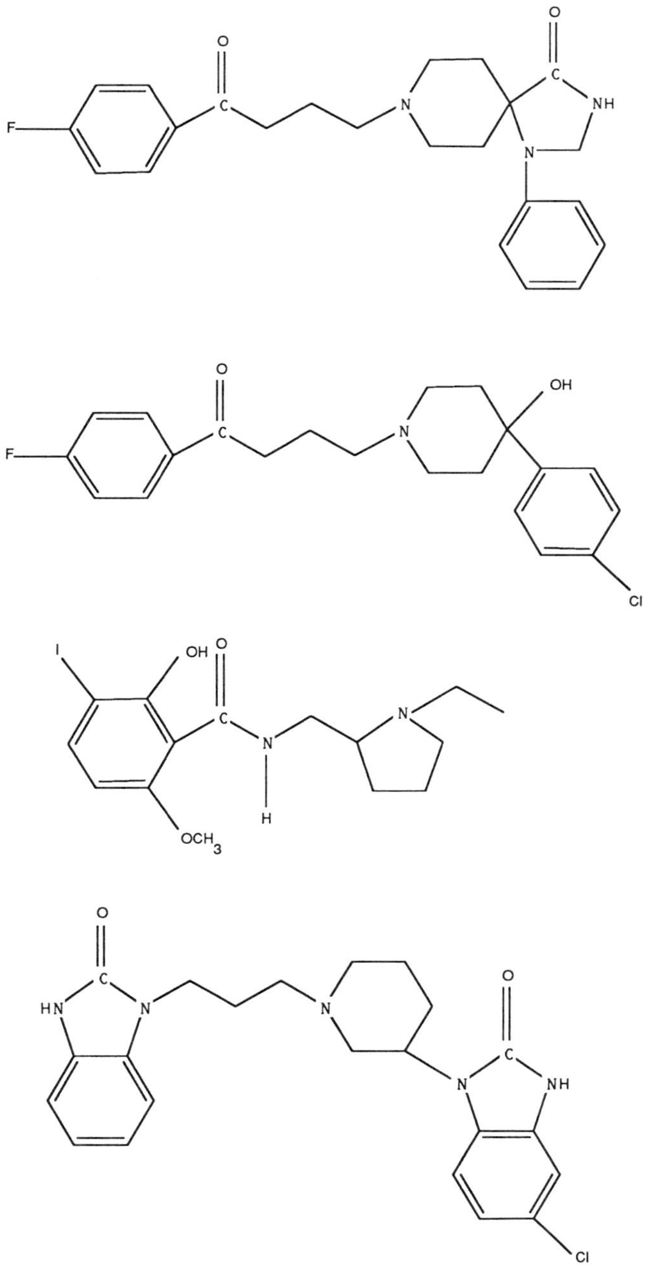

A

B

C

D

Figure 5. Structural formulas of the neuroleptic drugs: spiroperidol (A), haloperidol (B), iodobenzamide (C), and domperidone (D).

tended form of haloperidol also showed a low affinity for the dopaminergic agonist, dopamine, no correlation could be found in relative affinities of different haloperidol analogs for these antibodies and the receptor. This correlation could be found for the monoclonal antibodies recognizing the folded form, for the rigidly extended analog which shows the highest affinity for the dopamine D2 receptor. At least in the case of these antihaloperidol antibodies, no good candidate could be selected for raising anti-iodiotypic antibodies mimicking the receptor ligand (Sherman et al., 1986). Anti-idiotypic antihaloperidol antibodies inhibiting haloperidol binding to striatal membranes and immunoprecipitating spiperone-binding sites from solubilized membranes were, however, described by another group (Elazar et al., 1988). More investigations are needed to further characterize these anti-idiotypic antibodies.

The conclusions drawn from the pharmacological profiles of the five monoclonal antibodies described previously (Bolger et al., 1985) were further confirmed by prediction of the three-dimensional structure of the antibody-combining sites using the primary structures of the variable parts of the light and heavy chains, deduced from the sequence of the immunoglobulin mRNA (Sherman et al., 1988) and using the X-ray coordinates of the Fv regions of the antiphosphorylcholine myeloma protein McPC603, which shares the same framework with the five monoclonal antihaloperidol antibodies. Interestingly, the heavy chains of four of the five monoclonal antihaloperidol antibodies belonged to the J558 family, the same one highly expressed among antialprenolol antibodies (Nahmias et al., 1989). The two monoclonal antibodies recognizing the folded conformation of the hapten and for which a pocketlike-combining site was postulated display this conformation due to the deletion patterns in the hypervariable loops. The three monoclonal antibodies recognizing the extended conformation of the hapten showed a groovelike channel upon modelization of the Fv domains (Sherman and Bolger, 1988). Crystallization of the antibody-haloperidol complex will assess the validity of the predictions.

ANTIBENZODIAZEPINE ANTIBODIES

Benzodiazepines are the most widely prescribed psychoactive drugs in current therapeutic use. The pharmacological effects of benzodiazepines seem to be mediated through the γ-aminobutyric acid (GABA) receptor by increasing the duration of the Cl^- channel opening induced by GABA (Study and Barker, 1981). As for morphine, antibenzodiazepine antibodies could thus be used for the discovery of endogenous ligands with the same activity as the anxiolytic drugs.

The first radioimmunoassay for benzodiazepines was developed for the active component of Valium, diazepam (Fig. 6) (Peskar and Spector, 1973). Using 3-hemisuccinyloxy-clonazepam as hapten (Early et al., 1979), four monoclonal antibodies were obtained recognizing the agonist analogs of benzodiazepine but not the inverse agonists (β-carbolines) or the antagonists.

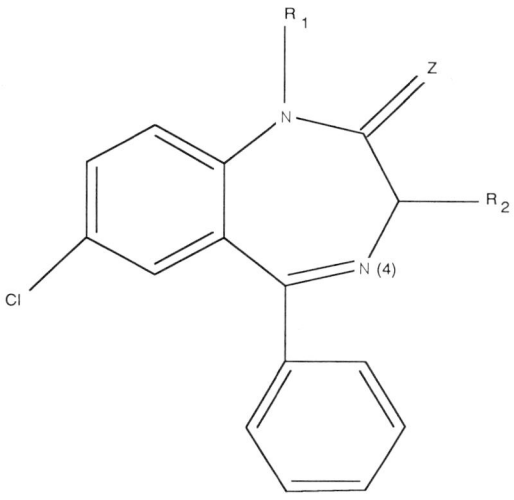

Figure 6. Structural formula of 1,4-benzodiazepines. Desmethyldiazepam is the "endogenous" benzodiazepine.

The pharmacological profile of these monoclonal antibodies shared more binding properties with the peripheral- than with the neuronal-type benzodiazepine receptors (DeBlas et al., 1985). These antibodies were used to purify benzodiazepine-like compounds from brain tissue. Immunoreactivity could be shown to be associated with macromolecules by immunocytochemistry and immunoblots. Benzodiazepine-like substances could also be purified as low-molecular weight compounds inhibiting binding of tritiated flunitrazepam to GABA receptors (Sangameswaran and deBlas, 1985). A similar approach led to the identification of the benzodiazepam-like substance as N-desmethyldiazepam. A major question, which until now has not been answered, concerns the biosynthesis of this "unnatural" compound. Although it was stated that immunoreactivity could be found in brain samples dating from 1940, before benzodiazepines were synthesized, N-desmethyldiazepam, a common metabolite of the benzodiazepine drugs, diazepam, chlordizepoxide, clorazepate, and prazepam could be of environmental origin. An alternative suggestion is that the benzodiazepine-like substances may be synthesized by microorganisms or plants and occur in the diet (Sangameswaran et al., 1986).

In analogy with antimorphine antibodies, which do not recognize the enkephalins, the antibenzodiazepine antibodies seem to mimic a binding site different from that for the endozepines, the neural peptides acting on the GABA receptor by shortening the opening of the Cl^- ion channel (Costa and Guidotti, 1985). Endozepines thus act as β-carbolines, inverse agonists which are not recognized by the antibenzodiazepine antibodies described so far (De Blas et al., 1985; Fry et al., 1987; Lange et al., 1987). The complex nature of the GABA receptor strengthens the hypothesis that it contains multiple binding sites whose occupancy can lead to different functional responses (Schofield et al., 1987). Antibodies raised against drugs with different activities on the receptor would only mimic their particular binding site on the receptor.

ANTICLONIDINE ANTIBODIES

An immunological approach has been used to test a specific pharmacological hypothesis to explain the hypotensive effect of imidazoline-type drugs. Based on binding studies with tritiated clonidine, the hypothesis was advanced that this hypotensive drug did not mediate its effect through the α-adrenoreceptors but through a specific imidazoline receptor (Bousquet et al., 1984). The existence of a putative ligand for the imidazoline receptor was proposed on the basis of the existence of a "clonidine-displacing substance" in brain extracts (Atlas and Burstein, 1984). Using polyclonal antibodies against clonidine, it could be shown that these extracts inhibited binding of tritiated p-aminoclonidine to anticlonidine antibodies (Dontenwill et al., 1987). Analysis of the fine specificity of the anticlonidine antibodies suggested the necessity for the "clonidine-displacing substance" to have at least an imidazolidine backbone (Dontenwill et al., 1988). Since the anticlonidine antibodies could be used to identify the "endogenous ligand" and to approach the "imidazoline receptor" by the anti-idiotypic pathway, a follow-up of the described results could be the first example of antibodies used to identify a new "neurotransmitter" ligand as well as a new "receptor". The substance has been isolated and displays the expected properties (Parini et al., 1989).

ANTITRICYCLIC ANTIDEPRESSANT ANTIBODIES

Tricyclic antidepressants are widely used in the treatment of depression. The difficulties inherent in the use of this class of drugs are the great variability of their metabolism among patients and the danger of cardiac and neurological toxicity by overdoses (Hollister, 1979). Rapid determination of plasma levels of these drugs was therefore essential and for this purpose rapid radioimmunoassays were established (Aherne et al., 1976). The tricyclic antidepressants, from a pharmacological point of view, are interesting molecules since they seem to interact with neurotransmitter receptors as different as the histamine H_1 and histamine H_2 receptors, α-adrenergic receptors, muscarinic acetylcholine receptor, opiate receptor, and its own specific binding sites in the brain. In order to verify whether antibodies against tricyclic antidepressants could mimic one of the binding sites of these pluripotent molecules, a monoclonal antibody against nortriptyline was evaluated for the fine specificity of its recognition characteristics. The antibody was able to discriminate between the Z and E conformation of doxepin which exists in two geometric isomeric forms due to the asymmetric presence of an oxygen atom in the central ring (Fig. 7) (Marullo et al., 1985). Since the Z isomer of doxepin displays antidepressant properties while the E isomer is responsible for its toxicity, and since the monoclonal antibody has a higher affinity for the E isomer, the binding properties of different analogs for the antibody-combining site and for the respective receptor targets of antidepressant drugs were compared. A remarkable correlation ($p < 0.005$) was found between binding of antidepressant drugs on the antibody and on the muscarinic acetylcholine receptor suggesting that the cardiotoxicity of this class of drugs could be due to interaction with the cardiac muscarinic receptor. Surprisingly, the tricyclic acetylcholine muscarinic receptor antagonist, pirenzepine, although it shares many structural features with the tricyclic antidepressants (Fig. 7), was not recognized by the antibody (Marullo et al., 1987). Competition binding experiments on the brain muscarinic acetylcholine receptor confirmed that the tricyclic antidepressants interacted noncompetitively with the receptor suggesting that they have a binding site on the receptor different from that of the acetylcholine-binding site (Marullo et al., 1987). Interestingly, although polyclonal antibodies against the tricyclic antidepressant imipramine (Fig. 7) seemed to have binding properties similar to the antidepressant site on the 5-hydroxytryptamine carrier in brain and platelets (O'Callaghan et al., 1987), the monoclonal antibody which was raised against the same molecule shared the properties of the antinortriptyline antibody described above, i.e., it mimics the antidepressant binding site on the muscarinic acetylcholine receptor (Ronayne et al., 1990). Unfortunately, the existence of monoclonal antibodies against muscarinic acetylcholine antagonists (Gainer and Nathanson, 1986) and especially against pirenzepine (Tanswell et al., 1986) has not yet been used to further probe the ligand-binding site of the acetylcholine receptor.

Analysis of the fine specificities of antibodies against another antidepressant drug, the tetracyclic compound oxaprotiline (Fig. 7), may help to understand the selection mechanisms underlying the heteroclitic response against enantiomeric haptens. When the racemic mixture of oxaprotiline was used as hapten, it appeared that, despite the heterogeneity of the immune response, the affinity for the (−)-enantiomer was always higher than for the (+)-enantiomer, showed a much higher affinity for the optically inactive oxaprotiline analog, maprotiline (Fig. 7). Using other oxaprotiline analogs, it

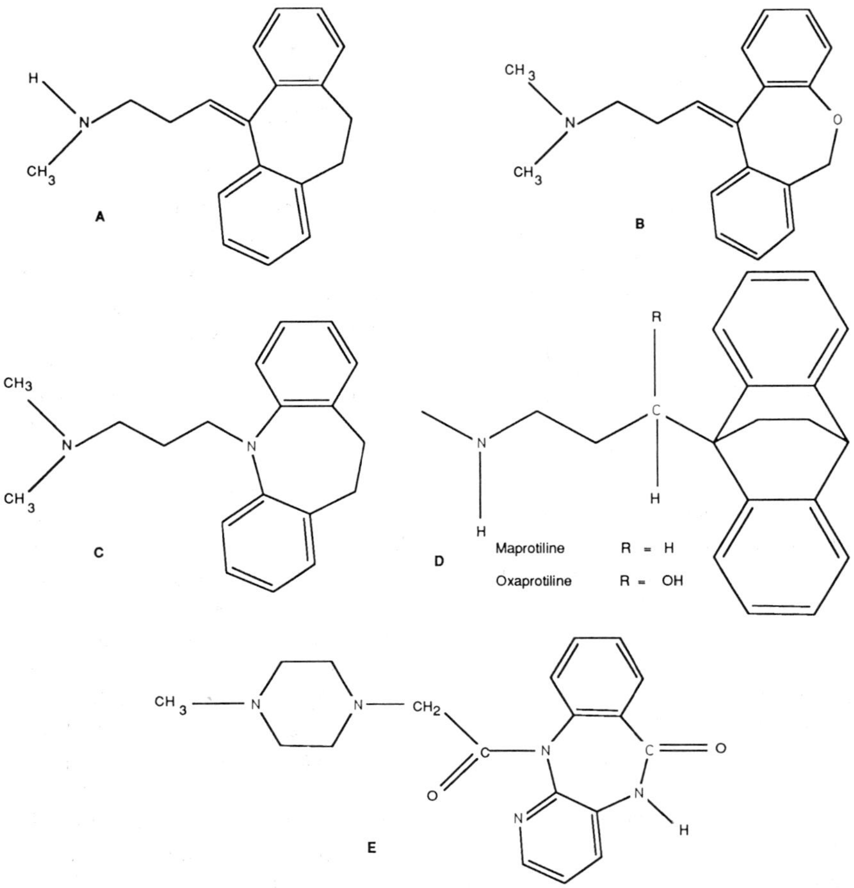

Figure 7. Structural formulas of antidepressants. Nortriptyline (A) and imipramine (C) have been used as haptens. Doxepin (B) has two *cis-trans* isomers, the *cis* isomer, which is therapeutically active and the *trans* isomer which is toxic. Oxaprotiline (D) has two stereoisomers, the (−) isomer which is therapeutically active and the (+) isomer which has a higher affinity for the monoclonal antibody. Pirenzepine (E) is a acetylcholine muscarinic antagonist with a tricyclic structure similar to that of the tricyclic antidepressants but which is not recognized by the monoclonal antibody.

could be shown that the preferential recognition of the (−)-enantiomer and maprotiline could be explained by the existence of a continuous hydrophobic surface on the (−)-enantiomer which was disrupted by the localization of the hydroxyl group in the (+)-enantiomer. This suggests that a continuous hydrophobic surface interacting with the antibody-combining site is more favorable than a discontinuous hydrophilic-hydrophobic surface (Chouchane et al., 1988).

ANTIHISTAMINIC ANTAGONIST ANTIBODIES

Although much effort has gone into developing radioimmunoassays or enzyme immunoassays for the quantitation of histamine, surprisingly little work has been done on the immunochemistry of antihistaminic drugs. The description of three classes of histamine receptors (Arrang et al., 1983; Ganellin and Persons, 1982), each possessing its own specific antagonists, has at least prompted one group to take an immunological approach to study the histamine H_1 receptor (Chatenoud et al., 1988). The most remarkable property of the polyclonal and monoclonal antibodies raised against the antagonist SK&F94461 was the high stereospecificity of recognition of the H_1 receptor antagonist chlorpheniramine, although the immunizing hapten lacked an asymmetrical carbon atom (Fig. 8). The d-enantiomer, which is the pharmacologically active enantiomer had at least 1000-fold higher affinity for the antibody than the ℓ-enantiomer. Surprisingly, when the antagonist brompheniramine was used, in which the Cl atom of chlorpheniramine has been replaced by a Br atom, only low-affinity binding could be observed. These results could be interpreted as suggesting that the antibody site interacting with the pyridinyl group of hapten and analogs is very shallow and does not allow binding of the bulkier chlorophenyl ring. Thus for d-chlorpheniramine both rings bind whereas for the ℓ-form only one ring binds and the other is held away from the binding site. The increase in size of the bromophenyl group in brompheniramine hinders the recognition of this ring and thus decreases its affinity to that of the ℓ-form of chlorpheniramine. Since the pharmacologically active form is recognized, it is tempting to speculate that the ligand-binding pocket on the H_1 receptor shares the same binding restrictions as those of the antibody. The induction of enantiomeric-sensitive antibodies by a hapten lacking an asymmetrical carbon atom is a unique example of the chiral character of biological molecules.

ANTIDIHYDROPYRIDINE CALCIUM CHANNEL BLOCKERS ANTIBODIES

The successful use of Ca^{2+} channel blockers and especially of the 1,4-dihydropyridine series in cardiovascular disease has focused attention on the voltage-dependent Ca^{2+} channels of cardiac, smooth, and skeletal muscles (Fleckenstein, 1983). Antibodies against 1,4-dihydropyridines were raised as models for the binding site of this group of drugs to the Ca^{2+} channel and as reagents to induce anti-idiotypic antibodies able to recognize this target. Two different methods of haptenizing the Ca^{2+} channel blockers were used: the nitro group of nifedipine (Fig. 9) was modified into an isothiocyanate reactive group (Campbell et al., 1986) and the ethylester of nitrendipine (Fig. 9) was modified to a n-butylaminoester (Thayer et al., 1986). This second choice yielded antibodies which were very selective for analogs in which the

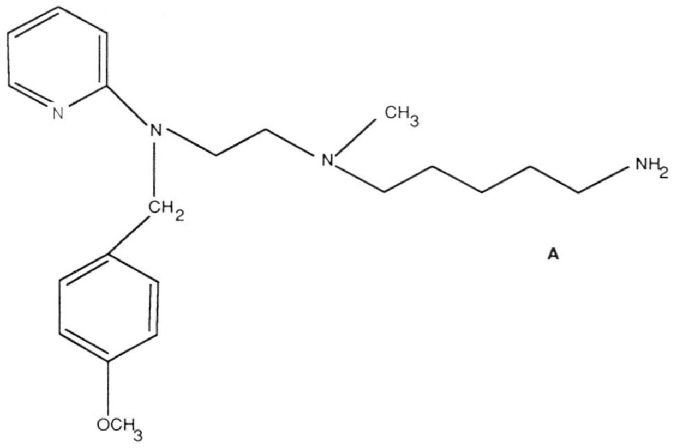

Figure 8. Structural formulas of histaminic H_1 receptor antagonists. SK&F94461 (A) was used for haptenization. Although the hapten does not contain an asymmetric carbon atom, the antibodies raised against it all showed a high stereospecificity towards the active d-enantiomer of chlorpheniramine (B).

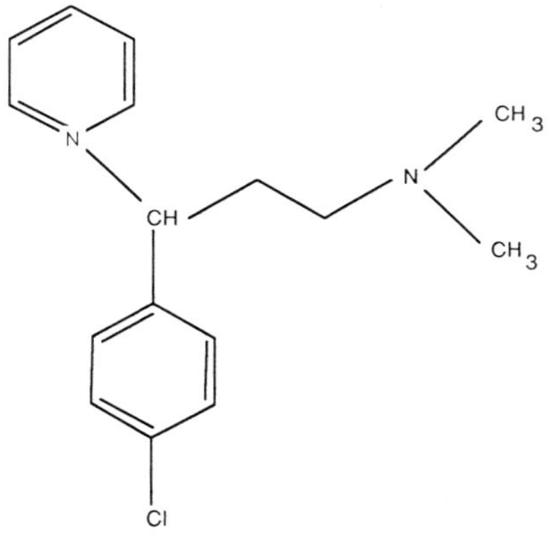

aryl group was modified compared to the properties of the antibodies raised by the isothiocyanated hapten which did not discriminate between aryl-substituted analogs. The latter antibodies had pharmacological profiles which better mimicked the binding site of 1,4-dihydropyridines on the Ca^{2+} channel. This is not surprising since it has been shown that bulky aryl substitutions are essential for receptor recognition while the ester group orientation and hydrophobic fit may control the availability of channel open and closed states (Langs and Triggle, 1985). As could be expected, the allosteric structurally unrelated Ca^{2+} channel antagonists diltiazem and verapamil were not recognized by the antinifedipine antibodies. Affinity-purified anti-1,4-dihydropyridine antibodies, recognizing hapten-protein conjugates able to bind to the

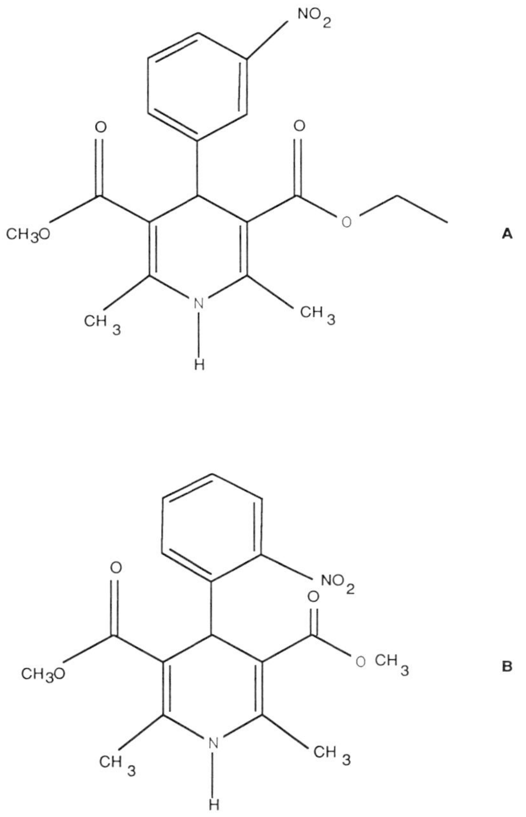

Figure 9. Structural formulas of the dihydropyridine Ca^{2+} channel blockers nitrendipine(A) and nifedipine (B). Nitrendipine was haptenized by prolongation to a butylamine of the ethylester group and nifedipine by modification of the nitro group to an isothiocyanate.

Ca^{2+} channel, could be useful in the identification of putative endogenous Ca^{2+} channel ligands, in the localization and determination of the receptor protein(s), and the production of anti-idiotypic antibodies against the same receptor (Sharp and Campbell, 1987).

ANTICYCLOSPORIN ANTIBODIES

Cyclosporin is a drug with powerful immunosuppressive properties commonly used to prevent graft rejection (Borel, 1986) whose target seems to be proline isomerase (Takahashi et al., 1989). As a neutral, hydrophobic cyclic undecapeptide, with a rigid structure as determined by X-ray crystallography

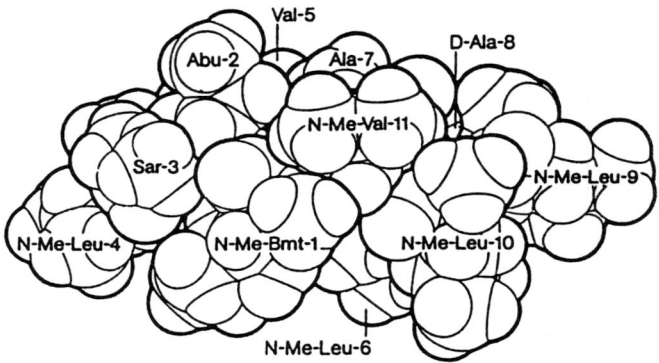

Figure 10. Structure of cyclosporin B according to X-ray crystallographic analysis and identification of the 11 amino acid residues. N-Me-Bmt, N-methyl-(4R)-4[(E)-2-butenyl]-4-methyl-L-threonine; Abu, L-α-aminobutyric acid; Sar, sarcosine. [According to Quesniaux, V. et al. (1987) *Mol. Immunol.* 24:1159—1168. With permission.]

and two-dimensional nuclear magnetic resonance (Fig. 10), it is an excellent model to study antigen-antibody interactions especially because hundreds of synthetic and natural cyclosporin analogs are available. The free peptide is only poorly immunogenic giving rise to low-affinity IgM antibodies while classical haptenization methods using carbodiimide induced the formation of anticarbodiimide antibodies more than anticyclosporin antibodies (Quesniaux et al., 1985). Using cyclosporin analogs modified at the 2 position (threonine instead of L-α-aminobutyric acid) or the 8 position (D-lysine instead of D-alanine), peptide-carrier conjugates could be produced which induced a specific anticyclosporin response (Quesniaux et al., 1987). As could be expected, the antisera raised against the Thr^2 analog were unable to recognize this residue but showed a high specificity toward the residues at positions 6 and 8, localized at the opposite part of the molecule, and a lesser affinity for the neighboring residues 1 and 3. The antisera raised against the D-Lys^8 analog was highly sensitive to residues 3 and 4, localized at the opposite side, and was less sensitive to their neighboring amino acids 1,2 and 5,6 (Quesniaux et al., 1990). Analysis of the fine specificity of the monoclonal antibodies obtained from mice immunized with the two different immunogens showed similar recognition profiles. With one exception, all monoclonal antibodies directed against the Thr^2 analog were highly sensitive to modifications at position 6, 8, and 9 and were less sensitive to modifications at position 1. Monoclonal antibodies against the D-Lys^8 analog were mostly specific for the sequence 1 to 6 and, in contrast with the monoclonal antibodies against the Thr^2 analog, were able to recognize the linear cyclosporin (Quesniaux et al., 1987). These results confirm in a quantitative way two empirical observations concerning antibodies against haptens: (1) the position of the residue coupled to the carrier protein will determine the specificity of hapten recognition and (2) the polyclonal antibody response is a good predictor of the specificity of the monoclonal antibodies. Furthermore, the monoclonal antibodies all showed high sensitivity to a maximum of four or five amino acid modifications. This number corresponds to the optimal size of the antibody-combining site (Kabat, 1966). The recent crystallization of a cyclosporin-Fab fragment complex will allow the analysis of the three-dimensional structure of one of the monoclonal antibodies described above (Altschuh et al., 1989). Correlation between the primary sequence of the heavy and light chains of seven monoclonal antibodies against cyclosporin with different specificities showed that the hypervariable regions of the heavy chain, in particular, determined the antigen specificity of the antibodies. A remarkable correlation was found between the extent of the HV_3 region and the size of the surface recognized on the cyclosporin molecule (Schmitter et al., 1990).

SUMMARY AND PERSPECTIVES

Table 2 summarizes our present knowledge of antidrug antibodies as models for pharmacological receptors. A first use of antidrug antibodies is the characterization of endogenous ligands and the production of antibody ligands by the anti-idiotypic route. In contrast with the successful determination of the structure of endogenous ligands which were purified by antidrug antibodies (digitoxin-like lignans, endogenous morphines, endogenous benzodiazepines), the anti-idiotypic approach has only rarely resulted in the structural characterization of the receptors. A recent report describes, however, the actual isolation and purification of a nicotinic receptor from rat brain using a monoclonal anti-idiotype raised against a monoclonal antibody specific for L-nicotine (Abood et al., 1987). One of the possible reasons could be that only a few monoclonal anti-idiotypic antibodies have been characterized and that several of them are of the IgM isotype; such antibodies because of their low affinity and their instability, are difficult to use as homogeneous reagents. Moreover, little effort has been invested in the detailed characterization of the interactions between idiotype and anti-idiotype. The recent development of the use of anti-idiotypic sequences to synthesize peptides which bind to the receptor (Pain et al., 1990; Vaux et al., 1990; Williams et al., 1989) will hopefully encourage structural studies on the idiotype-anti-idiotype interactions. One of the problems of the anti-idiotypic approach could be the existence of metatypes, i.e., conformations which are present on the antibody only in its liganded state (Voss et al., 1988). The kinetic results obtained with the antiaprenolol antibodies, indeed, suggest that the antibody-combining site could undergo conformational changes upon binding of haptens which do not have the optimal size corresponding to that predicted by Kabat (1966).

The three-dimensional structure of the complex drug-anti-drug Fab fragment could shed light on the atomic interactions between drug and antibody and, by extension, between drug and receptor. Although two complexes have been crystallized, no high-resolution analysis of the diffraction pattern has yet been published. It is remarkable that the two crystallized complexes are those of the voluminous drugs digitoxin and cyclosporin. Here again, the unfavorable free-energy state of complexes with drugs which do not occupy the optimal antibody-combining site could be a reason for the difficulty in crystallizing these complexes. Nuclear magnetic resonance measurements and modelization of antibody-combining sites, starting from the primary sequences of the variable domains of the light and heavy chains and using the canonical structures for the hypervariable regions (Chothia et al., 1989), could help in by-passing this bottleneck.

ACKNOWLEDGMENTS

Support for our work comes mostly from grants from the Centre National de la Recherche Scientifique, the INSERM, the Ministère de la recherche et de la Technologie, the Université Paris VII, the Ligue Nationale contre le Cancer, the Foundation pour le Recherche Médicale Française, the Association pour la Recherche sur le Cancer and by the Swedish Medical Research Foundation, the Swedish Life Insurance Company, the Swedish Association against Heart and Lung Diseases.

REFERENCES

Abood, L. G., Langone, J. J., Bjercke, R., Lu, X. and Banergee, S. (1987) Characterization of a purified nicotinic receptor from rat brain by using idiotypic and anti-idiotypic antibodies. *Proc. Natl. Acad. Sci. U.S.A.* 84:6587—6590.

Affolter, H., Hertel, C., Jaeggi, K., Portenier, M., and Staehelin, M. (1985) (−)-S-[^{3}H]CGP-12177 and its use to determine the rate constants of unlabeled β-adrenergic antagonists. *Proc. Natl. Acad. Sci. U.S.A.* 82:925—929.

Aherne, G. W., Piall, E. M., and Mark, D. (1976) The radioimmunoassay of tricyclic antidepressants. *Br. J. Clin. Pharmacol.* 3:561—565.

Altschuh, D., Kocher, H. P., Quesniaux, V. J. F., Schmitter, D., Van Regenmortel, M. H. V., and Thierry, J. C. (1989) Crystallization and preliminary X-ray investigation of a complex between a Fab fragment and its antigen: cyclosporine. *J. Mol. Biol.* 209:177—178.

Amzel, L. M., Poljak, R. J., Saul, F., Varga, J. M., and Richards, F. F. (1974) The three-dimensional structure of a combining site-ligand complex of immunoglobulin NEW at 3.5 Å resolution. *Proc. Natl. Acad. Sci. U.S.A.* 71:1427—1430.

Arrang, J. M., Garbarg, M., and Schwartz, J. C. (1983) Auto-inhibition of brain histamine release mediated by a novel class H_3 of histamine receptors. *Nature (London)* 302:832—837.

Atlas, D., and Burstein, Y. (1984) Isolation of an endogenous clonidine displacing substance from the rat brain. *FEBS Lett.* 170:387—390.

Blume, A. J., Shorr, J., Finberg, J. P. M., and Spector, S. (1977) Binding of the endogenous non-peptide morphine-like compound to opiate receptors. *Proc. Natl. Acad. Sci. U.S.A.* 74:4927—4931.

Bolger, M. B., Flurkey, K., Simmons, R. D., Linthicum, S. D., Laduron, P., and Michiels, M. (1985) Preparation and characterization of antisera and monoclonal antibodies to haloperidol. *Immunol. Invest.* 14:523—540.

Borel, J. F. (1986) Cyclosporin. *Prog. Allergy* 38.

Bousquet, P., Feldman, J., and Schwartz, J. (1984) Central cardiovascular effects of alpha-adrenergic drugs: differences between catecholamines and imidazolines. *J. Pharmacol. Exp. Ther.* 230:232—236.

Campbell, K. P., Sharp, A., Strom, M., and Kahl, S. D. (1986) High-affinity antibodies to the 1,4-dihydropyridine Ca^{2+} channel blockers. *Proc. Natl. Acad. Sci. U.S.A.* 83:2792—2796.

Cazaubon, S., Couraud, P. O., Hoebeke, J., Nahmias, C., Emorine, L., Gras-Masse, H., and Strosberg, A. D. (1988) Anti-HV3 peptide antibodies as probes for comformational changes in immunoglobulins. *J. Immunol. Meth.* 114:13—20.

Chamat, S., Hoebeke, J., Emorine, L., Guillet, J. G., and Strosberg, A. D. (1986) The immune response towards β-adrenergic ligands and their receptors. VI. idiotypy of monoclonal anti-alprenolol antibodies. *J. Immunol.* 136:3805—3811.

Chamat, S., Hoebeke, J., and Strosberg, A. D. (1984) Monoclonal antibodies specific for β-adrenergic ligands. *J. Immunol.* 133:1547—1552.

Chatenoud, L., Villemain, F., Hoebeke, J., Garbarg, M., Korner, M., Gros, C., Ruat, M., Cazenave, P. A., Ganellin, R. C., Bach, J. F., and Schwartz, J. C. (1988) Polyclonal and monoclonal antibodies directed against SK&F 94461, a specific H_1 histamine receptor ligand. *Mol. Pharmacol.* 34:136—144.

Chothia, C., Lesk, A. M., Tramontano, A., Smith-Gill, S. J., Air, G., Sheriff, S., Padlan, E. A., Davies, D., Tulip, W. R., Coleman, P. M., Spinelli, S., Alzari, P. M., and Poljak, R. J. (1989) Conformations of immunoglobulin hypervariable regions. *Nature (London)* 342:877—883.

Chouchane, L., Strosberg, A. D., and Hoebeke, J. (1988) Stereospecific immunorecognition of the tetracyclic anti-depressant oxaprotiline. *Mol. Immunol.* 25:1299—1308.

Collignon, A., Geniteau-Legendre, M., Sandre, C., Quero, A. M., and Labarre, C. (1988) Specific binding characteristics of high-affinity monoclonal anti-digitoxin antibodies. *Hybridoma* 7:355—366.

Contreras, M. L., Wolfe, B. B., and Molinoff, P. B. (1986) Kinetic analysis of the interactions of agonists and antagonists with β-adrenergic receptors. *J. Pharmacol. Exp. Ther.* 239:136—143.

Cook, C. E., and Drayer, D. E. (1988) Antibodies: a rich source of novel chemical agents for pharmacological studies. *Trends Pharmacol. Sci.* 9:373—375.

Costa, E., and Guidotti, A. (1985) Endogenous ligands for benzodiazepine recognition sites. *Biochem. Pharmacol.* 34:3399—3403.

De Blas, A. L., Sangameswaran, L., Haney, S. A., Park, D., Abraham, C. J. and Rayner, C. A. (1985) Monoclonal antibodies to benzodiazepines. *J. Neurochem.* 45:1748—1753.

Deguchi, T., and Yokoyama, E. (1985) Monoclonal antibody to enkephalins with binding characteristics similar to opiate receptor. *Biochem. Biophys. Res. Commun.* 126:389—396.

Dontenwill, M., Bricca, G., Molines, A., Belcourt, A., and Bousquet, P. (1987) A polyclonal antibody raised against clonidine: a model for the specific imidazoline receptor. *Eur. J. Pharmacol.* 137:143—144.

Dontenwill, M., Bricca, G., Molines, A., Bousquet, P., and Belcourt, A. (1988) Production and characterization of anti-clonidine antibodies not cross-reacting with catecholamines. *Eur. J. Pharmacol.* 149:249—255.

Early, J. V., Fryer, R. I. and Ning, R. Y. (1979) Quinazolines and 1,4-benzodiazepines. LXXXIX: haptens useful in benzodiazepine immunoassay development. *J. Pharm. Sci.* 68:845—850.

Erlich, P. (1900) On immunity with special reference to cell life. *Proc. R. Soc. London* 66:424.

Elazar, Z., Kanety, H., Schreiber, M., and Fuchs, S. (1988) Anti-idiotypes against a monoclonal anti-haloperidol antibody bind to dopamine receptor. *Life Sci.* 42:1987—1993.

Fagoo, M., Braquet, P., Robin, J. P., Eranne, A., and Godfraind, T. (1986) Evidence that mammalian lignans show endogenous digitalis-like activities. *Biochem. Biophys. Res. Commun.* 134:1064—1070.

Fleckenstein, A. (1983) Discovery and mechanism of action of specific calcium-antagonist inhibitors of excitation-contraction coupling in the mammalian myocardium, In *Calcium Antagonism in Heart and Smooth Muscle.* John Wiley & Sons, 34—108.

Fry, J. P., Rickets, C., and Martin, I. L. (1987) Polyclonal antibodies to agonist benzodiazepines. *Biochem. Pharmacol.* 36:3763—3770.

Gainer, M. W., and Nathanson, N. M. (1986) Recognition of muscarinic acetylcholine receptor ligands by monoclonal antibodies against propylbenzilylcholine mustard. *Biochem. Pharmacol.* 35:1209—1212.

Ganellin, C. R., and Persons, M. E., eds. (1982) *Pharmacology of Histamine Receptors.* John Wright, Bristol, United Kingdom.

Gintzler, A. R., Gershon, M. D., and Spector, S. (1978) A non-peptide morphine-like compound: immunocytochemical localization in the mouse brain. *Science* 199:447—448.

Gintzler, A. R., Levy, A., and Spector, S. (1976) Antibodies as a means of characterizing biologically active substances: presence of a non-peptide morphine-like compound in the central nervous system. *Proc. Natl. Acad. Sci. U.S.A.* 73:2132—2136.

Glasel, J. A. (1989) Nuclear magnetic resonance studies of flexible opiate conformations at monoclonal antibody binding sites. *J. Mol. Biol.* 209:747—761.

Glasel, J. A., and Borer, P. N. (1986) NMR studies of flexible opiate conformation at monoclonal antibody combining sites. I. Transferred nuclear Overhauser effects show bound conformation. *Biochem. Biophys. Res. Commun.* 141:1267—1273.

Glasel, J. A., and Pelosi, L. N. (1986) Morphine-mimetic anti-paratypic antibodies: cross-reactive properties. *Biochem. Biophys. Res. Commun.* 136:1177—1184.

Glasel, J. A., Bradbury, W. M., and Venn, R. F. (1983) Properties of murine anti-morphine antibodies. *Mol. Immunol.* 20:1419—1422.

Go, K., Kartha, G., and Chen, J. P. (1980) Structure of digoxin. *Acta Crystallogr.* B36:1811—1815.

Goldstein, A., Barrett, R. W., James, I. F., Lowney, L. I., Weitz, C. J., Knipmeyer, L. L., and Rapoport, H. (1985) Morphine and other opiates from beef brain and adrenal. *Proc. Natl. Acad. Sci. U.S.A.* 82:5203—5207.

Gramsch, C., Schulz, R., Kosin, S., and Herz, A. (1988) Monoclonal anti-idiotypic antibodies to opioid receptors. *J. Biol. Chem.* 263:5853—5859.

Gruber, K. A., Whitaker, J. M., and Buckalew, V. M. (1980) Endogenous digitalis-like substance in plasma of volume expanded dogs. *Nature (London)* 287:743—745.

Guillet, J. G., Kaveri, S. V., Durieu, O., Delavier, C., Hoebeke, J., and Strosberg, A. D. (1985) β-adrenergic agonist activity of a monoclonal anti-idiotypic antibody. *Proc. Natl. Acad. Sci. U.S.A.* 82:1781—1784.

Haddy, F. J., and Overbeck, H. W. (1976) The role of humoral agents in volume expanded hypertension. *Life Sci.* 19:935—948.

Herz, A., Gramsch, C., Höllt, V., Meo, T. and Riethmüller, G. (1982) Characteristics of a monoclonal β-endorphin antibody recognizing the N-terminus of opioid peptides. *Life Sci.* 31:1721—1724.

Hilschman, N., and Craig, L. C. (1965) Aminoacid sequence studied with Bence-Jones proteins. *Proc. Natl. Acad. Sci. U.S.A.* 53:1403—1409.

Hoebeke, J., Vauquelin, G., and Strosberg, A. D. (1978) The production and characterisation of antibodies against β-adrenergic antagonists. *Biochem. Pharmacol.* 27:1527—1532.

Hoebeke, J., Engelborghs, Y., Chamat, S., and Strosberg, A. D. (1987) The immune response towards β-adrenergic ligands and their receptors. VII. Equilibrium and kinetic binding studies of l-alprenolol to a monoclonal anti-alprenolol antibody. *Mol. Immunol.* 24:621—629.

Hoffman, B. F., and Bigger, J. T. (1985) Digitalis and allied cardiac glycosides. In *The Pharmacological Basis of Therapeutics* (A. G. Gilman, L. S. Goodman, T. W. Rall, and F. Murad, eds.), 7th Ed, MacMillan, NY, 716—747.

Hollister, L. E. (1979) Monitoring tricyclic antidepressant plasma concentrations. *J. Am. Med. Assoc.* 241:2530—2533.

Homcy, C. J., Rockson, S. G., and Haber, E. (1982) An antidiotypic antibody that recognizes the β-adrenergic receptor. *J. Clin. Invest.* 69:1147—1154.

Huston, J. S., Levinson, D., Mudgett-Hunter, M., Tai, M. S., Novotny, J., Margolies, M. N., Ridge, R. J., Bruccoleri, R. E., Haber, E., Crea, R., and Oppermann, H. (1988) Protein engineering of antibody binding sites: recovery of specific activity in an anti-digoxin single-chain Fv analogue produced in *Escherichia coli*. *Proc. Natl. Acad. Sci. U.S.A.* 85:5879—5883.

Kabat, E. A. (1966) The nature of an antigenic determinant. *J. Immunol.* 97:1—11.

Killian, A. K., Schuster, C. R., House, J. T., Sholl, S., Connors, M., and Wainer, B. H. (1981) A non-peptide morphine-like compound from brain. *Life Sci.* 28:811—817.

Köhler, H. D., and Milstein, C. (1975) Continuous cultures of fused cells secreting antibodies of predefined specificity. *Nature (London)* 256:495—496.

Kojima, I., Yoshihara, S., and Ogata, E. (1982) Involvement of endogenous digitalis-like substance in genesis of deoxycorticosterone-salt hypertension. *Life Sci.* 30:1775—1781.

Lange, M., Abecassis, P. Y., and Hunt, P. F. (1987) Monoclonal antibodies specific for 1-4 benzodiazepines. *Biochem. Pharmacol.* 36:2037—2040.

Langone, J. J. (1989) Antibodies, antigens and molecular mimicry. *Meth. Enzymol.* 178:1.

Langley, J. N. (1906) Croonean lecture, 1906, on nerve endings and on special excitable substances in cells. *Proc. R. Soc. London* 78:170—194.

Langs, D. A., and Triggle, D. J. (1985) Conformational features of calcium channel agonist and antagonist analogs of nifedipine. *Mol. Pharmacol.* 27:544—548.

Lebrun, E., Davoust, D., Hennig, Ph., Strosberg, A. D., and Van Rapenbusch, R. (1991) Proton assignment and conformational analysis of the Hv3 peptide segment from monoclonal anti-alprenolol antibody 37A4. *Peptide and Protein Res.* (in press).

Lechat, P., Midgett-Hunter, M., Margolies, M. N., Haber, E., and Smith, T. W. (1984) Reversal of lethal digoxin toxicity in guinea-pigs using monoclonal antibodies and Fab fragments. *J. Pharmacol. Exp. Ther.* 229:210—213.

Loo, J. C. K., Beaulieu, N., Jordan, N., Brien, R., and McGilveray, I. J. (1987) A specific radio-immunoassay for salbutamol in human plasma. *Res. Commun. Chem. Pathol. Pharmacol.* 55:283—286.

Luedtke, R. R., Korner, M., Neve, K. A., and Molinoff, P. B. (1988) Monoclonal antibodies with high affinity for spiroperidol. *J. Neurochem.* 50:1253—1262.

Luedtke, R. R., Bush, M., Mach, R. H., Ehrenkaufer, R. E., Kung, H. F., and Molinoff, P. B. (1990) Antibodies with high affinity for spiroperidol. II. Cross reactivity with iodobenzamide and domperidone. *Mol. Immunol.* 27:667—677.

Marullo S., Hoebeke, J., Guillet J. G. and Strosberg A. D. (1985) Structural analysis of the epitope recognized by a monoclonal antibody against tricyclic antidepressants. *J. Immunol.* 135:471—477.

Marullo, S., Hoebeke, J., Guillet, J. G., André, C., and Strosberg, A. D. (1987) Immunological mimicry by a monoclonal antibody of the tricyclic anti-depressants' binding site on muscarinic acetylcholine receptors. *J. Immunol.* 138:524—526.

Meo, T., Gramsch, C., Inan, R., Höllt, V., Weber, E., Herz, A., and Riethmüller, G. (1983) Monoclonal antibody to the message sequence Tyr-Gly-Gly-Phe of opioid peptides exhibits the specificity requirements of mammalian opioid receptors. *Proc. Natl. Acad. Sci. U.S.A.* 80:4084—4088.

Michiels, L. J. M., Heykants, J. J. P., Knaeps, A. G., and Janssen, P. A. J. (1975) Radioimmunoassay of the neuroleptic drug pimozide. *Life Sci.* 16:937—942.

Miller, A., and Glasel, J. A. (1989) Comparative sequences and immunochemical analyses of murine monoclonal anti-morphine antibodies. *J. Mol. Biol.* 209:763—778.

Mudgett-Hunter, M., Margolies, M. N., Ju, A., and Haber, E. (1982) High-affinity monoclonal antibodies to the cardiac glycoside, digoxin. *J. Immunol.* 129:1165—1172.

Mudgett-Hunter, M., Anderson, W., Haber, E. and Margolies, M. N. (1985) Binding and structural diversity among high-affinity monoclonal anti-digoxin antibodies. *Mol. Immunol.* 22:477—488.

Myers, W. E., and Glasel, J. A. (1986) Subclass specificity of anti-idiotypic antiopiate receptor antibodies in rat brain, guinea pig cerebellum and neuroblastoma x glioma (NG108-15). *Life Sci.* 38:1783—1788.

Nahmias, C., Strosberg, A. D., and Emorine, L. J. (1988) The immune response towards β-adrenergic ligands and their receptors. VIII. Extensive diversity of V_H and V_L genes encoding anti-alprenolol antibodies. *J. Immunol.* 140:1304—1311.

Nahmias, C., Cazaubon, S., and Strosberg, A. D. (1989) A rabbit antiserum detects a V_H J558 subgroup marker highly expressed among anti-alprenolol antibodies. *J. Immunol.* 142:871—876.

Ng, D. S. S. and Isom, G. E. (1984) Binding of antimorphine anti-idiotypic antibodies to opiate receptors. *Eur. J. Pharmacol.* 102:187—190.

Ng, D. S. S., and Isom, G. E. (1985) Anti-morphine anti-idiotypic antibodies: opiate receptor binding and isolated tissue responses. *Biochem. Pharmacol.* 34:2853—2858.

Noda, M., Takahashi, H., Tanabe, T., Toyosato, M., Furutami, Y., Hirose, T., Asai, M., Inamaya, S., Miyata, T., and Numa, S. (1982) Primary structure of alpha-subunit precursor of *Torpedo californica* acetylcholine receptor deduced from cDNA sequence. *Nature (London)* 299:793—797.

Novotny, J., Bruccoleri, R. E., and Haber, E. (1990) Computer analysis of mutations that affect antibody specificity. *Prot. Struct. Funct. Genet.* 7:93—98.

O'Callaghan, A. M., Phillips, O. M., and Williams, D. C. (1987) Antisera raised against the drug imipramine. *J. Neurochem.* 49:1091—1095.

Oka, K., Kantrowitz, J. D., and Spector, S. (1985) Isolation of morphin from toad skin. *Proc. Natl. Acad. Sci. U.S.A.* 82:1852—1854.

Oliver, G. C., Brasfield, D., Parker, B. M., and Parker, C. W. (1966) A sensitive radioimmunoassay for digitalis. *J. Lab. Clin. Med.* 68:1002—1003.

Pain, D., Murakami, H., and Blobel, G. (1990) Identification of a receptor for protein import into mitochondria. *Nature (London)* 347:444—449.

Parini, A., Coupry, I., Graham, R. M., Uzielli, I., Atlas, D., and Lanier, S. M. (1989) Characterization of an imidazoline/guanidinium receptive site distinct from the alpha2-adrenergic receptor. *J. Biol. Chem.* 264 (20):11874—11878.

Panka, D. J., and Margolies, M. N. (1987) Complete variable region sequences of five homologous high affinity anti-digoxin antibodies. *J. Immunol.* 139:2385—2391.

Panka, D. J., Mudgett-Hunter, M., Parks, D. R., Peterson, L. L., Herzenberg, L. A., Haber, E., and Margolies, M. N. (1988) Variable region framework differences resulting in decreased or increased affinity of variant anti-digoxin antibodies. *Proc. Natl. Acad. Sci. U.S.A.* 85:3080—3084.

Peskar, B., and Spector, S. (1973) Quantitative determination of diazepam in blood by radioimmunoassay. *J. Pharmacol. Exp. Ther.* 186:167—172.

Pincus, S. H., Watson, W. A., Harris, S., Ewing, L. P., Stocks, C. J., and Rollins, D. E. (1984) Phenotypic and genotypic characterization of monoclonal anti-digoxin antibodies. *Life Sci.* 35:433—440.

Quesniaux, V., Himmelspach, K., and Van Regenmortel, M. H. V. (1985) An enzyme immunoassay for the screening of monoclonal antibodies to cyclosporin. *Immunol. Lett.* 9:99—104.

Quesniaux, V. F. J., Reet, T., Schreier, M. H., Wenger, R. M. and Van Regenmortel, M. H. V. (1987) Fine specificity and cross-reactivity of monoclonal antibodies to cyclosporin. *Mol. Immunol.* 24:1159—1168.

Quesniaux, V. F. J., Schmitter, D., Schreier, M. H., and Van Regenmortel, M. H. V. (1990) Monoclonal antibodies to cyclosporin are representative of the major antibody populations present in antisera of immunized mice. *Mol. Immunol.* 27:227—236.

Rockson, S. G., Homcy, C. J., and Haber, E. (1980) Anti-alprenolol antibodies in the rabbit: a new probe for the study of β-adrenergic receptor interaction. *Circ. Res.* 46:808—813.

Ronayne, L., McInerney, M., Phillips, O. M., Regan, C. M., and Williams, D. C. (1990) A monoclonal anti-imipramine antibody with antidepressant binding properties similar to the muscarinic receptor. *Biochem. Pharmacol.* 39:507—511.

Rose, D. R., Seaton, B. A., Petsko, G. A., Novotny, J., Margolies, M. N., Locke, E., and Haber, E. (1982) Crystallization of the Fab fragment of a monoclonal anti-digoxin antibody and its complex with digoxin. *J. Mol. Biol.* 165:203—206.

Sangameswaran, L., and de Blas, A. L. (1985) Demonstration of benzodiazepine-like molecules in the mammalian brain with a monoclonal antibody to benzodiazepines. *Proc. Natl. Acad. Sci. U.S.A.* 82:5560—5564.

Sangameswaran, L., Fales, H. M., Friedrich, P., and de Blas, A. L. (1986) Purification of a benzodiazepine from bovine brain and detection of benzodiazepine-like immunoreactivity in human brain. *Proc. Natl. Acad. Sci. U.S.A.* 83:9236—9240.
Sawutz, D. G., Sylvestre, D., and Homcy, C. J. (1985) Characterization of monoclonal antibodies to the β-adrenergic antagonist alprenolol as models of the receptor binding site. *J. Immunol.* 135:2713—2718.
Sawutz, D. G., Kourny, R., and Homcy, C. J. (1987) Enhanced antigen-antibody binding affinity mediated by an anti-idiotypic antibody. *Biochemistry* 26:5275—5282.
Sawada, J. I., Janejai, N., Nagamatsu, K., and Terao, T. (1988) Production and characterization of high-affinity monoclonal antibodies against morphine. *Mol. Immunol.* 25:937—943.
Schofield, P. R., Darlison, M. G., Fujita, N., Burt, D. R., Stephenson, F. A., Rodriguez, H., Rhee, L. M., Ramachandran, J., Reale, V., Glencorse, T., Seeburg, P. H., and Barnard, E. A. (1987) Sequence and functional expression of the GABA$_A$ receptor shows a ligand-gated receptor super-family. *Nature (London)* 328:221—227.
Schmitter, D., Poch, O., Zeder, G., Heinrich, G. F., Kocher, H. P., Quesniaux, V. F. J., and Van Regenmortel, M. H. V. (1990) Analysis of the structural diversity of monoclonal antibodies to cyclosporine. *Mol. Immunol.* 27:1029—1038.
Schreiber, A. B., Couraud, P. O., André, C., Vray, B., and Strosberg, A. D. (1980) Anti-alprenolol anti-idiotypic antibodies bind to β-adrenergic receptors and modulate catecholamine-sensitive adenylate cyclase. *Proc. Natl. Acad. Sci. U.S.A.* 77:7385—7389.
Schreiber, M., Fogelfeld, L., Souroujon, M. C., Kohen, F., and Fuchs, S. (1983) Antibodies to spiroperidol and their anti-idiotypes as probes for studying dopamine receptors. *Life Sci.* 33:1519—1526.
Sege, K., and Peterson, P. A. (1978) Use of anti-idiotypic antibodies as cell-surface receptor probes. *Proc. Natl. Acad. Sci. U.S.A.* 75:2443—2447.
Sharp, A. H., and Campbell, K. P. (1987) Affinity purification of antibodies specific for 1,4-dihydropyridine Ca^{2+} channel blockers. *Circ. Res.* 61:I-37—I-45.
Sherman, M. A., and Bolger, M. B. (1988) Haloperidol binding to monoclonal antibodies. Predictions of three-dimensional combining site structure via computer modeling. *J. Biol. Chem.* 263:4064—4074.
Sherman, M. A., Linthicum, D. S., and Bolger, M. B. (1986) Haloperidol binding to monoclonal antibodies: conformational analysis and relationship to D-2 receptor binding. *Mol. Pharmacol.* 29:589—598.
Sherman, M. A., Deans, R. J., and Bolger, M. B. (1988) Haloperidol binding to monoclonal antibodies. Hypervariable region aminoacid sequence determination. *J. Biol. Chem.* 263:4059—4063.
Shorr, J., Foley, K., and Spector, S. (1978) Presence of a non-peptide morphine-like compound in human cerebro-spinal fluid. *Life Sci.* 23:2057—2062.
Shulz, R., and Gramsch, C. (1985) Polyclonal anti-idiotypic opioid receptor antibodies generated by the monoclonal β-endorphin antibody 3E-7. *Biochem. Biophys. Res. Commun.* 132:658—665.
Smith, T. W., and Skubitz, K. M. (1975) Kinetics of interactions between antibodies and haptens. *Biochemistry* 14:1496—1502.
Smith, T. W., Butler, V. P., and Haber, E. (1970) Characterization of antibodies of high affinity and specificity for the digitalis glycoside digoxin. *Biochemistry* 9:331—337.

Smith, T. W., Butler, V. P., Haber, E., Fozzard, H., Marcus, F. I., Bremmer, W. P., Shulman, I. C., and Philips, A. (1982) Treatment of life-threatening digitalis intoxication with digoxin-specific Fab fragments: experience in 26 cases. *N. Engl. J. Med.* 307:1357—1362.

Spector, S. (1982) Radioimmunoassay for morphine. *Meth. Enzymol.* 84:551—554.

Spector, S., and Parker, C. W. (1970) Morphine: radioimmunoassay. *Science* 168:1347—1348.

Strader, C. D., Sigal, I. S., and Dixon, R. A. F. (1989) Structural basis of β-adrenergic receptor function. *FASEB J.* 3:1825—1832.

Study, R. E., and Barker, J. L. (1981) Diazepam and (−)-pentobarbital: fluctuations analysis reveals different mechanisms for potentiation of gamma-butyric acid responses in cultured central neurons. *Proc. Natl. Acad. Sci. U.S.A.* 78:7180—7184.

Tai, M. S., Mudgett-Hunter, M., Levinson, D., Wu, G. M., Haber, E., Oppermann, H., and Huston, J. S. (1990) A bifunctional fusion protein containing Fc-binding fragment B of Staphylococcal protein A amino terminal to antidigoxin single-chain Fv. *Biochemistry* 29:8024—8030.

Takahashi, N., Hayano, T., and Suzuki, M. (1989) Peptidyl-prolyl *cis-trans* isomerase is the cyclosporin A binding protein cyclophilin. *Nature (London)* 337:473—475.

Tanswell, P., Kasper, W., and Zahn, G. (1986) Automated monoclonal radioimmunoassay for pirenzepine, a selective muscarinic receptor antagonist, in plasma and urine. *J. Immunol. Meth.* 93:247—258.

Thayer, S. A., Pham, D. H., Schultz, C. M., Minaskanian, G., and Fairhurst, A. S. (1986) An antibody to dihydropyridine calcium entry blockers. *Biochem. Pharmacol.* 35:4479—4485.

Tiselius, A., and Kabat, E. A. (1939) Electrophoretic study of immune serum and purified antibody preparations. *J. Exp. Med.* 69:119—131.

Vaux, D., Tooze, J., and Fuller, S. (1990) Identification by anti-idiotype antibodies of an intracellular membrane protein that recognizes a mammalian endoplasmic reticulum retention signal. *Nature (London)* 345:495—502.

Voss, E. W., Miklasz, S. D., Petrossian, A., and Dombrink-Kurzman, M. A. (1988) Polyclonal antibodies specific for liganded active site (metatype) of a high affinity anti-hapten monoclonal antibody. *Mol. Immunol.* 25:751—759.

Wang, L., Chorev, M., Feingers, J., Levitzki, A., and Inbar, M. (1986) Stereospecific antibodies to propranolol. *FEBS Lett.* 199:173—178.

Williams, W. V., Weiner, D. B., Cohen, J. C., and Greene, M. I. (1989) Development and use of receptor binding peptides derived from antireceptor antibodies. *Biotechnology* 7:471—475.

Wu, T. T. E., and Kabat, E. A. (1970) An analysis of the sequences of the variable regions of Bence-Jones proteins and myeloma light chains and their implications for antibody complementarity. *J. Exp. Med.* 132:211—250.

Zimmering, P. E., Lieberman, S., and Erlanger, B. F. (1967) Binding of steroids to steroid-specific antibodies. *Biochemistry* 6:154—164.

Chapter
13
Snake Toxins as Antigens

André Ménez, Laurence Pillet, Michel Léonetti, François
Bontems, and Bernard Maillère
*Service de Biochimie des Protéines
Laboratoire d'Ingénierie des Protéines
CEN Saclay, Gif-sur-Yvette, France*

INTRODUCTION

Some snakes possess specialized exocrine glands that synthesize complex mixtures of proteins called venoms. The function of a venom is to provide snakes with a potent means for subduing their prey. It has been recognized for nearly one century that venoms affect neuromuscular function and blood coagulation (Calmette, 1907). During the last two decades various toxins responsible for these actions have been isolated, and some of them have been extensively studied (Ménez, 1989). Meanwhile, it has been shown that snake venoms are capable of several other toxic effects, including blocking of the nicotinic acetylcholine receptors from peripheral and central nervous system (Changeux, 1990; Loring and Zigmond, 1988; Vidal and Changeux, 1989), cardiotoxicity (Harvey, 1985; Ménez et al., 1990), and cardiovascular disorder (Bdolah et al., 1991; Kloog et al., 1988). Snake toxins constitute, therefore, a remarkable source of highly specific ''molecular lancets,'' which are of considerable help in identifying elements implicated in the function of various physiological processes. In this respect, curaremimetic toxins offer perhaps one of the best examples since they have proven to be an essential factor for the isolation of the nicotinic acetylcholine receptor (Changeux, 1990).

As early as 1907, Calmette developed antisera against various venoms, which proved to be of considerable help for protecting humans against snake bites. A similar approach is still being used today (Reid, 1979; Campbell,

1979). Subsequently, a number of authors examined the immunological properties of snake venoms not only with the view to improve the quality of existing antisera but also as a means to understand the antigenic relationships of snake venoms and to identify their essential toxic principles (as reviewed by Boquet, 1979). However, because of the heterogeneity of venoms these studies were difficult.

A number of pure snake toxins have been isolated and their primary and tertiary structures characterized (Ménez, 1989). These toxins are proteins of relatively small size which often comprise between 20 and 120 amino acid residues, making them readily amenable to chemical modifications (Endo and Tamiya, 1987). Their polypeptide chains tend to be highly structured (see below), with several disulfide bridges which provide snake toxins with a high stability toward denaturing conditions. Notwithstanding their small size, most snake toxins are immunogenic in several types of hosts. For all these reasons snake toxins appeared to be excellent models to investigate the immunological properties of a toxic protein, at a molecular level. Moreover, understanding of these properties should be of value in improving the quality of treatments against these clinically important toxins (Warrell, 1986).

The specificity and cross-reactivity of both polyclonal and monoclonal antibodies raised against various toxins isolated from snake venoms are currently being studied in a number of laboratories. These aspects, which have been recently reviewed (Ménez, 1991), are beyond the scope of the present chapter. Instead, the review will focus on the immunological properties of snake toxins that have been investigated at a molecular level, and on the underlying therapeutical aspects. Only curaremimetic toxins and, to some extent cardiotoxins, have been subjected to such analyses. The review will be divided into four parts: First, the main toxic components of snake venoms will be classified and their structural and biological properties briefly summarized. Second, identification of epitopes recognized by neutralizing antibodies, especially in the case of curaremimetic toxins, will be presented. Third, the possible mechanism(s) associated with neutralization of toxins by antibodies will be examined. Fourth, the immunogenic properties, including identification of T epitopes and the design of T-B synthetic immunogens will be described.

SNAKE TOXINS: MORPHOLOGY AND BIOLOGICAL FUNCTION

Animal venoms (snakes, scorpions, conus, spiders, etc.) share the common property of sheltering a diversity of biologically toxic functions. Strikingly, however, within a given class of animals, this functional heterogeneity is associated with a small number of structural patterns. As an illustration, Table 1 shows that 13 activities can be expressed by proteins belonging only to two structural classes.

Toxins with Three Finger-Shaped Structures

The mold designated as three finger-shaped structure corresponds to proteins having a backbone folded into three adjacent loops (designated I, II, and III), which contain only β-pleated sheet and β-turns. These loops emerge from a small globular core in which four invariant disulfide bonds are located. Plate 2* shows a schematic view of three finger-shaped structures. Because of the large sheet found in the three loops, these molecules are rather flat with two distinct sides. Drenth et al. (1980) have made the interesting observation that the unrelated agglutinin from wheat germ also adopts this type of architecture. It was demonstrated by both X-ray (Bourne et al., 1985; Corfield et al., 1989; Love and Stroud, 1986; Tsernoglou and Petsko, 1976; Walkinshaw et al., 1980) and high-field NMR spectroscopy (Basus et al., 1988; Labhardt et al., 1988; Laplante et al., 1990; Yu et al., 1990) that curaremimetic toxins isolated from venoms of most elapid and hydrophid snakes are folded (shown in Plate 2) with their C-terminal loop located on the side of the molecule, which is clearly convex (Low, 1979; Low and Corfield, 1987). Curaremimetic toxins block neuromuscular transmission by binding to the nicotinic acetylcholine receptor (AcChoR) (Changeux, 1990). The cardiotoxins, uniquely found in cobra venoms, are also folded into a three finger-shaped structure (reviewed in Ménez et al., 1990). Abundant crystallographic and NMR data have revealed that their three-dimensional structures nearly superimpose with those of curaremimetic toxins (Rees et al., 1987; Roumestand et al., 1990). The structural analogy of cardiotoxins and curaremimetic toxins is illustrated in Plate 3.* Cardiotoxins are capable of lysing a variety of cells (Boquet, 1970; Gatineau et al., 1987; Takechi et al., 1986) and provoking membrane depolarization (Harvey, 1985). Both effects possibly result from the same, still unknown, action on cell membranes. Other toxins are likely to adopt a three finger-shaped structure, as evidenced by amino acid (Ménez, 1989) and cDNA (Ducancel et al., 1991) sequence analogies and circular dichroism measurements (Ducancel et al., 1991 and unpublished data). This is the case with fasciculins, which block acetylcholinesterase in a noncompetitive manner (Karlsson et al., 1985) and muscarinic toxins, which inhibit the binding of radioactive quinuclidinyl benzylate to muscarinic receptors from rat cortex synaptosomal membranes (Adem et al., 1988). Both fasciculins and muscarinic toxins are isolated from venom of mamba snakes of the genus *Dendroaspis*. Crystals of fasciculins (Basu et al., 1989; Le Du et al., 1989; Ménez and Ducruix, 1990) and muscarinic toxins (Ménez, R. unpublished data) have been obtained and X-ray studies are now in progress. These studies together with NMR investigations should inform us in the near future about the detailed architecture of these toxins. Neuronal toxins are also likely to adopt this type of conformation as judged from their primary structure (reviewed in Loring and Zigmond, 1988; Vidal and Changeux, 1989) and circular dichroism spectra (unpublished data). They

*Plates 2 and 3 follow page 298.

TABLE 1.
Structural Classifications of Snake Toxins[a]

I Conformational Classes	II Modes of Action	III Current Names of Typical Toxins	IV Approximative Molecular Weight	V Number of Disulfides	VI Venom Origin, Snake Family
Three finger-shaped structure	Blockade of peripheral nicotinic acetylcholine receptor	Postsynaptic neurotoxins: Erabutoxin	6,800	4	Hydrophidae
		Naja nigricollis toxin α	6,800	4	Elapidae
		α-Bungarotoxin	7,800	5	
	Blockade of neuronal nicotinic acetylcholine receptor	Neuronal toxins: Toxin F or k bungarotoxin	7,300	5	Elapidae (kraits)
	Depolarization of membrane of excitable cells	Cardio(cyto)toxin: *Naja nigricollis* toxin γ	6,800	4	Elapidae (cobras)
	Lysis of cells	Cardio (cyto) toxin: *Naja nigricollis* toxin γ	6,800	4	Elapidae (cobras)
	Blockade of acetylcholinesterase	Fasciculins	6,800	4	Elapidae (mambas)
	Blockade of muscarinic receptor	Muscarinic toxin	7,000	4	Elapidae (mambas)
	Binding to tachykinin receptor	α-bungarotoxin	7,800	5	Elapidae
PLA$_2$-like structure	Blockade of acetylcholine release	β-bungarotoxin	One subunit: 13,500 One subunit: 7,000	10[b]	Elapidae
	Myotoxicity	Notexin	13,600	7	Elapidae
		Notexin	13,600	7	
	Action on coagulation system	Basic PLA$_2$: Nigexine	13,000	7	Elapidae
	Cytotoxicity	Nigexine	13,000	7	Elapidae
	Initiation of platelet aggregation	Aggregoserpentin	14,000	nd[c]	Viperidae

	No specific name			
Inhibition of platelet aggregation	Dendrotoxin	7,000	3	Elapidae (mambas)
Facilitation of acetylcholine release	Sarafotoxin	2,500	2	Atractaspididae (Atractaspis)
Action on cardiovascular system	Myotoxin a	4,600	3	Viperidae[d]
Myotoxicity	Echistatin	5,400	4	Viperidae[d]
Inhibition of platelet aggregation	Ancrod	35,000	nd[c]	Viperidae[d]
Action on coagulation system	Babroxobin	32,000	nd[c]	
	Crotalase	32,000	nd[c]	

BPTI-like structure / Endothelin-like structure / nd[c] / nd[c] / nd[c]

[a] Biological and some biochemical properties are indicated. Note that "toxin" may not be correct in the strict sense. Indeed, all proteins listed here are extracted from venoms, but their lethal potency has not always been determined.
[b] The heavier and lighter subunits possess six and three disulfides, respectively, and are linked by an additional disulfide.
[c] Not determined, nd.
[d] Includes both viper and crotal snakes.

possess the interesting ability of recognizing particular cholinergic receptors in autonomic ganglia and or the central system. Other toxins of the same structural group are capable of inhibiting the binding of radioactive substance P and eledoisin, suggesting that they interact with rat brain tachykinin receptors (Utkin et al., 1989).

Toxins with PLA$_2$-Type Structures

The structural folding of phospholipase A$_2$ (PLA$_2$) is another pattern observed to express various types of toxic activities in snake venoms. There is evidence, based on comparison of protein (Dufton et al., 1983) or cDNA (Ducancel et al., 1989, 1991) sequences, secondary structure prediction (Dufton et al., 1983), and spectroscopic data, including circular dichroism (Dufton et al., 1983) and NMR (Endo et al., 1987) which indicates that toxic PLA$_2$ from snake venoms are folded like nontoxic PLA$_2$ from snake venom (Brunie et al., 1985; Renetseder et al., 1985; White et al., 1990) or pancreatic PLA$_2$ (Dijkstra et al., 1981). The PLA$_2$ pattern is schematically represented in Plate 2. This is the overall architecture of the essential subunit of the most potent toxins found in snake venoms, e.g., the presynaptically acting toxins. These venom components block release of acetylcholine from nerve endings and may recognize voltage-dependent K$^+$ channels, at least during one of their three phases of action (reviewed in Harvey et al., 1990). Presynaptically acting toxins sometimes comprise a single PLA$_2$ polypeptide chain. This is the case of notexin from venom of the Australian elapid snake, *Notechis scutatus scutatus* (Halpert and Eaker, 1975). They can also be composed of two subunits. This is the case with β-bungarotoxin from venom of the Asian kraits, *Bungarus multicinctus* (Kondo et al., 1982) and crotoxin from venom of the South American rattlesnake, *Crotalus durissus terrificus* (Aird et al., 1986, 1989, 1990; Bouchier et al., 1988). These two toxins possess a PLA$_2$ component and one additional subunit. In β-bungarotoxin the additional component is covalently linked to the PLA$_2$ and chemically analogous to the bovine pancreatic trypsin inhibitor (Kondo et al., 1978). In crotoxin, the additional component is noncovalently associated to the PLA$_2$ subunit and is composed of three small peptides cross-linked to each other by seven disulfides. These three peptides are likely to result from a postranslational hydrolysis of a PLA$_2$, as revealed by examination of the cDNA encoding its precursor (Bouchier et al., 1988). Presynaptically acting PLA$_2$ can even be more complex with three or four subunits like taipoxin and textilotoxin, respectively isolated from venoms of the Australian elapids, *Oxyuranus scutellatus scutellatus* (Fohlman et al., 1976) and *Pseudonaja textilis* (Tyler et al., 1987). For all these toxins, it was established that the PLA$_2$ component is capable of hydrolyzing, at least to some extent, 3-*sn* phospholipids by removing fatty acids at the second position (Slotboom et al., 1982). It is clear, however, that the enzymatic activity is necessary but not sufficient for a complete expression of the toxic function (Rosenberg, 1986).

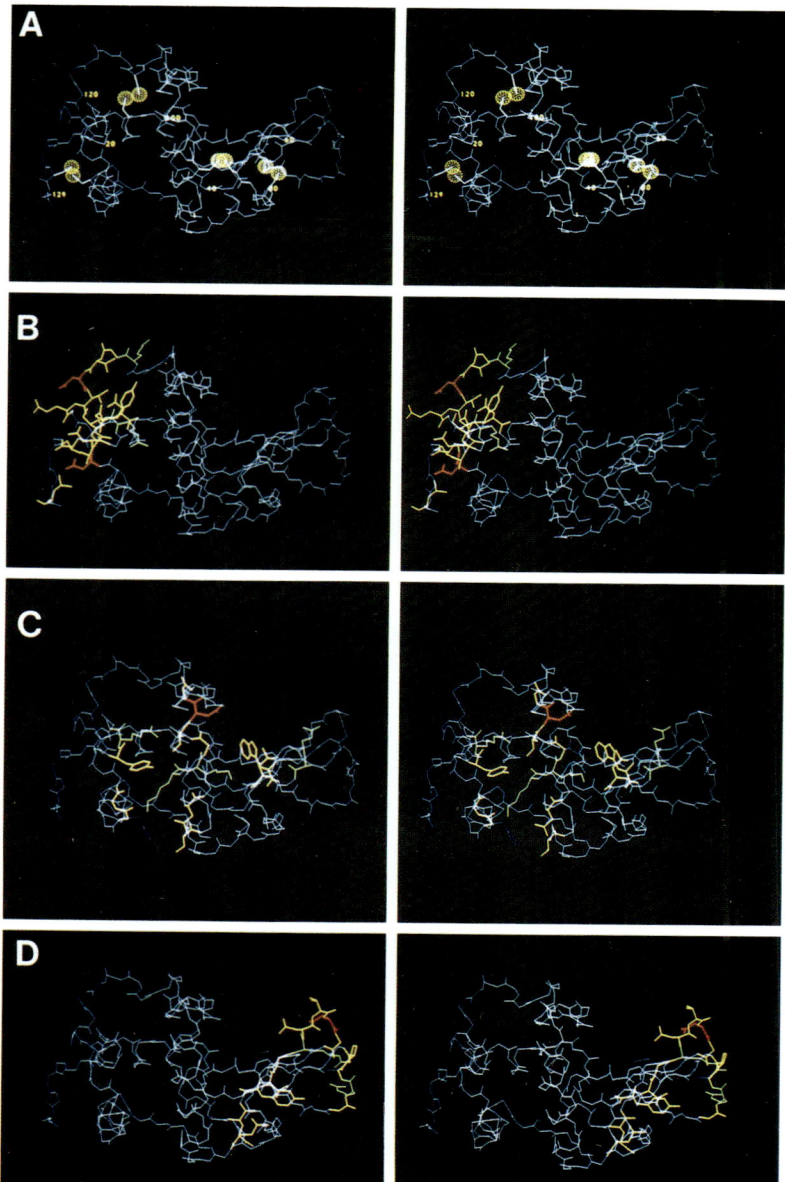

Plate 1. (A) Stereodrawing of the main chain atoms of hen egg white lysozyme. The four disulfide bridges (between cysteines 6 and 127, 30 and 115, 64 and 80, and 76 and 94) are depicted as yellow, dotted spheres. The N- and C-termini are labeled, as are the positions of every 20th residue. (B) The epitope for antibody D1.3. The side chains of the residues which contact the antibody are included; acidic residues are shown in red, basic residues are green. (C) The epitope for antibody HyHEL-10. (D) The epitope for antibody HyHEL-5.

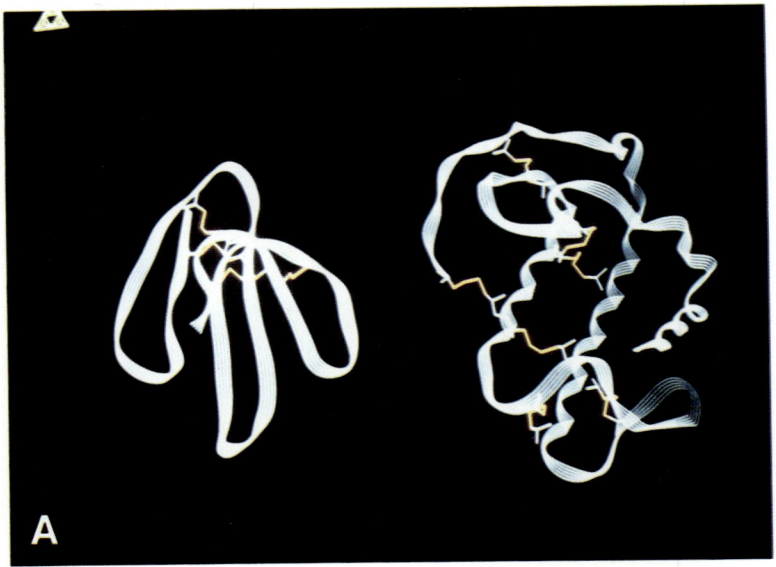

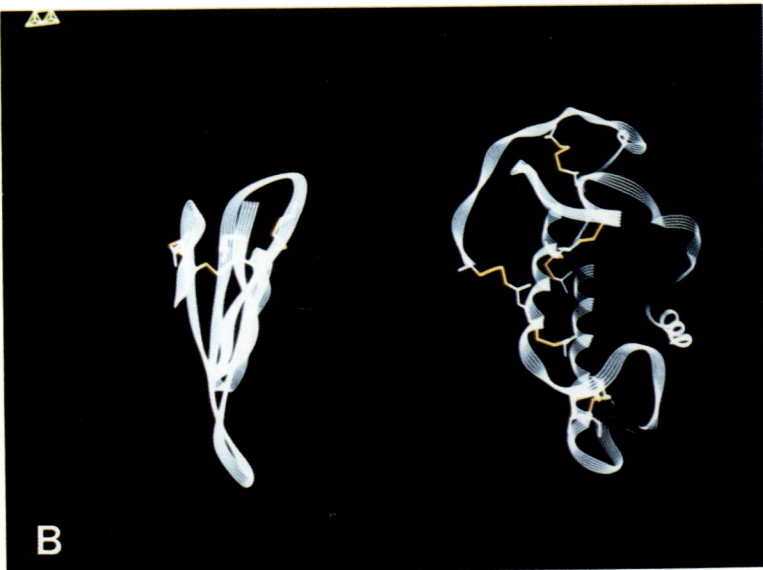

Plate 2. (A) Schematic conformation of toxic proteins. The polypeptide chain on the left adopts a "three finger-shaped structure", the one on the right a phospholipase A_2-like structure; both are derived from X-ray data depicting the three-dimensional structure of erabutoxin b [From Bourne, P. E. et al. (1985) *Eur. J. Biochem.* 153:521—527. With permission.] and phospholipase A_2 from *Crotalus atrox* [From Brunie, S. et al. (1985) *J. Biol. Chem.* 260:9742—9749. With permission.] (B) The two structures are turned by 90°.

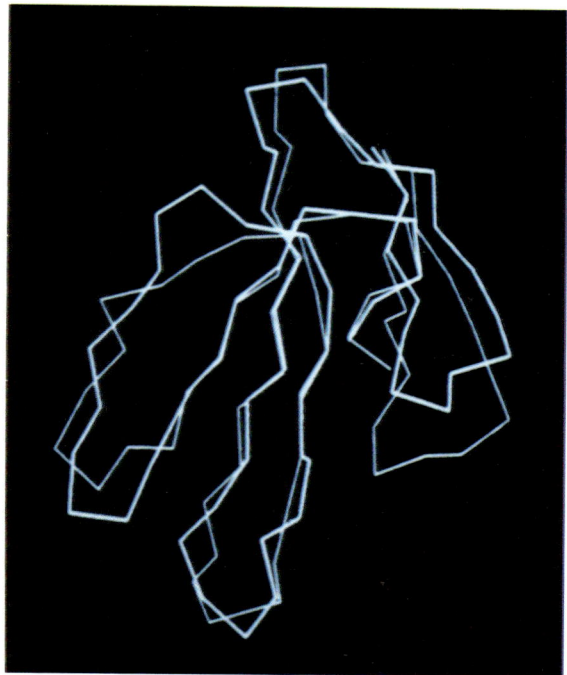

Plate 3. Superimposed three-dimensional structures of the curaremimetic toxin erabutoxin b from venom of *Laticauda semifasciata* and the cardiotoxin V_4^{II} from venom of *Naja mossambica mossambica*. Note that the representation is different from that in Plate 2, with the first loop being here on the right side. [From Rees, B. et al. (1987) *Proc. Natl. Acad. Sci. U.S.A.* 84: 3132—3136. With permission.]

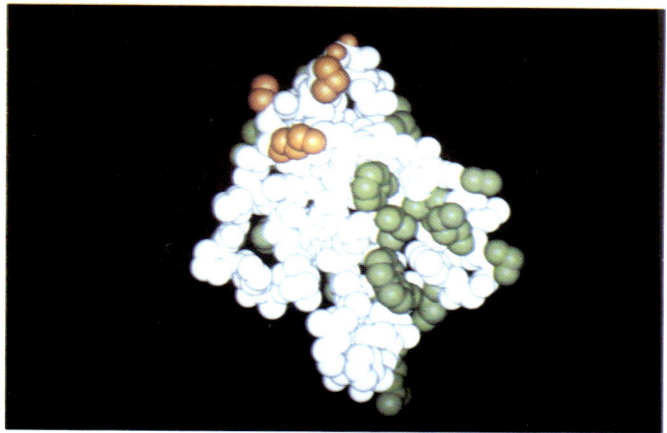

Plate 4A

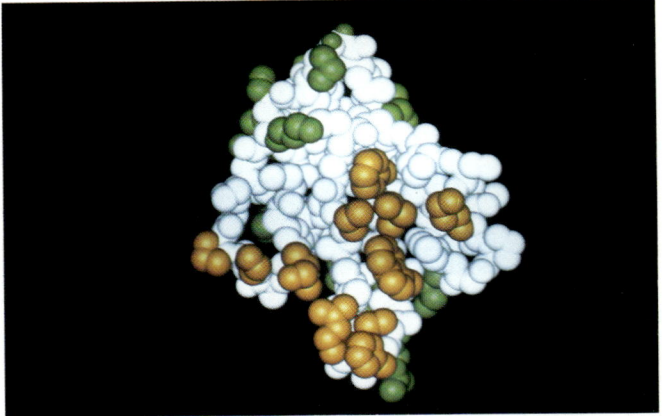

Plate 4B

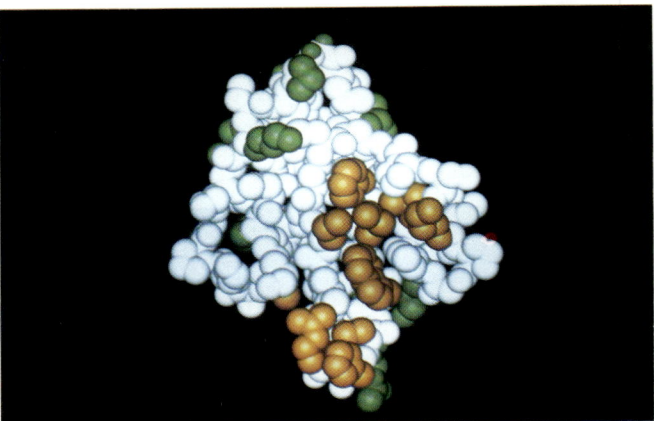

Plate 4C

Plate 4. Delineation of two "neutralizing" epitopes (A and B) and AcChoR binding site (C) of a snake venom curaremimetic toxin. The structure of toxin α from *Naja nigricollis* has been modeled from the X-ray structure of erabutoxin b (Bourne et al., 1985). The modeled structure is represented as in Plate 2 (left), with the first loop on the left side. Note that the concave side points toward the viewer. Residues in green and orange have been modified by chemical or genetic means in toxin α and erabutoxins, or substituted in a natural analogue. Changes at residues in orange were accompanied by a decrease in affinity of the toxin for the monoclonal antibodies Mᾱ1 (A), Mᾱ2-3 (B), or AcChoR (C). Changes at residues in green did not affect the affinities of the toxin. Residues in white remain to be tested. Chemical changes have already been published (see text), whereas genetic modifications will be reported elsewhere [Pillet et al. (1991) in preparation.]

Presynaptically acting toxins seem, therefore, to shelter discrete regions, perhaps topographically different from the catalytic region, which may recognize specific membranar targets, perhaps K^+ channels. It is possible that toxic PLA_2 bind first to their receptors and then locally express their enzymic activity, a mechanism that may account for their specific action on the neuromuscular presynaptic side. The PLA_2-type structure also serves as a basic pattern for the expression of several other activities of snake venoms (Table 1). These include: (1) myotoxins (Mebs and Ownby, 1990) the mode of action of which remains obscure, although the plasma membrane appears to be their primary site of action; (2) toxins with anticoagulant activity on platelet poor plasma (Kornalik, 1985); (3) initiators of platelet aggregation (Takagi et al., 1988); (4) inhibitors of platelet aggregation (Kini and Evans, 1988; Li et al., 1985); and (5) cytotoxins, like nigexine (Chwetzoff et al., 1989), which provoke the lysis of various nucleated cells *in vitro*, including some tumor cells, apparently independently from the PLA_2 activity. In contrast, the enzymatic activity of nigexine seems to be necessary to achieve the lysis of erythrocytes (Chwetzoff, 1990).

There are also a number of newly discovered proteins with extremely interesting properties. They are listed in Table 1, and belong to different structural classes. So far only one toxic function has been assigned to each of these groups. They are briefly discussed here.

Presynaptic Facilitatory Toxins

Mamba venoms contain proteins chemically analogous to Kunitz-type serine protease inhibitors which evoke release of acetylcholine at the neuromuscular junction and block selectively the f_1K^+ current at nodes of Ranvier of frog motor nerves (Benoit and Dubois, 1986; Dreyer, 1990; Harvey et al., 1990). Dendrotoxin, isolated from the venom of the eastern green mamba snake, *Dendroaspis angusticeps,* is probably the best documented of these molecules (reviewed in Harvey and Anderson, 1985; Harvey et al., 1990). It is a 59-amino acid polypeptide cross-linked by three disulfide bonds. Several dendrotoxin-like proteins have been isolated from other mamba venoms (reviewed in Harvey and Anderson, 1985). The architecture of dendrotoxins is likely to be similar to that of bovine pancreatic trypsin inhibitor (BPTI), as determined from comparison of amino acid compositions, primary structures (Joubert and Taljaard, 1980), and, for some dendrotoxins, circular dichroism spectra (Hollecker and Larcher, 1989). Other Kunitz-type serine protease inhibitors have been found in venoms of Elapidae *(Naja naja naja)* (Shafqat et al., 1990) and Viperidae (Ritonja et al., 1983); however, no toxic functions have, as yet, been ascribed to these proteins.

Sarafotoxins

Sarafotoxins have been isolated from the venom of the burrowing asps of the genus *Atractaspis* (reviewed in Bdolah et al., 1991). They are 21-

amino acid peptides having a strong effect on the cardiovascular system. They induce acute vasospasms probably by interfering with the second-messenger system, the phosphoinositide cycle (Kloog et al., 1988). The most striking feature of sarafotoxins is their high similarity with endothelins. Both types of peptides possess 21 amino acids and can have in common up to nearly 50% amino acids, among which four half-cystines are localized at identical places in the sequences (Bdolah et al., 1991). The presence of these common disulfides as well as the sequence similarities suggest that both sarafotoxins and endothelins share a similar spatial organization. Endothelin peptide chains are likely to comprise a loop region from residues 4-6 to 8-9, followed by a helical segment in the 9 to 16 region, as indicated by various NMR analysis (Brown et al., 1990; Endo et al., 1989; Kobayashi, 1990; Saudek et al., 1989). Sarafotoxins and endothelins have similar functions: both compete for the same receptors in the heart (Kloog et al., 1988) and induce phosphoinositide hydrolysis. In addition, cDNAs encoding receptors of endothelins and thereby presumably of sarafotoxins have been recently reported (Arai et al., 1990; Sakurai et al., 1990).

Myotoxic Peptides

Myotoxic peptides are found in venoms of crotalid snakes. They consist of 43 to 45 amino acids with three disulfides (reviewed in Mebs and Ownby, 1990). They clearly cause changes in skeletal muscle cells, inducing, in particular, vacuolation which seems to be due to dilatation of sarcoplasmic reticulum. The mechanism of myotoxicity induced by these peptides is still unclear. Some studies indicated that myotoxins act on the sodium channel of the plasma membrane of mammalian skeletal muscle cells and thereby increase the resting membrane permeability to sodium (Chang et al., 1983; Hong and Chang, 1985). Other studies suggest that myotoxic peptides might act on the Ca^{2+}-ATPase of sarcoplasmic reticulum from skeletal muscles (Volpe et al., 1986). The three-dimensional architecture of these peptides is still unknown. However, various spectroscopic experiments suggest that the polypeptide chains of myotoxic peptides comprise β-sheet and β-turns with some helicity (Bailey et al., 1979). A more recent NMR investigation indicated that the N-terminal region is mostly in helical conformation (Henderson et al., 1987).

Platelet-Aggregation Inhibitors

A family of platelet-aggregation inhibitors has been identified and sequenced (Dennis et al., 1989; Gan et al., 1988; Huang et al., 1987; Ouyang and Huang, 1983). Their sizes range from 47 to 83 amino acid residues, with 4 to 7 disulfide bonds, and they possess a conserved Arg-Gly-Asp recognition sequence, found in many adhesion proteins. One of them, called echistatin is now overproduced in *E. coli* (Gan et al., 1989). Evidence was provided that these small proteins bind to a platelet-integrin receptor, the membrane glycoprotein IIb-IIIa. The three-dimensional structure of these compounds remains to be elucidated.

Miscellaneous Toxins

Snake venom enzymes that act on the coagulation system are abundant, as reviewed by Kornalik (1985). A number of thrombic proteases are present in venoms of Crotalidae family. Among others, ancrod, batroxobin, and crotalase have been extensively studied. They are single-chain glycoproteins of 32,000 to 35,000 MW. The nucleotide sequence of cDNA encoding batroxobin was described by Itoh et al. (1987). The three-dimensional structure of these enzymes is still unknown.

This brief overview clearly shows that snake venoms contain a variety of components with widely different functions. Several of them are expressed by proteins which are conformationally related. It is also striking that a given type of snake toxin can express several unrelated biological activities. Thus, curaremimetic toxins have been recently recognized to be also capable of competing specifically with a hormone for binding to tachykinin receptors (Utkin et al., 1989). A similar situation is encountered with toxins having a PLA_2 structure. Thus, notexin from *Notechis scutatus scutatus* not only acts presynaptically but also as a potent myotoxin (Mebs and Ownby, 1990). It was also proposed that the regions responsible for these different functions may be topographically distinct from each other; the residues located in the C-terminal region are more specifically involved in the presynaptic action of notexin (Mollier et al., 1989). From all these observations it is tempting to speculate that the structural patterns of snake toxins undergo intense evolutionary pressure. They possibly evolve from a structurally related protein which has no toxic function, as illustrated by the observation that nontoxic proteins with three finger-shaped structure, PLA_2-like structure, or BPTI-like conformation are known (see above). So far, the routes followed by evolution to make one conformation adapted to a diversity of functions remain poorly understood. However, it is clear that these routes scrupulously respect the conservation of several elements indispensable to preserve the basic architecture including, in particular, disulfide bonds. It is then tempting to anticipate that structures for which only one biological action is currently recorded, can in fact express several other activities which remain, however, to be discovered.

EPITOPES RECOGNIZED BY NEUTRALIZING ANTIBODIES

Epitopes of Short-Chain Curaremimetic Toxins

Nearly 80 snake curaremimetic toxins have been isolated and their amino acid sequences identified (Endo and Tamiya, 1987). These compounds can be classified into two categories according to their sequence length. Short-chain toxins possess between 60 and 62 amino acids and 4 invariant disulfides (see Fig. 1), whereas long-chain toxins possess between 66 and 74 residues and, in addition to the previous 4 invariant disulfides, generally possess an extra disulfide located at the tip of the central loop. All toxins recognize AcChoR with specificity and high affinity ($K_d = 2$ to 10×10^{-11} M). In fact, two molecules of toxin bind to one molecule of AcChoR, and a model representing this complex has been recently proposed (Chatrenet et al., 1990). Once bound to their receptor, the toxins block neuromuscular transmission and, in particular, induce a paralysis of the diaphragm. Death occurs by respiratory failure. Approximately 1 to 2 μg of toxin injected intravenously kills a 20-g mouse.

Cross-reactivity studies using polyclonal antibodies raised against short-chain curaremimetic toxins (Abe and Tamiya, 1979; Boquet, 1979; Boulain 1979; Ménez et al., 1979), suggested that antigenically dominant areas were located in the core region and on the convex side of the toxins. In contrast, conserved residues, which are located on the concave face of the toxins, did not appear to be highly antigenic. Screening for MAbs recognizing either the hypervariable or the conserved regions of short-chain curaremimetic toxins was successively achieved using two antigenic variants presenting similar structure and function but appropriate sequence differences (Boulain et al., 1982; Trémeau et al., 1986). The two variants were toxin α isolated from venom of the African spitting cobra, *Naja nigricollis,* and erabutoxins a, b, or c isolated from venom of the sea snake, *Laticauda semifasciata.* The erabutoxin a sequence differs from erabutoxins b and c by a single substitution, at positions 26 and 51, respectively. Toxin α and erabutoxins have a highly similar, three finger-shaped structure, as indicated by various spectroscopic analyses (Ménez et al., 1978; Thiéry et al., 1980), including NMR (Zinn-Justin et al., in preparation). They also have similar affinities for AcChoR from *Torpedo marmorata* (Ishikawa et al., 1977; Trémeau et al., 1986). The lethal potencies of erabutoxins are only twofold lower than that of toxin α (Ishikawa et al., 1977). Toxin α and erabutoxins, however, possess 61 and 62 amino acids, respectively, and 17 amino acid differences (Fig. 1). The additional residue in erabutoxins is located at position 18 in the large turn that joins loops I and II within the globular core of the toxins, whereas several substitutions are distributed on the convex side of the sheet that encompasses the three loops of the toxin (Low, 1979). In contrast, the concave and functional side is nearly occupied by identical residues in both toxins. In short, toxin α and erabutoxins can be grossly regarded as functionally similar variants having a similar flat three finger-shaped structure, in which the concave sides are similar but the cores and the convex sides exhibit major amino acid differences.

Among a series of MAbs (Köhler and Milstein, 1975) raised against native (not detoxified) toxin α, one MAb, called Māl, recognized toxin α but none of the erabutoxins (Boulain et al., 1982), whereas another MAb,

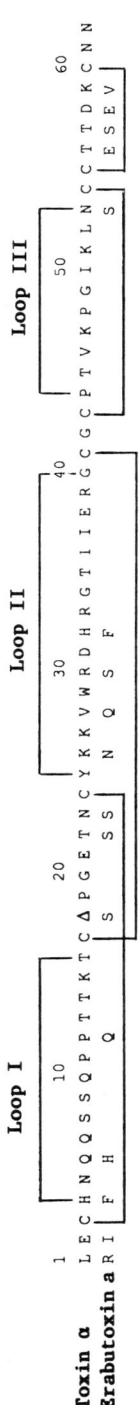

Figure 1. Amino acid sequence of toxin α from venom of *Naja nigricollis* and differences found in the sequence of erabutoxin a from venom of *Laticauda semifasciata* (Δ means deletion); disulfide pairings are indicated. Residues belonging to the three loops organized in β-pleated sheet are also shown.

called Mᾱ2-3, recognized both toxin α and erabutoxins (Trémeau et al., 1986). *In vitro,* both MAbs prevented binding of ³H-labeled toxin α to AcChoR in a dose-dependent manner. *In vivo,* however, Mᾱ1 was potent at neutralizing toxicity, whereas Mᾱ2-3 only delayed lethality. This differential behavior might result from the different affinities of the MAbs toward the antigen: Mᾱ1-toxin α and Mᾱ2-3-toxin α complexes are characterized by equilibrium dissociation constants equal to 0.4 and 9 n*M,* respectively (Boulain et al., 1982; Trémeau et al., 1986).

Several attempts were made to identify residues involved in the epitopes recognized by either antibody. In particular, crystallization of the toxin-Fab complexes (Guillon, 1985) has been attempted but no three-dimensional structures have emerged from these studies as yet. Furthermore, synthetic toxin fragments were investigated regarding their ability to bind the MAbs but no specific binding was detected, suggesting that the epitopes are discontinuous rather than continuous, as in most proteins (Barlow et al., 1986). Delineation of epitopes was, therefore, investigated by chemical and genetic mapping, an approach that turned out to be quite informative. The principle of the procedure is simple, though somewhat tedious. Most residues of the antigen are changed, one at a time, and the consequences of these changes on the affinity of the antigen for the antibody are examined. Two cases can be encountered. First, the modified and native antigens have the same affinity for the antibody. It is then concluded that the modification is not implicated in the complex formation. The residue is considered as being excluded from the antigenic site. Second, the modified antigen has a different affinity, usually lower, as compared to that of the native antigen. In this case, one can meet two situations: First the modification had not altered the conformation of the antigen outside the site of modification. One can then safely conclude that the modified residue is implicated in or in close proximity to the epitope. Second, the modification had perturbed the structure of the antigen. In this case, no conclusion can be drawn as to the possible implication of the modified residue in the epitope.

Delineations of Mᾱ1 and Mᾱ2-3 epitopes were initially attempted using derivatives of toxin α and erabutoxins a and b, chemically modified at a single residue (Tables 2 and 3). The three-dimensional structure of most of these derivatives was examined by various spectroscopic approaches including, far-UV circular dichroism, fluorescence (Faure et al., 1983), and electron-spin resonance (ESR) (Rousselet et al., 1984), and for some acetylated derivatives by X-ray crystallography (Sato, A., Ménez, A., and Tamiya, N. unpublished data). No change in the toxin structure could be seen upon any chemical modification. Affinity of antibodies for chemical derivatives was determined on the basis of competition experiments between ³H-labeled toxin α (Ménez et al., 1971) used as a radioactive tracer, and each derivative toward both MAbs, using a reproducible liquid-phase radioimmunoassay (Boulain et al., 1982). Tables 2 and 3 show that the stability of the Mᾱ2-3-toxin complex was altered after modifications of residues located on the concave side of the

TABLE 2.
Relative Dissociation Constants of Monoderivatives of Toxin α for Mα̃1

Modified Residue	Introduced Modification	Relative K_d[a]
Terminal-NH_2-α	Acetylation[b]	29
NH_2-ε-Lys[15]	Acetylation[b]	11
Tyr[25]	Nitration	1
NH_2-ε-Lys[27]	Acetylation[b]	1
Trp[29]	NPS[c]	1
NH_2-ε-Lys[47]	Acetylation[b]	1
NH_2-ε-Lys[51]	Acetylation[b]	1

[a] The dissociation constant of ^{3}H-labeled toxin α for Mα̃1 is equal to 0.4 nM (Boulain et al., 1982).
[b] Other chemical modifications performed on the same amino group are reviewed by Ménez et al. (1991).
[c] Introduction of a nitrophenyl thioether moiety on C_2 of the indole side chain.

TABLE 3.
Relative Dissociation Constants of Monoderivatized Toxins for Mα̃2-3

Modified Residue	Introduced Modification	Modified Toxin	Relative K_d[a]
Terminal-NH_2-α	Acetylation[b]	Toxin α	1
15-NH_2-ε-Lys	Acetylation[b]	Toxin α	1
		Erabutoxin b	1
25-Tyr	Nitration	Toxin α	5
27-NH_2-ε-Lys	Acetylation[b]	Toxin α	7
		Erabutoxin b	7,5
29-Trp	NPS[c]	Toxin α	19
47-NH_2-ε-Lys	Acetylation[b]	Toxin α	9
		Erabutoxin b	30
51-NH_2-ε-Lys	Acetylation[b]	Toxin α	1
		Erabutoxin b	1

[a] Kd values for toxin α and erabutoxin a are 9 and 2 nM, respectively (Trémeau et al., 1986).
[b] Other chemical modifications performed on the same amino group are reviewed by Ménez et al. (1991).
[c] Introduction of a nitrophenyl thioether moiety on C_2 of the indole side chain.

toxin, within loops II (residues 25, 27, and 29) and III (residue 47), but remained unchanged after modifications at positions 1, 15, and 51. In contrast, stability of the Mα̃1-toxin complex was affected by changes at residues located near the core (N-terminus) and at the edge of the concave side, within loop I (Lys[15]), but not by modifications at positions 25, 27, 29, 47, and 51. More information was subsequently obtained using natural variants. Thus, Boulain et al. (1982) showed that Mα̃1 did not recognize toxins possessing an additional residue at position 18, like the erabutoxins, or toxins having a proline residue at position 18, like *Naja naja oxiana* toxin α. However, its affinity was not affected by multiple substitutions occurring in the concave or convex sides of 61 amino acid-containing toxins like *Naja haje* toxin α, leaving little doubt that the core region was the target of this antibody. Recently, Pillet et al. (unpublished data) deleted Ser[18] in erabutoxin a by site-directed mutagenesis in its cDNA (Ducancel et al., 1989; Tamiya et al., 1985). The resulting mutant had the same affinity as native toxin α for Mᾱ1. This result shows that the epitope was completely generated by a single amino acid deletion in the initially unrecognized erabutoxin a, and gives clear confirmation that the antigenic site recognized by Mᾱ1 involves residues located in the turn that joins loops I and II. It should be noted that the deletion generated an identical stretch of 10 residues, between positions 13 and 22, in (Δ^{18})-erabutoxin a and toxin α (Fig. 1). Furthermore, the result indicates that the several residues that differ between toxin α and the (Δ^{18})-erabutoxin a mutant are not implicated in the epitope. Residues whose modification altered the affinity of Mᾱ1 for the toxin are shown in orange in Plate 4A,* whereas residues whose change had no effect on stability of the toxin-Mᾱ1 complex are indicated in green. Complete delineation of the contact surface is not achieved as yet, as illustrated by the untested residues colored in white. New mutants of (Δ^{18})-erabutoxin a, which are currently prepared in our laboratory, should be of great help in this respect.

In contrast to Mᾱ1 which only recognizes 61 residue-containing toxins, Mᾱ2-3 binds to all short-chain curaremimetic toxins that have been tested so far, indicating that its epitope involves conserved residues. In particular, it binds to *L. colubrina* toxin d with the same affinity as toxin α, despite the presence of as many as 17 mutations, including one insertion, between the two toxins. A detailed analysis of mutations that occurred in several variants (Trémeau et al., 1986) indicated that changes at the tip of the first loop (Gln[7], Gln[10], and Pro[11]) affected the binding of Mᾱ2-3 to the toxin, whereas multiple changes occurring on the convex side or in the core of the molecule had little, if any, effect on this binding. Several genetic mutants of erabutoxin a have been constructed (Pillet et al., in preparation), which proved to be valuable for further delineating the epitope recognized by Mᾱ2-3 (Table 4). In particular, the role of the tips of the first and second loops was evidenced by mutations at position 8 and positions 31, 32, 33, and 34, respectively. In addition, changes at side chains pointing toward the concave side of the molecule, like at positions 27, 29, and 38 affected Mᾱ2-3 binding affinity, whereas changes on the convex side, like at positions 26 or 51, had no effect. Furthermore, the core region was excluded from the epitope as judged from preservation of MAb affinity after deletion and/or several mutations in the region 18 to 23. Thus defined, the epitope recognized by Mᾱ2-3 is represented in Plate 4B. It is clearly better delineated, compared with the epitope recognized by Mᾱ1, even though not completely identified as yet.

*Plate 4 follows page 298.

TABLE 4.
Relative Dissociation Constants of Genetically Engineered or Natural Mutants of Erabutoxin a for $M\bar{\alpha}_{2-3}$, as Estimated from Competition Experiments

Mutated Residue(s)	Introduced Residue	Relative K_d^a
Ser[8]	Gly	9
Ser[18]	Δ^b	1
Ser[18], Pro[19], Gly[20]	Δ^b, Δ^b, Arg	1
Asn[26]	His[c]	1
Lys[27]	Glu	21
Trp[29]	Phe	44
	His	860
Asp[31]	His	184
Phe[32]	Leu	20
Arg[33]	Lys	10
Gly[34]	Ser	4
Glu[38]	Gln	130
	Lys	1890
Gly[49]	Val	1
Lys[51]	Asn[d]	1
Leu[52]	Ala	1

[a] Reference K_d value of erabutoxin a was equal to 2 nM.
[b] Deletion.
[c] Natural mutation (erabutoxin b).
[d] Natural mutation (erabutoxin c).

The epitopes recognized by Mᾱ1 and Mᾱ2-3 are topographically different. Not a single genetic or chemical change concomitantly affected stability of both complexes, suggesting that contact regions have no common boundaries. One of them recognizes the core region, whereas the other recognizes the conserved concave side of the toxin. Both epitopes are clearly topographical, being composed of residues apart from each other in the sequence but brought together in space as a result of protein folding, a situation that seems to predominate among protein epitopes (Barlow et al., 1986).

Epitopes at Surfaces of Other Toxins

Epitopes of other snake toxins have been tentatively identified, but at present none have been delineated as precisely as those shown in Plate 4. Two different MAbs directed against α-bungarotoxin, a long-chain curaremimetic toxin, have been shown to recognize fragments mimicking the tip of the toxin central loop (Chuang et al., 1989; Kase et al., 1989). Charpentier et al. (1990) described one MAb that recognized the tip of the central loop of another long-chain toxin, using chemically derivatized toxins. The authors also found a MAb that binds at the base of the second loop. A number of cardiotoxin epitopes have also been studied (Grognet et al., 1986; Mourier et al., 1989). Thus, one MAb was shown to recognize the edge of the first loop of toxin γ from *Naja nigricollis* on the basis of competition data with natural mutants, chemical derivatives, and synthetic peptides. Another toxin γ-specific MAb recognizes the loops II and III of toxin γ (Grognet et al., 1986), but delineation of its epitope remains to be determined. MAbs directed to toxic phospholipases or other snake toxins have been prepared, but no corresponding epitopes have, as yet, been identified (Ménez, 1991).

NEUTRALIZATION MECHANISMS OF SNAKE TOXINS BY ANTIBODIES

Neutralization of a toxic function implies that the site, called the "toxic" site, by which the toxin exerts its action is no longer able to recognize its physiological target. A priori, one can anticipate that this effect, when created subsequently to the binding of an antibody molecule, is associated with at least one of the following: (1) a complete masking of the toxic site by the paratopic surface; (2) a steric hindrance due to the size of the antibody molecule; and (3) a structural deformation of the toxic site. Clearly, identification of the functional residues of a toxic protein is a prerequisite to understanding the mechanisms of neutralization by antibodies.

The toxic site of curaremimetic toxins has been extensively studied with various techniques, including chemical modifications (reviewed in Endo and Tamiya, 1987) and site-directed mutagenesis experiments (Pillet et al., in preparation). Plate 4C shows residues whose modification (chemical or genetic) induced a decrease in the affinity of the toxin for AcChoR, as well as residues whose change did not affect toxin action. Functionally critical residues are mostly located on loops II and III with their side chains pointing toward the concave side of the toxin. Our experimental data, which will be described in detail elsewhere, generally agree with previous proposals of the AcChoR-binding site of short-chain curaremimetic toxins, based on the examination of conserved amino acid residues (Low, 1979; Ménez et al., 1984). The surface shown in Plate 4C obviously overlaps the epitope recognized by Mᾱ2-3 (see Plate 4B). As additional evidence that the epitope includes the toxic site, it has been shown that Mᾱ2-3 elicits anti-idiotypic antibodies that specifically bind to AcChoR (unpublished result). The toxic site and the epitope, however, are not strictly identical. The epitope largely encompasses the tip of the loop I, whereas only Ser^8 has been so far included in the toxic site. Nevertheless, in view of the great overlap between the two sites, there is no doubt that inhibition of toxin binding to AcChoR in the presence of Mᾱ2-3 is based on a mutual exclusion mechanism. That is, the toxin cannot bind simultaneously to both the receptor and antibody. Since the paratope of Mᾱ2-3 mimics the toxin-binding site in AcChoR, the antibody has the remarkable ability of recognizing and neutralizing, at least *in vitro,* all tested short-chain curaremimetic toxins (Trémeau et al., 1986).

With Mα1, the situation is more complicated. It certainly prevents the binding of the toxin to the receptor *in vitro* and *in vivo* (Boulain et al., 1982). However, none of the toxic residues currently examined belonged to the epitope. In contrast, the epitope is composed of residues that are located within the core of the molecule and at the edge of loop I. At present, five residues have been identified in the antigenic site recognized by Mα1. However, many additional residues should be involved in the site, as judged from X-ray data of other protein-antibody complexes (reviewed by Janin and Chothia, 1990). Since numerous residues on the concave side and convex side of loops II and III were excluded from the epitope, loop I appears to be the most likely region where Mα1 can make contact with the toxin. Interestingly enough, a recent model of the toxin-receptor complex revealed that in the bound state, the convex side of the loop I remains accessible from outside (Chatrenet et al., 1990). Considering the relative size of the receptor (250 kDa), the Fab fragment (50 kDa), and the toxin (7 kDa), it is tempting to anticipate that the inhibition results from an exclusion mechanism due to steric hindrance effects. However, a series of observations suggested that Mα1 may exert its neutralizing potency by a different mechanism. Thus, it was shown that an excess of Mα1 (or Fab fragment) accelerates *in vitro* the kinetics of dissociation of ^{3}H-labeled toxin-AcChoR complex, as compared to the kinetics determined in the presence of an excess of unlabeled toxin or under high dilution conditions (Boulain and Ménez, 1982). No such effect was seen with Mα2-3. Subsequently, Gatineau et al., (1988) reported *in vivo* experiments which showed that rats intoxicated with toxin α and maintained in life by artificial respiration, returned to normal breathing approximately 12 times faster after injection of Mα1 (78 ± 8 min), as compared with control animals (940 ± 40 min) which received saline only. Conversely, an excess of receptor was unable to accelerate the dissociation of the toxin-antibody complex (Boulain et al., 1985). These data allowed us to propose a kinetic model which indicated that Mα1 binds to receptor-bound toxin, thus forming a transient ternary complex that destabilized the toxin-receptor complex (Boulain et al., 1985). To explain this destabilizing effect, it was proposed that binding of Mα1 altered the architecture of the free and receptor-bound toxin. In agreement with this proposal was the observation that selective acetylation of the antigenic Lys^{15} induced an alteration in the functionally critical loop II, that is, a decrease in the efficiency of transfer energy between Tyr^{25} and Trp^{29} (Faure et al., 1983). To gain further insight on the structure of toxin bound to Mα1, an electron spin resonance study was undertaken, using several toxin derivatives harboring a single nitroxide probe located in the epitope or in the toxic site (Rousselet et al., 1984). No significant mobility change between the free and bound toxin was detected apart from the toxin-antibody contact area, indicating that the conformational change occurring in the antibody-bound toxin is subtle.

Antiserum raised against toxin α was also capable of reversing receptor-bound toxin *in vitro* (Boulain and Ménez, 1982), *ex vivo,* and *in vivo* (Gatineau et al., 1988). A similar effect was observed in monkeys envenomated with sea snake venoms and subsequently treated with specific antivenin (Vick et al., 1975). However, not all antitoxin antisera share this reversing property (unpublished results). Certainly, it would be a considerable improvement to provide all existing antisera with antibodies having such curative properties.

Neutralization mechanisms based on recognition of the toxic site by an antibody have been observed with toxins other than short-chain curaremimetic toxins. These include long-chain toxins (Charpentier et al., 1990; Chuang et al., 1989; Kase et al., 1989) and toxin γ from *Naja nigricollis,* a cardio(cyto)toxin (Grognet et al., 1986; Mourier et al., 1989). The functional site of toxin γ, recently identified (reviewed in Ménez et al., 1990), incorporates residues of the first loop, including Trp[11] (Gatineau et al., 1987) and Lys[12] (Gatineau et al., 1990), and the second loop. This site is associated with the cytotoxic, depolarizing, and lethal properties of the toxin. In contrast, residues of the third loop seem excluded from the functional site. The MAb Mγ1 that recognizes residues of loop I and, in particular, Trp[11] (Mourier et al., 1989) binds to an antigenic site that overlaps the functional site, providing a simple explanation as to the mechanism associated with its neutralizing property.

In summary, two particularly interesting situations have been met. In one of them the antibody mimics the receptor and acts as a sort of decoy. It has the unique ability to recognize all functionally homologous toxins, irrespective of the numerous mutations that occur outside its epitope. This sort of antibody should be used preferably in preventive serotherapy. In the other situation, the neutralizing antibody recognizes a variable region of the toxin but also possesses the unique ability of dissociating the toxin bound to its receptor. This sort of antibody should preferably be used in curative treatment of envenomated patients. Clearly, therefore, not all antibodies are equivalent in terms of neutralizing capability.

IMMUNOGENIC PROPERTIES OF TOXIN α FROM *NAJA NIGRICOLLIS*

Since the mechanisms of neutralization seem to differ from one type of antibody to another, it would be ideal to be capable of orientating an immune response against a given protein toward the production of antibodies having desired specificities. One way to approach this possibility consists of using synthetic peptides that mimic the appropriate antigenic areas. To be immunogenic, however, the peptides have also to stimulate specific T cells (Kishimoto and Hirano, 1989; Mitchison, 1971). This difficulty is currently overcome by coupling the peptide to carrier molecules. Now, however, it is clear that comparable effects can be obtained by linking B epitopes to T cell-stimulating fragments (Francis et al., 1987; Good et al., 1987; Leclerc et al., 1987).

Recently, Léonetti et al. (1990) investigated the regions of toxin α that were capable of stimulating T cells from BALB/c mice (H-2^d haplotype). Five peptides, 1 to 25, 15 to 30, 24 to 41, 32 to 49, and 39 to 62 that encompass the whole toxin sequence (Figure 1) were assayed for their ability to stimulate *in vitro* T cells harvested from mice primed with the toxin. Only the fragment 24 to 41 substantially stimulated T cells in a dose-dependent manner. Its stimulating potency was even higher compared with that of the whole toxin. Conversely, when mice were primed with each fragment, only T cells from animals primed with fragment 24 to 41 could be stimulated by the priming peptide and to a weaker extent by the toxin. Confirmation that this region contains T epitopes was recently shown by Maillère et al. (unpublished data), who prepared toxin-specific T hybridoma which recognized the fragment 24 to 41.

The five free toxin fragments described above were injected in BALB/c mice, in the presence of Freund's adjuvant, and the resulting antisera were examined. In agreement with the current view that stimulation of T-helper cells is a prerequisite for B-cell proliferation and thereby for antibody production (Roy et al., 1989), it was found that only the fragment 24 to 41 elicited specific antisera. The fragment 24 to 41, therefore, possesses all required elements to trigger an immune response in BALB/c mice (H-2^d haplotype). This observation was all the more interesting as this region corresponds to the second loop of the toxin which, as aforementioned, contains numerous residues that are conserved in the whole family of short-chain curaremimetic toxins. Examination of the antibody specificity, as determined by enzyme-linked immunosorbent blocking assay (ELISA), revealed that the immunizing fragment 24 to 41 as well as the unfolded toxin (the four disulfides were reduced and the thiol groups carbamidomethylated) were both recognized by the antisera. In sharp contrast, the antisera failed to recognize the native toxin and, accordingly, also failed to inhibit the binding of the toxin to its receptor. These results suggested that conformation of the free fragment 24 to 41 was more similar to the one that takes place in the unfolded toxin than in the native toxin. In an attempt to reverse this situation, the peptide was cyclicized by introducing a disulfide between residues 24 and 41. The cyclic peptide remained capable of stimulating T cells and elicited antisera that recognized the cyclic peptide and still the unfolded toxin. In addition, however, a substantial proportion of antibodies recognized the native toxin. Furthermore, these antisera were capable of inhibiting specifically the binding of the toxin to AcChoR. We found it striking, however, that the antisera raised against the cyclic peptide had a relatively low titer and weak neutralizing potency, as compared to antisera raised against the whole native toxin. Similar observations have commonly been reported for various other synthetic immunogens (Palmenberg, 1987). This indicates that the B-cell receptors selected by the peptides do not adequately complement the architecture of the whole native antigen, suggesting that the free peptides and their counterpart in the whole protein have distinct conformations. Accordingly, circular dichroism analysis (Léonetti et al., 1990) and preliminary NMR studies (Cuniasse et al., unpublished data) indicated that even though it was not completely disorganized, the free cyclic peptide 24 to 41 did not adopt a dominant β-sheet conformation in aqueous solution in contrast to what was observed in the whole native toxin (see Plate 4). Presumably, a major challenge in the forthcoming years for the design of efficient synthetic immunogens will be to provide them adequate T-cell stimulating ability and appropriate structural constraints for optimizing their conformational mimicry of their counterpart in the native antigen.

Therefore, the synthetic approach appears to be a little more complex today compared with what was believed a few years ago. However, this approach remains extremely promising because it offers a unique possibility for orientating at will the immune response toward the production of antibodies having expected neutralizing properties. Thus, it was observed that the antisera raised against the cyclic fragment 24 to 41 recognized several homologous short-chain toxins, including toxin α and erabutoxin. This is an interesting observation because these toxins display weak cross-reactivity toward polyclonal antisera raised against the whole toxins (Boulain, 1979; Ménez et al., 1979). However, since they are not directed to the core region, they are unlikely to possess the curative properties found for Mᾱ1 (see above). Orientation of the immune response of BALB/c mice to produce antisera having such properties should, in principle, be achieved with a peptide comprising the T-cell stimulating region 24 to 41 associated to the epitope recognizing Mᾱ1. This approach is currently under investigation.

CONCLUSION

The present review has shown that snake venoms contain a number of proteins of small size which possess a variety of functions expressed at the surface of a small number of structural patterns. These proteins are extremely well-suited models for immunological studies, as exemplified in the case of short-chain curaremimetic toxins. In particular, they proved of considerable help in investigating the mechanisms associated with the neutralization of a toxic protein by antibodies and providing evidence in favor of curative effects of some antibodies. They also enabled Léonetti et al. (1990) to show that a valuable approach for designing a synthetic immunogen consists of identifying a T-cell-stimulating peptide and to provide it directly with appropriate B-cell specificity. These studies finally show that one of the most challenging aspects in the design of synthetic immunogen is to provide the adequate architecture to the peptide fragment. Since the fundamental principles associated with the humoral immune response are now understood, it seems that the difficulties to be overcome in the preparation of an efficient synthetic immunogen are more of a chemical than immunological nature.

REFERENCES

Abe, T., and Tamiya, N. (1979) Immunological studies on erabutoxin b, a sea snake toxin. Attempts to locate the amino acid residues determining antigenicity. *Toxicon* 17:571—582.

Adem, A., Asblom, A., Johansson, G., Mbugua, P. M., and Karlsson, E. (1988) Toxins from the venom of the green mamba *Dendroaspis angusticeps* that inhibit the binding of quinuclidinyl benzilate to muscarinic acetylcholine receptors. *Biochim. Biophys. Acta* 968:340—345.

Aird, S. D., Kaiser, I. I., Lewis, R. V., and Kruggel, W. G. (1986) A complete amino acid sequence for the basic subunit of crotoxin. *Arch. Biochem. Biophys.* 249:296—300.

Aird, S. D., Yates, J. R., Hunt, D. F., and Kaiser, I. I. (1989) Amino acid sequence of crotoxin's acidic subunit B chain. *Toxicon* 27:29.

Aird, S. D., Yates, J. R., Martino, P. A., Shabanowitz, J., Hunt, D. F., and Kaiser, I. I. (1990) The amino acid sequence of the acidic subunit B chain of crotoxin. *Biochim. Biophys. Acta* 1040:217—224.

Arai, H., Hori, S., Aramori, I., Ohkubo, H., and Nakanishi, S. (1990) Cloning and expression of a cDNA encoding an endothelin receptor. *Nature (London)* 348:730—732.

Bailey, G. S., Lee, J., and Tu, A. T. (1979) Conformational analysis of myotoxin a (muscle degenerating toxin) of prairie rattlesnake venom. Predictions from amino acid sequence, circular dichroism and Raman spectroscopy. *J. Biol. Chem.* 254:8922—8926.

Barlow, D. J., Edwards, M. S., and Thornton, J. M. (1986) Continuous and discontinuous protein antigenic determinants. *Nature (London)* 322:747—748.

Basu, S. P., Hannick, L. I., and Ward, K. B. (1989) Preliminary characterization of single crystals of Fasciculin 2 suitable for X-ray diffraction analysis. *Toxicon* 27:832.

Basus, V. J., Billeter, M., Love, R. A., Stroud, R. M., and Kuntz, I. D. (1988) Structural studies of α-bungarotoxin. 1. Sequence-specific ^{1}HNMR resonance assignments. *Biochemistry* 97:2763—2771.

Bdolah, A., Wollberg, Z., and Kochva, E. (1991) Sarafotoxins: a new group of cardiotoxic peptides from the venom of *Atractaspis*. In *Snake Toxins*, (A. L. Harvey, ed.), Pergamon Press, NY (in press).

Benoit, E., and Dubois, J. M. (1986) Toxin I from the snake *Dendroaspis polylepis polylepis:* a highly specific blocker of one type of potassium channel in myelinated nerve fiber. *Brain Res.* 377:374—377.

Boquet, P. (1970) Action de la toxine γ du venin de *Naja nigricollis* sur les cellules KB cultivées in vitro. *C. R. Acad. Sci. Paris* 271:2422—2425.

Boquet, P. (1979) Immunological properties of snake venoms. In *Snake Venoms, Handbook of Experimental Pharmacology*, Vol. 52, (C. Y. Lee, ed.), Springer-Verlag, Berlin, 751—824.

Bouchier, C., Ducancel, F., Guignery-Frelat, G., Bon, C., Boulain, J.-C., and Ménez, A. (1988) Cloning and sequencing of cDNAs encoding the two subunits of crotoxin. *Nucleic Acids Res.* 16:9050.

Boulain, J.-C. (1979) Etude de la structure antigénique d'une neurotoxine courte: la toxine α de *Naja nigricollis*. Thèse de 3ème cycle. Université P. et M. Curie, Paris.

Boulain, J.-C., and Ménez, A. (1982) Neurotoxin-specific immunoglobulins accelerate dissociation of the neurotoxin-acetylcholine receptor complex. *Science* 217:732—733.

Boulain, J.-C., Ménez, A., Couderc, J., Faure, G., Liacopoulos, P., and Fromageot, P. (1982) Neutralizing monoclonal antibody specific for *Naja nigricollis* toxin α: preparation, characterization and localization of the antigenic binding site. *Biochemistry* 21:2910—2915.

Boulain, J.-C., Fromageot, P., and Ménez, A. (1985) Further evidence showing that neurotoxin-acetylcholine receptor dissociation is accelerated by monoclonal neurotoxin-specific immunoglobulin. *Mol. Immunol.* 22:533—556.

Bourne, P. E., Sato, A., Corfield, P. W. R., Rosen, L. S., Birken, S., and Low, B. W. (1985) Erabutoxin b. Initial protein refinement and sequence analysis at 0.140-nm resolution. *Eur. J. Biochem.* 153:521—527.

Brown, S. C., Donlan, M. E., and Jeffs, P. W. (1990) Structural studies of endothelin by CD and NMR. In *Peptides, Chemistry, Structure and Biology. Proc. 11th Am. Pep. Symp.* (J. E. Rivier, and G. R. Marshall, eds.), Leiden, the Netherlands, 595—597.

Brunie, S., Bolin, J., Gewirth, D., and Sigler, P. B. (1985) The refined crystal structure of dimeric phospholipase A_2 at 2.5 Å. Access to a shielded catalytic center. *J. Biol. Chem.* 260:9742—9749.

Calmette, A. (1907) *Les Venins. Les Animaux Venimeux et la Sérothérapie Antivenimeuse.* Masson et Cie, Paris.

Campbell, C. H. (1979) Symptomatology, pathology, and treatment of the bites of elapid snakes. In *Snake Venoms, Handbook of Experimental Pharmacology,* Vol. 52, (C. Y. Lee, ed.), Springer-Verlag, Berlin, 898—921.

Chang, C. C., Hong, S. J., and Su, M. J. (1983) A study of the membrane depolarization of skeletal muscles caused by a scorpion toxin, sea anemone toxin II and crotamine and the interactions between toxins. *Br. J. Pharmacol.* 79:673—680.

Changeux, J. P. (1990) Functional architecture and dynamics of the nicotinic acetylcholine receptor: an allosteric ligand-gated ion channel. In *Fidia Research Foundation Neuroscience Award Lectures,* Vol. 4, Raven Press, NY.

Charpentier, I., Pillet, L., Karlsson, E., Couderc, J., and Ménez, A. (1990) Recognition of the acetylcholine receptor binding site of a long-chain neurotoxin by toxin-specific monoclonal antibodies. *J. Mol. Recognition* 3:74—81.

Chatrenet, B., Trémeau, O., Bontems, F., Goeldner, M. P., Hirth, C. G., and Ménez, A. (1990) Topography of toxin-acetylcholine receptor complexes by using photoactivatable toxin derivatives. *Proc. Natl. Acad. Sci. U.S.A.* 87:3378—3382.

Chuang, L.-Y., Lin, S.-R., Chang, S.-F., and Chang, C.-C. (1989) Preparation and characterization of monoclonal antibody specific for α-bungarotoxin and localization of the epitope. *Toxicon* 27:211—219.

Chwetzoff, S. (1990) On the mode of action of basic phospholipase A_2 from *Naja nigricollis* venom. *Biochim. Biophys. Acta* 1045:285—290.

Chwetzoff, S., Tsunasawa, S., Sakiyama, F., and Ménez, A. (1989) Nigexine, a Phospholipase A_2 from cobra venom with cytotoxic properties not related to esterase activity. *J. Biol. Chem.* 264:13.289—13.297.

Corfield, P. W. R., Lee, T.-J., and Low, B. W. (1989) The crystal structure of erabutoxin a at 2.0-Å resolution. *J. Biol. Chem.* 264:9239—9242.

Dennis, M. S., Henzel, W. J., Pitti, R. M., Lipari, M. T., Napier, M. A., Deisher, T. A., Bunting, S., and Lazarus, R. A. (1989) Platelet glycoprotein IIb-IIIa protein antagonists from snake venoms: evidence for a family of platelet-aggregation inhibitors. *Proc. Natl. Acad. Sci. U.S.A.* 87:2471—2475.

Dijkstra, B. W., Kalk, K. H., Hol, W. G. J., and Drenth, J. (1981) Structure of bovine pancreatic phospholipase A_2 at 1.7 Å resolution. *J. Mol. Biol.* 147:97—123.

Drenth, J., Low, B. W., Richardson, J. S., and Wright, C. S. (1980) The toxin-agglutinin fold. A new group of small protein structures organized around a four-disulfide core. *J. Biol. Chem.* 255:2652—2655.

Dreyer, F. (1990) Peptide toxins and potassium channels. *Rev. Physiol. Biochem. Pharmacol.* 115:93—136.

Ducancel, F., Guignery-Frelat, G., Tamiya, T., Boulain, J.-C., and Ménez, A. (1989) Postsynaptically-acting toxins and proteins with phospholipase structure from snake venoms: Complete amino acid sequences deduced from cDNAs and production of a toxin with staphylococcal protein A gene fusion vector. In *Natural Toxins, Characterization, Pharmacology and Therapeutics, Proc. of the 9th World Congress on Animal, Plant and Microbial Toxins,* Stillwater, Oklahoma, August 1988 (C. L. Ownby, and G. V. Odell, eds.), Pergamon Press, Oxford, 79—93.

Ducancel, F., Rowan, E. G., Cassar, E., Harvey, A. L., Ménez, A., and Boulain, J.-C. (1991) Amino acid sequence of a muscarinic toxin deduced from the cDNA nucleotide sequence. *Toxicon* 29:516—520.

Dufton, M. J., Eaker, D., and Hider, R. C. (1983) Conformational properties of phospholipases A_2. Secondary-structure prediction, circular dichroism and relative interface hydrophobicity. *Eur. J. Biochem.* 137:537—544.

Endo, T., and Tamiya, N. (1987) Current view on the structure-function relationship of postsynaptic neurotoxins from snake venoms. *Pharmacol. Ther.* 34:403—451.

Endo, T., Oya, M., Tamiya, N., and Miyazawa, T. (1987) Proton nuclear magnetic resonance characterization of phospholipase A_2 from *Laticauda semifasciata*. *J. Biochem.* 101:795—804.

Endo, S., Inooka, H., Ishibashi, Y., Kitada, C., Mizuta, E., and Fujino, M. (1989) Solution conformation of endothelin determined by nuclear magnetic resonance and distance geometry. *FEBS Lett.* 257:149—154.

Faure, G., Boulain, J.-C., Bouet, F., Montenay-Garestier, T., Fromageot, P., and Ménez, A. (1983) Role of indole and amino groups in the structure and function of *Naja nigricollis* toxin α. *Biochemistry* 22:2068—2076.

Folhman, J., Eaker, D., Karlsson, E., and Thesleff, S. (1976) Taipoxin, an extremely potent presynaptic neurotoxin from the venom of the Australian snake taipan *(Oxyuranus s. scutellatus)*. Isolation, characterization, quaternary structure and pharmacological properties. *Eur. J. Biochem.* 68:457—469.

Francis, M. J., Hastings, G. Z., Syred, A. D., Mc Ginn, B., Brown, F., and Rowlands, D. J. (1987) Non-responsiveness to a foot-and-mouth disease virus peptide overcome by addition of foreign helper T-cell determinant. *Nature (London)* 300:168—170.

Gan, Z.-R., Gould, R. J., Jacobs, J. W., Friedman, P. A., and Polokoff, M. A. (1988) Echistatin: a potent platelet aggregation inhibitor from the venom of the viper, *echis carinatus*. *J. Biol. Chem.* 263:19827—19832.

Gan, Z.-R., Condra, J. H., Gould, R. J., Zivin, R. A., Bennett, C. D., Jacobs, J. W., Friedman, P. A., and Polokoff, M. A. (1989) High-level expression in *Escherichia coli* of a chemically synthetized gene for [Leu-28] echistatin. *Gene* 79:159—166.

Gatineau, E., Toma, F., Montenay-Garestier, T., Takechi, M., Fromageot, P., and Ménez, A. (1987) Role of tyrosine and tyrptophan residues in the structure-activity relationships of a cardiotoxin from *Naja nigricollis* venom. *Biochemistry* 26:8046—8055.

Gatineau, E., Lee, C. Y., Fromageot, P., and Ménez, A. (1988) Reversal of snake neurotoxin binding to mammalian acetylcholine receptor by specific antiserum. *Eur. J. Biochem.* 171:535—539.

Gatineau, E., Takechi, M., Bouet, F., Mansuelle, P., Rochat, H., Harvey, A. L., Montenay-Garestier T., and Ménez, A. (1990) Delineation of the functional site of a snake venom cardiotoxin: preparation, structure, and function of monoacetylated derivatives. *Biochemistry* 29:6480—6489.

Good, M. F., Lee Maloy, W., Lunde, M. N., Margalit, H., Cornette, J. L., Smith, G. L., Moss, B., Miller, L. H., and Berzofsky, J. A. (1987) Construction of synthetic immunogen: use of new T-helper epitope on malaria circumsporozoite protein. *Science* 235:1059—1062.

Grognet, J.-M., Gatineau, E., Bougis, P., Harvey, A. L., Couderc, J., Fromageot, P., and Ménez, A. (1986) Two neutralizing monoclonal antibodies specific for *Naja nigricollis* cardiotoxin: preparation, characterization and localization of the epitopes. *Mol. Immunol.* 23:1329—1337.

Guillon, V. (1985) Purification et cristallisation du fragment Fab de l'anticorps monoclonal anti-neurotoxine et du complexe neurotoxine-Fab anti-neurotoxine. D.E.A. Université, Paris.

Halpert, J., and Eaker, D. (1975) Amino acid sequence of a presynaptic neurotoxin from the venom of *Notechis scutatus scutatus* (Australian tiger snake). *J. Biol. Chem.* 250:6990—6997.

Harvey, A. L. (1985) Cardiotoxins from cobra venoms: possible mechanisms of action. *J. Toxicol. Toxin Rev.* 4:41—69.

Harvey, A. L., and Anderson, A. J. (1985) Dendrotoxins: snake toxins that block potassium channels and facilitate neurotransmitter release. *Pharmacol. Ther.* 31:33—55.

Harvey, A. L., Anderson, A. J., Marshall, D. L., Pemberton, K. E., and Rowan, E. G. (1990) Facilitatory neurotoxins and transmitter release. *J. Toxicol. Toxin Rev.* 9:225—242.

Henderson, J. T., Nieman, R. A., and Bieber, A. L. (1987) Assignment of the aromatic 1H-NMR resonances of myotoxin a isolated from the venom of *Crotalus viridis viridis*. *Biochim. Biophys. Acta* 914:152—161.

Hollecker, M., and Larcher, D. (1989) Conformational forces affecting the folding pathways of dendrotoxins I and K from black mamba venom. *Eur. J. Biochem.* 179:87—94.

Hong, S. J., and Chang, C. C. (1985) Electrophysiological studies of myotoxin a isolated from prairie rattlesnake *(Crotalus viridis viridis)* venom, on murine skeletal muscles. *Toxicon* 23:927—937.

Huang, T. F., Holt, J. C., Lukasiewicz, H., and Niewiarowski, S. (1987) Trigramin. A low molecular weight peptide inhibiting fibritinogen interaction with platelet receptors expressed on glycoprotein IIb-IIIa complex. *J. Biol. Chem.* 262:16157—16163.

Huang, T. F., Holt, J. C., Kirby, E. P., and Niewiarowski, S. (1989) Trigramin: primary structure and its inhibition of von Willebrand factor binding to glycoprotein IIb/IIIa complex on human platelets. *Biochemistry* 28:661—666.

Ishikawa, Y., Ménez, A., Hori, H., Yoshida, H., and Tamiya, N. (1977) Structure of snake toxins and their affinity to the acetylcholine receptor of fish electric organ. *Toxicon* 15:477—488.

Itoh, N., Tanaka, N., Mihashi, S., and Yamashina, I. (1987) Molecular cloning and sequence analysis of cDNA for Batroxobin, a thrombin-like snake venom enzyme. *J. Biol. Chem.* 262:3132—3135.
Janin, J., and Chothia, C. (1990) The structure of protein-protein recognition sites. *J. Biol. Chem.* 265:16027—16030.
Joubert, F. J., and Taljaard, N. (1980) The amino acid sequence of two proteinase inhibitor homologues from *Dendroaspis angusticeps* venom. *Hoppe-Seyler's Z. Physiol. Chem.* 361:661—674.
Karlsson, E., Mbugua, P. M., and Rodriguez-Ithurralde, D. (1985) Anticholinesterase toxins. *Pharmac. Ther.* 30:259—276.
Kase, R., Kitagawa, H., Hayashi, K., Tanoue, K., and Inagaki, F. (1989) Neutralizing monoclonal antibody specific for α-bungarotoxin: preparation and characterization of the antibody, and localization of antigenic region of α-bungarotoxin. *FEBS Lett.* 254:106—110.
Kini, R. M., and Evans, H. J. (1988) Correlation between the enzymatic activity, anticoagulant activity and platelet effects of phospholipase A_2 isoenzymes from *Naja nigricollis* venom. *Thromb. Haemos.* 60:170—173.
Kishimoto, T., and Hirano, T. (1989) B Lymphocyte activation, proliferation, and immunoglobulin secretion. In *Fundamental Immunology* (W. E. Paul, ed.), Raven Press, NY, 385—411.
Kloog, Y., Ambar, I., Sokolovsky, M., Kochva, E., Wollberg, Z., and Bdolah, A. (1988) Sarafotoxin, a novel vasoconstrictor peptide: phosphoinositide hydrolysis in rat heart and brain. *Science* 242:268—270.
Kobayashi, Y. (1990) Solution conformation of endothelin. In *Peptides, Chemistry, Structure and Biology. Proc. 11th Am. Pep. Symp.* (J. E. Rivier, and G. R. Marshall, eds.), 552—556.
Köhler, G., and Milstein, C. (1975) Continuous cultures of fused cells secreting antibody of predefined specificity. *Nature (London)* 256:495—497.
Kondo, K., Narita, K., and Lee, C.-Y. (1978) Amino acid sequences of the two polypeptide chains in β_1-bungarotoxin from the venom of *Bungarus multicinctus* (Formosan banded krait). *J. Biochem.* 83:101—115.
Kondo, K., Toda, H., Narita, K., and Lee, C.-Y. (1982) Amino acid sequences of three β-bungarotoxins (β_3-, β_4- and β_5-bungarotoxins) from *Bungarus multicinctus* venom. Amino acid substitutions in the A Chains. *J. Biochem.* 91:1531—1548.
Kornalik, F. (1985) The influence of snake venom enzymes on blood coagulation. *Pharmacol. Ther.* 29:353—405.
Labhardt, A. M., Hunziker-Kwik, E.-H., and Wüthrich, K. (1988) Secondary structure determination for α-neurotoxin from *Dendroaspis polylepis polylepis* based on sequence-specific ^{1}H-nuclear-magnetic-resonance assignments. *Eur. J. Biochem.* 177:295—305.
Laplante, S. R., Mikou, A., Robin, M., Guittet, E., Delsuc, M., Charpentier, I., and Lallemand, J.-Y. (1990) Rapid determination and NMR assignments of anti-parallel sheets and helices of a scorpion and a cobra toxin. *Int. J. Pept. Prot. Res.* 36:227—230.
Leclerc, C., Przewlocki, G., Schutze, M.-P., and Chedid, L. (1987) A synthetic vaccine constructed by copolymerization of B and T cell determinants. *Eur. J. Immunol.* 17:269—273.
Le Du, M. H., Marchot, P., Bougis, P. E., and Fontecilla-Camps, J. C. (1989) Crystals of fasciculin 2 from green mamba snake venom. Preparation and preliminary X-ray analysis. *J. Biol. Chem.* 264:21401—21402.

Léonetti, M., Pillet, L., Maillère, B., Lamthanh, H., Frachon, P., Couderc, J., and Ménez, A. (1990) Immunization with a peptide having both T cell and conformationally restricted B cell epitopes elicits neutralizing antisera against a snake neurotoxin. *J. Immunol.* 145:4214—4221.

Li, Y.-S., Liu, K.-F., Wang, Q.-C., Ran, Y.-L., and Tu, G.-C. (1985) A platelet function inhibitor purified from *Vipera russelli siamensis* (Smith) snake venom. *Toxicon* 23:895—903.

Loring, R. H., and Zigmond, R. E. (1988) Characterization of neuronal nicotinic receptors by snake venom neurotoxins. *TINS* 11:73—78.

Love, R. A., and Stroud, R. M. (1986) The crystal structure of α-bungarotoxin at 2.5 Å resolution: relation to solution structure and binding to acetylcholine receptor. *Prot. Eng.* 1:37—46.

Low, B. W. (1979) The three dimensional structure of postsynapic snake neurotoxins: consideration of structure and function. In *Snake Venoms, Handbook of Experimental Pharmacology*, Vol. 52, (C. Y. Lee, ed.), Springer-Verlag, Berlin, 213—257.

Low, B. W., and Corfield, P. W. R. (1987) Acetylcholine receptor: α-toxin binding site — theoretical and model studies. *Asia Pacific J. Pharm.* 2:115—127.

Mebs, D., and Ownby, C. L. (1990) Myotoxic components of snake venoms: their biochemical and biological activities. *Pharmac. Ther.* 48:223—236.

Ménez, A. (1989) Les principales toxines des venins des serpents Elapidae et Hydrophiidae. Structure et mode d'action. In *Serpents, Venins, Envenimations*. Edition Fondation Marcel Merrieux, Lyon, France, 111—147.

Ménez, A. (1991) Immunology of snake toxins. In *Snake Toxins*, (A. L. Harvey, ed.), Pergamon Press, NY (in press).

Ménez, R., and Ducruix, A. (1990) Preliminary X-ray analysis of crystals of fasciculin 1, a potent acetylcholinesterase inhibitor from green mamba venom. *J. Mol. Biol.* 216:1—2.

Ménez, A., Morgat, J.-L., and Fromageot, P. (1971) Tritium labelling of the α-neurotoxin of *Naja nigricollis*. *FEBS Lett.* 17:333—335.

Ménez, A., Langlet, G., Tamiya, N., and Fromageot, P. (1978) Conformation of snake toxic polypeptides studied by a method of prediction and circular dichroism. *Biochimie* 60:505—516.

Ménez, A., Boulain, J.-C., and Fromageot, P. (1979) Attempts to define the antigenic structure of *Naja nigricollis* toxin α. *Toxicon* 17 (Suppl.):123.

Ménez, A., Boulain, J.-C., Bouet, F., Couderc, J., Faure, G., Rousselet, A., Trémeau, O., Gatineau, E., and Fromageot, P. (1984) On the molecular mechanisms of neutralization of a cobra neurotoxin by specific antibodies. *J. Physiol. (Paris)* 79:196—206.

Ménez, A., Gatineau, E., Roumestand, C., Harvey, A. L., Mouawad, L., Gilquin, B., and Toma, F. (1990) Do cardiotoxins possess a funcitonal site? Structural and chemical modification studies reveal the functional site of the cardiotoxin from *Naja nigricollis*. *Biochimie* 72:575—588.

Mitchison, N. A. (1971) The carrier effect in the secondary response to hapten-protein conjugates. II. Cellular cooperation. *Eur. J. Immunol.* 1:18—27.

Mollier, P., Chwetzoff, S., Bouet, F., Harvey, A. L., and Ménez, A. (1989) Tryptophan 110, a residue involved in the toxic activity but not in the enzymatic activity of notexin. *Eur. J. Biochem.* 185:263—270.

Mourier, G., Gatineau, E., Ménez, A., and Nicolas, P. (1989) Identification of a topographic epitope at the surface of a cardiotoxic protein. In *Peptides 1988, Proc. 20th Eur. Pep. Symp.* (G. Jung, and E. Bayer, eds.), Walter de Gruyter, Berlin, New York, 721—723.

Ouyang, C., and Huang, T.-F. (1983) Potent platelet aggregation inhibitor from *trimeresurus gramineus* snake venom. *Biochim. Biophys. Acta* 757:332—341.

Palmenberg, A. (1987) A vaccine for the common cold? *Nature (London)* 329:668—669.

Rees, B., Samama, J. P., Thierry, J. C., Gilibert, M., Fischer, J., Schweitz, H., Lazdunski, M., and Moras, D. (1987) Crystal structure of a snake venom cardiotoxin. *Proc. Natl. Acad. Sci. U.S.A.* 84:3132—3136.

Reid, H. A. (1979) Symptomatology, pathology and treatment of the bites of sea snakes. In *Snake venoms, Handbook of Experimental Pharmacology*, Vol. 52, (C. Y. Lee, ed.), Springer-Verlag, Berlin, 922—955.

Renetseder, R., Brunie, S., Dijkstra, B. W., Drenth, J., and Sigler, P. B. (1985) A comparison of the crystal structures of phospholipase A_2 from bovine pancreas and *Crotalus atrox* venom. *J. Biol. Chem.* 260:11627—11634.

Ritonja, A., Turk, V., and Gubensek, F. (1983) Serine proteinase inhibitors from *Vipera ammodytes* venom. Isolation and kinetic studies. *Eur. J. Biochem.* 133:427—432.

Rosenberg, P. (1986) The relationship between enzymatic activity and pharmacological properties of phospholipases in natural poisons. In *Natural Toxins. Animal, Plant and Micriobial* (J. B. Harris, ed.), Clarenton Press, Oxford, 129—174.

Roumestand, C., Gatineau, E., Gilquin, B., Ménez, A., and Toma, F. (1990) Site-directed chemical modifications as an aid for the three-dimensional structure studies of the toxic site of a cardiotoxin using proton NMR and distance geometry calculations. In *Peptides, Chemistry, Structure and Biology, Proc. 11th Am. Symp.* (J. E. Rivier, and G. R. Marshall, eds.), Leiden, The Netherlands, 622—624.

Rousselet, A., Faure, G., Boulain, J.-C., and Ménez, A. (1984) The interaction of neurotoxin derivatives with either acetylcholine receptor or a monoclonal antibody. An electron-spin-resonance study. *Eur. J. Biochem.* 140:31—37.

Roy, S., Scherer, M. T., Briner, T. J., Smith, J. A., and Gefter, M. L. (1989) Murine MHC polymorphism and T cell specificities. *Science* 244:572—575.

Sakurai, T., Yanagisawa, M., Takuwa, Y., Miyazaki, H., Kimura, S., Goto, K., and Masaki, T. (1990) Cloning of a cDNA encoding a non-isopeptide-selective subtype of the endothelin receptor. *Nature (London)* 348:732—735.

Saudek, V., Hoflack, J., and Pelton, J. T. (1989) 1H-NMR study of endothelin, sequence-specific assignment of the spectrum and a solution structure. *FEBS Lett.* 257:145—148.

Shafqat, J., Zaidi, Z. H., and Jörnvall, H. (1990) Purification and characterization of a chymotrypsin Kunitz inhibitor type of polypeptide from the venom of cobra *(Naja naja naja)*. *FEBS Lett.* 275:6—8.

Slotboom, A. J., Verheij, H. M., and De Haas, G. H. (1982) On the mechanism of phospholipase A_2. *Phospholipids*, Vol. 4, (J. N. Hawthorne, and G. B. Ansell, eds.), Elsevier Biomedical, Amsterdam, 359—434.

Takagi, J., Sekiya, F., Kasahara, K., Inada, Y., and Saito, Y. (1988) Venom from southern copperhead snake *(Agkistrodon contortix contortrix)*. II. A unique phospholipase A_2 that induces platelet aggregation. *Toxicon* 26:199—206.

Takechi, M., Tanaka, Y., and Hayashi, K. (1986) Binding of cardiotoxin analogue III from formosan cobra venom to FL cells. *FEBS Lett.* 205:143—146.

Tamiya, T., Lamouroux, A., Julien, J.-F., Grima, B., Mallet, J., Fromageot, P., and Ménez, A. (1985) Cloning and sequence analysis of the cDNA encoding a snake neurotoxin precursor. *Biochimie* 67:185—189.

Thiéry, C., Nabedryk-Viala, E., Ménez, A., Fromageot, P., and Thiéry, J. M. (1980) Hydrogen exchange kinetics and dynamic structure of erabutoxin b from [¹H] NMR and infrared spectrometry. *Biochem. Biophys. Res. Commun.* 93:889—897.

Trémeau, O., Boulain, J.-C., Couderc, J., Fromageot, P., and Ménez, A. (1986) A monoclonal antibody which recognized the functional site of snake neurotoxins and which neutralizes all short-chain variants. *FEBS Lett.* 208:236—240.

Tsernoglou, D., and Petsko, G. A. (1976) The crystal structure of a postsynaptic-neurotoxin from sea snake at 2.2 Å resolution. *FEBS Lett.* 68:1—4.

Tyler, M. I., Barnett, D., Nicholson, P., Spence, I., and Howden, M. E. H. (1987) Studies on the subunit structure of textilotoxin, a potent neurotoxin from the venom of the Australian common brown snake *(Pseudonaja textilis). Biochim. Biophys. Acta* 915:210—216.

Utkin, Y. N., Lazakovich, E. M., Kasheverov, I. E., and Tsetlin, V. I. (1989) α-Bungarotoxin interacts with the rat brain tachykinin receptors. *FEBS Lett.* 255:111—115.

Vick, J. A., Von Bredow, J., Grenan, M. M., and Pickwell, G. M. (1975) Sea snake antivenin and experimental envenomation therapy. In *The Biology of Sea Snake* (W. A. Dunson, ed.), University Park Press, Baltimore, MD, 463—485.

Vidal, C., and Changeux, J.-P. (1989) Phamacological profile of nicotinic acetylcholine receptors in the rat prefrontal cortex: an electrophysiological study in a slice preparation. *Neuroscience* 29:261—270.

Volpe, P., Damiani, E., Maurer, A., and Tu, A. T. (1986) Interaction of myotoxin a with the Ca^{2+}-ATPase of skeletal muscle sarcoplasmic reticulum. *Arch. Biochem. Biophys.* 246:90—97.

Walkinshaw, M. D., Saenger, W., and Maelicke, A. (1980) Three-dimensional structure of the "long" neurotoxin from cobra venom. *Proc. Natl. Acad. Sci. U.S.A.* 77:2400—2404.

Warrell, D. A. (1986) Tropical snake bite: clinical studies in southeast Asia. In *Natural Toxins. Animal, plant and microbial* (J. B. Harris, ed.), Clarenton Press, Oxford, 25—45.

White, S. P., Scott, D. L., Otwinowski, Z., Gelb, M. H., and Sigler, P. B. (1990) Crystal structure of cobra-venom phospholipase A_2 in a complex with a transition-state analogue. *Science* 250:1560—1563.

Yu, C., Lee, C.-S., Chuang, L.-C., Shei, Y.-R., and Wang, C. Y. (1990) Two-dimensional NMR studies and secondary structure of cobrotoxin in aqueous solution. *Eur. J. Biochem.* 193:789—799.

Chapter

14

Antibody Subclasses

Roy Jefferis
The University of Birmingham
School of Medical Science
Division of Immunology
Edgbaston, Birmingham, U.K.

INTRODUCTION

The earliest studies of antibodies, or immunoglobulins, revealed physicochemical and functional heterogeneity. The availability of homogeneous paraproteins in humans (myeloma proteins) and mice (plasmacytomas) allowed the structural basis for this heterogeneity to be revealed and the Ig classes and subclasses to be defined. The WHO criteria for the definition of an Ig class or subclass, now collectively referred to as isotypes, is the antigenic uniqueness of the heavy polypeptide chains (Ballieux et al., 1964; Terry and Fahey, 1964; Grey and Kunkel, 1964; World Health Organization, 1966). At the time it was not fully appreciated that this criterion could depend critically on the species combination used to raise antisera, which was usually the rabbit at that time and followed later by sheep. Fortunately, these original designations have been confirmed by later serological and structural analysis and the isotypes so defined are now known to be products of distinct immunoglobulin genes (Honjo, 1983; Rathbun et al., 1989).

A complete understanding of the unique contribution that each of the nine human Ig isotypes makes to immune protection is essential if we are to advance the development of effective vaccines and reveal the cellular and molecular basis for humoral immune deficiencies. Until recently study of the humoral immune response focused on polyclonal antibody specific for whole organisms or macromolecular antigens. However, experience with murine and human monoclonal antibodies has taught us that immune protection or therapeutic benefit may be obtained with a single antibody species if it is of the correct isotype and epitope specificity. It is this knowledge that provides the theoretical justification for seeking to develop peptide vaccines. However, it will not be sufficient simply to provoke an antibody response but it will also be necessary to present the antigen so that the most efficacious isotype is produced and memory induced. We need therefore to elucidate and understand regulation of immune responses at the levels of both the B and T cells. Therapeutic *in vivo* applications may appear more straightforward as short-term objectives are sought. However, here also there exists the potential for new and far-reaching developments, using genetic engineering techniques to produce customized antibody molecules having a predetermined profile of effector functions (Bruggemann et al., 1987; Duncan et al., 1988).

COMPARISONS BETWEEN SPECIES

Humoral immunity in the lower vertebrates is provided by a single IgM-like antibody isotype. Multiple isotypes are first seen in amphibia and the five classes in the higher mammals and aves. The emergence of subclasses would appear to offer the possibility of further functional specialization, although the number of IgG isotypes is very variable. Whereas the human, mouse, and rat have four subclasses, bovids and ungulates have two and the rabbit only one. There is evidence that the subclasses arose in humans and the mouse after speciation, and there is no reason to suppose that we can identify equivalent IgG isotypes between these two species. This is an important consideration when deciding which murine or rat monoclonal antibody isotype may be optimal for *in vivo* diagnostic or therapeutic applications. The many problems, anticipated and experienced, arising from treatments with heterologous reagents have led to the development of various strategies for the "humanization" of antibodies (Bruggemann et al., 1987; Steplewski et al., 1988). For the purposes of this chapter, I shall anticipate a future in which only human antibodies are relevant to human disease and its treatment, and consequently restrict my discussion to the human antibody subclasses.

Immune protection requires the development of a specific response that prevents potentially infective microorganisms from colonizing or penetrating body tissues. In the intact individual (without skin or body lesions), the sites most vulnerable to infection are at mucosal surfaces, which present living tissue bathed in fluid, and at body temperature to an essentially external environment. Immune protection is afforded by the mucosal system which is predominantly mediated through the IgA1 and IgA2 subclass antibodies. When this barrier fails and there is overt infection, antibody is required not only to bind antigens but also to remove, inactivate, or kill target microorganisms. This requires the activation of one or more of a wide range of effector mechanisms mediated by IgG antibodies. For clarity, these two antibody classes and their subclasses shall be considered separately before commenting on their interrelationships.

TABLE 1.
Biological Activities of Human IgG

Fab Mediated	Fc Mediated
Antigen binding	huFcγRI recognition
C3b, 4b binding	huFcγRII recognition
	huFcγRIII recognition
	C1 activation
	Placental transfer
	Catabolism
	Rheumatoid factor binding
	Protein A ⎱ binding of viral and
	Protein G ⎰ bacterial "Fc" receptors

IgG — THE MULTIFUNCTIONAL MOLECULE

The activities of IgG are determined by different functional regions of the molecule. The Fab (fragment antigen binding) regions determine antigen binding specificity and are prime sites for covalent binding of C3b and C4b. The multiple effector functions mediated by this isotype are determined by Fc (fragment crystallizable) structure, together with regulation and hemostatic control (Table 1). However, these diverse activities may only be expressed if an essential flexibility in overall structure is possible, and this is ensured by the hinge-region sequence. (For a comprehensive review of the human subclasses see Shakib, 1990; Jefferis, 1990a, 1990b; Jefferis and Kumararatne, 1990.)

Since the antigen-binding site is the product of variable-region gene segments and has been discussed in detail in Chapter 3, I shall restrict myself to the observation that, although there is very clear evidence that IgG antibody to certain antigens is restricted in its distribution between the subclasses (Table 2), this is not necessarily evidence that there is restriction in the expression of V-region gene segments with C-region genes. At immunological maturity it may be anticipated that the entire repertoire of antigen-recognition specificity is expressed within the B cell population and, hence, through surface IgM and IgD. The site at which a B cell is stimulated by antigen will determine the local environmental factors to which it may be exposed. This, in turn, may determine the pattern of C-region gene switching and hence the isotype of the predominant antibody product. The influence of the local environment on isotype expression is well illustrated by the mucosal immune system with the predominant production of IgA. Our understanding of regulatory mechanisms determining IgG subclass production is at an elementary level but parameters to be included for future study are the following:

1. The nature of the antigen, e.g., thymus dependent or independent
2. The antigen-presenting cell
3. The site at which the antigen is presented
4. Cytokines released as a result of antigen presentation to reactive cells

TABLE 2.
Subclass Profile of Specific Antibody Responses

Antigen	IgG1	IgG2	IgG3	IgG4
Tetanus toxoid	+++	+	+	++
Polysaccharides	+	+++	+	(+)
Rhesus-D	+++	−	+++	−
Factor VIII	−	−	−	+++
Phospholipase A_2	+++	+	+	+
Phospholipase A_2[a]	+	+	+	+++

[a] Following long-term (chronic) antigenic stimulation in bee-keepers who are constantly stung.

TABLE 3.
Human Immunoglobulin Allotypes

	Heavy Chains					Light Chains
Isotype/type	IgG1	IgG2	IgG3	IgA	IgE	K
Allotypes	G1m	G2m	G3m	A2m	Em	Km(Inv)
	a(1)	n(23)	g1(21), g5(28)	1	1	1
	x(2)		b0(11), b1(5)	2		2
	f(3)		b3(13), b4(14)			3
	z(17)		b5(10), s(15)			
			t(16), c3(6)			
			c5(24), u(26)			
			v(27)			

HEAVY CHAIN CONSTANT REGIONS

Immunoglobulin heavy chains are encoded by rearranged V-region gene segments and the isotype-specific invariant gene segments. However, there is polymorphism within human populations and many allotypic variants have been defined (Table 3). The functional role of the C_{H1} domain, in association with the C_L domain of the light chain, is unclear. However, it does act as an enzyme-resistant "spacer" between the antigen-binding site and the Fc region, which may facilitate access to the multiple ligand-binding sites expressed by this protein moiety. Thus, although bacteria may engage each of the antigen-binding sites, the Fc region is still able to engage an Fc receptor on the surface of a monocyte. The Fab regions of all antibody isotypes, with the exception of IgD, are relatively resistant to proteolysis. This requires that Cκ and Cλ domains pair with nine different C_H domains to form globular enzyme-resistant structures. Whereas it is established that the Fab forms a primary site for deposition of C3b and C4b, it is not clear whether this is due to the presence of a specific acceptor site for these reactive species or whether they are generated and released in the vicinity of the Fab regions (Law and Reid, 1988). The interaction site is not clearly defined, but there is no evidence for differential reactivity between the subclasses.

TABLE 4.
Recognition Specificity of huFcγR

huFcγ	IgG1	IgG2	IgG3	IgG4
RI	+++	−	+++	++
RII	+	−	+	−
RIII	+	−	+	−

THE HINGE AND Fc REGION

Maximal sequence differences between the IgG subclasses is evident in the hinge region (Jefferis, 1990a). The number of residues and interheavy chain disulfide bridges constituting the hinge influences the relative mobility of the Fc and Fabs, with respect to each other, and, consequently, the accessibility of Fc effector sites. The multiple disulfide bridges of the extended IgG3 hinge region is thought to act as a semirigid spacer, allowing unrestricted access to Fc effector sites, thus accounting for the relative efficiency of IgG3 in activating complement, etc. Reduction of hinge-region disulfide bridges does not result in loss of IgG structural integrity since there are multiple noncovalent interactions between the C_{H3} domains.

It will be apparent from Tables 2 and 4 that the IgG subclass profile of an antibody response will determine the effector functions that may be activated to neutralize and eliminate infective microorganisms. Similarly, the outcome of *in vivo* administration of human, or murine, monoclonal antibodies will be determined, in part, by the isotype. Furthermore, if the amino acid residues directly determining biological function are identified, it may be possible, using protein engineering techniques, to modulate selected functions and produce "customized" antibody molecules (Duncan and Winter, 1988; Duncan et al., 1988; Ward et al., 1989). Essential to the study of all aspects of the biological activity of these antibodies is the availability of specific serological reagents.

HETEROLOGOUS ANTIBODIES TO IgG SUBCLASSES

Since there is >95% sequence homology between the IgG subclasses, immunization with any subclass paraprotein provokes the production of antibodies cross-reactive between the subclasses. Extensive absorption allows the preparation of specific polyclonal reagents that can be applied in relatively insensitive techniques. Secure reagents have become widely available through the development of monoclonal antibodies specific for each IgG subclass (Lowe et al., 1982; Reimer et al., 1984). The specificity and reactivity of a panel of 54 monoclonal antibodies of putative subclass specificity was evaluated in a WHO/IUIS (World Health Organization, International Union of Immunological Societies) collaborative study (Jefferis et al., 1985). As a result, a panel of WHO specificity reference reagents was established (Jefferis et al., 1987), and most of these antibodies are now commercially available.

There are subclass specific residues in the CH1 domain of IgG1, IgG2, and IgG4, and monoclonal antibodies have been produced that recognize subclass-specific epitopes expressed in the Fab fragments of proteins of these subclasses (Jefferis, 1986). The hinge region of IgG3 was shown to be very immunogenic, and most IgG3 subclass-specific antibodies (monoclonal and polyclonal) were shown to recognize epitopes located in the hinge region. These epitopes are lost on reduction of the interheavy chain disulfide bridges and have been used as sensitive probes for structural change in the hinge region resulting from free radical attack (Jose et al., 1987). These epitopes are also destroyed by most immunofixation protocols. However, antibodies have been produced to synthetic hinge-region peptides that react preferentially with denatured forms of IgG3 (Boersma et al., 1989). Antibodies have similarly been produced to synthetic peptides representative of IgG2 hinge-region sequences that are reactive with the native IgG2 molecule (Boersma et al., 1989).

It is of particular interest to consider the antigenicity of the Fc regions of the IgG subclasses in relation to their primary amino acid sequences and profiles of effector functions. Monoclonal antibodies have been produced that recognize epitopes specific for a given subclass, epitopes expressed on two of the four subclasses only, three of the four, etc. (Lowe et al., 1982; Reimer et al., 1984; Bird et al., 1984). These reactivity profiles may parallel those of effector function so that an antibody and a ligand, or receptor molecule, may have apparently identical specificities and one can be used as a probe for the other (Sarmay et al., 1985; Partridge et al., 1986). Since the primary structure of each Fc is known, sequence correlates for epitopes and effector sites may be identified. Thus, an antibody reactive with IgG1, IgG3, and IgG4 but not IgG2 proteins has the same reactivity profile as the human FcγRI receptor, and it inhibits the binding of the IgGs to the receptor. Examination of sequence reveals identity for IgG1 and IgG2 in the C_{H3} domain, but a unique sequence for IgG2 proteins at residues 233 to 236 (the lower hinge region) suggesting these residues to be the sequence correlates for FcγRI binding in IgG1 and the epitope recognized by the monoclonal antibody specific for IgG1, IgG3, and IgG4 proteins (non-IgG2) (Woof et al., 1986). These residues in IgG2 are the sequence correlates for an IgG2-specific epitope recognized by several monoclonal antibodies.

A further comparison relevant to antigenicity is the species combination. For many years the rabbit was used to generate polyclonal antihuman IgG Fc reagents, whereas the majority of murine monoclonal antibodies produced have been of the murine IgG1 isotype. The sequence homology between human IgG1, mouse IgG1, and rabbit Fcs is 71 and 73%, respectively. It may be anticipated that regions with maximal sequence differences will be candidates for epitopes. Thus, human IgG1 has the single subclass-specific CH2 domain amino acid residue Lys.[274] Examination of the rabbit and murine Fcs reveals that they have glutamine at this position and also differ in sequence at residues 268, 269, 276, 278, and 279, which are on the same exposed β strand (Kabat et al., 1987). It might appear, therefore, that the rabbit and murine antibodies are recognizing the same epitope. However, it is likely that Lys^{274} forms a focus for a series of overlapping nonidentical epitopes. Evidence in favor of this hypothesis is provided by two monoclonal antibodies we have produced, which are specific for IgG1-subclass proteins and exhibit mutual inhibition of binding. However, there is clear evidence for differences in fine specificity which determines their usefulness in some assay protocols. Thus, when human IgG1 is coupled to red cells, each antibody agglutinates the cells to very high titer, but when the human IgG1 is absorbed to an ELISA plate, only one antibody is able to react with the antigen presented in this way. We believe that immobilization in the ELISA protocol results in a structural change in the antigen with loss of the epitope recognized by one antibody but not the other (Jefferis, 1986).

The presence of subclass-specific residues for each subclass in the C_{H2} domain correlates with the production of antibodies having specificity for epitopes expressed in this domain. Subclass-specific epitopes in the C_{H3} domain have only been demonstrated for IgG_4, which is in accord with the presence of subclass-specific residues in the C_{H3} domain of this isotype. It has been a common experience for all groups producing subclass-specific monoclonal antibodies that IgG3- and IgG4-specific reagents are quite readily obtained, whereas IgG1 and IgG2 specificities are very difficult. Of the WHO/IUIS reagents (Jefferis et al., 1987), the anti-IgG2 are the least satisfactory, and it is hoped that better reagents can be added to the panel in the future. A second WHO/IUIS collaborative study is now complete and candidate reagents have been identified.

Other antibody specificities of interest are those that recognize epitopes expressed on only three of the four subclasses. They have been successfully applied to the purification of polyclonal IgG of a single subclass and have potential for application within quantitative assays (Bird et al., 1984; Persson, 1987; Parkes et al., 1990). Thus, where IgG2 responses are of interest, the non-IgG_2 component could be quantitated in a single assay using a monoclonal antibody reactive with IgG1, IgG3, and IgG4, that is, having non-IgG2 specificity. Our experience accords with that documented by Sarnesto (1983) that the most frequent specificities produced following immunization with IgG1, IgG2, or IgG4 are antibodies having non-IgG3 reactivity. We further demonstrated that the non-IgG3 specificity was restricted to IgG3 proteins of the G3m(u) allotype and that they did recognize IgG3 proteins of the G3m(s,t) allotype. This allows the presence of arginine at residue 435 to be identified as the sequence correlate for the non-G3m(u) specificity (Jefferis et al., 1984; Jefferis and Mageed, 1989). A similar specificity has been revealed for rheumatoid factors and "Fc receptors" produced by a wide range of bacterial and viral species (Jefferis et al., 1985; Woof and Burton, 1990). The interaction site for each of the "ligands" is mapped to the inter-C_{H2}/C_{H3} domain region and has been definitively described for the interaction of staphylococcal protein A (subfragment B) with IgG1, Fc (Diesenhofer, 1981).

HUMAN ANTIBODIES TO IgG, INCLUDING AUTOANTIBODIES

The human allotypic forms of IgG are defined by human antibodies, and the typing reagents in routine use are all of human origin. Murine monoclonal reagents have recently been produced but few have the uncomplicated specificity of the human reagents (Jefferis et al., 1985; de Lange, 1989; Nelson et al., 1990). This finding provides a further insight into the subtleties of antibody recognition. I suggest that the human reagent "sees" the allotype specific residue in the context of subclass-specific residues and fine structural differences characteristic of the subclass. Heterologous reagent "sees" the allotype-specific residue in the context of amino acid residues differing from those of its own IgG but common to those of the human IgG subclasses. The level of antigenic discrimination that can be achieved with human reagents can be illustrated by example. Thus, the anti-G1m(z) anti-allotype reagent recognizes Arg^{214} in the context of IgG1-specific residues, whereas the anti-non-G1m(z) reagent recognizes the same residue in the context of residues common to IgG1, IgG3, and IgG4 and defines an isoallotypic specificity. The source of the human reagents is there multiparous women who may be sensitized with fetal IgG when there is an allotype disparity between the parents. Another source is there individuals who have received multiple transfusions. Donors and recipients are not allotype matched for transfusion and hence the production of alloantibodies. However, the titers of anti-allotype antibodies produced are low and do not result in transfusion reactions.

Anti-allotype responses are relevant to the development of human antibodies for *in vivo* diagnostic and therapeutic applications. If there is an allotype disparity between the patient and the reagent, an anti-allotype response may be induced that will enhance elimination of the reagent following further therapy. In addition, the induction of an anti-idiotypic response may be enhanced when there is also an allotype disparity.

Rheumatoid factors are, by definition, autoantibodies having specificity for the Fc region of IgG (for a review, see Jefferis and Mageed, 1989); they were first identified in the serum of patients with rheumatoid arthritis. The presence and titer of these autoantibodies are one of the diagnostic criteria of the disease; the titer corresponds to disease activity. It is established that both rheumatoid factor and its antigen (IgG) are produced by plasma cells within the synovium of rheumatoid patients, and hence immune complexes may be formed *in situ* that activate complement and contribute to the inflammatory reactions characteristic of the disease. Since the immune complexes may also be potent immunogens, it is possible that rheumatoid factor plays a central role in generating a self-perpetuating inflammatory reaction. An interesting feature of autoimmunity is that there is a selective loss of self-recognition, so that one or a few molecular features of the autoantigen become autoimmunogenic. It is obviously of central importance to define the autoimmunogenic structure if one is to attempt to elucidate the lesion in the regulatory network of self-, nonself recognition.

Study of the specificity of the rheumatoid factor present in the serum of a rheumatoid patient (code named Ga) revealed a subclass reactivity profile of IgG1, IgG2, and IgG4 and no reactivity with IgG3 proteins tested (Allen and Kunkel, 1966). Subsequently it was shown that this was the dominant specificity for rheumatoid factors from a majority of rheumatoid patients. Recent studies have localized the epitope recognized by RF to the inter-C_{H2}/C_{H3} domain region and defined the molecular specificity more precisely. The Ga specificity was originally described using IgG3 proteins of G3m(u) allotype only. However, when proteins of the G3m(s,t) allotype were used, two specificity profiles emerged. Some RF did not bind any of the IgG3 proteins, whereas others bound the G3m(s,t) but not the G3m(u) proteins (Jefferis and Mageed, 1989). The critical amino acid interchange determining these specificities is Arg/His[435] (Jefferis et al., 1984). A parallel reactivity profile has been demonstrated for SpA binding, and His[435] is known to be a contact residue for this ligand. The overlapping specificity of RF and SpA is further demonstrated by the ability of SpA to inhibit RF binding to IgG (Nardella et al., 1988). Rheumatoid factor can be detected in the serum of normal individuals, and its induction has been observed as a normal consequence of an immune response. It is of particular interest to note that RF present in the serum of individuals without RA has been shown to be the product of germ line genes. The RF from RA patients shows evidence of somatic mutation and thus appears to be an autoantigen driven process (Shokri et al., 1990).

COMPLEMENT ACTIVATION

Complement activation by the classical pathway is a property of the IgG1 and IgG3 subclasses only; in most review articles a weak activity is usually also accorded to IgG2. However, most studies in the literature have used heterologous rather than homologous complement and assessed complement binding rather than activation. A recent study employing chimeric anti-NIP antibodies of each of the IgG subclasses demonstrated lysis of sensitized erythrocytes by IgG1 and IgG3 antibody molecules only (Bruggemann et al., 1987). A similar study using chimeric antidansyl hapten antibodies demonstrated fixation of human complement by IgG1 and IgG3 molecules only (Dangl et al., 1988). Interestingly, the IgG2 antibodies were shown to bind rabbit complement weakly, and this is probably the activity that results in most reviews ascribing a weak complement binding activity to IgG2. All studies conclude that IgG4 does not bind or activate complement.

Following a comprehensive exercise in the generation of antibody molecules, each having a single-site mutation within the C_{H2} domain, Duncan and Winter identified a motif comprising residues 318, 320, and 322 that could constitute the C1q binding site (Duncan and Winter, 1988). Although these studies were based on the mouse IgG2b molecule, it is suggested that this motif represents a general requirement for complement activation and therefore provides a route to modulate antibody function and generate noncomplement-fixing IgG1 and IgG3 molecules. A further mutant, Asp/Ala at residue 297, is of particular interest since it removes the acceptor site for glycosylation and results in the production of an aglycosylated molecule which has a threefold lower association constant for C1q and does not activate C1. Our studies suggest that aglycosylation results in very localized protein structural changes in the lower hinge region (Lund et al., 1990) distant from the identified motif.

Fc RECEPTORS

It is apparent from the different effector cell types that express Fc receptors (Pound and Walker, 1990) and the wide range of antigen elimination processes which they can trigger, that Fc receptor recognition is of fundamental significance. It is clear from virtually all published studies that the IgG1 and IgG3 isotypes are recognized by all of the receptors currently characterized. The data for IgG2 and IgG4 are incomplete and, in some instances, contradictory. It is important to establish the protective role of these isotypes and hence their Fc receptor-recognition specificity. I shall discuss the recognition specificity of each receptor in turn, and adopt the nomenclature huFcγRX, where hu denotes human, γ denotes heavy chain recognized, and X denotes the number assigned to the receptor.

huFcγRI

This receptor has been widely studied because its high affinity allows its specificity to be investigated in direct binding studies. IgG1 and IgG3 each have a K_{ass} 5 × 10^{-8} L mol^{-1} and IgG4 five- to tenfold lower, while no measurable binding activity is observed for IgG2 (Woof et al., 1986; Walker et al., 1988; Walker et al., 1989a). This isotype specificity has been confirmed, using chimeric antibodies, in the more sensitive rosette assay technique which allows low-affinity interactions to be detected (Walker et al., 1989b). In our own laboratory, we have further demonstrated that the IgG1, IgG3, and IgG4 isotypes can trigger a superoxide burst from the monocytic cell line U937 (Pound, J. D., Lund, J., and Jefferis, R., 1991). No activity was observed for IgG2.

Comparison of the primary amino acid sequences of the IgG subclasses reveals that IgG1 and IgG2 have identical sequence in the C_{H3} domain, but there are radical differences within the C_{H2} domain in the hinge-link region, embracing residues 233 to 237. In IgG4, there is a Leu/Phe interchange at residue 234 which might account for the lowered association constant observed for this isotype. Evidence from a series of indirect approaches to definition of the molecular specificity of huFcγRI led us to propose that residues 233 to 237 are crucial to recognition, and one or more may be contact residues (Woof et al., 1986). More direct evidence has been obtained with a panel of IgG3 chimeric antibodies, each having a single amino acid interchange in the proposed sequence. Complete loss of rosette formation was observed for Leu/Ala and Leu/Glu mutants at residue 235. These studies confirmed and extended the work of Duncan and Winter (1988), who showed that mutation of mouse IgG2b to effect a Glu/Leu interchange at residue 235 resulted in the production of a molecule that bound huFcγRI with an association constant equal to that observed for mouse IgG2a and the human IgG1 and IgG3 isotypes (Duncan et al., 1988). Glycosylation of the IgG molecule has also been shown to be essential for huFcγRI recognition (Walker et al., 1989b). Structural studies suggest that the oligosaccharide is not sterically available to contribute directly to FcγR binding but influences the tertiary structure of the C_{H2} domain to allow access of FcγR to the interaction site. Aglycosylation leads to a minor protein conformation change with loss of accessibility to this site (Lund et al., 1990). Since it is possible to generate many different glycoforms of an immunoglobulin, there may exist considerable potential to modulate FcγR activity through changes in the oligosaccharide structure (Rademacher et al., 1988).

huFc RII

Recent studies in our laboratory suggest that huFcγRII recognizes the IgG1 and IgG3 isotypes only (Table 4). This conclusion is based on experiments using chimeric antibodies and the huFcγRII expressing cell lines Daudi and K562 in rosette assays (Walker et al., 1988; Walker et al., 1989a). Other studies reported in the literature conclude that huFcγRII also recognizes IgG2 and IgG4. Thus, using paraprotein dimers, van de Winkle and Anderson (1991) observe the binding specificity IgG1, IgG2, and IgG3, while Simmons and Seed (1988) reported that huFcγRII expressed on COS cells exhibited an order of binding IgG1 > IgG2 = IgG4 > IgG3. This profile of subclass specificity would be appropriate for the placental huFcγR receptor since all four subclasses are actively transported from mother to fetus. In view of the wide range of cell types expressing huFcγRII and the biological effector mechanisms triggered through this receptor, it is important for these discrepancies to be resolved.

From our own data it would be consistent to argue that the interaction site for huFcγRII is determined by C_{H2} domain structure (see huFcγRI above). It is gratifying, therefore, that we have been able to demonstrate loss of huFcγRII recognition by IgG3 molecules having point mutations within residues 233 to 237. Maximal reduction in rosette formation was observed for the Leu/Ala^{234} and Gly/Ala^{237} mutants (J. Lund, pers. commun.). Reduced rosette formation was also observed for aglycosylated IgG1 and IgG3, thus extending the parallel between huFcγRI and huFcγRII recognition specificity.

huFc RIII

There is agreement from most binding (rosette) studies that huFcγRIII has recognition specificity for IgG1 and IgG3 only. This specificity profile has also been observed for lymphocyte-mediated killing of tumor cells (Steplewski et al., 1988) or NIP-sensitized cells by chimeric antibodies (Bruggemann et al., 1987). Evidence has been presented for the direct involvement of both the C_{H2} and C_{H3} domains in recognition of IgG by huFcγRIII (Sarmay et al., 1985). It was suggested that the C_{H3} domain may be essential for the formation of a receptor-ligand (IgG) bond, while a second interaction site determined activation of the cell bearing the huFcγRIII receptor. The activation site would also contribute to ligand-receptor binding energy in such a way that binding through the C_{H3} domain alone may be too weak to be observed in most systems.

Bacterial and Viral "Fc Receptors"

We are very familiar with the Fc-binding properties of staphylococcal protein A (SpA) and its exploitation as a second antibody. However, many bacterial species, and recently certain viral species, have been shown to express an Fc receptor (Woof and Burton, 1990). Since the microorganisms expressing Fc receptors are pathogenic in humans, it is likely that they facilitate infection. It has been suggested that by binding host IgG the microorganisms evade recognition by the immune system. Alternatively, if the host cellular FcγR site is still available on the bound IgG, it could provide a strategy for effecting entry into FcγR-expressing host cells. The molecular specificity of SpA is well defined from the studies of Diesenhofer (1981) of a crystalline complex of IgGFc, and a univalent fragment of SpA (fragment B) was determined by X-ray crystallography. The fragment was shown to make contacts with residues within the inter-C_{H2}/C_{H3} domain region, contributed to by both domains. Streptococcal protein G binds all four human IgG isotypes and is likely to replace SpA as universal second antibody for IgG. It has been shown to compete with SpA for binding to IgG and therefore its specificity is believed to be for a nonidentical overlapping site. Similar molecular specificities are indicated for other bacterial and viral Fc receptors. The similarities in specificity of hetero- and alloantibodies and bacterial and viral "Fc receptors" for this confined region of the IgG molecule suggest an interrelationship and a deeper significance than we can, at present, appreciate.

IgA AND MUCOSAL IMMUNITY

IgA present in the blood is the product of plasma cells of the bone marrow and is produced as part of the systemic immune response, while secretory IgA is produced by plasma cells present in the secretory glands and tissues (for reviews, see Mestecky and Russell, 1986; Underdown and Schiff, 1986; Crago and Tomasi, 1987). The two subclasses of IgA, designated IgA1 and IgA2, and the allotypic variants of IgA2 were defined by the unique antigenicity of their heavy chains in a manner similar to that described for the IgG proteins. Subsequent biochemical studies have revealed the structural basis for antigenic differences and demonstrated that the two isotypes are products of distinct genes. Allotypy is only observed for IgA2 molecules and the allotypic forms are designated A2m(1) and A2m(2). Although IgA is present in blood predominantly as a monomer, in secretions it is a dimer composed of two IgA molecules complexed with the polypeptides J chain and secretory component.

The IgA subclass proteins are structurally more dissimilar to each other than are the IgG subclass proteins. This suggests that duplication of the gene encoding for IgA is an earlier event than the duplication of the IgG gene(s). There are 20 amino acid substitutions between the constant regions and a deletion of 13 residues in the hinge region of IgA2 molecules. There are differences in the number of N-linked glycosylation sites, IgA1 having two, A2m(1) four, and A2m(2) five, and there are five O-linked oligosaccharide chains in the hinge region of IgA1 (Mestecky and Russell, 1986). Despite these structural differences, it has been difficult to produce reliable polyclonal antisera for routine qualitative and quantitative studies. The situation is considerably more complex for the secretory forms of IgA. Monoclonal reagents are now available but are subject to the same reservations expressed for the IgG subclasses. An international collaborative study to evaluate a large panel of such reagents is in progress, under the auspices of the IUIS Human Ig Subcommittee (Chairman, R. Jefferis).

SECRETORY IgA

Plasma cells producing secretory IgA also synthesize the 15-kDa protein J chain, resulting in the formation, intracellularly, of an IgA dimer composed of molecules of identical sequence and antigen specificity. The antibody product has four antigen-binding sites, although it is not certain that they can all function to bind a macromolecular antigen simultaneously. The formation of dimer IgA can result in the loss of epitopes expressed on monomer IgA, the generation of new epitopes specific to alpha chains in the dimer form, and the expression of J chain epitopes. Reagents specific for free J chains can also be produced, so that differential studies are possible. These reagents are important for the study and enumeration of IgA-producing plasma cells in tissue specimens.

To mediate its protective role, the dimer IgA must gain access to mucosal surfaces and therefore cross the epithelial barrier. This is achieved by complex formation between dimer IgA and the poly-Ig receptor expressed on the surface of the epithelial cells. This complex is internalized, transported across the cell, and reexpressed on the external surface. A proteolytic enzyme then cleaves the poly-Ig receptor with the release of the IgA dimer covalently bound to a 70-kDa component of the receptor, which is referred to as the secretory piece (Underdown and Schiff, 1986). Although expressing epitopes unique to its own structure, the presence of a secretory piece results in alterations in the epitopes expressed by the alpha and J chains. This allows for further opportunities to develop reagents specific to each molecular form and subsequent analysis of normal and pathological patterns of IgA synthesis.

The IgA2 subclass comprises only 10 to 25% of the systemic IgA response, but may comprise 30 to 60% of the IgA present in secretions. This is reflected in the proportions of IgA1- and IgA2-producing plasma cells present in the underlying tissue. IgA2 is most abundant in secretions present on the large intestine which is colonized by bacteria that produce enzymes capable of specifically degrading IgA1 molecules. It is interesting to note that these enzymes cleave at sites within the hinge region of IgA1 that is deleted from IgA2 molecules. It would appear that deletion of the hinge from IgA2 was a fortuitous evolutionary event that maintained an essential balance between the human host and commensal bacteria. Considering all of the evolutionary "coincidental" events that were required for the emergence of the mucosal immune system, it is paradoxical that selective IgA deficiency is the most common of all immunodeficiencies and is usually asymptomatic. This is due, in part, to the fact that IgM can function as a secretory immunoglobulin.

CONCLUDING OBSERVATIONS

The observation that initiated and has maintained interest in the IgG subclasses is selective IgG2 subclass deficiency and its association with recurrent chest and upper respiratory tract infection (Jefferis and Kumararatne, 1990). However, we may expect that protection at these sites should primarily be effected by secretory IgA. The accumulated clinical experience suggests that there is a critical interface between humoral and mucosal immunity at these local sites. It may be revealing that IgA deficiency combined with IgG2 or IgG2 and IgG4 deficiency is particularly associated with recurrent infection.

Immune responses are initiated at local sites where microenvironments may determine the isotype profile of the antibodies produced; this is evidently so for the mucosal immune response. To understand normal and pathological responses it will be necessary to investigate responses within local environments either *in vivo* or *in vitro* by the development of improved culture techniques for the maintenance of biopsy material. Such studies can only be as good as the reagents available. It is essential, therefore, that the development of reagents and assay techniques progress in parallel.

REFERENCES

Allen, J. C., and Kunkel, H. G. (1966) Hidden rheumatoid factors with specificity for native globulins. *Arthritis Rheum.* 9:758.

Ballieux, R. E., Bernier, G. M., Tominaga, K., and Putnam, F. W. (1964) Gammaglobulin antigenic types defined by their heavy chain determinants. *Science* 145:168—170.

Bird, P., Lowe, J., Stokes, R. P., Bird, A. G., Ling, N. R., and Jefferis, R. (1984) The separation of human IgG into subclass fractions by immunoaffinity chromatography and assessment of specific antibody activity. *J. Immunol. Meth.* 71:97.

Boersma, W. J. A., Deen, C., Gerritse, K., Zegers, N. D., Haaijman, J. J., and Claassen, E. (1989) Anti-peptide antibodies as subclass specific reagents: epitope mapping of human IgG2. *Protides Biol. Fluids* 36:161.

Boersma, W. J. A., Deen, C., Haaijman, J. J., Radl, J., and Claasen, E. (1989) Antibodies to a short synthetic peptide related to the hinge segment of human IgG3 recognizes Thermally or fixative induced conformational changes in the human IgG3 molecule. *Immunology* 68:427.

Bruggemann, M., Williams, G. T., Bindon, C. I., Clark, M. R., Walker, M. R., Jefferis, R., Waldmann, H., and Neuberger, M. S. (1987) Comparison of the effector functions of human immunoglobulins using a matched set of chimeric antibodies. *J. Exp. Med.* 166:1351.

Crago, S. S., and Tomasi, T. B. (1987) Mucosal antibodies. In *Food Allergy and Intolerance* (J. Brostoff and S. J. Challacombe, eds.), Bailliere and Tindall, Eastbourne, U.K.

Dangl, J. L., Wensel, T. G., Morrison, S. L., Stryer, L., Herzenberg, L. A., and Oi, V. T. (1988) Segmental flexibility and complement fixation of genetically engineered chimeric human, rabbit and mouse antibodies. *EMBO J.* 7:1989.

Diesenhofer, J. (1981) Crystallographic refinement and atomic models of a human Fc fragment and its complex with fragment B of protein A of *Staphylococcus aureus* at 2.9Å- and 2.8Å-resolution. *Biochemistry* 20:2361.

de Lange, G. G. (1989) Polymorphism of human immunoglobulins: Gm, Am, Em and Km. *Exp. Clin. Immunogen.* 6:7—17.

Duncan, A. R., and Winter, G. (1988) The binding site for C1q on IgG. *Nature (London)* 332:738.

Duncan, A. R., Woof, J. M., Partridge, J. M., Burton, D. R., and Winter, G. (1988) Localization of the binding site for the high-affinity Fc receptor on IgG. *Nature (London)* 332:563.

Grey, H. M., and Kunkel, H. G. (1964) H-chain subgroups of myeloma proteins and normal 7S g-globulin. *J. Exp. Med.* 120:253—266.

Isenman, D. E., Dorrington, K. J., and Painter, P. H. (1975) The structure and function of immunoglobulin domains. II. The importance of inter-chain disulphide bonds and the possible role of molecular flexibility in the interaction between immunoglobulin G and complement. *J. Immunol.* 114:1726.

Jefferis, R. (1986) Human IgG subclass epitopes recognized by murine monoclonal antibodies. *Monogr. Allergy* 19:71—85.

Jefferis, R. (1987) WHO/IUIS Programme for the standardisation of immunological reagents: availability of mouse monoclonal antibodies McAb to human IgG subclasses. *Scand. J. Immunol.* 26:459.

Jefferis, R. (1990a) The molecular structure of the IgG subclasses. In *Human IgG Subclasses — Molecular Analysis of Structure, Function and Regulation* (F. Shakib, ed.), Pergamon Press, Oxford, 15—29.

Jefferis, R. (1990b) Structure/function relationships of IgG subclasses. In *Human IgG Subclasses — Molecular Analysis of Structure, Function and Regulation* (F. Shakib, ed.), Pergamon Press, Oxford, 93—108.

Jefferis, R., and Kumararatne, D. S. (1990) Selective IgG subclass deficiency: quantification and clinical relevance. *Clin. Exp. Immunol.* 81:357.

Jefferis, R., and Mageed, R. A. (1989) The Specificity and Reactivity of Rheumatoid Factors with human IgG. *Monogr. Allergy* 26:45.

Jefferis, R., Nik Jaafar, M. I., and Steinitz, M. (1984) A human rheumatoid factor having specificity for a discontinuous epitope determined by histidine/arginine interchange as residue 435 of immunoglobulin G. *Immunol. Lett.* 7:191.

Jefferis, R., Reimer, C. B., Skvaril, F., de Lange, G., Ling, N. R., Lowe, J., Walker, M. R., Phillips, D. J., Aloisio, C. H., Wells, T. W., et al., (1985) Evaluation of monoclonal antibodies having specificity for human IgG subclasses: results of an IUIS/WHO collaborative study. *Immunol. Lett.* 10:223—252.

Jose, S. A., Lunec, J., Griffiths, H., Mageed, R. A., and Jefferis, R. (1987) Denaturation of human IgG3 by free radicals. *Mol. Immunol.* 4:1145.

Hondo, T. (1983) Immunoglobulin genes. *Ann. Rev. Immunol.* 1:499.

Kabat, E. A., Wu, T. T., Reid-Miller, M., Perry, H. M., and Gottsman, K. S. (1987) Sequences of immunological interest. 4th edition U.S. Dept. of Health Human Services Publication.

Law, S. K. A., and Reid, K. B. M. (1988) Complement. In *Focus Series* (D. Male, ed.), I.R.L. Press, Oxford.

Lowe, J., Bird, P., Hardie, D., Ling, N. R., and Jefferis, R. (1982) Monoclonal antibodies to determinants on human gamma chains: properties of antibodies showing subclass restriction or subclass specificity. *Immunology* 47:329.

Lund, J., Tanaka, T., Takahashi, N., Sarmay, G., Arata, Y., and Jefferis, R. (1990) A protein structural Change in aglycosylated IgG3 correlates with loss of huFc RI and huFc RII binding and/or activation. *Mol. Immunol.* 27:1145.

Mestecky, J., and Russell, M. W. (1986) IgA Subclasses. *Monogr. Allergy* 19:277.

Nardella, F. A., Oppliger, I. R., Stone, G. C., Sasso, E. H., Mannick, M., Sojquist, J., Schroder, A. K., Christensen, P. J. H., and Bjorck, L. (1988) Fc Epitopes for human rheumatoid factors and the relationship of rheumatoid factors to the Fc binding proteins of micro-organisms. *Scand. J. Rheumatol. (Suppl.)* 75:190.

Nelson, P. N., Fletcher, S. M., de Lange, G. G., van Leeuwen, A. M., Goodall, D. M., and Jefferis, R. (1990) Evaluation of monoclonal antibodies with putative specificity for human IgG allotypes. *Vox. Sang.* 59:190.

Parkes, A. B., Howells, R. D., Mower, J., and Hall, R. (1990) A primary standard for the ELISA of thyroglobulin and microsomal autoantibody IgG subclass associated activity. *J. Clin. Lab. Immunol.* (in press).

Partridge, L., Jefferis, R., Hardie, D., Ling, N. R., and Richardson, P. (1984) Subclasses of IgG on the surface of human lymphocytes: A study with monoclonal antibodies. *Clin. Exp. Immunol.* 56:167—174.

Partridge, L. J., Woof, J. M., Jefferis, R., and Burton, D. R. (1986) The use of anti-IgG monoclonal antibodies in mapping the monocyte receptor on IgG. *Mol. Immunol.* 23:1365.

Persson, M. A. A. (1987) Preparation of human sera containing one single subclass using affinity chromatography. *J. Immunol. Meth.* 8:91.

Pound, J. D., and Walker, M. R. (1990) Membrane Fc receptors for IgG subclasses. In *Molecular Aspects of Immunoglobulin Subclasses* (F. Shakib, ed.), Pergamon Press, Oxford.
Rademaker, T. W., Parekh, P. B., and Dwek, R. A. (1988) *Ann. Rev. Biochem.* 57:785.
Rathbun, G., Berman, J., Yancopoulos, G., and Alt, F. W. (1989) Organization and expression of the mammalian heavy-chain variable-region locus. In *Immunoglobulin Genes* (J. Honjo, F. W. Alt, and T. H. Rabbitts, eds.), Academic Press, New York.
Reimer, C. B., Philips, D. J., Aloisio, A. J., Moore, D. D., Galand, G. G., Wells T. W., Black, C. M., and McDougal, J. S. (1984) Evaluation of thirty-one monoclonal antibodies to human IgG epitopes. *Hybridoma* 3:263.
Sarmay, G., Jefferis, R., Klein, E., Benzcur, M., and Gergely, J. (1985) Mapping the functional topography of Fc with monoclonal antibodies: localization of epitopes interacting with the binding sites of Fc receptor on human K cells. *Eur. J. Immunol.* 15:1037.
Sarnesto, A. (1983) Monoclonal antibodies reacting with isotypic and/or allotypic determinants of human IgG. *Med. Biol.* 61:126.
Shakib, F. (1990) *Human IgG Subclasses — Molecular Analysis of Structure, Function and Regulation,* Pergammon Press, Oxford.
Shokri, F., Mageed, R. A., Tunn, E., Bacon, P. A., and Jefferis, R. (1990) Qualitative and quantitative expression of V_{HIII} associated cross-reactive idiotopes within IgM rheumatoid factor from patients with early synovitis. *Ann. Rheum. Dis.* 49:150.
Simmons, D., and Seed, B. (1988) The Fc receptor of natural killer cells is a phospholipid-linked membrane protein. *Nature (London)* 333:568.
Steplewski, Z., Sun, L. K., Shearman, C. W., Ghrayeb, J., Daddona, P., and Kaprowski, H. (1988) Biological activity of human and mouse IgG1, IgG2, IgG3 and IgG4 chimeric monoclonal antibodies with tumor specificity. *Proc. Natl. Acad. Sci. U.S.A.* 85:4852.
Terry, W. D., and Fahey, J. L., (1964) Subclasses of human g2-globulin based on differences in the heavy polypeptide chain. *Science* 145:400—401.
Underdown, B. J., and Schiff, J. M. (1986) Immunoglobulin A: strategic defense initiative at the mucosal surface. *Annu. Rev. Immunol.* 4:389.
van de Winkle, J. G. J., and Anderson, C. L. (1991) Biology of human immunoglobulin g Fc receptors. *J. Leuk. Biol.* 49:511.
Walker, M. R., Kumpel, B. M., Thompson, K., Woof, J. M., Burton, D. R., and Jefferis, R. (1988) Binding of human anti-D-antibodies to the monocyte-like U937 cell line. *Vox. Sang.* 55:222—228.
Walker, M. R., Lund, J., Thompson, K. M., and Jefferis, R. (1989a) Aglycosylation of human IgG1 and IgG3 monoclonal antibodies can eliminate recognition by human cells expressing FcRI and/or FcRII receptors. *Biochem. J.* 259:347.
Walker, M. R., Woof, J. M., Bruggemann, M., Burton, D. R., and Jefferis, R. (1989b) Interaction of human chimeric antibodies with human FcR1 and FcR11 receptors: Requirements for Antibody-mediated host-cell/target cell interactions. *Mol. Immunol.* 26:403—411.
Ward, E. S., Gussow, D., Griffiths, A. D., Jones, P. T., and Winter, G. (1989) *Nature (London)* 341:544.

Woof, J. M., and Burton, D. R. (1990) The nature of the interaction of bacterial Fc receptors and IgG. In *Bacterial Immunoglobulin Binding Proteins*. (M. D. P. Boyle, ed.), Academic Press, New York.

Woof, J. M., Partridge, L., Jefferis, R., and Burton, D. R. (1986) Localization of the monocyte-binding domain(s) on human immunoglobulin G. *Mol. Immunol.* 21:523.

WHO, World Health Organization (1966) *WHO Tech. Ser. Rep* No.35:953.

Chapter
15
Histocompatibility Antigens*

*Béatrice Perarnau, Hélène Gournier, and
François A. Lemonnier*
Unité INSERM 152
Institut Cochin de Génétique Moléculaire
Paris, France

Claude Barra and Razqallah Hakem
Centre d'Immunologie de Marseille-Luminy
INSERM-CNRS
France

INTRODUCTION

The graft of a tissue from one individual (the donor) to another individual (the recipient) usually elicits an immune response which results in the rejection of the graft. The molecules on the grafted tissue which are responsible for this phenomenon are the histocompatibility antigens. One distinguishes major and minor histocompatibility antigens by the rapid (few days) or slow (from weeks to years) kinetics of the rejection. Major histocompatibility antigens are cell surface-expressed molecules encoded in highly allopolymorphic genes clustered in a unique DNA segment — the major histocompatibility complex

---

* Definition of key words. Allopolymorphism indicates the existence at a given locus of several genes coding for structurally distinguishable products. The term is further restricted to variants found in the population with a reasonable ($> 0.1\%$) frequency. An HLA (or H-2 haplotype) designates a set of histocompatibility class I and class II genes which usually segregate together. HLA (or H-2) restriction indicates that specific recognition of antigens by T lymphocytes is dependent upon the expression by the antigen-presenting cells of the same histocompatibility molecules as those expressed by the animal from which the T lymphocytes were derived.

(MHC). The MHC is also designated from the name of each species. For example, the HLA complex stands for human leukocyte antigen complex and the SLA complex for swine leukocyte antigen complex. H-2 is, for historical reasons, an exception to this rule and corresponds to the mouse leukocyte antigen complex. Histoincompatibility (a phenomenon identified in the early 1900s) is a nonphysiological consequence of the recently understood biological function of the MHC molecules, which is to present partially degraded (processed) self- and foreign antigens to T lymphocytes. By contrast, antibodies and B lymphocytes have little histocompatibility function and recognize native antigens independent of MHC molecules. Two classes of MHC molecules have been identified which have related, but clearly different, immunological functions. Major class I histocompatibility molecules are ubiquitously expressed and present intracellularly encoded proteins to CD8+ cytolytic T lymphocytes. Major class II histocompatibility molecules have a more restricted tissue distribution and present extracellular proteins (following endocytosis and acidic proteolysis) to CD4+, usually helper, T lymphocytes. Notice that among the multiple class I MHC genes and to a lesser extent class II MHC genes, only some, for reasons which will be analyzed later on, encode for molecules with well-identified immunological functions and thus are called major histocompatibility antigens. These are the human HLA-A, -B, -C, and the HLA-DP,-DQ,-DR class I and class II molecules, respectively, and the mouse H-2-K,-D,-L and H-2-A,-E class I and class II molecules. MHC compatibility between donor and recipient is necessary but not usually sufficient for graft acceptance. Structural differences between the allelic products of other genes located anywhere in the genome can trigger immune responses leading to graft rejection. Minor histocompatibility antigens are either intracellular, cell surface-expressed or secreted molecules. In most cases, however, minor histocompatibility antigens have not yet been biochemically identified. As opposed to major histocompatibility antigens, minor histocompatibility antigens are not recognized per se but as small peptides presented to the immune system by the major histocompatibility molecules.

We will successively consider class I, class II, and minor histocompatibility antigens. For the purpose of clarity, we will focus on the human histocompatibility complex. We will not consider the class III histocompatibility antigens. These antigens are encoded by genes within the four megabase DNA segment which contains the MHC complex but they are structurally and, for most of them, functionally unrelated to class I and class II histocompatibility antigens.

HLA CLASS I HISTOCOMPATIBILITY ANTIGENS

The HLA-A2 Molecule

The HLA-A2 molecule (initially named MAC 1) was the first major histocompatibility antigen identified in the human species (Dausset, 1958).

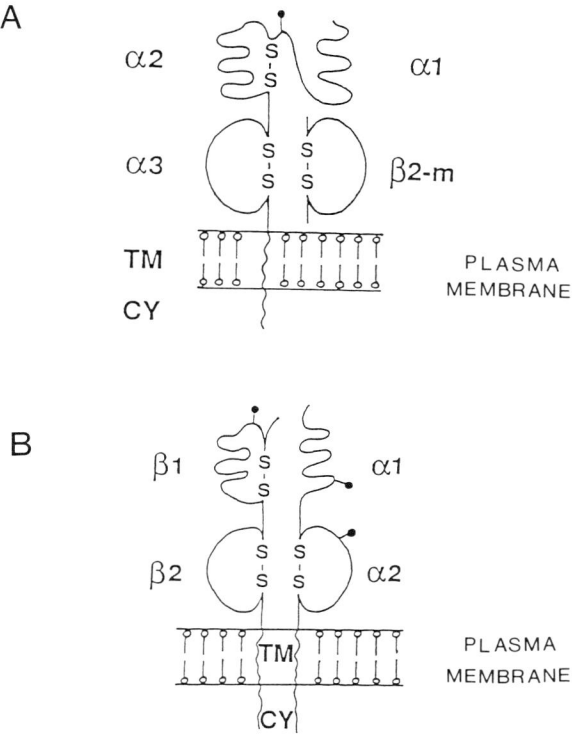

Figure 1. Schematic representation of HLA class I (A) and HLA class II (B) histocompatibility molecules. The closed circles represent the N-linked glycosyl residues: TM, transmembrane; CY, cytoplasmic domains.

It is an externally oriented plasma membrane-associated glycoprotein formed by the noncovalent association of a 45,000-Da membrane-anchored polypeptide heavy chain and a 12,000-Da light chain called β-2 microglobulin. The HLA class I heavy chain consists in three extracellular (α1, α2, and α3) NH_2-terminal domains of 90 amino acids each (Fig. 1A). The α1 and α3 domains contain a cysteine disulfide bridge; the α1 domain also has an N-linked glycosylation site at Asp^{86}. The HLA-A2 molecule is anchored to the cell surface by a 20-amino acid long hydrophobic sequence which spans the plasma membrane and by a short intracellular hydrophylic segment which contains potential (serine and threonine) phosphorylation sites. β-2 microglobulin is a nonpolymorphic globular 99-amino acid long nonglycosylated molecule (Cunningham et al., 1973; Orr et al., 1979).

The HLA-A2 and β-2 Microglobulin Genes

The HLA-A2 gene is contained in a 5.7-kb DNA fragment located on the short arm of chromosome 6. It has an intron/exon organization reflecting the domain structure of the protein (Fig. 2B). Exon 1 contains the 5'-untranslated region and codes for the leader sequence; exons 2, 3, and 4 code for the α1, α2, and α3 domains, respectively; exon 5 encodes the transmembrane segment; exons 6, 7, and 8 (initial part) code for the intracytoplasmic domain; the remainder of exon 8 corresponds to the 3'-noncoding sequence (Koller and Orr, 1985). The human β-2 microglobulin gene is located on the long arm of chromosome 15 and is included in a 7.2-kb DNA fragment. It consists of four exons (Fig. 2B). Exon 1 contains the 5'-untranslated region and codes for the leader sequence and the first two amino acids of the final polypeptide chain; exon 2 codes for the largest part (93 amino acid residues) of the β-2 microglobulin molecule; exon 3 codes for the last four amino acids of the polypeptide chain and contains the stop signal codon; exon 4 corresponds to the 3'-untranslated region (Güssow et al., 1987).

The HLA-A2 Three-Dimensional Structure

The three-dimensional structure of the HLA-A2 molecule has been defined (Bjorkman et al., 1987) and is illustrated in Fig. 3. The two (α1, and α2) domains form a pocketlike structure. The floor of the pocket is an antiparallel β-sheet formed by the central part of eight β-strands provided by both the α1 and α2 domains. The sides of the pocket are formed by two α-helices: one provided by residues 50 to 84 of the α1 domain and the other by residues 138 to 180 of the α2 domain. The pocket is probably the peptide-binding site, as suggested by the existence at this level of a poorly defined crystallographic structure likely to correspond to an heterogeneous population of bound peptides. Fourteen out of seventeen polymorphic amino acids of the HLA-A2 molecule (these are variable amino acid residues compared to an HLA class I consensus sequence) are located in the peptide-binding site, five on the α1-α2 β-sheet, pointing up between the two α-helices, six on the side of the helices facing into the site, and three on the top faces of the α-helices. The highly conserved α3 and β-2 microglobulin domains are organized around a cysteine disulfide bridge and have a structure similar to that of an immunoglobulin constant domain. A striking, however anticipated observation, in that β-2 microglobulin interacts tightly with both the α1 and α2 domains of the HLA-A2 molecule (Ferrier et al., 1985).

Diversity and Polymorphism of HLA Class I Genes and Molecules

The HLA-A2 is the most frequently found class I histocompatibility molecule. There are, however, about 100 different HLA class I molecules identified. This is due to the large number (diversity) of HLA class I genes per haploid genome and to the large number of alleles (polymorphism) at certain loci.

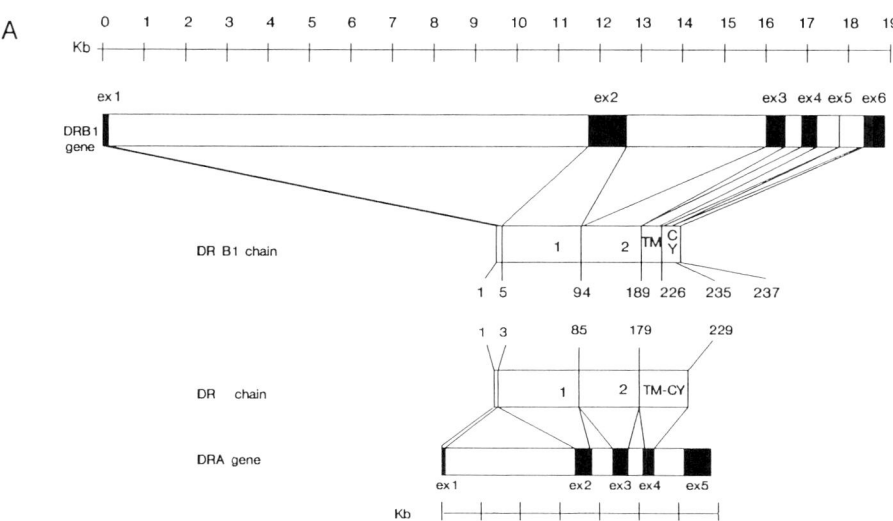

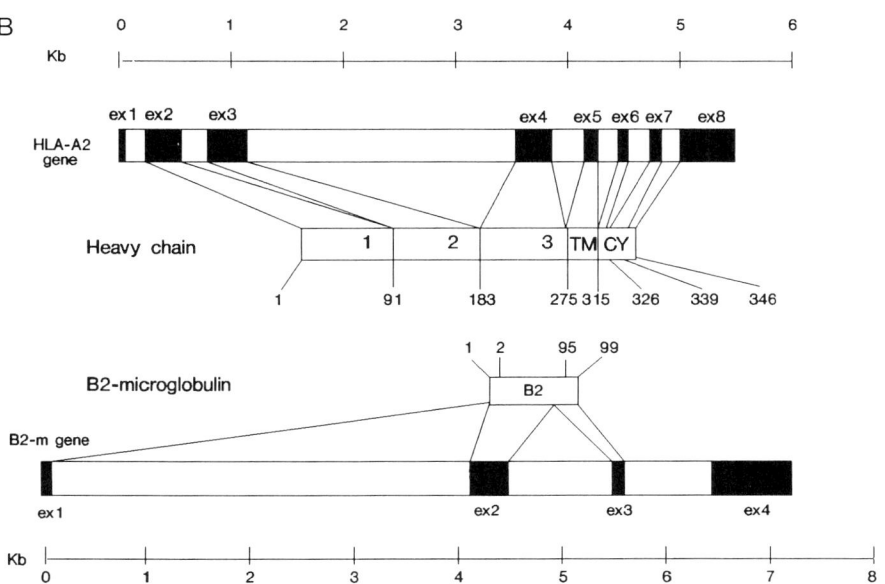

Figure 2. (A) Structure of the HLA class II β and α genes and corresponding to the mature proteins. (B) Structure of the HLA class I heavy chain and β2-microglobulin genes corresponding to the mature proteins. The last exon of each gene codes for the 3'-nontranslated RNA.

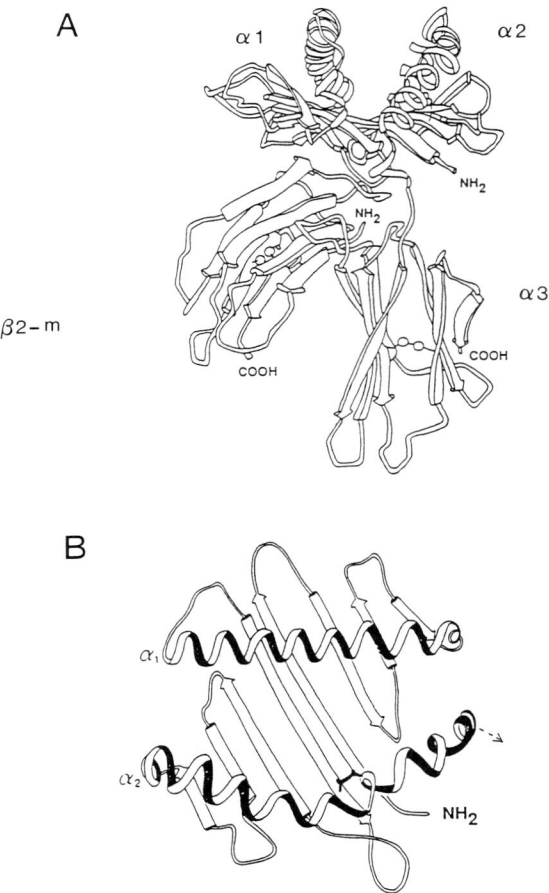

Figure 3. (A) Three-dimensional structure of the HLA-A2 molecule. (B) Detail of the putative peptide-binding site formed by the α1 and α2 domains of the heavy chain.

Diversity

There are about 16 different class I gene-related sequences per human haploid genome (Fig. 4). Their relative position on chromosome 6 has not yet been completely determined. However, by combining both the formal genetic analysis of intra-HLA recombinant families with the latest molecular biology techniques (pulsed-field electrophoresis, for example), it has been possible to position the most important HLA class I loci (Koller et al., 1989). From the centromeric to the telomeric sides of the HLA complex, one finds the HLA-B,-C,-E,-A,-F, and -G loci, which encode bona fide full-size HLA class I molecules. Loci B, C, and A encode ubiquitously expressed class I molecules, while the products of others (E, F, and G) have, apparently, a

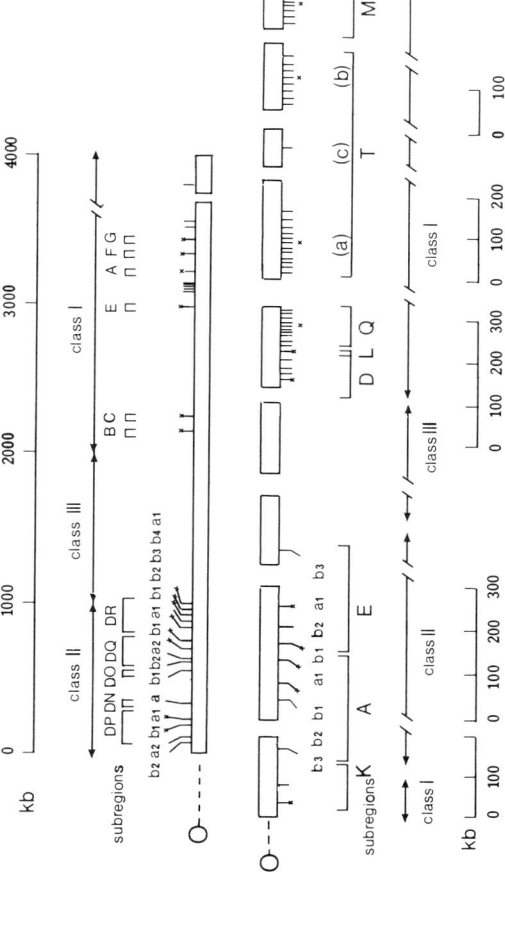

Figure 4. (A) HLA region and subregions on chromosome 6. The vertical symbols represent functional ('f) or pseudo (l)genes. The open circle denotes the centromere. (B) H-2 region and subregions. Due to the number of genes in the Q, T, and M subregions, and to variation in the number of genes from one strain of mice to another, the functional and pseudogenes in these subregions are not precisely identified on the figure. The class III genes (21-steroid hydroxylase, tumor necroting factor, C2, C4, factor B, etc.) are not represented.

more limited tissue distribution (the HLA-G is only expressed on the choriotrophoblast). Other class I-related genes have structural defect(s) and do not, at least in the few individuals in which they have been studied, encode complete HLA class I molecules. These pseudogenes are intermingled among the main loci. For example, the HLA-12-4 pseudogene (which was the first sequenced HLA gene, Malissen et al., 1982) is located between the HLA-A and -E loci.

Polymorphism

The HLA class I genes represent the most polymorphic genetic system in humans. This polymorphism was initially analyzed with human alloantisera, resulting in the identification of HLA class I specificities. The availability of monoclonal antibodies, cloned cytotoxic T lymphocytes, isoelectrofocusing techniques and, finally. DNA sequencing, have further refined (and will continue to refine) the definition of this polymorphism. A list of the HLA class I alleles which have been identified by DNA or protein sequencing is given in Table 1 and the corresponding HLA class I specificities are indicated. Note that, for some specificities, the corresponding gene has not yet been isolated and that the same serologically defined specificity can correspond to several genes. The HLA class I gene polymorphism is unequally distributed among the different loci. At the present time, the HLA-B locus has 42 specificities and 32 identified alleles, the HLA-A has 20 specificities and 25 alleles, and the HLA-C has 10 specificities and 11 alleles (Bodmer et al., 1990). By contrast, no polymorphism has been observed for the genes at the HLA-E, -G, and -F loci. This polymorphism has arisen by both point mutations (there is no evidence that the frequency of such mutations is higher in the HLA class I complex than elsewhere in the genome) and by gene conversion, that is exchange during abortive unequal crossing-over of a short stretch of nucleotides between a donor and an acceptor gene (Schulze et al., 1983). The multiple class I genes can, therefore, be viewed as a reservoir of potential polymorphism for the immunologically relevant HLA-B,-C, and -A genes. It is usually believed that fixation in the species of the structural modifications of interest was the result of some immunologically mediated selective pressure. In fact, two studies comparing the polymorphism of genetically related populations submitted to different pathogens support this hypothesis, as some HLA specificities are under- or overrepresented in relation to the pathological history of these populations (De Vriess et al., 1989; Piazza et al., 1972). It is at this point of crucial importance to reemphasize that most of the polymorphic residues are located in the peptide-binding pocket resulting, as documented by a comparative study of the HLA-A2 and HLA-28 three-dimensional structures, in substantial variations in the shape of the pocket which are likely to modify peptide binding (Garret et al., 1989). Comparative analysis of histocompatibility class I molecules in humans and chimpanzees has established that, in many instances, acquisition of polymorphic amino acid residues had occurred prior to speciation and was subsequently transmitted

TABLE 1.
HLA-A, -B, and -C Alleles and Specificities

HLA Alleles	HLA Specificities	HLA Alleles	HLA Specificities	HLA Alleles	HLA Specificities
A*0101	A1	B*0701	B7	Cw*0101	Cw1
A*0201	A2	B*0702	B7	Cw*0201	Cw2
A*0202	A2	B*0801	B8	Cw*0202	Cw2
A*0203	A2	B*1301	B13	Cw*0301	Cw3
A*0204	A2	B*1302	B13	Cw*0501	Cw5
A*0205	A2	B*1401	B14	Cw*0601	Cw6
A*0206	A2	B*1402	Bw65(14)	Cw*0701	Cw7
A*0207	A2	B*1501	Bw62(15)	Cw*1101	Cw11
A*0208	A2	B*1801	B18	Cw*1201	—
A*0209	A2	B*2701	B27	Cw*1301	—
A*0210	A2	B*2702	B27	Cw*1401	—
A*0301	A3	B*2703	B27		
A*0302	A3	B*2704	B27		
A*1101	A11	B*2705	B27		
A*2401	A24(9)	B*2706	B27		
A*2501	A25(10)	B*3501	B35		
A*2601	A26(10)	B*3701	B37		
A*2901	A29(w19)	B*3801	B38(16)		
A*3001	A30(w19)	B*3901	B39(16)		
A*3101	A31(w19)	B*4001	Bw60(40)		
A*3201	A32(w19)	B*4002	B40		
A*3301	Aw33(w19)	B*4101	Bw41		
A*6801	Aw68(28)	B*4201	Bw42		
A*6802	Aw68(28)	B*4401	B44(12)		
A*6901	Aw69(28)	B*4402	B44(12)		
		B*4601	Bw46		
		B*4701	Bw47		
		B*4901	B49(21)		
		B*5101	B51(5)		
		B*5201	Bw52(5)		
		B*5701	Bw57(17)		
		B*5801	Bw58(17)		

Note: Alleles are designated by a letter corresponding to the name of the HLA locus: A, B, Cw. The letter is followed by four numbers. The first two numbers correspond to the serologically defined specificity; the last two correspond to the allele. Specificities at the A and B loci are designated by a serial number. For example, A3 was the third serologically defined HLA-class I specificity. The number is preceded by a letter to indicate to which locus it corresponds. New specificities are given "w numbers," until a definitive agreement is reached at which point the w designation is dropped. The number in parentheses corresponds to split specificities; for example, the original HLA-A9 specificity has been subsequently subdivided into HLA-A23 (9) and -A24 (9). HLA-C specificities are exceptions to this rule. They are numbered independently and the w designation is kept to avoid confusion with complement components. The genes corresponding to the following specificities have not yet been isolated: HLA-A23 (9), -w34 (10), -w36, -w43, -w66 (10), -w47 (w19); HLA-B5, -B12, -B16, -B17, -B21, -Bw22, -B45 (12), -Bw48, -Bw50 (21), Bw53, -Bw54 (w22), -Bw56 (w22), -Bw59, Bw60 (40), -Bw61 (40), -Bw62 (15), -Bw63 (15), -Bw64 (14), -Bw65 (14), -Bw67, -Bw75 (15), -Bw76 (15), -Bw77 (15); HLA-Cw8, -Cw9, -Cw10(w3).

to both species. Furthermore, it has become evident that at each locus, a large number of ancestral alleles were transmitted to both species during speciation (Figueroa et al., 1988; Lawlor et al., 1988). This obliges us to consider that speciation has been a complex phenomenon simultaneously involving several individuals of the ancestral species. HLA-class I polymorphism has undoubtedly been used by the human species to overcome diseases caused by newly evolved pathogens. At the same time, alleles have been fixed, which favor the emergence of autoimmune diseases. For example, ankylosing spondylitis is strongly associated with HLA-B27. HLA class I polymorphism is therefore the actual, but transient, result of the adaptation of the human species to various pathogens, such adaptation being limited by the risk of disrupting self-tolerance.

Regulation of Expression of HLA Class I Molecules

Cell surface expression of HLA class I molecules is a complex phenomenon which depends on several parameters: abundance of HLA class I heavy chains, abundance of β-2 microglobulin, and availability of stabilizing peptides. Cell surface expression of HLA class I molecules can be up- or downregulated at different levels in various physiological and pathological situations.

Abundance of HLA Class I Heavy Chains

HLA class I heavy chain genes are transcribed by the RNA polymerase II. HLA class I transcripts are found in most tissues; however, important differences in the level of transcription have been documented. For example, germinal and early embryonic cells do not express HLA class I genes. The absence of expression at the feto-maternal interface (syncytiotrophoblast) might limit the risk of immune rejection of the implanted fetus. In adult tissues, HLA class I heavy chains are similarly not expressed or are expressed at very low levels in brain, muscles, and hepatic cells. This might be of importance for tolerance to self-antigens only expressed in such tissues. By contrast, lymphocytes, monocytes, and thymic epithelial cells constitutively express large amounts of HLA class I molecules. Constitutive expression of HLA class I gene can, furthermore, be upregulated by cytokines such as $INF\alpha$, $-\beta$, or $TNF\alpha$ or, conversely downregulated during some viral infections or tumorogenesis. The molecular basis of such regulation is currently being investigated. Various regulatory sequences associated with HLA class I promoters and regulatory factors interacting with them, have already been identified (Friedman and Stark, 1985; Kieran et al., 1990; Kimura et al., 1986; Miyazaki et al., 1986). We will not consider in detail these studies, which are beyond the scope of this review. It suffices to say that upregulation facilitates the recognition of virally infected cells but also can disrupt self-tolerance, whereas downregulation of HLA class I gene transcription, such as that mediated by the adenovirus E1 A or the c-myc gene products, will allow the infected or transformed cells to escape immune detection (Signäs et al., 1982; Versteeg et al., 1989).

Association of HLA Class I Heavy Chain with β-2 Microglobulin in the Endoplasmic Reticulum

As for most membrane-associated proteins, translation of both HLA class I heavy chain and β-2 microglobulin transcripts is intimately associated with export in the endoplasmic reticulum. There, class I heavy chains are rapidly glycosylated and associate with β-2 microglobulin. Attempts to reproduce such association *in vitro* has usually failed. The reason for these failures has recently been understood with the discovery that, to be stably associated with β-2 microglobulin, HLA-class I heavy chains usually need to bind a short (about 10 amino acids long) stabilizing peptide (Townsend et al., 1985; 1989; 1990). Mutant cells, defective for histocompatibility class I expression, were of key importance for this discovery. These cells present the following phenotype: absence (or considerable reduction) of cell surface expression of HLA class I molecules, absence of abnormalities of the heavy and light chain class I genes, correct transcription of these genes, and correct translation of heavy and light chain mRNA, as attested by the presence of normal amounts of both class I heavy and light chains in the endoplasmic reticulum. However, these chains do not associate and the glycosyl residue of the heavy chain remains sensitive to endo-H glucosidase, implying that they have not passed through the Golgi apparatus. Further studies have shown that addition of exogenous peptides (selected for their ability to bind and be presented by the heavy chains under study) during biochemical synthesis results in efficient heavy and light chain association (Townsend et al., 1990). Altogether, these results suggest that the mutant cells have a defect in a molecule which enables peptides, probably produced in the cytosol, to penetrate the endoplasmic reticulum. Interestingly, the defective gene is included in the MHC complex (Cerundolo et al., 1990). Therefore, MHC class I molecules are heterotrimers formed by the association, in the endoplasmic reticulum, of class I heavy chains, β-2 microglobulin, and short peptides, which bind to the polymorphic part of the heavy chain. As a consequence of the heavy chain structural polymorphism, these peptides are usually different from one heavy chain to another. In spite of the fact that there are exceptions to this rule (few histocompatibility molecules can reach the cell surface in the absence of either β-2 microglobulin or stabilizing peptides, (Allen et al., 1986), there is no strong evidence that such incomplete MHC class I molecules are immunologically functional. Again, the process of association and transport of MHC class I molecules to the cell surface can be up- or downregulated. Interferon has been found to enhance the transport, from the endoplasmic reticulum to the cell surface, of HLA class I heterodimers (Klar and Hömmerling, 1989). Certain adenoviruses can interact noncovalently with the $\alpha 1/\alpha 2$ domains of MHC class I molecules by synthesizing E3/19 proteins which possess a Lys-Asp-Glu-Leu endoplasmic reticulum retention sequence (Signös et al., 1982). In tumor and cytomegalovirus-infected cells, MHC class I cell surface expression can also be reduced by lowering the amount of available β-2 microglobulin either by deletion or mutation of the β-2 microglobulin gene (tumor cells) or by competing with heavy chains, in the endoplasmic reticulum, for binding to β-2 microglobulin (cytomegalovirus, Browne et al., 1990).

Main Function of HLA Class I Molecules

The main function of HLA class I molecules is to present immunogenic foreign or self-peptides to CD8+, usually cytolytic, T lymphocytes. The presentation of foreign peptides results in HLA class I restriction of the recognition and destruction of target cells, while the presentation of self-peptides results in tolerance to self. Recognition of HLA class I molecules and target cell destruction by cytolytic T lymphocytes was first identified by analysis of T lymphocyte-mediated cytolytic responses to allopolymorphic heterologous MHC class I molecules. If one cocultures two populations of lymphocytes from two individuals (mixed lymphocyte culture) which express different HLA class I molecules, one usually obtains cytolytic T lymphocytes which recognize and destroy target cells that express HLA class I specificities identical to either the HLA-B, -C, or -A molecules expressed by the stimulating cells. A key observation for the understanding of the function of the class I histocompatibility antigens was that the recognition of virally infected target cells, by CD8+ T lymphocytes, was not only specific for the strain of virus but was further restricted by the histocompatibility molecules of the stimulating cells (Zinkernagel and Doherty, 1974). This indicates that the cytolytic T lymphocytes can only recognize virus-infected cells expressing the same MHC class I molecules as themselves. For example, infection of C57BL/6 mice (H-2^b) by leukochoriomeningitis virus (LCM) generates cytolytic T lymphocytes recognizing only H-2^b-LCM-infected target cells. This double restriction phenomenon reflects the fact that the T-cell receptor of the effector cytolytic T lymphocytes recognizes a composite structure formed by the association of a short virally derived peptide in association with the H-2^b class I molecules. This peptide has been bound in the endoplasmic reticulum of the infected cells by virtue of the fact that it has the same stabilizing effect as some other, but naturally provided, endogeneous peptides. It has at this point to be noticed that the development of a cytolytic response is influenced by additional parameters. The interaction of T lymphocytes (including CD8+ T lymphocytes) with target cells is usually of relatively weak affinity (Schneck et al., 1989). It must be stabilized by accessory interactions (Fig. 5). Some of these interactions involve the LFA-1/I-CAM and CD2/LFA-3 molecules, the LFA-1 and CD2 being expressed on lymphocytes and the I-CAM and LFA-3 on target cells (Krensky et al., 1984). These interactions are not specific for CD8+ HLA class I-restricted T lymphocytes as will be seen later. An additional interaction, specific to HLA class I-restricted T lymphocytes (which in most cases are cytolytic cells), involves the CD8 molecule. The CD8 molecule is a transmembrane glycoprotein formed by the association of a 34,000-Da α chain and a 38,000-Da β chain. The CD8 molecule belongs to the immunoglobulin superfamily and is expressed at the surface of immature

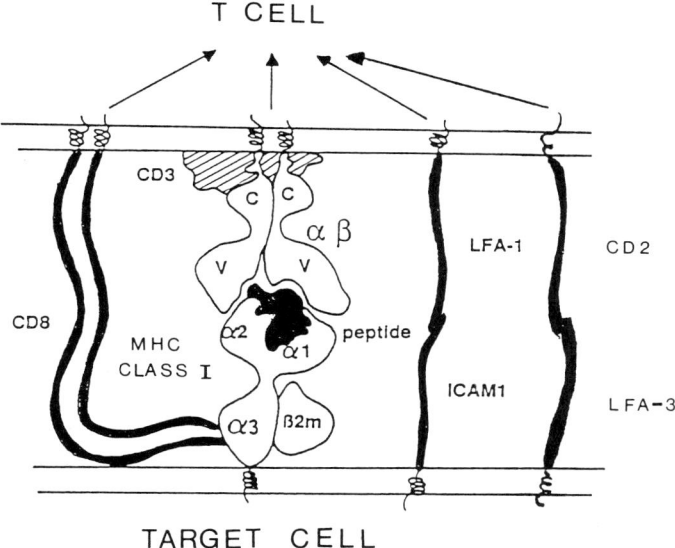

Figure 5. Schematic representation of the interaction of a CD8+ T lymphocyte with its target. The αβCD3 complex represents the T-cell receptor. Arrows indicate activating signals transduced across the plasma membrane.

thymocytes and in 40% of peripheral T lymphocytes. It is a specific marker of HLA class I-restricted T lymphocytes and stabilizes the interaction of T lymphocytes with HLA class I molecules by interacting with the α3 domain of the HLA class I heavy chain (Swain and Panfili, 1979). Following contact with the target cell, the CD8 molecule also transduces activating signals across the plasma membrane of the cytolytic T lymphocytes. If the recognition of foreign antigens and destruction of target cells is of importance to eradicate pathogens, it must be selective for abnormal (infected or transformed) cells. As already discussed, certain self-peptides can bind to and stabilize HLA class I heterodimers. Such peptides are potentially immunogenic. For example, as will be seen later, females can develop potent immune cytolytic responses against syngeneic male cells. Since syngeneic males and females share (at the genomic level) the same immunological potentialities (the T-cell receptor genes are located on autosomes), this observation implies that in males there is some mechanism to make them tolerant to male antigens. Tolerance to self-antigens is an absolute prerequisite. It can be acquired by CD8+ T lymphocytes in different ways: thymic deletion of autoreactive clones (Kappler et al., 1987; Kisielow et al., 1988), peripheral inactivation (T cell anergy; Ramsdell and Fowlkes, 1990), and downregulation of the expression of accessory molecules (for example, CD8). Like cytolysis, tolerance has to be selective and limited to T lymphocytes expressing T-cell receptors able to recognize self-antigens presented by HLA class I molecules. It has effectively been observed that tolerance of CD8+ T lymphocytes is HLA class I restricted (Kisielow et al., 1988).

Other Functions of HLA Class I Molecules

HLA class I molecules have been associated with various other roles. They have been found to be associated with hormonal receptors (insulin, glucagon, epidermal growth factor, etc.) and it has been claimed that in the absence of expression of histocompatibility class I molecules, the cell surface expression of at least some of these receptors was reduced (Due et al., 1986). β-2 Microglobulin is associated with some other cell surface-expressed molecules, members of the immunoglobulin superfamily, such as the intestinal immunoglobulin receptor, and the CD1 T lymphocyte molecules (Kefford et al., 1984; Simister and Mostov, 1989). β-2 Microglobulin has also chemiotactic properties for prothymocytes and might guide their homing to the thymus (Dargemont et al., 1989). In fact, the recent isolation of histocompatibility class I-deficient mice (by destruction of the mouse β-2 microglobulin gene by homologous recombination) suggests that these functions are not of prime importance for the whole development of the animal and for thymic colonization by prothymocytes (Koller et al., 1990; Zilstra et al., 1990). By contrast, histocompatibility class I molecules markedly and negatively influence the function of natural killer (NK) cells. In brief, these cells will kill any cell which does not express HLA class I molecules (Piontek et al., 1985). This observation, which has been reported by many different groups, might be, to some extent, influenced by the type of HLA class I molecules expressed (the HLA-B have a more pronounced inhibitory effect than the HLA-A molecules). However, the molecular basis of this phenomenon is not yet understood. Nevertheless, it illustrates the complementarity of two types of effector cells of the immune system. Natural killer cells control the proliferation of undifferentiated cells (for example, undifferentiated bone marrow stem cells) and that of cells which, following viral infection or tumoral transformation, have lost expression of HLA class I molecules, whereas cytolytic T lymphocytes eliminate HLA class I positive cells, expressing abnormal proteins.

HLA CLASS II HISTOCOMPATIBILITY ANTIGENS

HLA class II histocompatibility antigens were discovered in the 1970s by the analysis of CD4+ T-cell proliferative responses and extra (non-class I)-serological reactivities of anti-HLA sera from multiparous women.

Biochemistry and Gene Structure

HLA class II molecules are externally oriented, plasma membrane-associated glycoproteins, formed by the noncovalent association of two transmembrane polypeptide chains (Fig. 1B). The β chain of 26 to 29,000 Da consists of two domains (β1 and β2) of 80 to 95 amino acids, each organized around a disulfide bridge. The α chain of 31 to 34,000 Da consists of two domains (α1 and α2) of 80 to 95 amino acids with only the α2 domain containing a disulfide bridge. The β and α chains span the plasma membrane and have a short hydrophilic cytoplasmic tail which, in the case of the α chain, can be phosphorylated. The β (at position 19) and the α (at positions 81 and 119) have glycosylated asparagine residues. Both chains can also be acylated (Larhammar et al., 1985; Lee et al., 1982; Spies et al., 1985). The HLA class II β and α genes have, like the HLA class I heavy chain gene, an intron/exon organization which reflects the domain organization of the final polypeptide chain (Fig. 2A). The organization of both HLA class I and II molecules in four domains (the HLA class II α chain corresponds to the α1 and β-2 microglobulin domains of HLA class I molecules), the association of both types of molecules with short (usually 10 amino acids long), sometimes identical peptides (Babbits et al., 1985; Hickling et al., 1990; Perkins et al., 1989), and the documented usage of identical variable segments to build the antigenic receptors of class I-interacting and class II-interacting T lymphocytes (Rupp et al., 1985), have led to the expectation that the overall three-dimensional structure of these two types of histocompatibility molecules would be very similar. Based on the HLA-A2 three-dimensional structure, a structure of the HLA class II molecule has been predicted which, however, still awaits crystallographic confirmation (Brown et al., 1988).

Diversity and Polymorphism of HLA Class II Genes and Molecules

The genes coding for the α and β chains of the class II histocompatibility antigens are located on the centromeric side of the HLA class I genes on the short arm of chromosome 6 (Fig. 4). Three subregions (DP, DQ, and DR moving from the centromere toward the telomere) of the human MHC complex have been identified which each contain one α and at least one functional β class II gene. The DR subregion in certain haplotypes contains only one functional β gene at the DR B1 locus whereas in other haplotypes additional, functional β chains are encoded by genes at the DR B3, DR B4, and DR B5 loci (Rollini et al., 1985). The DQ subregion contains two sets of α and β genes. Those located at DQ A1 and DQ B1 code for cell surface-expressed DQ class II histocompatibility antigens, whereas those located at the DQ A2 and DQ B2 do not (Jonsson et al., 1987). The DP subregion codes for cell surface-expressed class II histocompatibility antigens corresponding to the DP A1 and DP B1 loci (Gustafsson et al., 1987). Preferential association between the β or α chains of each subregion is usually observed. However, transfection experiments and biochemical studies of normal human cells have demonstrated the possibility of intersubregion cis-complementation (DRα–DQβ, for example) which increases HLA class II diversity (Lotteau et al., 1987). Additional class II subregions (DN and DO) have been identified which contain α (DN)- and β (DO)-related sequences. However, the products of these genes are not expressed in significant amounts at the cell surface.

Considering the number of functional α and β HLA class II genes per human haploid genome, the tight genetic linkage of these genes, the limited tissue distribution of these molecules, and the association of α with β chain from different subregions, it is easy to see why the definition of the polymorphism of the HLA class II gene products has been laborious. The polymorphism of the HLA class II was, for practical reasons, first analyzed serologically. This resulted in the identification of HLA-DR, HLA-DQ, and HLA-DP specificities. The HLA class II polymorphism was later analyzed with HLA class II-restricted T lymphocytes resulting in the identification of HLA-Dw specificities. More recently, the HLA class II polymorphism has been analyzed by DNA sequencing resulting in the identification of alleles at the α and β loci of each HLA-DR, HLA-DQ, and HLA-DP subregion. A list of the HLA class II alleles, and the serologically and cellularly defined specificities is given in Table 2. Sixteen different serologically defined HLA class II specificities have been associated with HLA-DR, seven with HLA-DQ, and six with HLA-DP subregions. However, DNA sequencing data clearly indicate that the degree of polymorphism evaluated serologically, was underestimated. To date, 34 different alleles have been identified for the only DR B1 locus. Extensive polymorphism is also associated with the DQ B1 (13 alleles) and DP B1 (19 alleles) loci. Moderate polymorphism is associated with the DQ A (8 alleles), DP A (4 alleles), DR B3 (4 alleles), and DR B5 (4 alleles) loci. Conversely, the DR B4 and DR A loci are not polymorphic. This extensive polymorphism, at the species level, of the HLA class II antigens is further increased by the possible association of α and β chains from different subregions (cis-complementation already mentioned) and from the same subregion but from different chromosomes (transcomplementation) which results in the expression of hybrid molecules with distinct serological and functional properties (Charron et al., 1984).

Regulation of Expression of HLA Class II Molecules

The basic function of HLA class II molecules, namely association with short peptides and presentation to the immune system, is the same as that of HLA class I molecules. However, differences in the regulation of transcription, association of α/β heterodimers with the invariant chain in the endoplasmic reticulum targeting the resulting heterotrimers to endosomal vesicles, and, finally, usage of CD4 accessory molecules to stabilize the interaction with T lymphocytes with HLA class II molecules result in profound functional differences.

Regulation of Transcription

HLA class II molecules have a more restricted tissue distribution than HLA class I molecules. They are constitutively expressed on monocytes, dendritic cells, and B lymphocytes. They can be induced on mature macrophages and epithelial cells following treatment with interferon and are also expressed on activated T lymphocytes. Regulation of expression is controlled by several nucleotide sequences in their promoter known as the X, Y, and Z boxes, with which several factors interact (Benoist and Mathis, 1990). Removal or mutations of these sequences profoundly modify the tissue distribution of HLA class II molecules (Van Ewijk et al., 1988). A comprehensive picture of the overall regulation of expression of these genes is not yet at hand; however, three aspects should be stressed: (1) the HLA-DP, -DQ, and -DR genes are largely coregulated; (2) HLA class II gene expression is essentially an inductive phenomemon, which is possibly important in the development of autoimmune diseases; and (3) HLA class II gene expression can be abolished in several ways by interfering negatively with regulatory factors. There are currently four to five regulatory factors in the process of identification and this analysis should result in an understanding of the molecular basis of a congenital immune deficiency known as the Bare lymphocyte syndrome in which class II genes are not expressed (Reith et al., 1988).

Association in the Endoplasmic Reticulum

HLA class II β and α chains associate in the endoplasmic reticulum. Furthermore, in this cellular compartment, they are noncovalently associated with a nonpolymorphic (invariant) 31,000-Da transmembrane glycosylated polypeptide chain, encoded by a gene located on chromosome 5 (Charron and McDewitt, 1973). The invariant chain has an inverted orientation compared to other transmembrane molecules, (the NH_2-terminus is cytosolic). It targets the HLA class II α and β chains to a post-Golgi endosomal compartment. Once the α, β, and invariant chain trimeric complex has reached this compartment, the invariant chain is proteolytically degraded and the α/β chain heterodimer becomes available to bind peptides provided by the acidic degradative endolysosomal pathway (Bakke and Dobberstein, 1990; Guagliardi et al., 1990; Peterson and Miller, 1990; Roche and Cresswell, 1990). The invariant chain appears, therefore, as a class II-specific chaperone molecule and prevents association of HLA class II molecules with peptides in the endoplasmic reticulum. It is difficult to evaluate whether peptide association is limited to neosynthetized class II molecules or also involves class II molecules already expressed on the cell surface. HLA class II molecules, as well as class I molecules, are internalized, which leaves open the possibility of peptide association with previously expressed and recycled class II molecules (Reid and Watts, 1990).

Function of HLA Class II Molecules

The same general rules govern the interaction of HLA class I and class II molecules with T lymphocytes. There is first specific recognition by HLA class II-restricted T lymphocytes of a trimolecular complex formed by the HLA class II α and β chains associated with a short peptide. Note that both HLA class I- and class II-restricted T lymphocytes can interact with T-cell receptors with similar variable region for such interaction. As for HLA class I-restricted T lymphocytes, the class II-T cell interaction is stabilized by LFA-

TABLE 2. HLA-DR, -DQ, and -DP Alleles and Specificities

HLA Alleles	HLA-DR Specificities	HLA-Dw-Associated (T-Cell Defined) Specificities	HLA Alleles	HLA-DQ Specificities	HLA-Dw-Associated (T-Cell Defined) Specificities
DRB1*0101	DR1	Dw1	DQA1*0101	—	Dw1, w9
DRB1*0102	DR1	Dw20	DQA1*0102	—	Dw2,w21,w19
DRB1*0103	DR'BR'	Dw'BON'	DQA1*0103	—	Dw18, w12, w8
DRB1*1501	DRw15(2)	Dw2			Dw'FS'
DRB1*1502	DRw15(2)	Dw12	DQA1*0201	—	Dw7,w11
DRB1*1601	DRw16(2)	Dw21	DQA1*0301	—	Dw4, w10,w13
DRB1*1602	DRw16(2)	Dw22			w14, w15, w23
DRB1*0301	DRw17(3)	Dw3	DQA1*0401	—	Dw8,Dw'RSH'
DRB1*0302	DRw17(3)	Dw'RSH'	DQA1*0501	—	Dw3,w5,w22
DRB1*0401	DRw18(3)	Dw4	DQA1*0601	—	Dw8
DRB1*0402	DR4	Dw10			
DRB1*0403	DR4	Dw13	DQB1*0501	DQw5(w1)	Dw1
DRB1*0404	DR4	Dw14			
DRB1*0405	DR4	Dw15	DQB1*0502	DQw5(w1)	Dw21
DRB1*0406	DR4	Dw'KT2'	DQB1*0503	DQw5(w1)	Dw9
DRB1*0407	DR4	Dw13	DQB1*0601	DQw6(w1)	Dw12,w8
DRB1*0408	DR4	Dw14	DQB1*0602	DQw6(w1)	Dw2
			DQB1*0603	DQw6(w1)	Dw18,Dw'FS'
DRB1*1101	DRw11(5)	Dw5	DQB1*0604	DQw6(w1)	Dw19
DRB1*1102	DRw11(5)	Dw'JVM'	DQB1*0201	DQw2	Dw3,w7
DRB1*1103	DRw11(5)	—			
DRB1*1104	DRw11(5)	Dw'FS'	DQB1*0301	DQw7(w3)	Dw4,w5,w8
DRB1*1201	DRw12(5)	Dw'DB6'			w13
DRB1*1301	DRw13(w6)	Dw18	DQB1*0302	DQw8(w3)	Dw4,w10,w13
DRB1*1302	DRw13(w6)	Dw19			w14
DRB1*1303	DRw13(w6)	Dw'HAG'	DQB1*0303	DQw9(w3)	Dw23,w11
DRB1*1401	DRW14(w6)	Dw9	DQB1*0401	DQw4	Dw15
			DQB1*0402	DQw4	Dw8,Dw'RSH'

Allele	DR	Dw	Allele	DPw
DRB1*1402	DRw14(w6)	Dw16	DPA1*0101	—
DRB1*0701	DR7	Dw17	DPA1*0102	—
DRB1*0702	DR7	Dw'DB1'	DPA1*0103	—
DRB1*0801	DRw8	Dw8.1	DPA1*0201	—
DRB1*0802	DRw8	Dw8.2		
DRB1*0803	DRw8	Dw8.3		
DRB1*0901	DR9	Dw23	DPB1*0101	DPw1
DRB1*1001	DRw10	—	DPB1*0201	DPw2
			DPB1*0202	DPw2
DRB3*0101	DRw52a	Dw24	DPB1*0301	DPw3
DRB3*0201	DRw52b	Dw25	DPB1*0401	DPw4
DRB3*0202	DRw52b	Dw25	DPB1*0402	DPw4
DRB3*0301	DRw52c	Dw26	DPB1*0501	DPw5
			DPB1*0601	DPw6
DRB4*0101	DRw53	Dw4,Dw10,Dw13	DPB1*0801	—
		Dw14,Dw15,Dw17	DPB1*0901	DP'Cp63'
		Dw23	DPB1*1001	—
			DPB1*1101	—
DRB5*0101	DRw15(2)	Dw2	DPB1*1301	—
DRB5*0102	DRw15(2)	Dw12	DPB1*1401	—
DRB5*0201	DRw16(2)	Dw21	DPB1*1501	—
DRB5*0202	DRw16(2)	Dw22	DPB1*1601	—
			DPB1*1701	—
			DPB1*1801	—
			DPB1*1901	—

Note: Same legend as Table 1. Note, however, the following: the serological specificities are referred to subregions (DR, DQ, DP) since it is usually impossible with certitude to discriminate between the products of closely linked class II genes before direct analysis at the DNA level. Designation of alleles refers, by contrast, to the loci where the functional genes are located (for example, DR B1, DR B3, etc.). Several specificities could not be discriminated serologically but were differentiated with alloreactive T lymphocytes and are designated Dw, without reference to the corresponding subregion. Finally, in most instances, DNA sequencing data have resulted in the association of several alleles with a single serologically defined specificities, illustrating the limits of the serological approach. However, only serological detection of the molecule on the cell surface gives the certitude that the product of an HLA class II histocompatibility gene is expressed on cell surfaces, is biologically relevant, and is the only way to detect the hybrid molecules resulting from cis or trans inter- and intrasubregion α/β complementation.

1/I-CAM and CD2/LFA3 interactions. The key difference between HLA class I- and class II-restricted T lymphocytes is a differential usage of the CD4 and CD8 molecules. These molecules play an essential role for the stabilization of the T lymphocytes' interaction with other cells. For that purpose, HLA class II-restricted T lymphocytes use CD4 and HLA class I-restricted T lymphocytes use CD8 molecules. CD4 molecules are monomeric transmembrane glycoproteins of 55,000 Da which belong to the immunoglobulin superfamily. CD4 molecules are coexpressed with CD8 molecules on the surface of immature thymocytes; however, thymic differentiation results in mutually exclusive expression of CD4 and CD8 molecules: 60% of peripheral T lymphocytes are CD4+ and the other 40% are CD8+. CD4 molecules bind to HLA class II molecules. This binding (which might involve a conserved Arg-Phe-Asp-Ser sequence of the α1 domain) is essential for the intercellular contact of CD4+ T lymphocytes with the few types of cells (macrophages, dendritic cells, and B lymphocytes) which express HLA class II antigens. Since both CD4 and CD8 molecules can transduce activating signals across the plasma membrane, it is tempting to speculate that CD4 or CD8 interactions in the thymus direct the functional differentiation of T lymphocytes. CD4+ T lymphocytes are usually helper cells which secrete various cytokines (including interleukin 2) and stimulate both the multiplication and terminal differentiation of other cells as long as these cells express the appropriate cytokine receptors. Thus, CD4+ T lymphocytes play a key role in the control of the development of immune responses. In fact, most of the Ir genes (a generic name for the genes which control immune responses) identified in the 1970s were associated with the HLA-D region. Accordingly, most association of HLA haplotypes with autoimmune diseases implicate HLA class II molecules.

HLA and Disease Association

Susceptibility to various diseases, listed in Table 3, has been associated with the HLA region. These diseases predominantly affect the joints, endocrine glands, or the skin and have a strong autoimmune component. Type I diabetes provides a good illustration of HLA association with susceptibility to certain diseases and, in the early stages of this diabetes, the pancreatic Langerhans islets are infiltrated by T lymphocytes. In the rat, diabetes can be transmitted by injection of T lymphocytes which infiltrates the pancreatic Langerhans islets. In humans, coexpression of the HLA-DR3 and HLA-DR4 haplotypes is associated with an increased relative risk of developing type I diabetes. Stronger association was later documented with the DQ B1 locus. Sequence comparisons of human and mouse class II genes have led to the proposal that susceptibility to diabetes might be due to the replacement at position 57 of an aspartic acid residue by a neutral amino acid (Todd et al., 1987). The expression of this neutral amino acid is predicted to modify the peptide-binding pocket of HLA class II molecules and to allow the binding of exogeneous and/or endogeneous peptides which can stimulate autoreactive

TABLE 3.
Association between HLA and Some Diseases

Disease	HLA Specificities	Relative Risk[a]
Nasopharyngeal carcinoma	DR2/4	21
IgA deficiency	A1	13
Idiopathic thrombocytopenic purpura	DR3	72
Ankylosing spondylitis	B27	88
Reiter's syndrome	B27	37
Rheumatoid arthritis	DR4	19
Goodpasture's syndrome	DR2	16
Acute anterior uveitis	B27	10
Bird shot retinochoroidopathy	A29	50
Psoriasis vulgaris	Cw6	13
Phemphigus	DR4	14
Dermatis herpetiformis	DR3	15
Behcet's disease	B51	10
Insulin-dependent diabetes (type 1)	DR3/4	47
Subacute thyroiditis	B35	14
Narcolepsia	DR2	135
Celiac disease	DR3/7	60

[a] The relative risk indicates how many times more frequently a disease occurs in individuals expressing a given HLA antigen compared to the frequency of the same disease in individuals who do not express it. It is calculated according for the following formula:

$$RR = \frac{(a \times d)}{(b \times c)}$$

in which a is the number of patients expressing the allele, b is the number of patients lacking the allele, c is the number of controls expressing the allele, and d is the number of controls lacking the allele.

T lymphocytes. However, there are exceptions to the "57 rule", suggesting that other structural modifications of the peptide-binding pocket can result in similar disruption of self-tolerance to some pancreatic-specific antigens, as suggested recently, as well as the existence of additional susceptibility genes mapping outside the MHC. Identification of the self-derived T-cell antigenic determinant will be of key importance not only to understand the pathogenesis of this frequent disease but also to prevent it.

HISTOCOMPATIBILITY ANTIGENS OF OTHER SPECIES

Histocompatibility class I and class II genes and molecules have been found in all vertebrate species studied. Phylogenic analysis of these genes and molecules is of great interest since it illustrates the different strategies which have evolved in different species to cope with pathogens. They will further give insights into the mechanisms which have been at work to immunologically select important class I molecules, and fix them in the species, and will illuminate the selective pressures which have been coexerted on the different molecules (heavy chain, β-2 microglobulin, CD8 accessory molecules, T-cell receptor chains, and intracellular machinery which provides the stabilizing peptides) to keep them working together. Interesting differences in some aspects of MHC genes and molecules have already been noted. In addition to variation in the number of class I genes (Fig. 4), variations in the degree of polymorphism have been observed. There are up to 100 alleles at the K and D loci in the mouse but only two in the syrian hamster and few other species (Darden and Streilein, 1984). Ontogenic differences of interest have also been documented. For example, in batracien (frog) species, histocompatibility class I molecules are only expressed following adult morphogenesis — perhaps class II molecules, which are expressed much earlier in this species, compensate the absence of class I molecules (Flajnik and DuPasquier, 1990).

MINOR HISTOCOMPATIBILITY ANTIGENS

Minor histocompatibility antigens were first identified in the mouse. It was observed that genetic identity at the MHC complex was not sufficient to prevent graft rejection which occurred at a slower pace. Genetic analysis of this phenomenon has identified 45 different loci in mice versus 6 in humans (Voogt et al., 1988). It is, however, clear that more minor histocompatibility loci exist in both humans and mice since a single amino acid difference between two allelic products can suffice to trigger an immune response. Minor histocompatibility antigens are, however, still poorly defined. Most probably correspond to allelic variation resulting in structural polymorphism of certain gene products (Loveland et al., 1990). It is important to bear in mind the large number of inherited recessive diseases and to realize that any structural alteration of any molecule, even alteration without functional consequences for the modified molecule, can be immunogenic. Other minor histocompatibility antigens might arise from gene duplication or deletion in multigene families in which case gene deletion or gene duplication frequently occur as a result of unequal crossing-over. Finally, minor histocompatibility antigens can correspond to the acquisition of new coding sequences by retroviral insertion (in fact retrovirus-related sequences are often found in close association with minor histocompatibility loci; Rossomando and Meruelo, 1986).

One of the minor histocompatibility loci has been mapped to the H-Y chromosome. The gene at this locus is responsible for the rejection by females of male skin grafts and such a female antimale response has been observed in both mouse and human (Goulmy et al., 1977; Wachtel et al., 1973). This rejection depends on both CD4+ T helper cells and CD8+ cytolytic T lymphocytes. Direct evidence for the recognition of a male-specific peptide has been recently obtained (Rötzscke et al., 1990). It seems unlikely that this peptide is derived from the recently identified testis differentiation factor (Sinclair et al., 1990), since this molecule is only encoded in testis germinal centers. More likely, this peptide(s) derives from the products of genes expressed in other tissues, but whose transcription is controlled by the testis differentiating factor. Another type of minor histocompatibility antigen was recently described in mouse (Perarnau et al., 1990). The mouse β-2 microglobulin gene is polymorphic — seven different alleles have been identified which differ either at one (alleles a, b, and c) or several, amino acid positions. The results reported in this case, using cells differing only at the a and b allele, indicate that the cytolytic T lymphocyte response, which was elicited by cells expressing the b allele, is not due to the presentation of a β-2 microglobulin-derived peptide. In fact, association of a given heavy chain with the different forms of β-2 microglobulin modifies its affinity for peptides resulting in the association and presentation to the immune system of a partially different set of peptides.

Therefore, a molecule, which associates noncovalently to histocompatibility heavy chains can modify their peptide-presenting capacities. Whether this observation will be extended to other noncovalent interactions is still an open question. Another implication of these results is that polymorphic residues, distal from the peptide-binding pocket, can influence peptide binding. This might indicate that the conformation of the heavy chain during peptide loading is substantially different from the structure defined by crystography. Other parameters could also influence peptide production and presentation. A better definition of the various proteases involved, of their tissue distribution, of their possible intra- and interspecies polymorphism, of their subcellular localization, and a better understanding of the T-cell receptor interactions with histocompatibility class I and class II molecules are important for a more rational development of future vaccines and for a better understanding of autoimmune diseases.

ACKNOWLEDGMENTS

The authors acknowledge Dr. Johan Breyer for careful reading of the manuscript and Mrs. Sandrine Vitteaud for excellent secretarial assistance.

REFERENCES

Allen, H., Fraser, J., Flyer, D., Calvin, S., and Flavell, R. (1986) β2-microglobulin is not required for cell surface expression of the murine class I histocompatibility antigen H-2D^b or of a truncated H-2D^b. *Proc. Natl. Acad. Sci. U.S.A.* 83:7447—7451.

Babbits, B. P., Allen, P. M., Matsueda, G., Haber, E., and Unanue, E. R. (1985) Binding of immunogenic peptides to Ia histocompatibility molecules. *Nature (London)* 317:359—361.

Bakke, O. and Dobberstein, B. (1990) MHC class II-associated invariant chain contains a sorting signal for endosomal compartments, *Cell* 63:707—716.

Benoist, C., and Mathis, D, (1990) Regulation of major histocompatibility complex class II genes: X, Y and other letters of the alphabet. *Annu. Rev. Immunol.* 8:681—715.

Bjorkman, P. J., Saper, M. A., Samraoui, B., Bennett, W. S., Strominger, J. L., and Wiley, D. C. (1987) Structure of the human class I histocompatibility antigen, HLA-A2. *Nature (London)* 329:506—518.

Bodmer, J. G., Marsh, S. G. E., and Albert, E. (1990) Nomenclature of the HLA system, 1989. *Immunol. Today* 11:3—10.

Brown, J. H., Jardetzky, T., Saper, M. A., Samraoui, B., Bjorkman, P. J., and Wiley, D. C. (1988) A hypotical model of the foreign antigen binding site of class II histocompatibility molecules. *Nature (London)* 332:845—850.

Browne, H., Smith, G., Beck, S., and Minson, T. (1990) A complex between the MHC class I homologue encoded by human cytomegalovirus and β2-microglobulin. *Nature (London)* 347:770—772.

Cerundolo, V., Alexander, J., Anderson, K., Lamb, C., Cresswell, P., McMichael, A., Gotch, F., and Townsend, A. (1990) Presentation of viral antigen controlled by a gene in the major histocompatibility complex. *Nature (London)* 345:449—452.

Charron, D., and McDewitt, H. O. (1979) Analysis of HLA-D region associated molecules with monoclonal antibody. *Proc. Natl. Acad. Sci. U.S.A.* 76:6567—6571.

Charron, D. J., Lotteau, V., and Turmel, P. (1984) Hybrid HLA-DC antigens provide molecular evidence for gene trans-complementation. *Nature (London)* 312:157—159.

Cunningham, B. A., Wang, J. L., Beggard, I., and Peterson, P. A. (1973) The complete amino acid sequence of β2-microglobulin. *Biochemistry* 12:6811—6822.

Dausset, J. (1958) Iso-leuco-anticorps. *Acta Hematol.* 20:156.

Darden, A. G., and Streilein, J. W. (1984) Syrian hamsters express two monomorphic class I major histocompatibility complex molecules. *Immunogenetics* 20:603—622.

Dargemont, C., Dunon, D., Deugnier, M. A., Denoyelle, M., Girault, J.-M., Lederer, F., Ho Diep Lê, K., Godeau, F., Thierry, J.-P., and Imhof, B. A. (1989) Thymotaxin, a chemostatic protein, is identical to β2-microglobulin. *Science* 24:803—806.

De Vriess, R. R. P., Schrender, G. M. Th., Naipal, A., D'Amaro, J., and Van Rood, J. J. (1989) Selection by typhoid and yellow fever epidemies witnessed by the HLA-DR locus. In *Immunobiology of HLA*, Vol. 2: Immunogenetics and Histocompatibility B. Dupont, Ed. Springer-Verlag, NY, 461—462.

Due, C., Simonsen, M., and Olsson, L. (1986) The major histocompatibility complex class I heavy chain as a structural subunit of the human cell membrane insulin receptor: implications for the range of biological functions of histocompatibility antigens. *Proc. Natl. Acad. Sci. U.S.A.* 83:6007—6011.

Ferrier, P., Layet, C., Caillol, D. H., Jordan, B. R., and Lemonnier, F. A. (1985) The association between murine β2-microglobulin and HLA class I heavy chains results in serologically detectable conformational changes of both chains. *J. Immunol.* 135:1281—1287.

Figueroa, F., Günther, E., and Klein, J. (1988) MHC polymorphism pre-dating speciation. *Nature (London)* 335:265—267.

Flajnik, M. F., and DuPasquier, L. (1990) The major histocompatibility complex of frogs. *Immunol. Rev.* 113:47—63.

Friedman, R. L., and Stark, G. R. (1985) α-Interferon-induced transcription of HLA and methallothionein genes containing homologous upstream sequences. *Nature (London)* 314:637—639.

Garret, T. P. J., Saper, M. A., Bjorkman, P. J., Strominger, J. L., and Wiley, D. C. (1989) Specificity pockets for the side chains of peptide antigens in HLA-Aw68. *Nature (London)* 342:692—696.

Goulmy, E., Termijelen, A., Bradley, B. A., and VanRood, J. J. (1977) Y-antigen killing by T cells of women is restricted by HLA. *Nature (London)* 266:544.

Guagliardi, L. E., Koppelman, B., Blum, J. S., Marks, M. S., Cresswell, P., and Brodsky, F. M. (1990) Co-localization of molecules involved in antigen processing and presentation in an early endocytic compartment. *Nature (London)* 343:133—139.

Güssow, D., Rein, R., Ginjaar, I., Hochstewbach, F., Seemann, G., Kottman, A., and Ploegh, H. L. (1987) The human β2-microglobulin gene: primary structure and definition of the transcriptional unit. *J. Immunol.* 139:3132—3138.

Gustafsson, K., Widmark, E., Jonsson, A. K., Servenius, B., Sachs, D., Larhammar, D., Rask, L., and Peterson, P. A. (1987) Class II genes of the human major histocompatibility complex. Evolution of the DP region as deduced from nucleotide sequences of the four genes. *J. Biol. Chem.* 262:8778—8786.

Hickling, J. K., Fenton, C. M., Howland, K., Marsh, S. G. E., and Rothbard, J. B. (1990) Peptides recognized by class I restricted T cells also bind to MHC class II molecules. *Int. Immunol.* 2:435—441.

Jonsson, A. K., Hyldig-Nielsen, J. J., Servenius, B., Larhammar, D., Andersson, G., Jorgensen, F., Peterson, P. A., and Rask, L. (1987) Class II genes of the human major histocompatibility complex. Comparison of the DQ and DX and β genes. *J. Biol. Chem.* 262:8767—8777.

Kappler, J. W., Roehm, N., and Marrack, P. (1987) T cell tolerance by clonal elimination in the thymus. *Cell* 49:273—280.

Kefford, R. F., Calabi, F., Fearnley, I. M., Burrone, O. R., and Milstein, C. (1984) Serum β2-microglobulin binds to a T cell differentiation antigens and increases its expression. *Nature (London)* 308:641—642.

Kieran, M., Blank, V., Logeat, F., Vandekerckhove, J., Lottspeich, F., Le Bail, O., Urban, M. B., Kourilsky, P., Baeuerle, P. A., and Israël, A. (1990) The DNA binding subunit of NF-kB is identical to factor KBF1 and homologous to the rel oncogene product. *Cell* 62:1007—1018.

Kimura, A., Israël, A., Le Bail, O., and Kourilsky, P. (1986) Detailed analysis of the mouse H-2K^b promoter: enhancer-like sequences and their role in the regulation of class I gene expression. *Cell* 44:261—272.

Kisielow, P., Blüthmann, H., Staerz, U. D., Steinmetz, M., and Von Boehmer, H. (1988) Tolerance in T-cell-receptor transgenic mice involves deletion of nommature CD4+ 8+ thymocytes. *Nature (London)* 333:742—746.

Klar, D., and Hämmerling, G. J. (1989) Induction of assembly of MHC class I heavy chains with β2-microglobulin by interferon-y. *EMBO J.* 8:475—481.

Koller, B. H., and Orr, H. T. (1985) Cloning and complete sequence of HLA-A2 gene: analysis of two HLA-A alleles at the nucleotide level. *J. Immunol.* 134:2727—2733.

Koller, B. H., Geraghty, D. E., DeMars, R., Duvick, L., Rich, S. S., and Orr, H. T. (1989) Chromosomal organization of the human major histocompatibility complex class I gene family. *J. Exp. Med.* 169:469—480.

Koller, B. H., Marrack, P., Kappler, J. W., and Smithies, O. (1990) Normal development of mice deficient in β2-m class I proteins, and CD8+ T cells. *Science* 248:1227—1230.

Krensky, A. M., Robbins, E., Springer, T. A., and Burakoff, S. J. (1984) LFA-1, LFA-2 and LFA-3 antigens are involved in CTL-target conjugation. *J. Immunol.* 132:2180—2182.

Larhammar, D., Hämmerling, U., Rask, L., and Peterson, P. A. (1985) Sequence of gene and cDNA encoding murine major histocompatibility complex class II gene Aβ2. *J. Biol. Chem.* 260:14111—14119.

Lawlor, D. A., Ward, F. E., Ennis, P. D., Jackson, A. P., and Parham, P. (1988) HLA-A and B polymorphisms predate the divergence of humans and chimpanzees. *Nature (London)* 335:268—271.

Lee, J. S., Trowsdale, J., and Bodmer, W. (1982) cDNA clones coding for the heavy chain of human HLA-DR antigen. *Proc. Natl. Acad. Sci. U.S.A.* 79:545—549.

Lotteau, V. L., Teyton, L., Burroughs, D., and Charron, D. J. (1987) A novel HLA class II molecule (DR-DQβ) created by mismatched isotype pairing. *Nature (London)* 329:339—341.

Loveland, B., Wang, C. R., Yonekawa, H., Herzel, E., and Fischer-Lindahl, K. (1990) Maternally transmitted histocompatability antigen of mice: a hydrophobic peptide of a mitochondrial encoded protein. *Cell* 60:971—980.

Malissen, M., Malissen, B., and Jordan, B. R. (1982) Exon/intron organization and complete nucleotide sequence of an HLA gene. *Proc. Natl. Acad. Sci. U.S.A.* 79:893—897.

Miyazaki, J. I., Appella, E., and Ozato, K. (1986) Negative regulation of the major histocompatibility class I gene in undifferentiated embryonal carcinoma cells. *Proc. Natl. Acad. Sci. U.S.A.* 83:9537—9541.

Orr, H. T., Lopez de Castro, J. A., Lancet, D., and Strominger, J. L. (1979) Complete amino acid sequence of a papain-solubilized human histocompatibility antigen, HLA-B7: sequence determination and search for homologies. *Biochemistry* 18:5711—5720.

Pérarnau, B., Siegrist, C.-A., Gillet, A., Vincent, C., Kimura, S., and Lemonnier, F. A. (1990) β2-microglobulin restriction of antigen presentation. *Nature (London)* 346:751—754.

Perkins, D. L., Lai, M. Z., Smith, J. A., and Gefter, J. A. (1989) Identical peptides recognized by MHC class I and II restricted cells. *J. Exp. Med.* 170:279—290.

Peterson, M. and Miller, J. (1990) Invariant chain influences the immunological recognition of MHC class II molecules. *Nature (London)* 345:172—174.

Piazza, A., Belvedere, M. C., Bernoco, D., Conighi, C., Contu, L., Curton, E. S., Mattiuz, P. L., Mayz, W., Richiard, P., Scudeller, G., and Ceppellini, R. (1972) HLA variation in four sardinian villages under differential selective pressure by malaria. In *Histocompatibility Testing*, (P. I. Terasaki, ed.), Munksgaard, Copenhagen, 73—84.

Piontek, G. E., Taniguchi, K., Ljunggren, H.-G., Grönberg, A., Kiesling, R., Klein, G., and Kärre, K. (1985) YAC-1 MHC class I variants reveal an association between decreased NK sensitivity and increased H-2 expression after interferon treatment or in vivo passage. *J. Immunol.* 135:4281—4288.

Ramsdell, F., and Fowlkes, B. J. (1990) Clonal deletion versus clonal anergy: the role of the thymus in inducing self-tolerance. *Science* 248:1342—1348.

Reid, P. A. and Watts, C. (1990) Cycling of cell-surface MHC glycoproteins through primaquine-sensitive intracellular compartments, *Nature (London)* 346:655—657.

Reith, W., Satola, S., Herrero-Sanchez, C., Amaldi, L., Losiwska-Grospierre, B., Griscelli, C., Hadam, M. R., and Mach, B. (1988) Congenital immunodeficiency with a regulatory defect in MHC class II gene expression lacks a specific HLA-DR promoter binding protein, RF-X. *Cell* 53:897—915.

Roche, P. A. and Cresswell, P. (1990) Invariant chain association with HLA-DR molecules inhibits immunogenic peptide binding. *Nature (London)* 345:615—618.

Rötzscke, O., Falk, K., Wallny, H.-J., Faath, S., and Rammensee, H.-G., (1990) Characterization of naturally occurring minor histocompatibility peptides including H-4 and H-Y. *Science* 249:283—286.

Rollini, P., Mach, B. and Gorski, J. (1985) Linkage map of three HLA-DRβ-chain genes: evidence for a recent duplication event. *Proc. Natl. Acad. Sci. U.S.A.* 82:7197—7201.

Rossomando, A. and Meruelo, D. (1986) Viral sequences are associated with many histocompatibility genes. *Immunogenetics* 23:233—245.

Rupp, F., Acha-Orbea, H., Hengartner, H., Zinkernagel, R., and Joho, R. (1985) Identical V beta T-cell receptor genes used in alloreactive cytotoxic and antigen plus I-A specific helper T cells. *Nature (London)* 315:425—427.

Schneck, J., Maloy, W. L., Coligan, J. E., and Marguelis, D. H. (1989) Inhibition of allo-specific T cell hybridoma by soluble class I proteins and peptides: estimation of the affinity of a T cell receptor for MHC. *Cell* 56:47—55.

Schulze, D. H., Pease, L. R., Geier, S. S., Reyes, A. A., Sarmiento, L. A., Wallace, R. B., and Nathenson, S. (1983) Comparison of the cloned H-2K^{bm1} variant gene with the H-2K^b gene shows a cluster of seven nucleotide differences. *Proc. Natl. Acad. Sci. U.S.A.* 80:2007—2011.

Signäs, C., Katze, M. G., Persson, H., and Philipson, L. (1982) An adenovirus glucoprotein binds heavy chains of class I transplantation antigens from man and mouse. *Nature (London)* 299:175—178.

Simister, N. E., and Mostov, K. E. (1989) An Fc receptor structurally related to MHC class I antigens. *Nature (London)* 337:184—187.

Sinclair, A. H., Berta, P., Palmer, M. S., Hawkins, J. R., Griffiths, B. L., Smith, M. J., Foster, J. W., Frischauf, A.-M., Lowell-Badge, R., and Goodfellow, P. N. (1990) A gene from the human sex-determining region encodes a protein with homology to a conserved DNA-binding motif. *Nature (London)* 346:240—244.

Spies, T., Sorrentino, R., Boss, J. M., Okada, K., and Strominger, J. L. (1985) Structural organization of the DR subregion of the human major histocompatibility complex. *Proc. Natl. Acad. Sci. U.S.A.* 82:5165—5169.

Swain, S. L. and Panfili, P. R. (1979) Helper cells activated by allogenneic H-2K or H-2D differences have a Ly phenotype distinct from those responsive to I differences. *J. Immunol.* 122:383—391.

Todd, J. A., Bell, J. I., and McDewitt, H. O. (1987) HLA-DQβ gene contributes to susceptibility and resistance to insulin-dependent diabetes mellitus. *Nature (London)* 329:599—604.

Townsend, A. R. M., Gotch, F. M., and Davey, J. (1985) Cytotoxic T cell recognize fragments of the influenza nucleoprotein. *Cell* 42:457—467.

Townsend, A., Ohlen, C., Bastin, J., Ljunggren, H. G., Foster, L., and Karre, K. (1989) Association of class I major histocompatibility heavy and light chains induced by viral peptides. *Nature (London)* 340:443—446.

Townsend, A., Elliot, T., Cerundolo, V., Foster, L., Barber, B., and Tse, A. (1990) Assembly of MHC class I molecules analysed in vitro. *Cell* 62:285—295.

Van Ewijk, W., Ron, Y., Monaco, J., Kappler, J., Marrack, P., LeMeur, M., Gerlinger, P., Durand, B., Benoist, C., and Mathis, D. (1988) Compartmentalization of MHC class II genes expression in transgenic mice. *Cell* 53:357—370.

Versteeg, R., Krüse-Wolters, K. M., Plomp, A. C., Leeuwen, A. V., Stam, N. J., Ploegh, H. L., Ruiter, D. J., and Schrier, P. I. (1989) Suppression of class I human histocompatibility leukocyte antigen by c-myc is locus specific. *J. Exp. Med.* 170:621—635.

Voogt, P. J., Goulmy, E., Veenhof, W. F. J., Hamilton, M., Fibbe, W. E., VanRood, J. J., and Falkenburg, J. H. F. (1988) Cellularly defined minor histocompatibility antigens are differentially expressed on human hematopoietic progenitor cells. *J. Exp. Med.* 168:2337—2347.

Wachtel, S., Gasser, D. L., and Silvers, W. K. (1973) Male specific antigens: modification of potency by the H-2 locus in mice. *Science* 181:862.

Zilstra, M., Bix, M., Simister, N. E., Loring, J. M., Raulet, D. H. and Jaenish, R. (1990) β2-microglobulin deficient mice lack CD4-8+ cytolytic T cells. *Nature (London)* 344:742—746.

Zinkernagel, R. M. and Doherty, P. C. (1974) Restriction of *in vitro* T cell mediated cytotoxicity in lymphocyte choriomeningitis within a syngenic or semi-allogenic system. *Nature (London)* 248:701—702.

Chapter 16

Vaccine Antigens

Gordon L. Ada
Department of Immunology and Infectious Diseases
Johns Hopkins School of Hygiene and Public Health
Baltimore, MD

INTRODUCTION

Traditionally, vaccines have been developed to prevent disease by infectious agents and have been used mainly, though not solely, as a prophylactic measure. They are being developed today not only for this purpose but also as a prophylactic measure to control fertility for both human and animal use. This chapter will deal mainly with antigens of vaccines to infectious diseases.

Infectious agents occur in a wide range of shapes, sizes, and complexity. Among the simplest are the plant viroids and the agents of scrapie and Jacob-Kreutsfeld diseases. The viruses most studied vary from having multiple copies of few antigens, e.g., the picornaviruses, to the pox viruses which contain >100 different proteins, including a number of enzymes. In contrast to viruses which only replicate in cells, bacteria contain all the necessary components for extracellular life, although many infect eukaryotic cells. Infectious agents with the highest levels of complexity include the rickettsia and the different types of parasites from protozoa, which replicate in cells, to worms which live and replicate in body fluids.

The different components, the antigens, of infectious agents often have quite different roles in the life cycle of the agent. Particularly for those that live outside cells, the architecture of the organism and the properties of the surface components must be fashioned so that the organism can survive the destructive forces in the environment outside the body. The structure and properties of other agents that may be transmitted by more intimate means, such as body fluids, may be quite different. These considerations will affect the nature and the efficacy of a vaccine that can be developed against the different agents.

GENERAL PROPERTIES OF A VACCINE

A vaccine has two basic properties (Ada, 1990a). For human use, in particular, current vaccines must be very safe, that is, cause an acceptably low incidence of morbidity and especially mortality. Furthermore, a vaccine should not sensitize a recipient so that serious immunopathological reactions occur when the vaccinee is later exposed to the wild-type agent (Kapikian et al., 1969).

The second property of the vaccine is efficacy which depends almost entirely on the immune response generated by the vaccine. The vaccine should prime and activate the host's immune system so that, on exposure to the wild-type agent, there is an accelerated immune response which greatly decreases the infectious challenge and clinical disease does not occur. The following section will briefly summarize important aspects of the immune response to an antigen with particular attention to the stimulation and responses of T and B lymphocytes.

The Immune Response to Antigens

Most antigenic materials are either protein (polypeptide) or carbohydrate in nature. Carbohydrates sometimes represent a special situation, which will be discussed later; in this section, proteins are used to illustrate the major steps in immune recognition and cellular responses.

Historical Overview

An early indication that there were different mechanisms of antigen recognition was the finding by Gell and Benacceraf (1959) that if ovalbumin (OVA)-immune guinea pigs were challenged, only native OVA could induce anaphylaxis (an antibody-mediated reaction) whereas both native and denatured OVA could induce delayed-type hypersensitivity (DTH) reactions. DTH is one manifestation of a "cell-mediated" response which was subsequently shown to be mediated by T lymphocytes (Miller et al., 1976). In the next decade, experiments with synthetic antigens (Sela, 1969) led to the conclusion that the immunoglobulin (Ig) receptors on B lymphocytes predominantly recognized three-dimensional shapes or conformations. B cells could be inactivated by intact, radioactive antigen which bound to the Ig receptors (Ada and Byrt, 1969).

Studies on the fate of antigens (Nossal and Ada, 1971) implicated macrophages as a major cell type for handling antigen in the body. When the role of macrophages in presenting antigen to the lymphocyte was examined in detail in the early 1970s, it was found that major histocompatibility antigen complex (MHC) gene products were directly involved in three ways (Ada, 1989; Allen et al., 1987). Two of these ways involved interaction between macrophages (or related cells) and T cells, so that T-cell responses to the antigen could be defined as class I (mainly cytotoxic, Tc) reactions or class II (helper T, Th, or DTH T, Td cell)-restricted responses. Thus, the T-cell response was genetically controlled and this explained the considerable variation in immune responses often seen between individuals in an outbred population.

Pathways to T- and B-Cell Activation and Differentiation

These two pathways were elucidated as follows. In an antigen-presenting cell, such as a macrophage, proteins were nonspecifically endocytosed and degraded in lysosomes and some of the peptides produced bound specifically to class II MHC antigens and were transported to the plasma membrane (Buus et al., 1987). In contrast, if an agent, for example, a virus, *infected* the macrophage, some of the newly synthesized infectious viral proteins were degraded in the cytoplasm to peptides, but these peptides associated with class I MHC antigens and were transported to the plasma membrane (Townsend et al., 1985). The first pathway is called the *endosomal* pathway and the second, the *cytoplasmic* pathway. It is now clear that there are other ways whereby proteins can enter the cytoplasmic pathway, e.g., through fusion of a protein with the plasma membrane or by having a lipid "tail" (Deres et al., 1989), or by constructing immunostimulating complexes (ISCOMS) (Jones et al., 1988, Takahashi et al., 1990).

Suppressor T cells (Ts) can also be generated and are known to be important in some situations, but the pathway to their generation is not well understood. They may be class I or II MHC restricted. Suppressor effects can be mediated in different ways, such as prevention of helper or effector T-cell generation, or by prevention of effector cell function (Hodes, 1989; Simpson, 1988).

In addition to antigen recognition as described above, cells in the immune system interact through protein messengers, called cytokines or interleukins (ILs). These are produced mainly by T cells and a variety of nonlymphocytic cells, including macrophages, and act at short range via specific receptors on a wide variety of cells including T and B lymphocytes. The pattern of interleukin production by different cells and their action on cells is complex (Gillis, 1989) and will not be discussed further here. The processing of antigen and activation and differentiation of T cells is illustrated in Fig. 1 (Ada, 1990b). It was subsequently found that another class of cells, the dendritic cells including Langerhans cells, express high levels of class II MHC antigens and are very effective antigen presenters to T cells (Steinman et al., 1975). Sometimes, they may act in association with macrophages (Guidos et al., 1987).

The third mode of MHC antigen involvement in antigen presentation is illustrated in Fig. 2. An epitope on a simple antigen, or even on a more complex particle such as a virus, is recognized by the Ig receptor with the

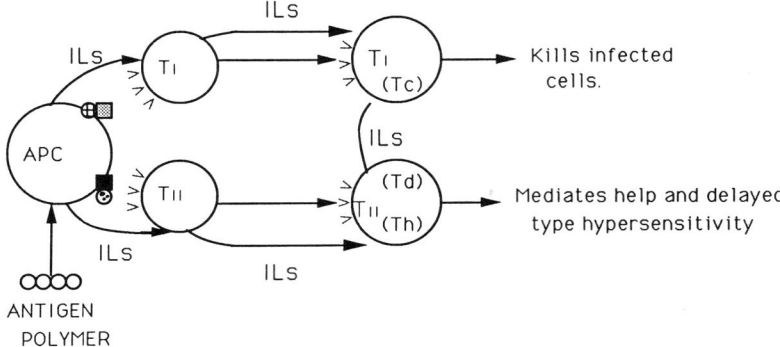

Figure 1. Processing of antigen and activation of T cells. Antigen-presenting cell (APC); class I (□) and II (■) MHC antigens; peptides from degraded antigen (○ ○) which bind to MHC antigens; T-cell receptors (>); class I- (TI) and class II (TII)–restricted T cells; interleukins (ILs); cytotoxic T cells (Tc); helper T cells (Th); T cells mediating delayed-type hypersensitivity (Td). [Reproduced from G. L. Ada (1990) *Sem. Virol.* 1:3—9. With permission.]

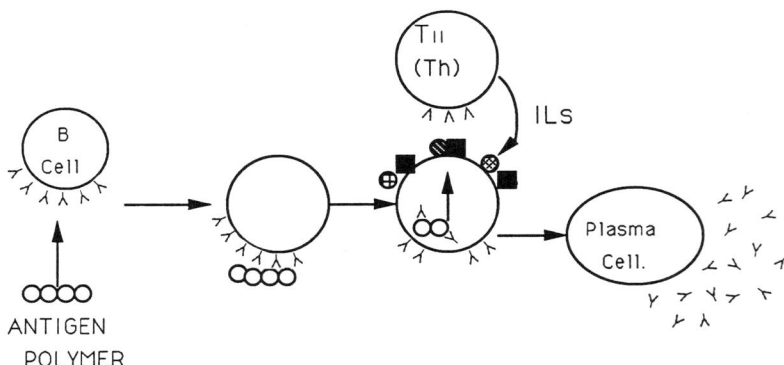

Figure 2. Antigen-presentation by B cells and their activation to become antibody-secreting (plasma) cells. B cell receptor, immunoglobulin (antibody) (Y); class II MHC antigens (■); peptides from processed antigen-receptor complexes (○ ○ ○); activated, class II MHC-restricted T helper cell (TII, Th); interleukins (ILs). [Reproduced from G. L. Ada (1990) *Sem. Virol.* 1:3—9 With permission.]

appropriate specificity on the B cell. The complex is endocytosed and is believed to be processed in much the same way as occurs with foreign proteins in the macrophage so that the peptide/MHC complexes expressed at the B cell surface are similar to those expressed by the macrophage (Lanzavecchia, 1987). Already activated Th cells which have T-cell receptors of the appropriate specificity recognize these complexes at the B cell membrane, and this induces the secretion by the T cell of other ILs which induce differentiation/

replication of the B cell to become an antibody-secreting cell (ASC), such as a plasma cell. The more complex the antigen taken up by the B cell, the greater the possibility of a variety of peptide/MHC complexes expressed at the cell surface which in turn allows Th cells with several different specificities to interact with an individual B cell.

In addition to these "primary" events, two other processes are important. The first is immunological memory, the generation of increased numbers of T and B cells with receptors of a given specificity. These cells are not identical to their "naive" precursors. T memory cells have increased levels of some cell surface antigens (Rajewsky, 1989) and, in humans, the antigen CD45RO is being increasingly seen as a reliable marker (Beverley et al., 1989). Memory B cells may express IgG or IgA receptors as well as IgM and IgD (Black et al., 1978). In addition, the requirements of Tc and B memory cells for T cell help for activation and differentiation seem to be less stringent.

The second event is antigen localization on the surface of dendritic follicular cells (DFC) in primary or secondary lymphoid follicles in lymphoid tissues, such as lymph nodes or spleen (Nossal and Ada, 1971). Antigen-antibody complexes attach via complement receptors to the surface of these cells and this is now seen as a mechanism for the recruitment of specific B memory cells to form ASCs (Skazal et al., 1989; van Rooijen, 1989). Depending on the nature of the antigen, these complexes can quickly disappear or they may persist for many months after antigen administration (Nossal and Ada, 1971).

Different Immune Responses Arise in a Time-Dependent Fashion

Figure 3 (Ada, 1990a) illustrates the response to an influenza virus infection in naive mice. Virus (curve A) replicates in the lungs, reaches maximum titers by day 4-5, and decreases thereafter, so that no infectious virus is detected after about day 12. Tc cell activity (curve B) peaks a few days after maximum virus levels and then decreases so that no activity is found after about 2 weeks. However, memory T cells reach their highest levels (20- to 100-fold increase in numbers) at about 2 weeks and remain high for the life of the mouse. In contrast, the numbers of ASCs, first detected at about day 6, rise to maximum levels at about 6 weeks (curve C) and then steadily decline, although some are detectable (in particular, ASCs secreting IgG) for at least 18 months. Maximum levels of B memory cells are found 10 to 15 weeks after infection and then decrease in number, although some are still found at 18 months (Jones and Ada, 1987).

The Role of Different Immune Responses

In the case of an acute infection, several different phases of the immune response can readily be identified (Ada, 1989). The situation is more complicated with agents that cause chronic, persisting infections, although the general principles remain the same.

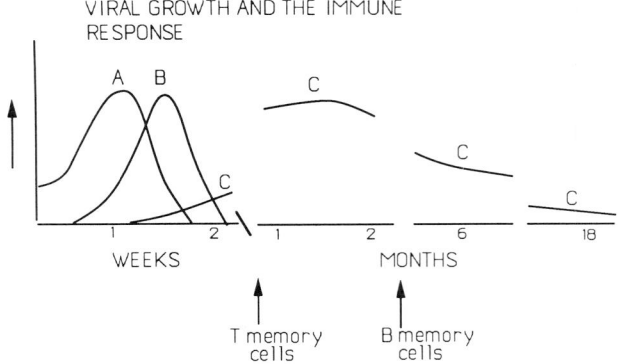

Figure 3. Time sequence of the infectious process and the subsequent immune response. Ordinate, increase in infectivity/effector cell numbers; abscissa, time after initiation of infection. (A) Growth and disappearance of infectious virus. (B) Appearance and disappearance of effector Tc cells. (C) Appearance and continuing presence of antibody-secreting cells. [Reproduced from *Lancet*, 335, 523 (1990). With permission.]

Prevention of Infection

Other than physical or chemical barriers, specific antibody is the only known method for preventing infection by an infectious agent. The generation of protective antibody has generally been the only criterion used by vaccine developers and is measured *in vitro* by the neutralization assay, and in experimental animal model systems by antibody transfer. Generally, such antibody reacts with a limited number of epitopes on one or a few antigens of the infectious agent.

Limitation of Replication

There are a number of nonadaptive and nonspecific responses which, shortly after infection, can limit replication of the agent. These include complement, a variety of cells such as natural killer (NK) cells, eosinophils, and cytokines, such as α- and β-interferon.

Recovery from Infection

Specific antibody can reduce titers of an agent through reactions such as antibody-dependent cellular cytotoxicity (ADCC) and complement-mediated lysis of infected cells. It is not clear whether these mechanisms, in the absence of effector T cells, will completely clear an infection.

For many viral infections and for some bacterial and parasitic infections, cellular responses are critical. This applies particularly to the generation of Tc cells which mainly, if not only, are mediated by class I MHC-restricted

TABLE 1.
Viral Vaccines

Type	Agent	
	Current	Under Trial
Live, attenuated	Vaccinia, measles, yellow fever, mumps, polio (OPV)[a], adenovirus[a], rubella, varicella zoster	Cytomegalovirus, hepatitis A, influenza (2), dengue, rotavirus (2), parainfluenza, Japanese encephalitis, polio (OPV)
Inactivated	Polio (IPV), influenza, rabies, Japanese encephalitis	Hepatitis A
Subunit	Hepatitis B, influenza	

[a] Administered orally.

reactions. The need for this class of cells is greatest if the "protective" external antigen(s) of the agent undergo marked antigenic variation so that antibody is largely or completely ineffective. In some situations, class II MHC-restricted T-cell responses may also be critical.

These considerations lead to the recognition that a vaccine should achieve four goals (Ada, 1990a):

1. Activation of antigen-presenting cells to initiate antigen processing and production of ILs;
2. Generation of a high yield of T and B memory cells;
3. Generation of Th and Tc cells to several epitopes so as to overcome the variation in the immune response due to MHC polymorphism;
4. Persistence of antigen on dendritic follicular cells in lymphoid tissues, where memory B cells are recruited to form ASCs so that there is continual production of antibody, because individual ASCs have a relatively short half-life.

CURRENT AND TRIAL VACCINES

Tables 1 and 2 list the viral and bacterial vaccines currently licensed for human administration and those candidate vaccines which are at an advanced stage of clinical testing. They will not be described in detail but some general points will be discussed.

1. Most of the diseases represented by the agents in these tables are acute infections, that is, in most infected people, a nonlethal infection is over and eliminated in a few weeks.
2. There are three types of vaccines: attenuated, live agent, inactivated whole agent, and subunit vaccine, composed of one or a very few antigens of the agent.

TABLE 2.
Bacterial Vaccines

Type	Agent Current	Under Trial
Live, attenuated	BCG	V. cholerae[a] S. typhimurium (Ty21a), S. typhimurium (aro A)
Inactivated	V. cholerae, B. pertussis, S. typhimurium	V. cholerae + subunit[a], M. leprae
Subunit	H. influenzae, N. meningitidis, S. pneumoniae	S. typhimurium (Vi polys.), H. influenzae-DT conjugate, B. pertussis
Toxoid	Tetanus, diphtheria	

[a] Administered orally.

3. Attenuated, live viruses have generally been highly successful as vaccines and, for those in Table 1, the level of efficacy is considered to be about 90% or higher. In contrast, the one bacterial vaccine of this type has given very variable protection levels, being as low as 27% in a major Indian trial (Frimodt-Moller et al., 1964).
4. Some inactivated whole viral vaccines, such as rabies, Japanese encephalitis, and polio, have been quite successful though 100- 1000-fold larger doses are needed compared to live preparations. The influenza vaccine is of limited efficacy, but the reason for this is the extensive antigenic variation to which this virus is subject. Bacterial vaccines in this category have given variable results: pertussis has been effective though having a high level of side reactions (Mortimer, 1988).
5. The hepatitis B vaccine represents a great achievement in this area and although it remains to be seen whether it will prevent primary liver cancer, it has a good efficacy with about 10% of vaccinees failing to respond. This may be overcome by using a product with more T-cell epitopes.
6. With the exception of the toxoids, bacterial vaccines have been less successful than their viral counterparts. The pertussis vaccine is effective but reactogenic and great effort is being expended to make a subunit vaccine which is less reactogenic (Edwards et al., 1986; Kimura and Kuno-Sakai, 1990). There is great interest in developing attenuated bacterial vaccines but this is proving to be more difficult than was found with viruses (Ada, 1989).
7. Many bacteria of great medical importance are encapsulated, i.e., they have an outer covering of polysaccharide which is often a major protective antigen. Though some vaccines composed of the polysaccharide component are variably effective in children over 2 years of

age and in adults (Gaillat et al., 1985; Riley et al., 1986), they are ineffective in infants (Fedson, 1989). These vaccines are discussed at greater length later in this chapter.

Special Properties of Vaccine Antigens
Dichotomy of Immune Recognition

With this information as a background, it is clear that if a vaccine is to be optimally successful, the antigens in the vaccine require special properties. The first feature for discussion is the implications for antigen structure arising from the dichotomy of immune recognition.

It is a feature of many biological structures that identical molecules are held together in a strict geometrical pattern, and sometimes as a small or large mosaic. Thus the flagella of motile bacteria are comprised of identical monomeric flagellin molecules held together by noncovalent bonds (Lowy and Hanson, 1965). The surface antigens of myxovirus exist as trimers of the hemagglutinin and tetramers of the neuraminidase (Murphy and Webster, 1985; Vargese et al., 1983). The surface pattern of a picornavirus, such as polio, consists of a set of different mosaics, each one consisting of closely packed identical (within a mosaic) molecules of the proteins VP1, VP2, or VP3 (Hogle et al., 1985). For such situations, it is frequently found that highly effective neutralizing antibodies recognize discontinuous epitopes composed of adjacent molecules so that such epitopes have a tertiary or quaternary conformation (Nestorowicz et al., 1985).

This antigenic structure must be preserved for two reasons: (1) so that B cells with the appropriate receptor specificity are selected to undergo a primary antibody response; and (2) so that a sufficient amount of antigen with the same structure can persist on the surface of dendritic follicular cells. Circulating B memory cells with the appropriate receptor specificity are "recruited" by this antigen and differentiate to antibody-secreting cells. Furthermore, as the concentration of antigen declines over time, mutant cells which may have higher affinity receptors can be selected (Skazal et al., 1989; van Rooijen, 1989). In this way advantage is taken of affinity maturation of B-cell receptors (Goidl et al., 1968). For this to occur, the persisting antigen should retain its conformation and this requires that it should be resistant to proteolysis. The carbohydrate side chains of glycoproteins can serve this function, as is discussed later. Recently, the addition of lipids, such as myristic acid, to polio virus was found not only to make the virus more heat stable but also to render the virus less susceptible to proteolysis (Dorval et al., 1989). It was postulated that the lipid penetrated a hydrophobic "canyon" in the VP1 viral antigen.

Although it can be postulated that idiotypic-antiidiotypic networks, in principle, may serve a similar function, there is some evidence (Nossal and Ada, 1971) of a correlation between prolonged persistence of antigen on dendritic follicular cells and prolonged antibody production, and no evidence (to this author's knowledge) for such a long-term (years) role for a network mechanism.

In complete contrast to the above requirement for retention of conformation *outside* the cell, such antigens usually have T-cell epitopes (Anders et al., 1981; Sterkers et al., 1985) as well as B-cell epitopes and these will only be available to the immune system if the protein can be readily degraded *inside* the cell by proteases to yield peptides. Two mechanisms are as follows:

1. When protein is taken up by the endosomal pathway, it enters the acidic (pH ca. 5) medium in lysosomes. This change is sufficient to expose certain sequences in a protein, e.g., influenza hemagglutinin (Skehel et al., 1982) and this may make it more susceptible to proteolytic degradation, leading to the production of at least some active peptides;
2. This mechanism is not available for the production of peptides to react with class I MHC antigens. The exact stage at which peptides are derived from newly synthesized protein in the cytoplasm is not clear, except that it happens before the protein passes through Golgi and is glycosylated (Townsend et al., 1989; Yewdell et al., 1985). It is likely that in a newly synthesized state and before the final conformation of a protein is adopted, e.g., by attachment of sugar residues, it is more susceptible to proteolytic breakdown. The role of carbohydrate side chains in this connection is discussed later.

Whether all the "potentially active" peptides in a protein are ever made available in either pathway is not known but it can be predicted that this is unlikely. It would be of interest to compare the natural occurring, cell-derived peptide specificities with those provided externally to the cell by a series of overlapping synthetic peptides covering the entire amino acid sequence of a protein (Geyson et al., 1986).

Surface vs. Internal Antigens

There are several ways in which a surface antigen can differ from an internal antigen in an infectious agent, including the degree of antigenic variability, the susceptibility to proteolytic degradation, and the content of T- and B-cell epitopes. The last two will be discussed first.

Particularly in the case of those viruses where there is a clear demarcation between external and internal antigens, as is the case with enveloped viruses, the internal antigens are shielded from potential hazards in the medium so that there might not be such a high premium on, for example, lack of susceptibility to proteases. Few internal viral antigens are glycosylated and this might make them more susceptible to enzymatic breakdown. The author is unaware of any systematic study of this aspect.

In principle, all proteins of an infectious agent are potential sources of T-cell epitopes. Few viruses have been examined in great detail, but evidence is accumulating to suggest this is generally the case. The influenza virus has a segmented RNA genome which codes for ten proteins, including two non-structural proteins. Each protein has now been shown to contain Tc-cell epitopes, although the contribution varies both according to and within the host species, e.g., human and mice (Ada and Jones, 1986). There is a general concensus that in the mouse, most Tc activity is specific for internal antigens and the nucleoprotein is a major target (Andrew et al., 1987; Kees and Krammer, 1984; Yewdell et al., 1985). Similarly, at least six of the major proteins of the human immunodeficiency virus (HIV) contain Tc-cell epitopes (Mills et al., 1989; M. McChesnick, 1989, pers. commun.) but the overall contribution of each has not been assessed. Most proteins of the flaviviruses have been shown to contain Tc-cell epitopes (Hill, 1990) and the internal antigen of LCM virus has been shown to be a major contributor of Tc-cell epitopes of that virus (Whitton, 1988). From these examples, it can be seen that the prediction noted above is likely to be generally correct. Although not examined yet to the same extent, the distribution of Th epitopes is likely to be similar. In fact, there is evidence (Perkins et al., 1989) that the same epitope can be functional with both class I and II MHC antigens.

Antigenic Variation — Serotypes vs. Antigenic Drift/Shift

A major feature of most infectious agents is antigenic variation and this may take three forms. The first, which is prevalent particularly with agents in which DNA is the sole genomic material, is different serotypes. A serotype is defined here as a genetically stable derivative with almost constant antigenicity. In contrast, antigenic drift is defined as the potential for sequential mutations to occur during successive viral replications and one or more of these to become dominant for one or other reason. Antigenic shift involves the reassortment of genomic material.

During the biosynthesis of nucleic acids, mutations and mistakes can occur at relatively high frequency. In the case of DNA, there are several effective cellular mechanisms for repairing errors in the nucleic base sequence so that the number of mistakes in the final product is so low as to be almost — but not quite — negligible (Drake et al., 1983). These mechanisms do not operate during RNA synthesis so that mistakes and mutations can persist (Holland et al., 1982).

Agents with a DNA genome can exist as a distinct and stable entity, such as vaccinia virus. For many such agents, however, there is a variable number of known serotypes (Field, 1985; Plotkin and Mortimer, 1988). The existence of multiple serotypes increases the difficulty of vaccine development. It is somewhat ameliorated if only a few are present or dominant in a given region, usually a country. Thus with pneumococcus, the 23-valent vaccine represents the dominant (ca. 90%) serotypes (of a total of >80 known serotypes) in the United States. Of the >40 serotypes of adenovirus, the vaccine contains only two, 4 and 7. Should similar vaccines be made for other regions of the world, the serotypes included in the vaccine would most likely be different.

The mutation frequencies of animal virus RNA genomes is 10^4- to 10^6-fold greater than the highly stable DNA genomes of viruses of similar complexity (Holland et al., 1982; Smith and Inglis, 1987; see also Temin, 1989). There are differences between different RNA viruses (Temin, 1989) but they are relatively minor compared to the observed differences in genetic stability of the different virions. Although antigenic mutants can be recovered from populations immunized with polio types 1, 2, and 3, these viruses are sufficiently stable for the TOPV and TIPV vaccines to be effective (Melnick, 1988). Vaccines against a number of other RNA viruses, such as measles, mumps, and rubella, have been highly successful. This is particularly the case with the measles vaccine which is effective independently of the source of the challenge virus (R. T. Johnson, 1990, pers. commun.). It would be of great interest to know in this case whether the neutralizing epitopes are conserved amino acid sequences in a surface glycoprotein which shows sequence variation in other regions; or whether glycoprotein molecules which show such variation are not incorporated into the virion. In contrast, viruses such as influenza, rhino, and human immunodeficiency show marked antigenic drift. It has been concluded that the mutation frequencies of the RNA genome of a virus does not reflect the rate of field variation observed (Smith and Inglis, 1987). There is much to be found out about this most important property of viral antigens.

Influenza and HIV are the best documented and the former will be mainly described, as currently no vaccines for rhinovirus or HIV are available. In influenza, antigenic drift occurs mainly in the surface glycoproteins, the hemagglutinin (HA) and the neuraminidase (NA). Both antigens have been examined in great detail. The HA contains five epitopes recognized by infectivity-neutralizing antibody (for review, see Ada and Jones, 1986). These were detected in two ways — by sequence analysis of mutant strains which showed that all sites were subject to amino acid substitutions, and by the use of monoclonal antibodies (MAbs) with high neutralizing activity. These were the only regions of substantial sequence variation in the molecule. A study of the binding of a panel of neutralizing MAbs specific for four of these regions (Nestorowicz et al., 1985) showed that MAbs to three sites bound preferentially to the trimeric molecular complex. For the fourth site, the MAbs bound well to both the monomer and the trimer. None of the MAbs bound to denatured HA. Despite extensive studies, antibodies to constant regions of the molecule have not been found to neutralize the infectivity of the virus (Lerner, 1982). In very large part, therefore, the epitopes important for antibody-mediated neutralization of influenza virus infectivity are conformational and nonlinear. In contrast, the internal antigens of the influenza virus show very little antigenic variation, e.g., the nucleoprotein has showed significant variation only once (Murphy and Webster, 1985).

Several neutralizing epitopes on polio virus are also conformational; one, on VP1 (aa sequence 91 to 104), is a linear sequence (Almond and Burke, 1990).

Due to the tremendous international research effort underway, our knowledge concerning HIV is in a continual state of flux. The surface antigen, env, is a glycoprotein of size 160 kda which is composed of an extramembrane component, gp120, and a molecule, gp41, which spans the viral membrane. Amino acid sequence variation in gp120 may amount to at least 26% (Saag et al., 1988). It is less for gp41 and substantially less for the internal viral antigens. There is a consensus that gp120 contains a principle neutralizing domain (PND); this is a disulfide-bonded linear amino acid sequence, aa 305—330, the V3 loop, in which certain residues are highly variable (Meloen et al., 1989).This sequence also contains a T-cell epitope (Takahashi et al., 1988). There are, however, reports of conserved sequences recognized by neutralizing antibody in both gp41 and gp120 (Shafferman et al., 1989; Veronese et al., 1989; Weiss et al., 1988). It is of interest that in a recent report (Berman et al., 1990) preparations of both gp120 and gp160 which were made by transfected Chinese hamster ovary cells, when used to immunize chimpanzees, induced rather similar levels of total antibody yet only the former protected the animals from a challenge with HIV. The former induced considerably higher levels of antibody to the PND compared to gp160!

Antigenic Variation — T-Cell Epitopes

Shortly after the discoveries of MHC antigen restriction of cytotoxic T cells (Zinkernagel and Doherty, 1974) and their formation during a murine influenza virus infection (Yap and Ada, 1977), the surprising finding was made that Tc cells to one strain of influenza A virus would react with any other influenza A virus, independently of the viral subtype (Doherty et al., 1977). As is clear from previous comments, the reason is that most epitopes derive from internal antigens which show little antigenic variation. This is now a general finding for viruses and, in fact, it has been proposed that this could be used as an additional means for viral classification (A. Mullbacher, 1985, pers. commun.). Current information indicates that HIV shows a similar pattern of cross-reactivity at this level (Chenciner et al., 1989). Current data on helper T-cell epitopes shows a similar pattern (Mills et al., 1989).

There seems a very good reason for this pattern of T cell crossreactivity. The most successful parasite causing an *acute* infection will not kill most hosts it infects. If, because of antigenic variation at the level of epitopes recognized by neutralizing antibody, a second infection by a mutant virus occurs, memory Th and Tc cells (from a first infection), which recognize conserved sequences on mainly internal antigens, will rapidly be mobilized, leading to recovery by most hosts from the infection. This has been observed in model systems (e.g., Zinkernagel, 1990). This is not so critical in the case of a chronic, persistent infection such as HIV when the interval between infection and disease (AIDS) may be more than 10 years. In addition, some persistent and chronic infections are often characterized by deficient or ineffective (in clearing virus) effector T-cell responses.

Chimeric Protein Molecules

Despite the success of most viral vaccines, there is reason to think that some improvements are possible. OPV administration, for example, causes paralysis in about 1/5 million doses. This is due to the type 3 vaccine strain reverting to virulence at a fairly high frequency (Evans et al., 1985). Furthermore, the type 3 strain is less immunogenic than types 1 and 2 so that the immune response to type 3 may be relatively low if there is interference between strains during infection. This is seen particularly in developing countries (Patriaca et al., 1990). Two ways to overcome this are being studied. One is to make "chimeric" viruses, i.e., to incorporate into the one virion antigenic molecules from one or more strains (Burke et al., 1988). A second approach, which appears more promising at present, is to make chimeric protein molecules. One of the several viral neutralizing epitopes on the VP1 antigen of polio virus is a linear amino acid sequence (aa) and constructs have now been made in which the corresponding sequence from strain 3 replaces the sequence from strain 2, which is the most immunogenic (Murray et al., 1988). This chimeric virus preparation is under investigation.

Further developments in this area are even more interesting. A construct has been made in which this 12 aa sequence in polio virus strain 1 has been replaced with an 18 aa conserved sequence from gp41 which is said to be a cross-neutralizing epitope between different HIV isolates (Dalgleish et al., 1988; Kennedy et al., 1986). This construct was immunogenic and, following a multiimmunization schedule in rabbits, induced low levels of HIV-neutralizing antibody, and also absorbed out some of this activity from anti-HIV sera (Evans et al., 1989). A number of other chimaeras have been made (Almond and Burke, 1990).

Although very innovative, this approach has limitations. To date, few neutralizing epitopes on viral proteins are linear which is required if this approach is to be generally used. Second, it may well be unusual for a single epitope like this one to be highly immunodominant. Nevertheless, further developments in this area are awaited with interest.

CARBOHYDRATE ANTIGENS

Carbohydrate antigens are of interest for two reasons. The first is as a component (the prosthetic groups) of glycoproteins, and second, as antigens in their own right.

Glycoproteins

With few exceptions, vertebrate cell plasma membrane-associated proteins are glycoproteins and some of the proteins of viruses which replicate in such cells are also glycosylated. This is especially the case with the surface antigens of enveloped viruses such as the myxo- and paramyxoviruses and lentiviruses, which bud from the plasma membrane of infected cells. Thus, both of the surface antigens of the influenza virus, HA and NA, have several carbohydrate side- chains (Ward, 1981, 1983) and the env antigen of HIV is heavily glycosylated — some 40% of the total weight. Several generalizations can be made about the carbohydrate groups:

1. They are poorly immunogenic in comparison with the protein component. Anti-carbohydrate antibodies are formed after infection but the important epitopes are peptide in nature. The surface antigen of hepatitis B virus, HBsAg, is glycosylated. The carbohydrate side chains of the plasma product and of the yeast-derived product differ, but the two preparations seem to be equally protective (Krugman, 1988).
2. As the structure of the carbohydrate side chains is determined largely by the cellular enzymes responsible for their synthesis, some cross-reactivity between antiviral and antihost glycoprotein antibodies would be expected and has been observed (Ward et al., 1981). If these components were more immunogenic, viral infection could induce autoimmunity and possibly disease, but this is not generally observed. The molecular mimicry observed using monoclonal antibodies has so far been located to amino acid sequences (Oldstone et al., 1986).
3. Extensive glycosylation could mask protease-susceptible bonds, as has been observed with influenza HA (Schwartz and Klenk, 1974; Skehel et al., 1984). There is also recent evidence that a similar situation occurs with a lentivirus; removal of sialic acids by neuraminidase treatment did not reduce infectivity but rendered the virus more susceptible to proteolysis (Huso et al., 1988).
4. Extensive glycosylation could be expected to contribute to the conformation of the molecule.

Oligo/Polysaccharides

Several bacterial pathogens causing acute invasive disease have carbohydrate capsules which generally serve as virulence factors, inhibiting antibody and complement-mediated phagocytosis (Easmon, 1987). They include *Streptococcus pneumoniae*, *Hemophilus influenzae*, and *Neisseria meningitidis*, which are major respiratory pathogens. The very young and the elderly are at risk from these infections. Group B streptococcus is a normal inhabitant of the gastrointestinal tract and the female lower genital tract. It is a major cause of neonatal septicemia and meningitis. *Escherichia coli* also has capsular K antigens and may also cause meningitis.

It has been a major task to develop vaccines against these organisms, a task not yet completed. Perhaps the most successful vaccine is to *H. influenzae*. Six antigenically distinct capsular polysaccharides have been identified but the type b, consisting of repeating polymers of ribosyl and ribitol phosphates, accounts for 95% of invasive disease cases. Furthermore, 85% of disease occurs in children under 5 years of age (Ward and Cochi, 1988). The critical period is between 6 and 24 months of age. It has been clearly shown that antibody to this polysaccharide protects against invasive disease and IgM and IgG1 and IgG2 subclasses, in conjunction with complement, appear to be the most effective.

The poor response of infants to this and other capsular polysaccharides has been a major cause for the development of vaccines more complex than the sugar alone. These polysaccharides are poorly immunogenic for T cells, in part, because of inefficient processing by macrophages; the main antibody produced is IgM. Shorter chains of the polysaccharides have been used in some preparations (Schneerson et al., 1987), possibly in an attempt to facilitate processing by macrophages. In addition, poor B cell memory is induced (Howard, 1987). Landsteiner in 1924 first showed that improved immunogenicity could be achieved by employing a hapten-carrier system in which the polysaccharide was the hapten. The first candidate conjugate vaccine was produced by Avery and Goebels in 1929 (Avery and Goebel, 1929). Great effort has been expended to determine the most effective kind of conjugate and several such vaccines are now available. The carrier protein may be diphtheria toxoid or a mutant preparation — tetanus toxoid or a group B outer membrane protein (OMP). Considerable ingenuity has been shown in exploring different ways to conjugate the polysaccharide to the protein (For details, see Schneerson et al., 1987.) Such vaccines generally elicit a much improved response in infants which is characterized by T-cell activation and a maturation of class-specific immunity composed mainly of IgG. Preimmunization with the carrier improves the response. It can be argued that use of the homologous OMP as a carrier is preferable as both T and B memory cells would be activated by subsequent infection by the organism.

In a ranking of diseases in developing countries by total disease burden, *S. pneumoniae* far outstripped all other infections (Institute of Medicine, 1986). Some 83 serotypes have so far been identified, and the vaccine currently available in the United States contains the capsular polysaccharides of the 23 types responsible for most disease. This achieves a 90% overall protective efficacy. Clearly, the formation of conjugate vaccines similar to current *H. influenzae* vaccines would be desirable for administration to infants, but this would require a very great effort.

The development of vaccines to *N. meningitidis* has been more difficult. Nine serotypes of this organism have been identified (Lepow, 1988). The capsular polysaccharides contain neuraminic acid, which is a universal sugar component. For example, group A polysaccharide is a polymer of *N*-acetyl-*O*-acetylmannosamine phosphate, whereas the group B polysaccharide is mainly *N*-acetylneuraminic acid itself, and therefore is poorly immunogenic, stimulating, at best, short-lived IgM responses of low affinity. Short oligosaccharides of sialic acid with a similar linkage to that of the group B polysaccharide have been found in newborn and fetal brain (Finne et al., 1983). In other words, it is likely that the host is largely tolerant of such structures. It is all the more remarkable, therefore, that one person has been found with a benign monoclonal gammopathy with 23 mg/ml of IgM anti-poly A(2-8)-NeuNAc. (Kabat et al., 1986), raising the possibility of obtaining cell lines to produce antibodies for adjunct treatment of group B meningococcal meningitis. Unfortunately, group B is the most prevalent cause of disease in the United States. Currently, the safety and efficacy of a tetravalent vaccine (types A, C, Y, and W-135) is being assessed (Lepow, 1988).

PEPTIDE-BASED VACCINES

In principle, vaccines composed of peptides should have several advantages (Brown, 1990). These include a chemically defined and stable product, inclusion of only the most appropriate epitopes (T and B cell), and exclusion of other segments such as suppressor sequences and those sequences which may induce infection-enhancing antibody. The preparation should be very safe. With an effective adjuvant, such preparations should be efficacious but this remains to be established. No vaccine like this has yet been developed and licensed, but several have undergone early clinical testing and two will be described here.

Human Fertility Control Vaccines

One step toward this goal is the development of a vaccine to control human fertility. Of the several approaches being tried, one uses portion of a critical hormone as the hapten. In this case, it is the 37 C-terminal amino acid sequence of the B subunit of the human chorionic gonadotropin hormone which is linked to diphtheria toxoid as the protein carrier (Stevens, 1986). The sequence of this segment is unique among human hormones. The rationale of this approach is the requirement for this hormone for implantation of the fertilized egg in the uterus; the presence of specific antibody prevents this from occurring. Phase 1 trials of this prototype vaccine in nonfertile women have demonstrated safety and immunogenicity (Jones et al., 1988) and phase 2 trials should shortly begin. In this application, activation of anti-self T cells, which may initiate autoimmune disease is to be avoided. For this reason, a foreign protein is used as carrier and the relatively short peptide should contain few if any T-cell epitopes (Ada, 1990c). As further development of such a vaccine occurs, it may be possible to devise a means of avoiding T cell involvement by the judicious use of selected interleukins, such as IL-6, to directly enhance a B-cell response.

Antimalaria Vaccines

Malaria remains one of the most serious and widespread of human infectious diseases; approximately one third of the human population on the earth are at risk of infection. There has been an intensive effort for more than 15 years, using the most recent technology, to develop a malaria vaccine. Due to the finding that some parasite antigens contain tandemly repeating amino acid sequences, the use of peptides at least as haptens could be successful as an approach to vaccine development.

All three stages of the malaria life cycle — sporozoite, merozoite, and gametocyte — are vaccine targets and the former will be used to illustrate both the progress and difficulties involved. Sporozoites, injected by feeding infected mosquitoes, rapidly enter the liver and infect hepatocytes. In model systems, irradiated sporozoites or high concentrations of anticircumsporozoite protein (CP) antibody can protect against infection. It has recently been found that irradiated sporozoites can protect humans from infection (D. Clyde, 1990, pers. commun.). There are three polymorphic regions of CS and the repetitive sequence of *P. falciparum* CS, NANP, is immunodominant and hence a good B-cell epitope for a vaccine. However, preparations of this sequence fused to nonmalarial protein polypeptides have provided poor levels of antibody and, consequently, of protection in humans (Ballou et al., 1987; Herrington et al., 1987). It is recognized that it is more desirable to use T-cell epitopes from CS or possibly other sporozoite proteins rather than unrelated proteins, as subsequent infection would then activate both memory T as well as B cells. However, the T-cell epitopes in CS have been found to be both antigenically variable and highly MHC restricted (Good et al., 1988), an effective combination of adverse properties for vaccine development. In addition, Tc cells secreting γ-interferon have been shown to effectively prevent progress from the sporozoite to the merozoite stage of infection (Romero et al., 1989). Although it has been recently demonstrated that peptides with a lipid tail can induce Tc-cell formation (Deres et al., 1989), this has yet to be shown to be a practical approach for vaccination. The use of ISCOMS may offer better prospects (Jones et al., 1988). Others have argued (Sinigaglia and Pink, 1990) that other CS epitopes should be evaluated as vaccine candidates. From our present knowledge, it can be argued that the irradiated sporozoite is effective because (1) more conserved and less MHC-restricted T-cell epitopes derived from sporozoite proteins other than CS induce both class I and II MHC-restricted responses, and (2) class I MHC responses occur because the irradiated sporozoites undergo an abortive replication cycle in liver cells, thus facilitating class I MHC-restricted responses. Although it has been reported that other peptides from *P. falciparum* are protective in humans (Patarroyo et al., 1988), this work has still to be repeated by other investigators.

The malaria example illustrates some of the difficulties that can face the development of simple peptide-based vaccines. These can best be overcome by a thorough study of the properties of the antigens of the infectious agent and an understanding of mechanisms of induction of the desired immune responses.

CONCLUSION

Vaccine efficacy is considered to depend primarily upon the immune response generated by the vaccine. There is a serious lack of information about the responses in humans given highly protective vaccines to viral or bacterial vaccines. This chapter reviews the nature of the immune response generated in model systems to viruses and, to a lesser extent, bacteria. This has led to an enumeration of the immune responses which a vaccine should induce to be successful and, in turn, to the particular properties vaccine antigens should possess in order to induce those responses.

REFERENCES

Ada, G. L. (1989) Vaccines. In *Fundamental Immunology* (W. E. Paul, ed.), 2nd ed., Raven Press, NY, 985—1032.

Ada, G. L. (1990a) The immune response to antigens; the immunological principles of vaccination. *Lancet* 335:523—6.

Ada, G. L. (1990b) The immunological basis of vaccine development. In *Seminars in Virology* Vol. 1, (F. Brown ed.) Saunders, Philadelphia, PA, 1, 3—10.

Ada, G. L. (1990c) Immunosafety aspects of fertility control vaccines. In *Gamete Interaction: prospects for Immunocontraception.* (N. Alexander, D. Griffin, J. M. Spieler, and G. M. H. Waites, eds.), 565—578.

Ada, G. L. and Byrt, P. (1969) Specific inactivation of antigen-reactive cells with ^{125}I-labeled antigen. *Nature (London)* 222:1291—2.

Ada, G. L., and Jones, P. D. (1986) The immune response to influenza infection. *Curr. Top. Microbiol. Immunol.* 128:1—54.

Allen, P. M., Babbitt, B. P., and Unanue, E. R. (1987) T-cell recognition of lysozyme: the biochemical basis of presentation. *Immunol. Rev.* 98:171—87.

Almond, J. W., and Burke, K. L. (1990) Poliovirus as a vector for the presentation of foreign antigens. *Semin. Virol.* 1:11—20.

Anders, E. M., Katz, J. M., Jackson, D. C., and White, D. O. (1981) *In vitro* antibody response to influenza virus. II. Specificity of helper T cells recognizing hemagglutinin. *J. Immunol.* 127:669—78.

Andrew, M. E., Coupar, B. E. H., Boyle, D. B., and Ada, G. L. (1987) The roles of influenza virus haemagglutinin and nucleoprotein in protection: analysis using vaccinia virus recombinants, *Scan. J. Immunol.* 25:21—28.

Avery, O. T., and Goebel, W. F. (1929) Chemico-immunological studies on conjugated carbohydrate proteins. II. Immunological specificity of synthetic sugar-protein antigens. *J. Exp. Med.* 50:533—50.

Ballou, W. R., Sherwood, J. A., Hoffman, S. L., et al. (1987) Safety and efficacy of a recombinant DNA *Plasmodium falciparum* sporozoite vaccine. *Lancet* 1:1277—81.

Berman, P. W., Gregory, T. J., and Riddle, L. (1990) Protection of chimpanzees from infection with HIV-1 after vaccination with recombinant gp120 but not gp160. *Nature (London)*, 345:622—625.

Beverley, P. C. L., Merkenschlager, M., and Wallace, D. L. (1989) Identification of human naive and memory T cells. In *Progress in Immunology*, VII. (F. Melchers, ed.), Springer Verlag, Berlin, 432—8.

Black, S. J., van der Loo, W., Loken, M. R., and Herzenberg, L. A. (1978) Expression of IgD by murine lymphocytes. Loss of surface IgD indicates maturation of memory B cells. *J. Exp. Med.* 146:984—996.

Brown, F. (1990) The potential of peptides as vaccines. *Semin. Virol.* 1:67—74.

Burke, K. L., Dunn, G., Ferguson, M., et al. (1988) Antigen chimaeras of poliovirus as potential new vaccines. *Nature (London)* 322:81—2.

Buus, S., Sette, A., and Grey, H. M. (1987) The interaction between protein-derived immunogenic peptides and Ia. *Immunol. Rev.* 98:115—42.

Chenciner, N., Michel, F., Dadaglio, G., et al. (1989) Multiple subsets of HIV-specific cytotoxic T lymphocytes in humans and in mice. *Eur. J. Immunol.* 19:1537—44.

Dalgleish, A. G., Chanh, T. C., Kennedy, R. C., et al. (1988) Neutralization of diverse HIV-1 strains by monoclonal antibodies raised against a gp41 synthetic peptide. *Virology* 165:209—15.

Deres, K., Schild, H., Wiesmuller, K. H., et al. (1989) *In vivo* priming of virus specific cytotoxic T lymphocytes with synthetic lipopeptide vaccine. *Nature (London)* 342:561—4.

Doherty, P. C., Effros, R. B., and Bennink, J. (1977) Heterogeneity of the cytotoxic response of thymus-derived lymphocytes after immunization with influenza virus. *Proc. Natl. Acad. Sci. U.S.A.* 74:1209—13.

Dorval, B. L., Chow, M., and Klibanov, A. M. (1989) Stabilization of poliovirus against heat inactivation. *Biochem. Biophys. Res. Commun.* 159:1177—1183.

Drake, J. W., Glickman, B. W., and Ripley, L. S. (1983) Updating the theory of mutation. *Am. Sci.* 71:621—30.

Easmon, C. S. F. (1987) Profiles of diseases caused by encapsulated bacteria. In *Towards Better Carbohydrate Vaccines*. (R. Bell and G. Torrigiani, eds.), John Wiley & Sons, NY, 155—67.

Edwards, K. M., Lawrence, E., and Wright, P. F. (1986) Diphtheria, tetanus and pertussis vaccine. A comparison of the immune response and adverse reactions to conventional and acellular pertussis components. *Am. J. Dis. Child.* 140:867—71.

Evans, D. M. A., Dunn, G., Minor, P. D., et al. (1985) Increased neurovirulence associated with a single nucleotide change in a noncoding region of the Sabin type 3 polio vaccine genome. *Nature (London)* 314:548—50.

Evans, D. J., McKeating, J., Meredith, J. M., et al. (1989) An engineered poliovirus chimaera elicits broadly reactive HIV-1 neutralizing antibodies. *Nature (London)* 39:385—8.

Fedson, D. S. (1989) Pneumococcal vaccine. In *Vaccines* (S. A. Plotkin, and E. A. Mortimer, eds.). W. B. Saunders, Philadelphia, PA, 271—299.

Field, B. N. (ed.), (1985) *Virology*. Raven Press, NY.

Finne, J., Leinonen, M., and Makela, P. H. (1983) Antigenic similarities between brain components and bacteria causing meningitis. Implications for vaccine development and pathogenesis. *Lancet* 2:355—7.

Frimodt-Moller, J., Thomas, J., and Parthasanathy, R. (1964) Observations on the protective effect of BCG vaccination in a South Indian rural population. *Bull. WHO* 30:545—74.

Gaillat, J., Zmirou, D., and Mallaret, M. R. (1985) Essai clinique du vaccin antipneumococcique chez des personnes agees vivant en Institution. *Rev. Epidemiol. Sante Publ.* 33:437—44.

Gell, P. D. H. and Benacerraf, B. (1959) Studies on hypersensitivity. II. Delayed hypersensitivity to denatured proteins in guinea pigs. *Immunology* 2:64—70.

Geyson, H. M., Rodda, S. J., and Mason, T. J. (1986) The delineation of peptides able to mimic assembled epitopes. In *Synthetic Peptides as Antigens*. Ciba Found. Symp., (R. Porter and J. Whelan, eds.), John Wiley & Sons, NY, 130—44.

Gillis, S. (1989) T cell-derived lymphokines. In *Fundamental Immunology* (W. E. Paul, ed.), Raven Press, NY, 621—38.

Goidl, E. A., Paul, W. E., Siskind, G. W., and Benacerraf, B. (1968) The effect of antigen dose and time after immunization on the amount and affinity of anti-hapten antibody. *J. Immunol.* 100:371—8.

Good, M. F., Kumar, S., and Miller, L. H. (1988) The real difficulties for malaria vaccine development: nonresponsiveness and antigenic variation. *Immunol. Today* 9:351—4.

Guidos, C., Sinha, A. A., and Lee, K. C. (1987) Functional differences and complementation between dendritic cells and macrophages in T cell activation. *Immunology* 61:269—76.

Herrington, D. A., Clyde, D. F., Losonsky, G., et al. (1987) Safety and immunogenicity in man of a synthetic peptide malaria vaccine against *Plasmodium falciparum* sporozoites. *Nature (London)* 328:257—9.

Hill, A. (1990) An analysis of the cytotoxic T cell response to flaviviruses using Kunjin-vaccinia virus recombinants. Ph.D. Thesis, Australian National University, Canberra.

Hodes, R. J. (1989) T-cell-mediated regulation: help and suppression. In *Fundamental Immunology* (W. E. Paul, ed.) Raven Press, NY, 587—620.

Hogle, J. M., Chow, M., and Filman, D. J. (1985) The three-dimensional structure of poliovirus at 2.9 Å resolution. *Science* 229:1358—63.

Holland, J., Spindler, K., and Horodyski, F., et al. (1982) Rapid evolution of RNA genomes. *Science* 215:1577—85.

Howard, J. G. (1987) T cell-independent responses to polysaccharides: their nature and delayed ontogeny. *Science* 215:221—9.

Huso, D. L., Narayan, O., and Hart, G. W. (1988) Sialic acids on the surface of caprine arthritis-encephalitis virus define the biological properties of the virus. *J. Virol.* 62:1974—80.

Institute of Medicine (1986) *New Vaccine Development: Establishing Priorities. Vol. II. Diseases of Importance in Developing Countries*. National Academy Press, Washington, D.C.

Jones, P. D., and Ada, G. L. (1987) Influenza-specific antibody-secreting cells and B cell memory in the murine lung after immunization with wild-type, cold-adapted variant and inactivated influenza viruses. *Vaccine* 5:244—8.

Jones, P. D., Tha Hla, R., Morein, B., and Ada, G. L. (1988) Cellular immune responses in the murine lung to local immunization with influenza A virus glycoproteins in micelles and ISCOMs. *Scand. J. Immunol.* 27:645—52.

Jones, W. R., Bradley, J., and Judd, S. J., et al. (1988) Phase I clinical trial of a World Health Organization birth control vaccine, *Lancet* 1:1295—8.

Kabat, E. A., Nickerson, K. G., and Liao, J., et al. (1986) A human monoclonal macroglobulin with specificity for a (2-8) linked poly-N-acetylneuraminic acid, the capsular polysaccharide of group B meningococci and *E. coli* K1 which cross-reacts with polynucleotides and with denatured DNA. *J. Exp. Med.* 164:642—54.

Kapikian, A. Z., Mitchell, R. H., and Chanock, R. M., et al. (1969) An epidemiological study of altered clinical reactivity to RSV virus infection in children previously vaccinated with an inactivated RSV vaccine. *Am. J. Epidemiol.* 89:405—21.

Kees, U., and Krammer, P. H. (1984) Most influenza A virus-specific memory cytolytic T lymphocytes react with antigenic epitopes associated with internal virus determinants. *J. Exp. Med.* 159:365—77.

Kennedy, R. C., Henkel, R. D., and Pauletti, D., et al. (1986) Antiserum to a synthetic peptide recognizes the HIV envelope protein. *Science* 231:1556—9.

Kimura, M., and Kuno-Sakai, H. (1990) Developments in pertussis immunisation in Japan. *Lancet* 336:30—2.

Krugman, S. (1988) Hepatitis B vaccine. In *Vaccines* (S. A. Plotkin, and E. M. Mortimer, eds.), Saunders, Philadelphia, PA, 458—74.

Lanzavecchia, A. (1987) Antigen uptake and accumulation in antigen-specific B cells. *Immunol. Rev.* 99:39—51.

Lepow, M. L. (1988) Meningococcal vaccines. In *Vaccines* (S. A. Plotkin, and E. A. Mortimer, eds.), W. B. Saunders Company, Philadelphia, 263—70.

Lerner, R. A. (1982) Tapping the immunological repertoire to produce antibodies of predetermined specificity. *Nature (London)* 299:593—6.

Lowy, J. and Hanson, J. (1965) Electron microscope studies of bacterial flagella. *J. Mol. Biol.* 11:293—302.

Melnick, J. L. (1988) Live, attenuated poliovirus vaccines. In *Vaccines* (S. A. Plotkin and E. A. Mortimer, eds.), Saunders, Philadelphia, PA, 115—157.

Meloen, R. H., Liskamp, R. M., and Goudsmit, J. (1989) Specificity and function of the individual amino acids of an important determinant of human immunodeficiency virus type 1 that induces neutralizing activity. *J. Gen. Virol.* 70:1505—1512.

Miller, J. F. A. P., Vadas, M. A., Whitelaw, A., and Gamble, J. (1976) Role of major histocompatibility complex gene products in delayed-type sensitivity. *Proc. Natl. Acad. Sci. U.S.A.* 73:2486—90.

Mills, K. H. G., Nixon, D. F., and McMichael, A. J. (1989) T-cell strategies in AIDS vaccines: MHC-restricted T-cell responses to HIV proteins. *AIDS*, 3:S101—10.

Mortimer, E. A. (1988) Pertussis vaccine. In *Vaccines* (S. A. Plotkin, and E. A. Mortimer, eds.), Saunders, Philadelphia, PA, 74—97.

Murray, M. G., Kuhn, R. J., and Arita, M., et al. (1988) Poliovirus type 1/type 3 antigenic hybrid virus constructed *in vitro* elicits type 1 and type 3 neutralizing antibodies in rabbits and monkeys. *Proc. Natl. Acad. Sci. U.S.A.* 85:3202—7.

Murphy, B. R., and Webster, R. G. (1985) Influenza viruses. In *Virology* (B. Fields, ed.), Raven Press, NY, 1179—1239.

Nestorowicz, A., Laver, G., and Jackson, D. C. (1985) Antigenic determinants of influenza haemagglutinin. X. A comparison of the physical and antigenic properties of monomeric and trimeric forms. *J. Gen. Virol.* 65:1687—95.

Nossal, G. J. V., and Ada, G. L. (1971) *Antigens, Lymphoid Cells and the Immune Response*. Academic Press, New York, 1—324.

Oldstone, M. B. A., Schwimmbeck, P., Dryberg, T., and Fujinami, R. (1986) Mimicry by virus of host molecules: implications for autoimmune disease. *Prog. Immunol.* 6:787—82.

Patarroyo, M. E., Amador, R., and Clarijo, P., et al. (1988) A synthetic vaccine protects humans against challenge with asexual blood stages of *Plasmodium falciparum* malaria. *Nature (London)* 332:156—8.

Patriaca, P. A., Wright, P. F., and John, T. J. (1990) Factors affecting the immunogenicity of oral polio vaccine in developing countries: a review. *W.H.O.* EPI/90/WP.12.

Perkins, D. L., Lai, M-Z., Smith, J. A., and Gefter, M. L. (1989) Identical peptides recognized by MHC class I- and II-restricted T cells. *J. Exp. Med.* 170:279—289.

Plotkin, S. A., and Mortimer, E. A., eds. (1988) *Vaccines.* Saunders, Philadelphia, PA, 1—633.

Rajewsky, K. (1989) Evolutionary and somatic immunological memory. In *Progress in Immunology,* Vol. VII. (F. Melchers, ed.), Springer-Verlag, Berlin, 397—403.

Riley, I. D., Lehmann, D., and Alpers, M. (1986) Pneumococcal vaccine prevents death from acute lower respiratory-tract infections in Papua New Guinean children. *Lancet* 2:877—81.

Romero, P. J. L., Maryanski, G., and Corradin, R. S., et al., (1989) Cloned cytotoxic T cells recognize an epitope on the CS protein and protect against malaria. *J. Exp. Med.* 341:323—5.

Saag, M. S., Hahn, B. H., Gibbons, J., et al. (1988) Extensive variation of human immunodeficiency virus type 1. *Nature (London)* 334:440—3.

Schneerson, R., Robbins, J. B., Szu, S. C., and Yang, Y. (1987) In *Towards better Carbohydrate Vaccines.* (R. Bell, and G. Torrigiani, eds.), John Wiley & Sons, NY, 307—34.

Schwartz, R., and Klenk, H-D. (1974) Inhibition of glycosylation of the influenza virus hemagglutinin. *J. Virol.* 14:1023—34.

Sela, M. (1969) Antigenicity: some molecular aspects. *Science* 166:1365—74.

Shafferman, A., Lennox, J., Grosfeld, H., Sadoff, J., Redfield, R. R., and Burke, D. S. (1989) Patterns of antibody recognition of selected conserved sequences from the HIV envelope in sera from different stages of HIV infection. *AIDS Res. Hum. Retrov.,* 5:33—9.

Simpson, E. (1988) Suppression of the immune response by cytotoxic T cells. *Nature (London)* 336:426.

Sinigaglia, F., and Pink, J. R. L. (1990) A way round the 'real difficulties' of malaria sporozoite vaccine development. *Parasitol. Today* 6:17—9.

Skazal, A. K., Kosko, M. H., and Tew, J. (1989) Microanatomy of lymphoid tissue during humoral immune responses: structure function relationships. *Annu. Rev. Immunol.* 7:91—110.

Skehel, J. J., Bayley, P. M., and Brown, E. B. (1982) Changes in the conformation of influenza virus hemagglutinin at the pH optimum of virus-mediated membrane fusion. *Proc. Natl. Acad. Sci. U.S.A.* 79:968—72.

Skehel, J. J., Stevens, D. J., and Daniels, R. S., et al. (1984) A carbohydrate sidechain on hemagglutinins of Hong Kong influenza viruses inhibits recognition by a monoclonal antibody. *Proc. Natl. Acad. Sci. U.S.A.* 81:1779—83.

Smith, D. B., and Inglis, S. C. (1987) The mutation rate and variability of eukaryotic viruses: an analytical review. *J. Gen. Virol.* 68:2729—40.

Steinman, R. M., Adams, J. C., and Cohn, Z. A. (1975) Identification of a novel cell type in peripheral lymphoid organs of mice. VI. Identification and distribution in mouse spleen. *J. Exp. Med.* 141:804—20.

Sterkers, G., Michon, J., Henin, Y., Gomard, E., Hannoun, C., and Levy, J. (1985) Fine specificity analysis of influenza-specific cloned T cell lines. *Cell Immunol.* 94:394—405.

Stevens, V. C. (1986) Use of synthetic peptides as immunogens for developing a vaccine against human chorionic gonadotrophin. In *Synthetic Peptides as Antigens*. Ciba Found. Symp., (R. Porter and J. Whelan, eds.), John Wiley & Sons, NY, 184—94.

Takahashi, H., Cohen, J., and Hosmalin, A., et al. (1988) An immunodominant epitope of the human immunodeficiency virus envelope glycoprotein gp160 recognized by class I major histocompatibility complex molecule-restricted murine cytotoxic T lymphocytes. *Proc. Natl. Acad. Sci. U.S.A.* 85:3105—9.

Takahashi, H., Takashita, T., and Morein, B., et al. (1990) Induction of CD8+ cytotoxic T cells by immunization with purified HIV-1 envelope protein in ISCOMS. *Nature (London)* 344:873—5.

Temin, H. (1989) Is HIV unique or merely different? *J. AIDS* 2:1—9.

Townsend, A. R., Rothbard, J., and Goth, R. M., et al. (1985) The epitopes of influenza nucleoprotein recognized by cytotoxic T lymphocytes can be defined with short synthetic peptides. *Cell* 44:959—9.

Townsend, A., Ohlen, C., and Bastin, J., et al. (1989) Association of class I major histocompatibility heavy and light chains induced by viral peptides. *Nature (London)* 340:443—448.

van Rooijen, N. (1989) Direct intrafollicular differentiation of memory B cells into plasma cells. *Immunol. Today* 11:154—7.

Vargese, J. N., Laver, W. G., and Colman, P. M. (1983) The structure of the influenza virus glycoprotein neuraminidase at 2.9f resolution. *Nature (London)* 303:35—40.

Veronese, F. D. M., Rahman, R., and Kalyanaraman, V. S. (1989) Monoclonal antibodies to $HTLVIII_{451}$ gp41: delineation of an immunoreactive conserved epitope in the transmembrane region of divergent isolates of HIV-1. *AIDS Res. Hum. Retroviruses* 5:479—486.

Ward, C. W. (1981) Structure of the influenza virus hemagglutinin. *Curr. Top, Microbiol. Immunol.* 94/95:1—74.

Ward, C. W., Brown, L. E., Downie, J. C., and Jackson, D. C. (1981) Antigenic determinants of influenza virus hemagglutinin. VII. The carbohydrate side chains of A/Memphis/102/72 hemagglutinin heavy chain which cross-react with host antigen. *Virology* 108:71—9.

Ward, C. W., Murray, J. M., Roxburgh, C. M., and Jackson, D. S. (1983) Chemical and antigenic characterization of the carbohydrate side chains of an Asian (N2) influenza virus neuraminidase. *Virology* 126:370—5.

Ward, J., and Cochi, S. (1988) *Hemophilus influenzae* vaccines. In *Vaccines* (S. A. Plotkin and E. A. Mortimer, eds.), Saunders, Philadelphia, PA, 300—32.

Weiss, R. A., Clapham, P. R., and McClure, M. O., et al. (1988) Human immunodeficiency viruses: neutralization and receptors. *J. Aids* 1:536—41.

Whitton, J. L. (1988) Analysis of the cytotoxic T cell responses to the glycoprotein and nucleoprotein components of lymphocytic choriomeningitis virus. *Virology* 162:321—7.

Yap, K. L., and Ada, G. L. (1977) Specific lysis of myxovirus-infected target cells by cytotoxic T cells. *Immunology* 32:151—9.

Yewdell, J. W. and Bennink, J. R. (1989) Brefeldin A specifically inhibits presentation of protein antigens to cytotoxic T lymphocytes. *Science* 244:1072—5.

Yewdell, J. W., Bennink, J. R., Smith, G. L., and Moss, B. (1985) Influenza A virus nucleoprotein is a major target antigen for cross-reactive anti-influenza A virus cytotoxic T lymphocytes. *Proc. Natl. Acad. Sci. U.S.A.* 83:1785—9.

Zinkernagel, R. M. (1990) Antiviral T-cell memory? *Curr. Top. Microbiol. Immunol.* 159:65—78.

Zinkernagel, R. M., and Doherty, P. C. (1974) Restriction of in vitro T cell mediated cytotoxicity in lymphocytic choriomeningitis virus within a syngeneic or semi-allogeneic system. *Nature (London)* 248:701—2.

INDEX

A

Ab anti-idiotopes
 definition of, 57
 relative affinities for antigen, 66–67
ABO blood group antigens, epitope location in, 194
absolute quantitation, of antibodies, 244, 246
acetylcholine receptor
 cDNA clones of, 262
 recognition by curaremimetic toxins, 302, 306–307
N-acetyldesmethylmuramyl-L-alanyl-D-isoglutamine (nor-MDP), as immunoadjuvant, 171
N-acetyldesmethylmuramyl-L-threonyl-D-isoglutamine (thr-MDP), as immunoadjuvant, 171, 172
N-acetylglucosamine residues, anti-idiotypic mimicry of, 58, 68, 69
N-acetylmuramyl-L-alanyl-D-isoglutamine (MDP), as immunoadjuvant, 160
N-acetylmuramyl-L-threonyl-D-isoglutamine, in Syntex Adjuvant Formulation, 168
acute anterior uveitis, HLA region association with, 359
adenovirus, serotypes of, 377
adrenaline, ligands of receptor for, 268
β-adrenergic drugs
 antibodies against, 268–272
 structure of ligands in, 268
adsorption
 nonspecific, 234, 235
 of peptides, for solid-phase immunoassay, 233
 of protein to synthetic polymers, 211
affinity
 high, effects on solid-phase immunoassay, 246
 low, problems caused by, 245
affinity chromatography
 antigens and antibodies in, 234–235
 development of, 221
affinity diffusion, for antigen-antibody precipitation, 188, 189–190

affinity electrophoresis, for antigen-antibody precipitation, 188, 189
affinity of antibodies, 112, 127–148, 149–150, 213, 242
 capture antibodies, 229, 239, 243, 244
 equilibrium reactions in, 128–133, 216
 increase of, by somatic mutations, 153–154
 intrinsic and functional types, 112, 113
 maturation of, 155
 measurement of, 127–148
 polyclonal and monoclonal compared, 116–117
 role in antigen-specific response, 152
 in solid-state immobilization, 219
 steady-state binding and, 142
affinity precipitation methods in gels, 188–190
affinity purification, use in immunology, 234, 235
agarose, use in affinity chromatography, 221, 234
agglutinates, sedimented, properties of, 192, 193
agglutination, 179–208
 active, 201
 automated methods for, 193
 on flat surfaces, 193
 in gels, 193
 inhibition of, 202
 mechanism of, 191
 mixed, 202
 passive, 201
 sensitivity of, 204
 types of, 201–202
 visualization of, 191–193
aggregates, adsorption of, in hydrophobic surface adsorption, 225
aggregoserpentin, mode of action and structure of, 296
AIDS, *see also* human immunodeficiency virus (HIV)
 immunoblotting assay detection of, 212

time lapse between infection and symptoms of, 379
albumin
  coadsorption of, 227
  polymerized, use in hemagglutination, 198
alcohol dehydrogenase I, MAb specific for, 73
algorithms, use in antigenicity prediction, 16
alkaline phosphatase (AP)
  induced expression of, 173
  as signal generator in antigen immunoassays, 211
allergic diseases, liposome-allergen system for treatment of, 167
allopolymorphism, definition of, 339
alloreactivity, molecular mimicry in, 56
allotypes, of IgG antibodies, in humans, 328–329
allotypic determinants, definition of, 56
alprenolol, antibodies against, 265, 268–272, 283
alum, as immunoadjuvant, 161–162, 165, 168, 172
A2m(1) and A2m(2), as allotypic forms of IgA2 molecules, 333
amino acids
  in D1.3 Fab-lysozyme complex, 31, 32
  hydrophobicity of, 102
  in HyHEL-5 Fab-lysozyme complex, 32, 33
  in HyHEL-10 Fab-lysozyme complex, 33–34
  in lysozyme, exposure patterns for, 36, 37
  in lysozyme epitopes, role in antigenicity, 38
  of NC41-neuraminidase complex, 35
  in peptide-antibody reaction, pepscan identification of, 13
  recognition of pairs, 5
  substitution of in idiotopes, 59, 60
  unnatural, in peptide mimics, 48
γ-aminobutyric acid (GABA) receptor, role in benzodiazepine activity, 274, 276
α-aminoisobutyric acid, peptide mimics containing, 48
amphipathic proteins, incorporation into immunostimulating complexes, 166
amphipathic structure, of T-cell recognized peptides, 85, 94

amphiphilicity, in stabilization of peptide conformation, 46–47, 49
analogs, in studies of epitope substitutions, 15
analyte, as ligand in solid-phase immunoassay, 211
ancrod, mode of action and structure of, 297, 301
animal toxins, structural similarity of, 294
ankylosing spondylitis, HLA region association with, 359
anti-allotypic reagent, sources and uses of, 328
antibodies, *see also* immunoglobulins
  abundance of, 229
  in affinity chromatography, 234–235
  affinity of, *see* affinity of antibodies
  antidrug, 261–291
    uses of, 265, 283
  antigen reactions with, *see* antigen-antibody interactions
  anti-idiotypic, *see* anti-idiotypic antibodies
  antipeptide, cross-reactivity studies on, 13–14
  combinatorial diversity of, 151
  combining sites of, 29
  comparison between species, 322
  complementarity determining regions of, 5
  cross-reactive binding properties of, 8
  discovery of, 261
  dissociation from interfaces, 215
  germ-line diversity of, 151, 152
  heterogeneity of, 110, 112
  immobilized, applications of, 234–244
  immunoassay of, 228
  immunochemical immobilization of, 229
  junctional diversity of, 151
  as molecular mimics, 72
  monoclonal, *see* monoclonal antibodies (MAbs)
  monovalent and divalent, binding by, 130
  nitrogen in, 182
  radioactive, use in quantitative hemagglutination, 201
  against snake toxins, 294
  solid-phase, 209–259
    in immunoassays, 236–238
    performance criteria for, 236–238

solubility of, 179–181
specific for denatured protein, 3
subclasses of, 321–338
valencies of, 99, 108, 181
   experimental determination, 139–140
V module of, 57, 58
antigen-antibody bonds
   Lifshitz-van der Waals forces in, 100–101, 106
   minimum equilibrium distance for, 101
   polar forces in, 101, 106, 119–120
antigen-antibody complexes
   cluster formation by, 217
   coagulative, 217
   cross-linking of, 217
   dissociation of, 215
   equivalent ratio of, 181, 183
   insolubilization mechanism of, 180
   precipitate line formation by, see precipitate lines
   solubility of, 179–181
antigen-antibody interactions, 99–125, 213
   Ab affinity and Ag affinity in, 112
   association-dissociation in, 117–122
   binding reaction of, 99–100
   bonds in, see antigen-antibody bonds
   calcium-bridging in, 105
   conformation changes in, 29–30
   electrostatic forces in, 104, 106–107
   energies of formation of, 113
   entropy in, 100
   equilibrium constants of, see equilibrium constant(s)
   hydrogen bonding in, 104
   hysteresis in, 110, 118–119
   in immunodiagnostics, 245–248
   interfacial, 213–221, 247, 248
   kinetics of, 112, 137–138, 214, 217
   models of, 9–10
   nonstoichiometry of, 99, 107, 181–183
   orders of magnitude for parameters of, 112–116
   primary bond formation in, 118–119
   reaction volume of, 213
   secondary bond formation in, 118–119
   on solid phases, 209–259
   thermodynamics of, 109–111, 113, 114–115
antigen-capture capacity (AgCC), of immobilized antibody, 229–230, 237, 238

antigenic determinants
   lysozyme amino acids and, 38
   variations in, 99, 112
antigenicity
   adsorption effects on, 227, 243
   alteration of, in solid-phase antigens, 238
   conformation role in, 44
   epitope mobility and, 117–118
   of immobilized peptides, 233
   of lysozyme, 38
   prediction of, 16, 18
   structural properties related to, 30
antigenic loop, of lysozyme, 37
antigenic selection, mutation recurrence by, 153
antigenic valency, of large, multivalent antigens, 130
antigenic variation, in infectious agents, 377–379
antigen-presenting cells (APC)
   in immune response, 159, 164
   macrophages as, 161
antigens
   in affinity chromatography, 234–235
   amphipathic character as step in processing of, 86–87
   avidity of, 112
   B cell activation by, 149
   carbohydrates as, 58, 68, 380–383
   delivery systems for, 164–169
   drugs as, 261–291
   epitope amino acids, in antibody-combining site, 38
   glycoproteins as, 379, 380–381
   histocompatibility type, see histocompatibility antigens
   immune response to, 368–369
   immunochemical immobilization of, 228–229
   immunoelectrophoresis of, 187–188
   immunogenic determinants in, 84
   mimicry of
      with anti-idiotypic antibodies, 55–79
      with synthetic peptides, 43–54
   molecular dissection of, 1–27
   multivalent, binding equilibria of, 129
   processed form of, T-cell recognition of, 56–57
   quantitation of, vs. antibody activity, 246

snake toxins as, 293-320
solid-phase
  in immunoassay, 238-244
  preparation of, 209-259
solubility of, 179-181
surface vs. internal, 376
of vaccines, 367-391
valencies of, 99, 108, 181
variable domains in, 262
antihistamine drugs, antibodies against, 279
anti-idiotypic antibodies
  advantages and uses of, 56, 74
  antigen mimicry with, 55-79
  classification of, 63
    problems, 67-68
  interaction with receptors, 262
  liposome delivery of, 167
  nomenclature of, 57
anti-idiotypic mimicry
  of carbohydrate antigens, 58, 68, 69
  disparities in magnitudes of different types of, 70
  functional, 66, 69
  fundamentals of, 65-71
  immunochemical, 55, 65-66
  of immunogenicity, 55-56, 66
  intracellular applications of, 72
  limitations of, 71-73
  neo-Darwinian perspective of, 55, 74
  potentials of, 71-73
  rationale for, 57-58
  in receptor isolation, 56
  relative affinities of anti-Id mimic and antigen in, 66-67
  structural, 65
  structural constraints of, 69-70
  T-cell recognition and, 56-57, 70-71
anti-idiotypic vaccines, 56, 74, 82
  alternatives to, 72
  obstacles for preparing, 72
antimalaria vaccines, 384
antipeptide antibodies, cross-reactivity studies on, 13-14
antisera, to snake toxins, 293-294, 310, 311, 312
antistreptolysine-O antibodies, detection by latex agglutination test, 202
antithyroglobulin, detection by latex agglutination test, 202
apoferrin, valency of, 109

aromatic amino acid residues
  in D1.3 Fab-lysozyme complex, 31, 32
  in HyHEL-5 Fab-lysozyme complex, 31, 32
  in HyHEL-10 Fab-lysozyme complex, 34
association, of antigen-antibody, conditions favoring, 120, 121
association constant
  of antigen-antibody interaction, 109-110, 142
  measurement of, 138
atractaspid snake venom toxins, 297, 299-300
Australia antigen, rheophoresis of, 187
autoantibodies, rheumatoid factors as, 328-329
autoimmune diseases, HLA region association with, 355, 358-359, 361
autoimmunity, 94, 155
  mechanism of, 329
  molecular mimicry in, 56, 81
  T cell role in control of, 150
avidin, immobilization of, 229
avidity
  of antigens, 112, 128
  of proteins for plastic membranes, 223
p-azobenzene arsonate haptens, thermodynamics of antibody reactions with, 114
p-azobenzoylamino-β-lactoside haptens, thermodynamics of antibody reactions with, 114
p-azophenylarsonate hapten, antibodies specific for, 152, 153
3-azopyridine, primary bond formation with antibodies, 118, 119

B

bacteria
  agglutination of, 201
  coagglutination of, 202-203
  immobilization of, 231
  lipids of, see lipopolysaccharides
  vaccines against, 374
Bare lymphocyte syndrome, lack of HLA class II histocompatibility gene expression in, 355
basophils, IgE binding to, 111
batroxobin, mode of action and structure of, 297, 301

B-cell receptors, 84
  anti-idiotypic mimicry and, 70
B cells
  activation and differentiation of, 149,
    369–371
  in germinal center, 154
  hypermutation role in differentiation of,
    152, 154
  in immune response, 159, 368
  maturation of, 151, 154
  memory cells from, 149, 154, 155, 371,
    375
  rosetting of, 203
  stimulation of, 172, 311, 323
  variable regions of, 151
Behcet's disease, HLA region association
    with, 359
benzoate hapten, reaction with anti-*p*-azo-
    benzoate antibody, 104
benzodiazepines
  antibodies against, 274–276, 283
  structural formulas of, 275
β-2 microglobulin
  association with HLA class I heavy
    chain, 349–350
  function of, 352
  gene for, 341–342, 343
  as light chain of HLA-A2 molecule, 341
  of mice, 352
β-pleated sheets
  formation in helix, 83, 85, 91
  in snake toxins, 295, 303
β-structure, in peptide mimics, 47, 48
β-turns, in snake toxins, 295
BIAcore™ system
  equilibrium constant assay by, 135–137
  kinetic measurements using, 138–141
bidimensional single diffusion in gels, for
    antigen-antibody precipitation,
    190–191
binding assays, for epitope identification,
    7, 8, 17–18
binding sites, size of, 108–109
biopolymers
  hypersoluble, 180
  solubility of, 179–180
Biosensor system, equilibrium constant
    assay using, 135–136
biotin, in protein-avidin-biotin-capture
    (PABC) system, 229
bird shot retinochoroidopathy, HLA region
    association with, 359

bisdiazobenzidine, use for carrier-peptide
    coupling, 162
blocking protein, effects on solid-phase
    immunoassay, 245
block polymers, as immunoadjuvants,
    167–168, 171
blood groups, passive agglutination use to
    study, 201
blotting tests, use for immunoassay, 202,
    211, 212, 228
Boltzmann's constant, 110, 180
bovine serum albumin
  antibody reactions with, 110, 115, 119
  in immunostimulating complexes, 165
BPTI-like structure, snake toxins character-
    ized by, 297, 301
bromelin, use to facilitate hemagglutina-
    tion, 196
Brownian motion, effects on antigen-anti-
    body interactions, 117–118
α-bungarotoxin, mode of action and struc-
    ture of, 296
β-bungarotoxin
  epitopes of, 307–308
  mode of action and structure of, 296,
    298
k bungarotoxin, mode of action and struc-
    ture of, 296
Bungarus multicinctus venom toxin, 298
butyrophenone drugs, antibodies against,
    272

C

calcium-bridging, in antigen-antibody reac-
    tions, 105
capture antibodies (CAb)
  engineered, 213
  immobilized, 217, 228–229
  performance criteria for, 238–239
  in solid-phase immunoassay, 236, 245
carbodiimide, use for carrier-peptide
    coupling, 162
carbohydrate antigens, 368, 380–383
  anti-idiotypic mimicry of, 58, 68
cardiac glycosides, antibodies against,
    262–265
cardiotoxins
  immunological properties of, 294
  in snake venoms, 293, 296, 299–300
  structure of, 295

carrier proteins
    immunogen preparation by peptide binding to, 162–163
    in solid-phase immobilization, 218
cations, plurivalent, use to facilitate hemagglutination, 196
CD45RO antigen, as marker for T memory cells, 371
celiac disease, HLA region association with, 359
cells, immobilization of, 231–232
cell-surface receptors, anti-idiotypic antibodies use in identification of, 55–75
cellular immune response, 149
cellular receptors, anti-idiotypic antibodies in studies of, 56
centrifugation, erythrocyte cellular distance reduction by, 196
chaotropic salts, effect on antigen-antibody dissociation, 120, 121
C_{H1} domain
    of IgG subclass antibodies, 326
    of immunoglobulin heavy chain, 324
C_{H2} domain
    of IgG isotypes, 332
    of IgG subclass antibodies, 327
    mutations affecting, 330
C_{H3} domain
    of IgG antibodies, 325
    of IgG isotypes, 332
        comparison, 330–331
        essentiality for huFcδRII recognition, 330–331
    of IgG subclass antibodies, 327
chimeric antibodies, as standards for specific antibody immunoassay, 213
chimeric protein molecules, use in vaccines, 380
chlordiazepoxide, structural formula of, 275
chlorpheniramine
    antibodies against, 279
    structural formula of, 280
cholesterol, in immunostimulating complexes, 165
chorionic gonadotropic hormone
    detection by latex agglutination test, 202
    use in fertility control vaccines, 383
chromosome 6, HLA region and subregions on, 344, 345, 353

circle-shaped precipitate lines, 185
circular dichroism, of T cell-presented peptides, 92
C_L domain, of immunoglobulin light chain, 324
clonidine, antibodies against, 270, 276
cluster formation
    in adsorbed proteins, 225, 243
    by antigen-antibody complexes, 217
coagglutination, bacterial characterization by, 202–203
coagulation, surface-induced, effect on Ag-Ab equilibrium constant, 215, 217
cobra venom toxins, 295, 296–297, 302
combinatorial diversity, of antibodies, 151
competitive binding assays, of idiotopes, 58
competitive enzyme-linked immunosorbent assay (CELIA), 238
complement activation, by IgG subclasses, 329–330
complementarity
    of HyHEL-10 Fab and lysozyme surfaces, 33
    of NC41 Fab and neuraminidase surfaces, 35
complementarity determining regions (CDRs)
    of antialprenolol antibodies, 271
    of antibodies, 5, 150
    of D1.3 antibody-lysozyme complex, 31, 32
    of HyHEL-5 Fab-lysozyme complex, 32, 33
    of HyHEL-10 Fab-lysozyme complex, 33
    of NC10 Fab-neuraminidase complex, 35
    of NC41-neuraminidase complex, 35
complement-mediated hemolysis, passive, 201
complex-forming substances
    antigen-antibody complexes as, 184
    nonstoichiometry of, 181
computer analysis, of antidigoxin antibody secondary structure, 264
computer modeling, of antigen-antigen interaction thermodynamics, 116
conformation
    of antigen, importance for antigenicity, 44
    of solid-phase reactants, 218

stabilization of, in synthetic peptides, 43
conformational changes
  in adsorbed proteins, 225, 227, 228
  in antigen-antibody binding, 29–30, 31, 283
conformational sequencing, of peptide mimics, 47
contactable surface area, of haptens, 117
contact angle measurements, of polar free energies, 102–103
contact residue, of epitope, 8
continuous epitopes
  antigenicity related to structure of, 10
  definition of, 1
  identification of, 5
  in peptides, 11
  prediction of, 16–17
  recognition of, 2, 5
  replacement studies of, 13
  as unfoldons, 2–3
Coombs test, mechanism and use of, 200, 202
copolymer L81, as immunoadjuvant, 168
copolymers, see block polymers
Coulombic forces, see electrostatic bonds
counterelectrophoresis, antigen-antibody convergence by, 187, 191
covalent bonds
  energies of formation of, 113, 116
  formation in immobilization, 231, 233
C1q binding site, on IgG2b, 330
C-reactive protein, detection by latex agglutination test, 202
cross-binding, of erythrocytes, with polymers, 197–199
crossing, of precipitate lines, 183
cross-reactive binding properties, of antibodies, 8, 17
cross-reactivity
  antigenic, 3–6, 11
    pepscan method in detection of, 13
    of peptides, 12, 44
  in antipeptide antibodies, 13–14
  irrelevant, 5
  between proteins and peptides, 3
  shared, 3
  of small peptides, 11
  true, 3–5
crotalase, mode of action and structure of, 297
crotalid snakes venom toxins, 297, 298, 300, 301

Crotalus durissus terrificus, toxin in venom of, 298
crotoxin, structure of, 298
crystallographic thermal factors, of lysozyme epitopes, 39
curaremimetic toxins
  cross-reactivity of, 302
  epitopes of, 301–307
  structures and properties of, 294, 295, 301–302
  use to isolate nicotinic acetylcholine receptor, 293
cyclic loop peptide, antigenicity of, 46
cyclization, of peptides, in antigenicity studies, 12
cyclosporin
  antibodies against, 270, 281–283, 284
  structure of, 282
cytochrome c, antigenic activity of, 14
cytomegalovirus
  -infected cells, MHC class I cell surface expression in, 349–350
  peptide, MHC reaction with, 70–71
cytoplasmic pathway, of antigen recognition, 369
cytotoxic T lymphocytes (CTL)
  in immune response, 159, 166, 172
  stimulation of, 164
cytotoxins, in snake venoms, 296, 299

D

dehydration, flocculation by, 180–181
dehydration-rehydration vesicles, preparation of, 166–167
delayed-type hypersensitivity (DTH), induction of, 160, 168, 368
DeLisi-Berzofsky method for identification of T cell-presented helices, 90
Dendroaspis spp. venom toxins, 295, 299
dendrotoxin, mode of action and structure of, 297, 299
de novo protein design, polypeptide synthesis by, 49
dermatitis herpetiformis, HLA region association with, 359
desetopes, MHC antigen-binding sites as, 83
desmethyldiazepam
  biosynthesis of, 275
  structural formula of, 275

detergents
    effect on protein adsorption on nitrocellulose, 226, 231–232
    use in immunochemical immobilization, 228, 241, 245
dextran
    -antibody reactions, 104, 108
    thermodynamics of antibody reactions with, 115
    use in affinity chromatography, 221
    use to facilitate hemagglutination, 197
D1.3 Fab
    -lysozyme complex, 30–31
    lysozyme epitope for, 36, 38, 39, 40
diabetes type I, HLA region association with, 358–359
diazepam
    antibodies against, 270, 274–275
    structural formula of, 275
diazotization, use in antigen-erythrocyte coupling, 201
dielectric constant, effect on antigen-antibody dissociation, 121
diffusion coefficients, of antigens and antibodies, 184, 185
digitoxin, antibodies against, 262–266, 270, 283, 284
digoxigenin, structural formula of, 264
digoxin
    antibodies against, 262–265
    kinetics of antibody reactions with, 113
dihydropyridine calcium channel blockers, antibodies against, 279–281
dimethyl sulfoxide (DMSO), 118
2,4-dinitrophenyl derivatives, antibody reactions with, 113, 114, 150
dipeptides, recognition of, 5–6
diphenylbutamine drugs, antibodies against, 272
discontinuous epitopes
    chemical methods for synthesis of, 49–50
    crystallographic identification of, 9
    definition of, 1–2
    of lysozyme, 37
    synthetic peptide mimics of, 48–49
discrimination potential, of antibody binding potential, 6
dissociation
    of antigen-antibody, 120, 121
    of ligands, 234
dissociation constant
    of antigen-antibody interaction, 109–110
    measurement of, 138
disulfide bonds
    inter-heavy chain type, breakage in IgG, 199–200
    loop peptide stabilization by, 45, 46
    in snake toxins, 296–297, 299, 301
DNA-anti-DNA complexes
    primary bond formation in, 119, 120
    salting out of, 181
domperidone
    antibodies against, 272
    structural formula of, 272
dopamine D2 receptor, binding site of, 272
double diffusion in gels, precipitation by, 183
doxepin
    antibodies to, 277
    structural formula of, 278
drugs
    as antigens, 261–291
    radioimmunoassays of, 265–266

E

echistatin, mode of action and structure of, 297
Edmundson wheel projection, 89
effector sites, of IgG subclasses, 326
egg albumin, valency of, 109
elapid snake venom toxins, 296–297, 298, 299
electrical surface potential, of proteins and polysaccharides, 179
electron-acceptor parameter, of polar free energies, 102
electron-donor parameter, of polar free energies, 102
electron-donor solvents, effect on antigen-antibody dissociation, 120, 121
electron microscopy, of idiotopes, 58, 61
electroosmotic backflow, 187
electrophoresis
    in antibody-containing gels, 190–191
    crossed-over, see counterelectrophoresis
electrostatic bonds
    in antigen-antibody reactions, 104, 107, 119
    exclusive occurrence of, 106
electrostatic interactions

free energies of, 104–105
  in protein adsorption onto plastics, 226
  rate of decay of, 105
electrosyneresis, *see* counterelectrophoresis
eledoisin, snake toxin binding of, 296
ELISA, 211
  of anti-toxin α antibody, 311
  dependence on affinity, 216
  homogeneous, 212
  of human IgG1, 327
  modifications of, 202, 212
  sandwich type, 228, 245
ellipsometry, kinetic rate measurements by, 137
endocrine gland disease, HLA region association with, 358
endoplasmic reticulum, association of HLA class II histocompatibility antigens in, 355
endorphins, antibody recognition of, 266, 267
endosomal pathway, of antigen recognition, 369
endothelins, sarafotoxin similarity to, 297, 300
endozepines, as β-carbolines, 276
energetic epitope, definition of, 8
energies of formation, of antigen-antibody interactions, 113–114, 116
enkephalins, antibody recognition of, 267, 276
enthalpy-entropy compensation, definition of, 116
enzyme immunoassay (EIA), *see* ELISA
enzyme-linked immunosorbent assay, *see* ELISA
enzymes
  as signal generators in immunoassays for antigens, 211, 220–221
  use to facilitate hemagglutination, 196
epinephrine, antibodies against, 269
epitopes, 55, 99, 160
  characterization of, 63–65
  conformational changes in, 227
  contact residues of, 8, 64
  continuous, *see* continuous epitopes
  crystallographic studies on, 64–65
  definition of, 1, 56, 63
  discontinuous, *see* discontinuous epitopes
  effects of substitution on, 15

energetic types, 8–9
energy measurements on, 103
hierarchical list of residues in, 64
identification in fusion proteins and peptides, 13
identification methods for, 7–16
immunochemical immobilization effects on, 229, 242–243
immunodominant, of globular proteins, 108
on immunoglobulins, 56
in immunostimulating complexes, 165
of lysozyme, 36–37
mobility of, 117–118
paratope interfaces with, 4
on pathogens, 232
relational concepts of, 9
segmental mobility of, 10
size of, 8, 108–109
of snake toxins, 294, 301–308
static surface accessibility of, 10
steric burying by passive adsorption, 217–219
steric hindrance of, 227–228, 235, 238, 243, 244
structure of, 36–40
synthetic immunogens from, 163–164
T-cell recognized, prediction of, 81–97
topographic mapping of, 15–16
epitope-specific suppression, 162
equilibrium, in specific antibody immunoassay, 241
equilibrium constant(s)
  of an antibody, 128, 238
  of antigen-antibody interactions, 109–110, 213, 214
  immunoassay of, 135–136
  measurement of, 133
  solid-phase assays of, 134
  solution-phase assays of, 133–134
equilibrium dialysis, use to measure thermodynamics of antigen-antibody interactions, 114–115
equivalence ratio, of antigen-antibody complex, 186
erabutoxins
  antibodies against, 304, 305
  mode of action and structure of, 296, 302–303
erythrocytes
  agglomeration of, 198

agglutination of, *see* hemagglutination
cross-linking of, 194
intercellular distance of, 194
intracellular distance reduction in, 196–199
rosetting of, 203
sedimentation rate of, 192
sonicated stromata from, 191, 193
spiculation induction on, 199
thermodynamics of antibody reactions with, 115
ethanol, as precipitant, 181
etorphine, recognition of, 267
euglobulins, erythrocyte adsorption of, 198
eurotoxins, in snake venoms, conformation of, 295, 298

F

Fab-anti-idiotypic Fab complex, structure of, 29, 283–284
Fab fragment(s)
of antibody isotypes, 324
-antigen complexes, crystallography of, 29
cyclosporin complex of, 283
detoxifying properties of, 265
functions of, 323
of IgG antibody subclasses, 326
fasciculins
mode of action and structure of, 296
toxic action of, 295
Fc receptors
bacterial and viral, 332
recognition of, 330–332
specificity of, 327–328
Fc regions
of IgG subclass antibodies, 326
structure of, 326
Fc structure
of antibody isotypes, 324
function of, 323
hinge region effects on, 325
females, rejection of male skin grafts by, 360–361
fertility control vaccines, 367, 383
α-fetoprotein, detection by latex agglutination test, 202
fibrinogen, use in hemagglutination, 198
flocculation, of antigen-antibody complexes, 180–181

flow calorimetry, use to measure thermodynamics of antigen-antibody interactions, 114–115
fluorescein, kinetics of antibody reactions with, 113
fluorescence quenching, use to measure thermodynamics of antigen-antibody interactions, 114–115
fluorescent labeling, of antibodies, 220
folding units, in model peptides, epitope grafting onto, 49
follicular dendritic cells, in germinal center, 154
foot-and-mouth disease virus, 71
immunoprecipitation of, 191
formaldehyde, use in coagglutination, 203
four-helix bundles, in synthetic model peptides, 49
Freund's adjuvants, use to increase immune response, 161–162
Freund's complete adjuvant (FCA), use to increase immune response, 160–161, 162, 163, 166, 168, 170, 172
Freund's incomplete adjuvant (FIA), 160, 171
fusion, of precipitate lines, 183
fusion proteins and peptides, antigenic studies on, 13

G

gas constant, 110
gastrointestinal virus, immobilized, use to measure antibodies, 231
gels
agglutination in, 193, 204
antibody-containing, electrophoresis in, 190–191
antigen-antibody precipitation in, 188–190
genetic engineering
for defective gene products, 73
use in immunoassay standardization, 212–213
germinal centers, immune response maturation in, 154–155
germ-line diversity, of antibodies, 151, 152
globular proteins, valencies of, 108
γ-globulin
early antibody studies on, 262
valency of, 109

glucan, as immunomodulator, 169, 173
glucose, as inhibitor of dextran-induced cross-binding, 198
glutaraldehyde
 facilitation of passive adsorption by, 227
 use for carrier-peptide coupling, 162
 use in passive agglutination, 201
glycans, see glucan
glycocalix, negatively charged sites on, 199
glycoproteins
 as antigens, 380–381
 immunochemical immobilization of, 229
 role in antigenic structure, 375
 in surface antigen of HIV, 379
glycosylation
 in IgA subclasses and allotypes, 333
 of IgG molecule, essentiality for huFcδRI recognition, 331
 in lower hinge region of IgG subclasses, 330
Goodpasture's syndrome, HLA region association with, 359

H

haloperidol
 antibodies against, 270, 272, 274
 structural formula of, 272
Hamaker coefficient, 100, 101
hapten-carrier-linked activity, interleukin mediation of, 161
haptens
 cospecific, effect on antigen-antibody dissociation, 121
 interactions with antihaptens, kinetics and thermodynamics of, 113
H chains, gene segments for, 151
heavy chains
 constant regions of, 324
 of HLA class I histocompatibility antigens, 348
helical sequences, in peptide mimics, 47
helix
 biophysics of formation of, 83
 structural, prediction in proteins, 90–91
 structure of, in T cell-presented epitope, 82
helix bundles, in synthetic model peptides, 49
helix structure, in peptide mimics, 47

hemagglutination, 194–201
 with IgM and IgG antibodies, 194
 inhibition of, 202
 intercellular distance in, 195
 quantitative, 200–201
 rouleau-formation type of, 197–198
 temperature of, 200
hemocyanin, valency of, 109
hemolytic disease, neonatal detection of, 200
Hemophilus influenzae
 coagglutination in typing of, 203
 vaccine, 374, 381–382
hen egg white lysozyme, see lysozyme
heparin, use in hemagglutination, 198
hepatitis A virus, specific antibody immunoassay of, 242
hepatitis B virus
 alum-mediated response to, 162
 -associated antigen, rheophoresis of, 187
 surface antigen
  anti-idiotope binding studies on, 66–67
  assembly with core proteins into viruslike particles, 163
  as glycoprotein, 381
 vaccine, 374
herpes simplex virus 1, immunoadjuvants for, 162, 167, 168, 170, 172
herpes simplex virus 2, immune responses to, 72
heteroclitic binding, see heterospecificity
heterospecificity, of antibodies, 4, 6, 9
hinge region
 in IgG subclasses, 325, 326
 sequence of, antibodies, 323
 synthetic peptides based on, 326
histocompatibility antigens, 339–366
 of non-human species, 359–360
histoincompatibility, definition of, 340
HLA-A2 molecule
 gene for, 341–342, 343
 structure of, 340–341
 three-dimensional structure of, 342, 344
HLA class I histocompatibility antigens, 340–352
 diversity and polymorphism of, 342–348
 functions of, 350–352
 heavy chains of, 348
 regulation of expression of, 348
 schematic representation of, 341

specificities of, 342–348
HLA class II histocompatibility antigens
   association in endoplasmic reticulum, 355
   biochemistry and gene structure of, 352–353, 356–357
   diversity and polymorphism of, 353–354
   function of, 355–358, 369
   invariant chain of, 355
   regulation of expression of, 354–355
   role in autoimmune disease, 355, 358–359
   schematic representation of, 341
   transcription regulation of, 354–355
HLA complex, definition of, 339, 340
HLA region
   on chromosome 6, 346
   disease association with, 358–359
homobody, Ab2-β as, 57
Hopp-Woods hydrophilicity plot, 86
horseradish peroxidase (HRP), as signal generator in antigen immunoassays, 211
HTLV III B envelope gp120, immunoadjuvant for, 172
huFcγR, recognition specificity of, 325
huFcδRI, IgG subclasses recognized by, 330
huFcδRII, IgG subclasses recognized by, 331–332
huFcδRIII, IgG subclasses recognized by, 331–332
human immunodeficiency virus (HIV), see also AIDS
   alum-mediated response to, 162
   antigenic drift in, 378, 379
   cross reactivity in, 378, 379
   epitopes on, 232, 379
   free core protein p24 of, 136
   glycoprotein antigen (env) of, 381
   gp120 of, 230, 379
   immune response to, 159, 379
   immunoadjuvants for, 166, 172
   -poliovirus chimera, 380
   surface antigen of, 378, 379
   Tc-cell epitopes on proteins of, 377
   viruslike particle expression of, 163
humoral immune response, 149, 322
   alum stimulation of, 161–162
hybridoma lines, antigen-specific, 150, 152
hybridoma technology, use in immunoassay standardization, 212–213

H-Y chromosome, minor histocompatibility loci on, 360–361
hydration, of biopolymers, 180
hydrogen bonds, 102
   in antigen-antibody reactions, 104, 120
   in D1.3 Fab-lysozyme complex, 31
   in HyHEL-5 Fab-lysozyme complex, 32
   in HyHEL-10 Fab-lysozyme complex, 34
hydrophid snake venom toxins, 296
hydrophilicity
   antigenicity and, 30
   of lysozyme epitopes, 39
   in solid-phase immobilization, 218, 247
hydrophilicity scale, of antigenicity prediction, 16
hydrophobic bond energy, increase of, in antigen-antibody interactions, 116
hydrophobic bonds, formation in protein-synthetic membrane surfaces, 224–225
hydrophobic core, of protein, 91
hydrophobic interactions, in antigen-antibody reactions, 102, 104
hydrophobicity, in solid-phase immobilization, 218, 221, 222, 247
hydrophobic patches, on biopolymers, 180
hydrophobic residues, restriction to longitudinal strip in helices, 91, 94, 95
hydrophobic surface, role in helix formation, 83, 84
(4-hydroxy-3-nitrophenyl) acetyl hapten, mutations in response to, 153
HyHEL-5 Fab
   -lysozyme complex, structure of, 31–32
   lysozyme epitope for, 37–40
HyHEL-10 Fab
   combining site of, 33
   -lysozyme complex, structure of, 32–33
   lysozyme epitope for, 36–40
hypermutation mechanism
   activation of, 152–153
   in maturation of immune response, 150, 154
hysteresis, in antigen-antibody reactions, 110, 118–120

I

idiopathic thrombocytopenic purpura, HLA region association with, 359

idiotopes, 55
  amino acid sequence correlates of, 59, 60, 63
  characterization of, 58, 63–65
  competition of corresponding anti-Ids by, 63
  competitive binding assays of, 58
  contact residue composition of, 62–63, 64
  definition of, 57
  electron microscopy of, 58
  mapping of, 58
  overlap of, 58–63
  size-exclusion chromatography of, 58
  spatial overlap of, 62
  topography of, 67
  X-ray crystallography of, 61
IgA antibodies
  deficiencies of, 334
    HLA region association with, 359
  dimers of, 333–334
  divalency of, 108
  induction of, 161, 167, 169, 323
  measurement using adsorbed virus, 231
  mucosal immunity and, 333
  passive adsorption of, 226, 227
  secretory type, 333–334
  specific antibody immunoassay of, 242
  subclasses of, 333
    human allotypes, 324
IgA1 subclass antibodies, 322
  hinge region of, 334
IgA2 subclass antibodies, 322
  allotypes of, 333
  hinge region of, 333
  in large intestine secretions, 334
IgD antibodies, 323
  divalency of, 108
IgE antibodies, 162, 163
  alum-augmented release of, 161
  binding to Fc receptors, 111
  detection by latex agglutination test, 202
  divalency of, 108
  solid-phase immunoassay of, 247
  specific antibody immunoassay of, 242
  subclasses of, human allotypes, 324
  suppression of, 167
IgG antibodies
  against alprenolol, 269–270
  antigen binding by, 134, 323
  biological activities of, 322, 323

  in coagglutination, 202–203
  complex formation by, 180
  cross-reactivity of, 5
  divalency of, 108
  hemagglutination with, 194, 196, 197, 198, 204
  hinge-region disulfide bridges of, 325
  human allotypes of, 328–329
  human antibodies to, 328–329
  immunoprecipitation methods for, 191
  induction of, 167
  isotypes of, 322
  in latex agglutination test, 202
  measurement using adsorbed virus, 231
  methods for extending the reach of, 199–200
  passive adsorption of, 226, 227
  protein A binding of, 230
  subclasses of
    amino acids sequences of, 330–331
    complement activation by, 329–330
    deficiencies, 334
    heterologous antibodies to, 325–328
    hinge region, 325
    human allotypes, 324
    responses to antigens, 324
  thermodynamics of antibody reactions with, 115
  tobacco mosaic virus binding by, 130, 131
IgG-anti-IgG systems, precipitation of, 185
IgG1 subclass antibodies, alum-augmented release of, 161, 163
IgG2 subclass antibodies
  FCA-augmented induction of, 161
  hinge region of, 326
IgG3 subclass antibodies
  hinge region in, 325
  hinge region of, 326
IgM antibodies, 323
  agglutination with, 194, 204
  antidrug type, 283
  cross-reactivity of, 5
  decavalency of, 108
  immunoprecipitation methods for, 191
  measurement using adsorbed virus, 231
imidazoline-like drugs, antibodies to, 276
imipramine
  antibodies to, 277
  structural formula of, 278
immune complexes, production in rheumatoid arthritis, 328–329

immune protection, mechanism of, 322
immune recognition, molecular basis of, 262
immune response
  cells interacting in, 159
  cellular, 149
  humoral, 149
  maturation of, 149–157
    in germinal centers, 154–155
  mucosal, 333, 334
  primary, 151–152, 155
  receptorlike molecule role in, 262
  role of, 371–372
  secondary, 154, 155
  tertiary, 155
  time dependence of, 371
  vaccine-generated, 368–369
immunoadjuvants, 159–177
  alum, 161–162
  Freund's adjuvants, 160–161
immunoassays
  of antigenic reactivity of peptides, 11
  automated procedures for, 182
  of equilibrium constant, 135–136
  heterogeneous, 220
  homogeneous, 220
  solid-phase type, see solid-phase immunoassay (SPI)
immunoblotting assays, 202, 211, 212, 228
immunodeficiency
  of IgA, 334
  of IgG2 and IgG4 subclasses, 334
immunodiagnostics
  of epitopes on pathogens, 232
  solid-phase immunoassay use in, 245–248
immunodominance, of antigen, epitope amino acids related to, 38
immunoelectroosmophoresis, see counter-electrophoresis
immunoelectrophoresis
  of antigens, 186–187
  crossed, 190
immunogenicity
  anti-idiotypic mimicry of, 70
  lessening of, therapeutic value, 82
  of short peptides, 44
immunogenic potential, of antigen, epitope amino acids related to, 38
immunogens
  artificial, 162–164, 312

  with B-cell and T-cell determinants, 163–164
immunoglobulins, see also antibodies
  discovery of, 261
  epitope types on, 56, 58
  heavy chains of, 324
  human allotypes of, 324
  human isotypes of, 321
immunological memory, of T and B cells, 149, 154, 155, 371, 375
immunoosmophoresis, see counterelectrophoresis
immunopathology, molecular mimicry in, 56
immunoprecipitation methods, sensitivity and limitations of, 191
immunorheophoresis, antigen-antibody convergence by, 187
immunostimulating complexes (ISCOMs), preparation and activity of, 164–166, 173, 369
induced fit mechanism, of antigen-antibody interaction, 9, 10
infectious agents
  antigenic variation in, 377–379
  immune response to, 371–373
influenza virus
  antigenic drift in, 378, 379
  detection of antibodies to, 202
  hemagglutinin, 376, 378, 381
    antigenic loop of, 46
    immunoadjuvant for, 168
    secondary immune response to, 154
  neuraminidase epitopes, crystallographic identification of, 9, 29
  nucleoprotein, artificial immunogen from, 164
  vaccines, 374
inhibition assays, of antigens, 210
inhibition curve, derivation in competitive immunoassay, 238
inhibitors
  of adsorption, 231, 238, 242, 243, 245
  peptides as competitors in immunoassay, 232
interaction energy
  of antigen, amino acid role in, 38
  polar component of, 103
interatomic contacts, in antigen-antibody binding, 30
inter-C_{H2}/C_{H3} domain region, of IgG subclasses, 328, 329

interfacial free energy of interaction, between polymer molecules, 179–180
interfacial interactions, see hydrophobic interactions
γ-interferon, production by T-helper cells, 161
interleukin 1
  alum-promoted release of, 161
  as immunoadjuvant, 169, 170
interleukin 2, production by T-helper cells, 161
interleukins
  recombinant, weakening of, 94
  role in antigen recognition, 369
  use in fertility control vaccines, 383
internal image, 69, 74
  of Ab2-β, 57
iodine, radioactive, use in early immunoassays, 220
iodobenzamide
  antibodies against, 272
  structural formula of, 273
ion exchangers, biomolecule substitution in, 210
ionic strength, effect on antigen-antibody dissociation, 120, 121
irradiation, use to introduce nucleophilic groups, 222
isoallotypic specificity, definition of, 328
isoproterenol, antibodies against, 269
isotypic determinant, definition of, 56

J

Japanese encephalitis virus vaccine, 374
J chain, secretion by plasma cells, 333
joint diseases, HLA region association with, 358
junctional diversity, of antibodies, 151

K

kappa L chain
  antibodies containing, 150, 151
  human allotype, 325
kinetic rate constants, of antigen-antibody interactions, 112, 137–138
kinetics, of snake toxin-antibody interaction, 309
krait venom toxins, 296–297, 298
Kunitz-type serine protease inhibitors, in snake venoms, 299

L

lactate dehydrogenase C_4, residues, in model peptides, 49
lambda L chain, antibodies containing, 150, 151
large-probe accessibility
  antigenicity and, 30
  of lysozyme epitopes, 39
latex agglutination, of antibody or antigen, 193, 204
latex agglutination test, 202
Laticauda spp. venom toxins, 302
L chains
  of B cells, 151
  gene segments for, 151
LCM virus, Tc-cell epitopes of, 377
lectins
  in affinity chromatography, 234–235
  use in noncovalent immobilization, 230
  use in specific antibody immunoassay, 242
Leishmania donovani, glucan as immunoadjuvant in vaccine for, 169
Liesegang rings, production in gels, 188
Lifshitz-van der Waals bonds
  combined with other bonds, 107
  exclusive occurrence of, 106, 119
Lifshitz-van der Waals forces
  attractive and repulsive, 101
  in erythrocytes, 194
  role in antigen-antibody bonds, 100–101
ligand, as soluble reactant, in solid-phase immobilization, 209, 234
light scattering, in automatic determination of agglutination, 193
lipids, as peptide carriers, 162
lipopolysaccharides, as immunomodulators, 170, 173
lipoproteins, use in immunogen preparation, 164
liposomes, as immunogen carriers, 162, 164, 166–167, 172, 173
lock-and-key model, of antigen-antibody interaction, 9, 10, 107
longitudinal hydrophobic strip, in T cell-presented epitope, 82
loops
  in complementarity determining regions, 71
  in proteins, synthetic peptide mimics of, 45–46
lung cancer tumor cells, interleukin as adjuvant for, 169
lysozyme
  -antibody complexes, structure of, 30–32, 68
  antigenicity of, structural parameters affecting, 39–40

antigenic loop of, 37, 45
epitopes, 36–37
   crystallographic identification of, 9, 29
   peptide mimics of, 49
   secondary structure, 38
   solvent-accessible surface of, 37
   structure, 36

M

M$\overline{\alpha}$1 and M$\overline{\alpha}$2-3 antibodies, raised against snake toxins, 302–307, 308–309
macrophages, alum effects on, 161
major class I histocompatibility antigens, activity of, 340, 369, 372–373
major class II histocompatibility antigens, activity of, 340, 369
major class III histocompatibility antigens, 340
major histocompatibility complex (MHC), 368–369, see also HLA histocompatibility antigens
   definition of, 339
   of non-human species, 359–360
   recognition by T-cell receptor, 57, 70–71, 82, 83–84, 86, 93, 150, 159, 369
malaria
   peptide-based vaccines for, 384
   peptide mimics of antigen of, 48
maleimidobenzo-N-hydroxysuccinimide ester, use for carrier-peptide coupling, 162
mamba venom toxins, 295, 296, 299
mass action law, applied to antibody-antigen binding, 128, 132
mass transport, in BIAcore™ system, 135
mast cells, IgE binding to, 111
matrix affinity, kinetics and, 142
maturation, of the immune response, 149–157
McPC603 protein, Fv regions of, 274
measles virus
   detection of antibodies to, 202
   vaccine, 373, 378
melittin, peptide mimics of, 47
membrane(s)
   interfacial, antigen-antibody interactions as models for, 247
   plastic and synthetic, protein adsorption onto, 223–228

receptors, anti-idiotypic antibody studies on, 262
memory cells, antigen-activated B cells as, 149, 154, 155, 371, 375
β-2 microglobulin
   association with HLA class I heavy chain, 349–350
   function of, 352
   gene for, 341–342, 343
   as light chain of HLA-A2 molecule, 341
   of mice, 352
microorganisms
   immobilization of, 231–232
   interaction with antibodies, 138
microparticles, as immunoadjuvants, 168–169, 173
mimotopes, definition of, 6, 48
minimum solubility product, of antigen-antibody complexes, 184
minor histocompatibility antigens
   activity of, 340
   gene analysis of, 360–361
MN antibodies, 201
mobility, of lysozyme epitopes, 39
molecular mimicry, principles and uses of, 55–56
monoazobenzene arsonate-N-tyrosine, as immunoadjuvant, 161
monoclonal antibodies (MAbs)
   affinity of, 116–117
   cross-reactivity in, 3
   development and uses of, 212–213, 321–322
   dipeptide recognition by, 5–6
   in solid-phase immunoassay, 246
   specificity of, 2
   in studies of epitopes, 15–16
monoclonal antibody 37A4, use in ligand-receptor studies, 269–270, 271
monodimensional single diffusion in gels, for antigen-antibody precipitation, 188
monophosphoryl lipid A (MPL), as immunoadjuvant, 170, 172
morphine
   antibodies against, 265–267, 270, 283
   receptor for, 266
   structural formula of, 267
mouse, antibody repertoire of, 151
mucosal immunity, 322
   IgA and, 333

multiple-antigen peptide (MAP) system, 14, 50
mumps virus vaccine, 373, 378
murabutide, as immunoadjuvant, 171
muramylpeptides, as immunoadjuvants, 170–173
muscarinic toxins, mode of action of, 295, 296
mutations
  in studies of epitope substitutions, 15
  in viruses, 378
myeloma protein
  lambda L chains of, 150
  three-dimensional structure of, 262
myoglobin, peptide analogs of, 45–46, 49
myohemerythrin-antibody complex, structure of, 10
myotoxin a, mode of action and structure of, 297
myotoxins, in snake venoms, 299, 300
myristic acid, addition to polio virus, 375

N

Naja naja naja, venom toxin of, 299
Naja naja oxiana toxin α, structure of, 306
Naja nigricollis toxin α
  antibodies against, 302–303, 305
  immunogenic properties of, 310–312
  mode of action and structure of, 296, 302, 303
Naja nigricollis toxin γ
  antibodies against, 302–303, 305
  mode of action and structure of, 296
naloxone, structural formula of, 267
naprotiline, antibodies to, 278
narcolepsy, HLA region association with, 359
nasopharyngeal carcinoma, HLA region association with, 359
NC10 Fab-neuraminidase complex, structure of, 35
NC41 Fab-neuraminidase complex, structure of, 34–35
Neisseria meningitidis
  coagglutination in typing of, 203
  vaccine, 374, 382–383
neuraminidase
  -Fab complexes, structural studies, 34–35, 36, 68
  use to facilitate hemagglutination, 196

neuroleptic drugs, antibodies against, 272–274
neurotoxins, in snake venoms, 293, 295, 296, 298
neurotransmitter receptors, tricyclic antidepressant interaction with, 277
NEW immunoglobulin, hypervariable regions in, 262, 263
nicotinic acetylcholine receptors, snake venom blockage of, 293
nicotinic receptor, isolation from brain, 283
nifedipine
  antibodies against, 270, 279–281
  structural formula of, 281
nigexine, mode of action and structure of, 296, 299
nitrendipine
  antibodies against, 279
  structural formula of, 281
nitrocellulose, protein adsorption onto, 226, 228, 231–232
p-nitrophenyl derivative, thermodynamics of antibody reactions with, 114
norepinephrine, antibodies against, 269
nortriptyline
  antibodies against, 270, 277
  structural formula of, 278
Notechis scutatus scutatus venom toxin, 301
notexin, mode of action and structure of, 296, 298, 301
nuclear magnetic resonance (NMR)
  of antibody-combining sites, 284
  two-dimensional
    of protein epitopes, 40
    of synthetic peptides, 46
nucleic acids, use in hemagglutination, 198

O

oligosaccharide moiety
  in IgA1 hinge region, 333
  of IgG, role in Fc receptor recognition, 331
oligosaccharides, as antigens, 381–383
opioid peptides, common tetrapeptide sequence in, 267
ouabain, kinetics of antibody reactions with, 113
oxaprotiline

antibodies to, 277–278
structural formula of, 278
Oxyuranus scutellatus scutellatus venom toxin, 298

P

palmitic acid, as peptide carrier, 162
papain
  induction of erythrocyte spiculation by, 199
  use to facilitate hemagglutination, 196
parabola-shaped precipitate lines, 185
parallelism, control of in solid-phase immunoassay, 243, 244, 246
paratopes, 55
  definition of, 1, 56
  epitope interfaces with, 4
  variations in, 99
parvovirus, immobilized, use to measure antibodies, 231
pepscan method, 6, 12–13
  in detection of amino acids in peptide-antibody reaction, 13
peptide hormones, amphipathic structure of, 85–86
peptide mimics, TASP approach to, 50
peptides
  antigenic cross-reactivity of, 12
  as antigenic probes, 11, 160
  conjugates of, as antigenic probes, 11–12
  cyclization of, 12
  in solid-phase immunoassay, 232–233
  solid-phase synthesis of, 43
  support-attached, antigenic activity of, 12–13
  synthetic
    as antigenic probes, 11, 43–54
    antigen mimicry with, 43–54
peptide vaccines, 93, 383–384
pesticides, interaction with antibodies, kinetics of, 138
pEX expression, use in antigenic studies, 13
pH, effect on antigen-antibody dissociation, 120, 121
phase separation
  flocculation by, 181
  in polymer-assisted hemagglutination, 197

phemphigus, HLA region association with, 359
phenothiazine drugs, antibodies against, 272
2-phenyloxazolone hapten, antibody response to, 153, 155
D-phenyl-(*p*-azobenzoylamino) derivative, thermodynamics of antibody reactions with, 114
PH-1.0 peptide, sheet projection of, 92–93
pilin, solid-phase immunoassay of, 214
pirenzepine
  antibodies to, 277
  structural formula of, 278
PLA_2-like structure, snake toxins characterized by, 296–297, 298–299, 301
plant viruses, antibody reactions with, 117
plasma cells, formation from B cells, 149
plasma membrane
  exposure of, in immobilization, 231
  as target of myotoxins, 299, 300
plasma proteins, radial immunodiffusion of, 190
Plasmodium falciparum sporozoites, mimic peptide cross-reactivity with, 48
plastic surfaces, protein adsorption on, 211, 223–228
platelet aggregation, snake toxins as initiators or inhibitors of, 299, 300–301
β-pleated sheets
  formation in helix, 83, 85, 91
  in snake toxins, 295, 303
pleiotropism, of muramylpeptides, 172
pluronic polymers, *see* block polymers
pneumococcus, serotypes of, 377
polar bonds
  exclusive occurrence of, 106
  in secondary antigen-antibody bonding, 119–120
polar forces
  in antigen-antibody bond, 102, 107
  attractive and repulsive types, 103
  exterior, use to reduce erythrocyte intercellular distance, 197
  rate of decay with distance, 103
polar free energies, in antigen-antibody bond, 102
polar intercellular repulsion, in erythrocytes, decrease of, 196–197
polar surface tension component, of polar free energies, 102

poliovirus
  antigenic mutants of, 378
  -HIV chimera, 380
  vaccines, 374, 375
polybrene, erythrocyte cross-binding by, 199
polyclonal antibodies, affinity of, 116–117
polyethylene glycol, as precipitant, 181
poly-Ig receptor, complex with IgA, 334
polylysine
  erythrocyte cross-binding by, 199
  facilitation of passive adsorption by, 227
polymerase chain reaction, studies of memory B cells using, 155
polymers
  cross-binding of, use in hemagglutination, 197–198
  protein adsorption on, 211
polymorphism, in HLA class I genes, 346
polysaccharides
  as antigens, 374–375, 381–383
  immunochemical immobilization of, 229
  interaction energy of epitopes on, 103
  specific antibody immunoassay of, 242
  use in passive agglutination, 201
polystyrene
  adsorption proteins to, 222, 224
  passive agglutination with, 202
postsynaptic neurotoxins, in snake venoms, 296
p24 protein, kinetic measurements using, 140, 143
prazepam, structural formula of, 275
precipitate lines, 183
  circle-shaped, 185
  crossing of, 183
  decay of, 183
  of first formation, 183–184
  fusion of, 183
  geometry of, 186
precipitation, 179–208
  by affinity precipitation in gels, 188–190
  by double diffusion in gels, 183–187
  by single diffusion in gels, 188–190
  in tubes, 181–183
pregnancy test, detection of urinary chorionic gonadotropic hormone in, 202
presynaptically facilitatory toxins, in snake venoms, 298–299
primary bonds, between epitopes and paratopes, 118–119

proline, spirocyclic, peptide mimic containing, 48
propranolol, antibodies against, 268, 269
protamine, erythrocyte cross-binding by, 199
protein A, see staphylococcal protein A
protein antigens, use in passive agglutination, 201
protein-avidin-biotin-capture (PABC) system, use in immmobilization, 229–230, 238
proteins
  adsorbed
    conformational changes in, 227, 228
    properties of, 227–228
  adsorption on plastic and synthetic membranes, 223–228
  antigenic determinants of, see epitopes
  as antigens, 358
  denatured vs. native
    antigenic recognition of, 14
    continuous epitopes in, 2–3
  interaction energy of epitopes on, 103
  loops in, synthetic peptide mimics of, 45–46
  prediction of structural helices in, 90–91
  solid-phase immobilization of, 217
protrusion index, of lysozyme epitopes, 39
prozoning, in specific antibody immunoassay, 241
Pseudonaja texilis venom toxin, 298
psoriasis vulgaris, HLA region association with, 359
pullulan, as peptide carrier, 162–163

Q

quaternary association
  of HyHEL-5 Fab, 31
  of HyHEL-10 Fab, 33
Quil A, as adjuvant in immunostimulating complexes, 164–165

R

rabbit antimouse (RAM), use in antibody-binding studies, 140, 145
rabies vaccine, 374
radial immunodiffusion, for antigen-antibody precipitation, 190, 191

radioactive antibodies, 201
radioimmunoassay (RIA), 211, 238
  conversion to enzyme immunoassay, 221
rattlesnake venom toxins, 297, 298, 300, 301
receptor(s)
  antidrug antibodies as analogs of, 262
  as capture reagent, in solid-phase immobilization, 209, 234
  concept of, 261–262
  for drugs, anti-idiotypic approach to, 283
recognition
  of continuous epitopes, 2
  immunological vs. chemical, 5
recombinant techniques, in epitope analysis, 13
Reiter's syndrome, HLA region association with, 359
relative affinities, of anti-Id mimic and antigen, 66–67
renin, peptide analogs of, 45–46
reovirus type 3, anti-idiotypic mimicry studies on, 70, 71, 74
replacement studies, of peptide-antibody reactions, 13
repulsive Brownian energy, 117
respiratory syncytical virus, artificial immunogen from, 164
respiratory tract infections
  associated with IgG2 subclass deficiency, 334
  from bacterial pathogens with carbohydrate capsules, 381
retrovirus-related sequences, association with minor histocompatibility loci, 360
Rh blood group antigens
  antibodies to, 199, 200, 201, 203
  epitope location in, 194
  immunoprecipitation of epitopes of, 191
rheophoresis, antigen-antibody convergence by, 187, 191
rheumatoid arthritis, HLA region association with, 359
rheumatoid factors
  as autoantibodies, 328–329
  detection by latex agglutination test, 202
  specificity of, 327–328
rhinoviruses, antigenic drift in, 378
Ribi adjuvant system, efficacy of, 170

ribonuclease, valency of, 109
RNA virus vaccines, 378
Rothbard-Taylor method for identification of T cell-presented helices, 90
rouleau-formation type of hemagglutination, 197–198
rubella virus
  detection of antibodies to, 202
  vaccine, 373, 378

S

salbutamol, antibodies against, 272
salt bridges
  in HyHEL-5 Fab-lysozyme complex, 32
  in HyHEL-10 Fab-lysozyme complex, 34
salting out, of antigen-antibody complexes, 180–181
Salvarsan, as first synthetic antibacterial agent, 261
sandwich immunoassays, capture antibodies in, 236, 245
sarafotoxins, mode of action and structure of, 297, 299–300
scanning electron microscopy (SEM), of protein adsorption onto membranes, 224
Scatchard plots, of equilibrium constants, 129
sea snake venom toxin, 302
secondary bonds, between epitopes and paratopes, 119–120
secondary minimum attraction, in hemagglutination using polymers, 197–198
secondary structure
  prediction algorithms, for antigenicity, 16
  of proteins, peptide mimics of, 46–48
secretory piece, IgA dimer bound to, 334
sedimentation rate, in agglutination, 191–192
segmental mobility, of epitopes, 10
segmental mobility scale, of antigenicity prediction, 16
Semliki Forest virus, immunogenicity of, 164
serotypes, of infectious agents, 377–379
serum albumin
  primary bond formation with antibodies, 110

thermodynamics of antibody reactions
with, 115
use to facilitate hemagglutination, 197
valency of, 109
shared cross-reactivity, 3
sheet projection, hydrophobic strip analysis
by, 89
silica, use in affinity chromatography, 221,
235
site occupancy, effects on solid-phase
immunoassay, 245
size-exclusion chromatography, of
idiotopes, 58
SK&F 94461
antibodies against, 270, 279, 280
structural formula of, 280
skin diseases, HLA region association
with, 358
snake toxins
antibodies against, 294
as antigens, 293–320
antisera against, 293–294, 310, 311,
312
epitopes of, 294, 301–308
immunogenic properties of, 294
isolation and characterization of, 294
morphology and biological function of,
294–301
neutralization mechanisms for, 294,
308–310
structural classification of, 298–299
with three finger-shaped structures,
295–298
solid-phase assays, 134
solid-phase immobilization
of antigens and antibodies, 209–259
biological properties of reactants in,
217–219
concentration and distribution of reactants in, 219–220
conformational changes in, 218
covalent, 218, 221–223
monolayers in, 219
retention of biological activity by, 219
solid-phase immunoassay (SPI), 134, 209,
see also enzyme immunoassay
(EIA)
antibodies in, 236–238
antigens in, 238–244
direct competitive type, 238
history of, 210–211

of immobilized peptides, 232–233
parallelism control in, 243, 244, 246
peptides in, 232
protein denaturation in, 14
reaction volume in, 247
reliability of, 246–247
sandwich type, 135, 236, 245
use in immunodiagnostics, 245–248
solid-phase technology, development of,
210
solution-phase assays, of equilibrium constant, 133–134
somatic mutations, increase of antibody
affinity by, 153–154
specific antibody immunoassay (SpAbI)
chimeric antibodies for use in, 213
ELISA-type, 244
interpretation of, 241–244
need for parallelism in, 243, 244
problems in, 241, 242
prozoning in, 242
solid-phase antigens in, 238–241, 248
titration plots from, 243
specificity, of antibody binding, 6
spiculation, induction in erythrocytes, 199
spiroperidol
antibodies against, 272
structural formula of, 272
squalene, in immunoadjuvants, 171
stabilizing protein, use in solid-phase
immobilization, 218
staphylococcal protein A
immobilization of, 229, 245
interaction with IgG, 328, 329
molecular specificity of, 332
use in typing, 203
staphylococci, coagglutination of, 202–203
static surface accessibility, of epitopes, 10
steady-state binding, affinity and, 142
steroids, antibodies against, 262
stoichiometric ratio, of antigen-antibody reaction, 99
Stokes' law, in calculation of sedimentation rate, 191–192
stomatocyticism, in erythrocytes, 199
streptavidin, immobilization of, 229, 230
streptococcal protein G, IgG isotype binding of, 332
streptococci, coagglutination in typing of,
203
Streptococcus mutans, immunoadjuvant
for, 167

Streptococcus pneumoniae vaccine, 374, 382
strip-of-helix hydrophobicity index (SOHHI), 83, 88, 94, 95
  algorithm for, 86, 87, 90
  structural helices algorithm (SHA) helix prediction by, 91
  SOHHI incorpration into, 88–89
β-structure, in peptide mimics, 47, 48
substance P, snake toxin binding of, 296
superoxide burst, triggered by IgG isotypes, 330
surface plasmon resonance (SPR), equilibrium constant assay by, 135
surface-stimulation peptides, antigenicity of, 49
Syntex Adjuvant Formulation (SAF), uses of, 168, 172
systemic lupus erythematosus, detection of anti-DNA antibodies in, 181

T

tachykinin receptors, snake toxin binding of, 296, 298
tannic acid, use to facilitate hemagglutination, 196–197, 201
T cell-presented peptides, helical coiling of, 91–92
T-cell receptor (TCR)
  antigen specificity of, 56
  anti-idiotypic mimicry and, 70
  reaction with antigen and MHC, 150
T cell-recognized epitopes, 379
  amphipathic structure of, 85
  in proteins
    prediction of, 81–97
    sequence selection, 83
    structure of, 81
    theory of, 82
T cells
  activation and differentiation of, 369–371
  autoreactive, role in type I diabetes, 358–359
  in immune response, 159, 368
  memory cells from, 371
  molecular mimicry and reactivity of, 56
  role in autoimmunity control, 150
  role in hypermutation process, 152–153
  rosetting of, 203

toxin α stimulation of, 310–312
T-dependent antigen (TD), Quil A enhancement of, 165
temperature, effect on antigen-antibody dissociation, 120, 121–122
template-assembled synthetic proteins (TASP), construction of, 50
tertiary structures, of model peptides, 49
testis differentiation factor, minor histocompatibility antigens and, 360–361
test tubes, precipitation in, 181–183
T-helper cells
  FCA stimulation of, 161
  in germinal center, 154
  in immune response, 159, 311
thermal mobility, antigenicity and, 30
three finger-shaped structures, snake toxins characterized by, 295–298, 301, 302
thrombic proteases, in snake venoms, 301
thyroglobulin, valency of, 109
thyroiditis, subacute, HLA region association with, 359
tobacco mosaic virus
  antibody binding data for, 130, 131
  in antibody valence studies, 139–140
  valency of, 109
tomato bushy stunt virus, valency of, 109
topographic mapping, of epitopes, 15–16
toxin F, mode of action and structure of, 296
transferred ^{1}H nuclear Overhauser enhancement (TRNOE), studies of morphine-antibody reaction using, 266
translational diffusion, in adsorbed proteins, 225
transport mechanisms, causing antigen and antibody to converge, 187
trehalose dimycolate, as immunoadjuvant, 170
tricyclic antidepressant drugs
  antibodies to, 276–278
  structural formulas of, 276–278
2,4,6-trinitrophenyl derivatives, kinetics of antibody reactions with, 113
Trypanosoma cruzi, glucan as immunoadjuvant in vaccine for, 169
T-suppressor cells, in immune response, 159
tumor cells

lysis by snake toxin, 299
MHC class I cell surface expression in, 349–350
β-turns, in snake toxins, 295
Ty-viruslike particles, formation by fusion proteins, 163

U

unfoldons, continuous epitopes as, 2–3

V

vaccines
  antigens used for, 367–391
    immune recognition, 375–376
  anti-idiotypic, see anti-idiotypic vaccines
  bacterial, 374
  chimeric protein molecule use in, 380
  current and trial types of, 373–380
  development of, 160, 232, 246, 321, 367–391
  general properties of, 368–373
  goals of, 373
  immune response generated by, 368–369
  peptide-based, 93, 383–384
  preparation with toxin-polysaccharide, 162–163
  uses of, 367
  veterinary, Quil A use in, 165
  viral, 373
vaccinia virus, DNA genome of, 377
valencies, of antibodies and antigens, 99, 107–108, 112
Valium, radioimmunoassay of, 274
van der Waals bonds, 106
  in D1.3 Fab-lysozyme complex, 31
  in HyHEL-5 Fab-lysozyme complex, 32
  in HyHEL-10 Fab-lysozyme complex, 34
van der Waals-Debye forces, 100
van der Waals forces, see Lifshitz-van der Waals forces
van der Waals-Keesom forces, 100
van der Waals-London forces, 100
viper venom toxins, 296–297, 299
viral chimeras, 380
  use in epitope analysis, 13
viral envelope antigens, efficacy of immunostimulating complexes against, 165–166
viral vaccines, 373
virosomes, as immunoadjuvants, 164
viruses
  characterization by inhibition of hemagglutination, 202
  glycoproteins in surface antigens of, 380–381
  immobilization of, 231
  immunization against, 3
  valencies of, 108, 109
viruslike particles, from fusion proteins, 163
vitamin K, binding of, 262, 263
V module, of antibody, 58, 59
  dimensions, 71

W

water of formation, release in antigen-antibody interactions, 116, 122
WHO specificity reference reagents, 326, 327

X

X-ray crystallography
  antibody-antigen studies using, 40
  epitope characterization by, 7–8, 29–42, 64–65
  of idiotopes, 61–62
  of protein-antigen complexes, 9–10, 17

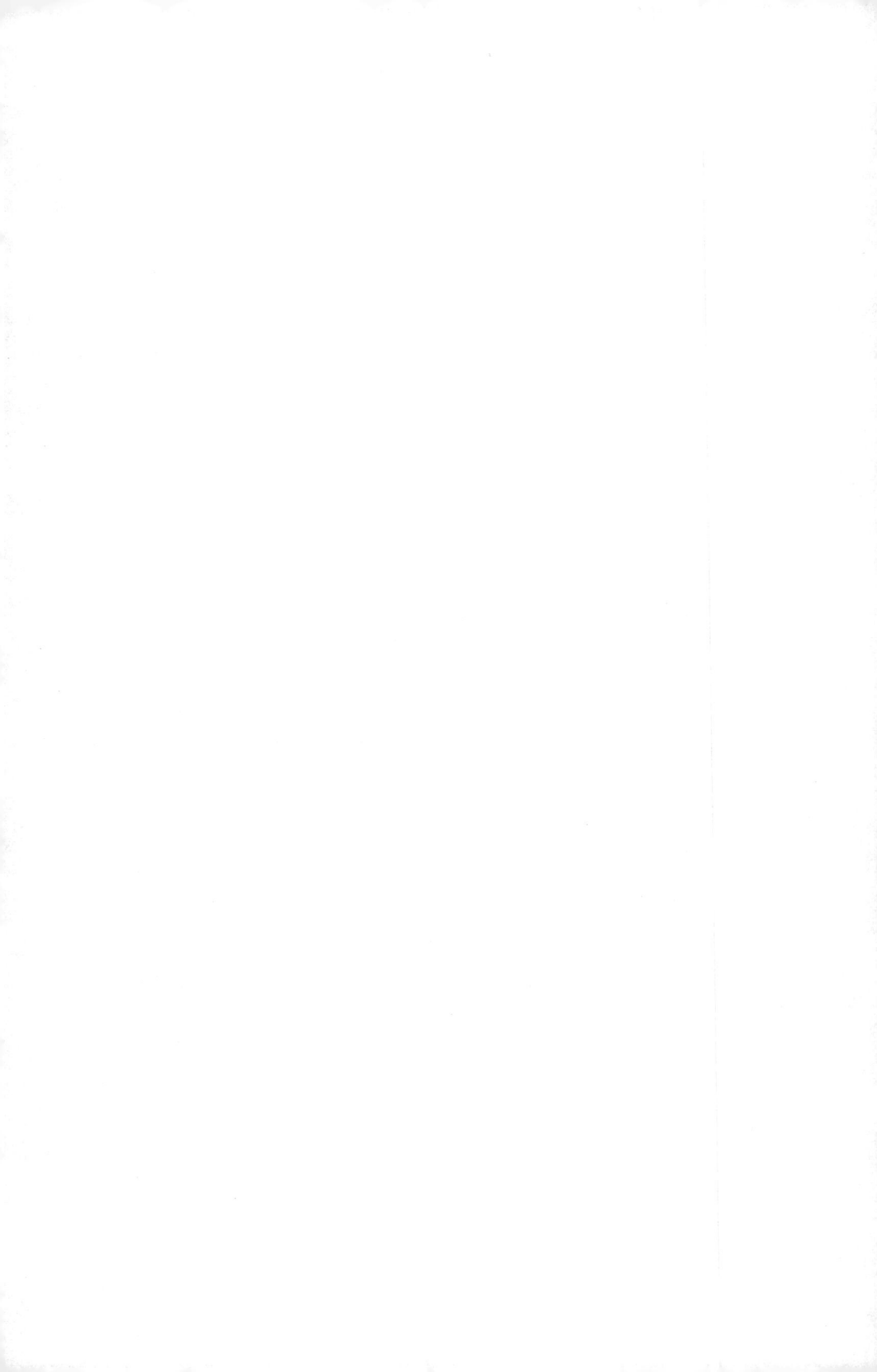